LONG

Aspects of Medical Care Administration

This volume is published as part of a long-standing cooperative program between the Harvard University Press and the Commonwealth Fund, a philanthropic foundation, to encourage the publication of significant and scholarly books in medicine and health.

Aspects of Medical Care Administration:

Specifying Requirements for Health Care

Avedis Donabedian, M.D., M.P.H.

A Commonwealth Fund Book
Harvard University Press, Cambridge, Massachusetts

This work is dedicated to three who have been most
influential in making it possible

FRANZ GOLDMANN, teacher and advisor,
whose sharp insights and masterly teaching
opened up for me the new and largely unexplored
field of medical care;

LEONARD S. ROSENFELD, mentor and coworker,
who introduced me to the rewards and rigors of
research, and set for me the highest standards
of scholarship;

WILLIAM H. MCBEATH, student and colleague,
who professed to see such merit in my teaching
that he encouraged me to make my work known
to a wider audience.

Preface

This book is an attempt to take a systematized view of certain aspects of medical care administration. It is constructed around the simple notion that the medical care administrator is often faced with certain responsibilities that he must discharge or tasks that he must perform. He may find it necessary, for example, to define his objectives, to assess the need for service, or to decide whether or not resources are adequate. These major tasks are accordingly the points of departure.

It is realized (and the reader must have this clearly in mind) that the medical care administrator in question is a hypothetical figure. He is an amalgam of all persons at all levels in the medical care system who are called upon to make decisions germane to the organization and delivery of medical care. Any particular administrator may perform only one aspect of any given task. But it is important for him to understand that the part he performs is a portion of a larger task and to see what relationships there might be between what he does and the larger activity.

The primary orientation of this work is therefore operational. It is meant to contribute to administrative competence, but only within a particular frame of reference. First, this is not a text on management. It deals with the medical care substance in managerial decisions. Second, this is not a manual of procedures tested or otherwise. On the contrary, the approach is conceptual and abstract. The object is to bring about a fundamental understanding of the phenomena in question and to foster a particular way of thinking about medical care problems. This objective represents a passionate conviction that only in this way can a person be prepared who is capable of imaginative, innovative action and of intellectual growth.

A major feature is the attempt at systematization. Knowledge in the field of medical care administration is now more in the nature of a vast collection of facts and fancies, strewn about like stones in a quarry. An attempt has been made to bring together these building blocks so that some semblance of a structure might emerge. The primary device is that of classification—the customary first step in any relatively primitive field. To this are added certain models that are meant to depict, in skeletal form, basic structural and functional relationships as I see them. It should be clear that these classifications, and these models, do not represent theory in medical care administration. They are, simply, categories and relationships that may be useful in the analysis of medical care phenomena. They should also prove useful in revealing deficiencies in present knowledge and in preparing the reader to appreciate the relevance of new information as it becomes available. In the text the reader will find illustrations of how the models have been used to demonstrate relationships, to reveal gaps in knowledge, and to suggest subjects that require further research.

It is clear from the above that the hypothetical medical care administrator is seen as a student of medical care phenomena. He differs from the scholar only in having the further responsibility of taking action on the basis of what he knows. It is therefore hoped that this book will be equally useful to the student, scholar, and researcher. Its particular contribution to the scholar and researcher may be in presenting a particular formulation that they may wish to challenge, or in revealing deficiencies in knowledge which they may want to rectify. The rsearcher who has been trained in a field other than medical care may find the presentation particularly helpful in summarizing present knowledge and in indicating more precisely those areas where his own expertise would be likely to make the greatest contribution toward the solution of operational problems in medical care administration.

In order to encourage further independent study, the titles in the bibliography have been arranged under subject headings rather than serially as they are cited in the text. This makes the bibliography partly independent of the text, allowing the inclusions of sources not cited specifically. It is believed that these advantages outweigh the minor inconvenience to the reader of not having the references appear in the order in which they are cited.

This monograph represents only the beginning of a larger enterprise that has no precise end point. Obviously, the aspects of administration included are only a few of the many tasks that the administrator has to perform. It is hoped that future publications will deal with additional tasks using an approach similar to that used in this text. A second volume that will deal with clients and professionals in medical care organizations is now under preparation with equal support from the Carnegie Corporation of New York and Milbank Memorial Fund.

Needless to say, I am fully aware of the magnitude of the task and of the limitations in my own background and preparation. These I feel most acutely when dealing with material from the social sciences that clearly have a bearing on medical care phenomena and, therefore, have to be included. Nevertheless, it appears necessary, as a step in the development of the field, to present a systematic view of its major features as seen by one scholar. The product is likely to have defects, especially where high levels of specialized knowledge are required to ensure complete accuracy. It is hoped that this is more than balanced by gains in coherence and consistency. It is further hoped that, through constructive criticism by other scholars, the present work will serve as a stepping-stone to something better. In this spirit I would welcome criticism and suggestions from all my readers.

Several colleagues have given help in the preparation of this volume. Sylvester Berki has attempted to instruct me in the rudiments of economics, probably with little success, through no fault of his own. Eugene Feingold has provided references on the subject of legislative intent. Rashid Bashshur and Gary Shannon have provided materials on spatial aspects of organization and have criticized that portion of the text. Robert de Vries has made useful suggestions, especially relating to features of hospital operations. These are in addition to the help, guidance, and inspiration I have received from many colleagues and students in the Department of Medical Care Organization at the University of Michigan School of Public Health. These have influenced my thinking so continuously, and in so many ways, that it is no longer possible for me to identify their separate contributions. I owe a debt of gratitude even to those colleagues and students who saw little merit in my work. They have impelled me to submit it to a larger jury of my peers.

. . . O

> the untrustworthiness of Egyptologists
> Who do not know their trips. Who was that
> dog-faced man? they asked, the day I rode
> from town.*

The preparation of a manuscript entails much unglamorous but necessary labor which the author alone cannot do. I was fortunate in having the help of several who worked with me superlatively well. Two of my students, Emily Bale and Barak Wolff, undertook the tedious task of verifying many of the references. Mary Bodley typed the manuscript for the last chapter; all the rest was typed by Elizabeth Plant. Susan

---

* Ishmael Reed, "I Am A Cowboy In The Boat Of Ra." From *The New Black Poetry*, edited by Clarence Major, International Publishers, 1969.

Keystone and Helen Heys did the secretarial work for the small, but numerous, revisions that have been made in the original manuscript. Barbara Black kept my accounts straight and saw to it that I came through financially solvent in the end. Finally, Kathleen Ahern, of the Harvard University Press, edited with sensitivity and awesome competence a difficult manuscript that was made even more exasperating by my frequent revisions.

The Medical Care Reference Collection at The University of Michigan has been an essential library resource without which I would probably not have had the courage to undertake this work. I am therefore indebted to the many devoted and farsighted people* who originated and nurtured this treasure trove of materials in our field. More immediately, I am grateful to the present staff, especially Jack Tobias and Lillian Fagin, who helped me trace elusive materials that too often I was able to describe only in vague or even misleading terms.

This monograph would not have been possible without a grant from the Commonwealth Fund and support during sabbatical leave by The University of Michigan. I am happy to acknowledge my indebtedness to these two institutions.

Finally, I would like to acknowledge unfailing support from my wife, who suffered through the preparation of this monograph even more than I did.

Ann Arbor, Michigan
May 1, 1972   A.D.

* In historical order, Nathan Sinai, Odin Anderson, Dorothy Paton, Jean Thorby, Solomon Axelrod, Charles Metzner, Jack Tobias and Eugene Feingold, among others.

Contents

Preface

I

Social Values

BASIC VALUES RELEVANT TO MEDICAL CARE ADMINISTRATION

Introduction and General Model

Social values permeate a society and all of its institutions. To a considerable degree such values are responsible for the forms that these institutions take and the directions along which they may be acceptably modified. The institutionalized forms for the provision of health services are no exception to this rule. Social values may, in fact, be more than usually relevant. This is because medical care touches upon the most vital concerns of people, involves intimate and intensely personal relationships, and is surrounded by a variety of moral and ethical proscriptions.

A characteristic of social values in a reasonably stable society is that they are largely implicit and that their influence on behavior may easily escape notice. This is true for administrative decisions as well. Even when such decisions appear to be largely technical, value preferences may have been critical, though concealed.

Another characteristic of pervasive social values is that they are acquired through a process of profound and lengthy socialization. They are accepted rather than reasoned. Any challenge to them is therefore likely to evoke a disproportionately heated response. Seemingly irreconcilable battle lines are rapidly drawn.

It follows from all this that the medical care administrator must learn to identify and appreciate the social value components in institutionalized forms for the delivery of personal health services, current and proposed. He must, in particular, understand his own value positions and the manner in which they influence his own choices among alternative courses of action. The purpose is not to disavow these values but to deal with them explicitly as relevant factors in arriving at decisions. This chapter is offered as a contribution to achieving these aims.

Very emphatically, it is not the purpose of this chapter to impose upon the administrator a particular value orientation espoused by the author, although the author's preferences will be made clear. Even if this were the objective, it would be fruitless to make the effort, since a genuine change in values is only possible over the long haul through personal reflection and adjustment. Nor is it the purpose of this chapter to attempt anything approaching a definitive analysis of social values relevant to medical care administration. Primarily, it is intended to be illustrative of an approach, thus pointing the way for further exploration to be undertaken by the administrator himself. In the process of doing so, this chapter will make explicit certain values that are implicit in the medical care system we now have; demonstrate relationships between these values and certain features of the system; and, it is hoped, illustrate how values can be dealt with systematically. In so doing, it will render such values less elusive, less threatening, and more subject to voluntary change.

As a framework for analysis we will assume a situation in which the issue is the acceptability of greater governmental responsibility for the provision of health services to a particularly vulnerable population group. We will also postulate that there are only two positions relevant to the issue under consideration. To avoid any prejudgments we shall identify these merely as positions, or viewpoints, A and B. We will also postulate that each of these positions is derived from a particular interpretation of the content and relevance of the same four social values. The major outlines of the presentation are indicated roughly in the following diagram, and in much greater detail in the summary that concludes this chapter.

Social	Positions, or Viewpoints,	
values	A	B
Personal responsibility		
Social concern		
Freedom		
Equality		

Personal Responsibility

VIEWPOINT A. This viewpoint places particular emphasis on the values of personal responsibility for achievement. It contends that nothing unearned should be given lest there be injury to the recipient of the gift as well as to society at large. The recipients of unearned rewards suffer through a diminution of the urge for personal achievement. All others are similarly dissuaded from personal effort since such effort does not lead to advantages in comparison to the advantages enjoyed by those who do not make a similar effort. It follows that every withdrawal of a commodity from the system of rewards weakens that system and threatens the motive force that assures economic well-being. More than that, it weakens moral well-being as well, since there is seen to be an intimate connection between moral excellence and the dedication to the personal effort to achieve. Thus, both the economic and moral well-being of the individual and of society are considered to depend on the integrity of a reward system that distributes goods and services in proportion to the magnitude and value of the individual effort expended to earn them.

Medical care services, in particular, should remain as part of the system of rewards, because they are among the most valuable rewards that a society can offer. Furthermore, there is little that is distinctive about medical care services to justify their selective exemption from the general rule linking individual rewards to personal effort.

This emphasis on personal responsibility for achievement and the system of rewards that nourishes it, is deeply rooted in our society. No wonder, since it represents a conjunction of two dominant strands of Western thought: the "Protestant Ethic" and the doctrines of classical laissez-faire economics (16, 17).* Later in the nineteenth century this position received additional support by absorbing yet another strand of thought, this time from the field of biology: Darwin's theory of evolution through natural selection (18). Social Darwinism, though no longer in vogue, is by no means extinct. Many still harbor the fear that allowing the physically and morally unfit to survive poses a distinct threat to future generations and to the progressive amelioration of the social order.

VIEWPOINT B. This viewpoint does not challenge in any fundamental way the value of personal responsibility for achievement. There is, as in Viewpoint A, a basic commitment to maintaining the system of rewards

---

* The numbers in parentheses within the text pertain to Readings and References at the end of each chapter.

and the link between rewards and effort. What is different is, first, a tendency to reject the equating of economic failure with moral failure. The failure to achieve is not so readily taken to connote moral depravity or social worthlessness, present or future. Second, there is emphasis on the need to remove from the reward system certain commodities to which all persons should be entitled by virtue of being members of any given society. Access to these commodities is more in the nature of a right than a reward. Medical care, in particular, is considered to be such a commodity by virtue of a host of distinctive characteristics that set it apart. An enumeration of these characteristics at this point in the discussion would require a lengthy digression that might obscure the overall design of this presentation. For that reason, this aspect of Viewpoint B will be presented separately in a later section of this chapter.

Social Concern

VIEWPOINT A. Concern for the welfare of the individual and of society as a whole is a value as deeply rooted in our culture as is the value of personal responsibility. To a large extent, however, the one is contrary to the other; hence the need to reconcile the two values if they are to be simultaneously held. There are a number of ways of achieving at least some degree of reconciliation. At one extreme, the Social Darwinist would contend that the true welfare of society, in the long run, requires a seemingly cruel indifference to the fate of those individuals who cannot make the grade. As William Graham Sumner put it, "a plan for nourishing the unfittest and yet advancing civilization, no man will ever find" (18, p.57). A less extreme, and therefore more prevalent, viewpoint is to hold, as did the classical economists, that each person pursuing single-mindedly his own interests thereby makes the greatest contribution to the collective good. Perhaps more congenial to the Judaeo-Christian tradition is a third formulation: that the true interests of the individual, in the moral and spiritual as well as in the more practical domains, require a seemingly disinterested concern for others. However, this is an argument that appears to rest on "egoistic reasons why a man should not be egoistic" (19). Therefore, most congenial to the Judaeo-Christian tradition, and perhaps most typical of Viewpoint A in our model, is to accept the moral legitimacy, even the moral imperative, of social concern for the individual, but to exercise this concern within boundaries so as to protect the twin principle of individual responsibility for personal welfare.

Under this formulation, Viewpoint A recognizes that the involuntary nature of disease, and other misfortunes, must temper the strict application of the principle of personal responsibility. It is recognized that not all who fail to achieve can be held guilty. There are, in fact the "worthy poor." This strengthens the case for those who would manifest concern on their behalf.

Under Viewpoint A, charity, individually or collectively expressed, preferably under private auspices, is the proper vehicle for implementing social concern for the individual. However, lest the availability of charity weaken the capacity and motivation to assume personal responsibility, in the recipient as well as in others, it is to be exercised under carefully prescribed conditions. The potential recipient is first encouraged to mobilize all personal and family resources. When these prove inadequate, arrangements are made to supplement these resources—without, however, being so generous as to make the recipient's position comparable to that of the self-supporting. The practical result is that standards of care are set at a low level and needs are usually not fully met. Furthermore, the circumstances and conditions under which services are provided are calculated to be unpleasant, uncomfortable, even humiliating. An element of chastisement, presumably rehabilitative, has not been considered foreign or inappropriate to the exercise of Christian charity.

All this is derived from the principle of "lesser eligibility," hallowed by usage, and designed to spur the recipient to efforts on his own behalf, as well as to buttress the determination of all others to remain self-supporting. The historical roots of "lesser eligibility" are perhaps best appreciated by quoting directly from the Reports of the Poor Law Commissions in England:

The fundamental principle with respect to the legal relief of the poor is, that the condition of the pauper ought to be, on the whole, less eligible than that of the independent laborer . . .

The only expedient, therefore, for accomplishing the end in view, which humanity permits, is to subject the pauper inmate of a public institution to such a system of labor, discipline, and restraint, as shall be sufficient to outweigh in his estimation, the advantages which he derives from the bodily comfort he enjoys" (Report of the Poor Law Commissioners, 1840. Quoted in ref. 20, pp. 132–133).

All poor law relief is given reluctantly. Every Guardian is told to give it reluctantly; every Poor Law Officer gives it reluctantly . . . poor people were dissatisfied with the medical relief they got from the Poor Law (because) it is given grudgingly . . . the man going to the Relieving Officer being put in the dock, questioned up hill and down dale, and treated as a thief" (Report of the Poor Law Commission, 1909. Quoted in ref. 21, p. 14).

Another argument in favor of charity as the appropriate expression of social concern is that its exercise is beneficial to the giver as well as to the recipient. To best serve this function charity would have to be voluntary and carried out in a manner that keeps personal involvement by the philanthropist in some way meaningful to him. In addition to private psychic returns to the individual philanthropist, the nourishing of the philanthropic impulse is regarded by some to make for a better society through creating opportunities for altruistic activities among its elites. This is an idea rather eloquently expressed by de Jouvenal as follows:

> It is clear enough that progress is linked with the existence of elites, the production and upkeep of which are costly, and the incomes of which could not be flattened out without great social loss . . . it is generally agreed that men fulfilling certain functions need considerable means, and eventual amenities which fit them to render their specific services . . . But the individual's value to society does not lie exclusively in the professional services he renders. It would be a sorry society in which men gave nothing to their contemporaries over and above the services for which they are rewarded and which enter into the computation of national income. Often enough one has a frightening vision of such a society, when one sees in some suburban train tired men travelling back from the day's toil to the small house in which they will shut themselves up to eat and sleep until they travel back to the factory or to the office. At these moments one treasures what is left of society: warm hospitality, leisured and far-ranging conversation, friendly advice, voluntary and unrewarded services. Culture and civilization, indeed the very existence of society depends upon such voluntary, unrewarded activities (Quoted in ref. 22, pp. 76 and 77).

Finally, charity recommends itself to those who would wish to keep intact the reward system. Charity, certainly if it is voluntary, but perhaps when exercised under the law, is seen to create less of an unchallenged entitlement to service. Provision of service, it would seem, is more by suffrance and less as a right.

VIEWPOINT B. This viewpoint does not differ radically from the modal position under Viewpoint A in accepting social concern as a moral imperative or, at the very least, as enlightened self-interest. Nor does it reject out-of-hand the charity approach to meeting social needs. It does maintain, however, that charity is probably the least desirable avenue for expressing social concern. This is because charity is often demeaning to the recipient and corrupting to both the institutions and the individuals charged with its application. Rather than being rehabilitative, institutionalized charity usually leads to further dependency, with atrophy of the capacity to exercise personal initiative and responsibility. A truer expression of social concern is to create a general environment and more specific mechanisms that reduce to a minimum the need for charity. Among these specific mechanisms is health insurance, voluntary or compulsory, which is infinitely to be preferred over public assistance medical care programs that embody the charity approach.

By placing the emphasis on the application of social mechanisms that create and maintain self-sufficiency, the adherents to Viewpoint B also seem to solve rather neatly the conflict inherent in the desire to foster personal responsibility on the one hand and provide charity on the other. It was persuant to this line of reasoning that Wilbur Cohen was able to declare social health insurance for the aged as "the conservative approach" even though it was to be compulsory (23). The fact that the scheme was based on the principle of self-help took precedence, in his opinion, over the fact that it was compulsory. As we shall see, the adherents of Viewpoint B would debate this interpretation.

Objections can also be raised concerning charity as a mechanism for meeting medical care needs on a number of other grounds, mainly technical or operational. Some of these will be referred to later in this chapter and discussed in greater detail in a subsequent volume under the rubric of eligibility determination.

Freedom

VIEWPOINT A. A basic value in our society is that nothing should be done to curtail freedom unnecessarily. Freedom is to be sought as a supreme good in itself. Furthermore, compulsion attenuates personal responsibility as well as individualistic and voluntary expressions of social concern. Those who adhere to Viewpoint A tend to emphasize in particular political freedom and danger of coercion through political means. Government, in particular, is seen to possess an inherent tendency to proliferate, and thus to encroach progressively upon individual freedom. Each new responsibility assigned to government becomes a step to the acquisition of still greater control unless the progression is checked by determined external opposition. Suspicion of government, in direct proportion to its distance from the local level, is characteristic of this viewpoint.

This position is further reinforced by the conviction that there is a self-balancing state, a "natural harmony," that becomes established only if freedom is maintained. In the economic field this is expressed in the doctrine of the "invisible hand" that brings about optimal allocations through the operations of a freely competitive marketplace. Similarly, among the tenets of Social Darwinism was the belief that if natural selection were not hampered by ill-advised, though well-meaning, interference, society would naturally evolve to ever higher levels of perfection.

The natural consequence of these beliefs is suspicion of centralized health planning and opposition to granting government a larger role in the financing and provision of health services. Compulsory health insurance, in particular, is seen as an unwarranted abridgment of the freedom of clients as well as of health professionals. In addition, many physicians, imbued with the central importance of their social role, appear to believe that private medicine is often the major bulwark of freedom in society and, hence, the initial target of those who would enslave it. Once medicine is "socialized," it is feared that the whole structure of freedom will inevitably crumble.

VIEWPOINT B. Once again, there is agreement on the validity of the basic value—in this case that a maximum of freedom is to be maintained. What is different about Viewpoint B is its definition of freedom and of the role of government in society.

Freedom is defined as the presence of real opportunities to make alternative choices. It is seen less as a single abstract principle and more in operative terms as composed of a multitude of freedoms, each representing a real opportunity for choice in any given situation. Tawney states it well:

> There is no such thing as freedom in the abstract, divorced from the realities of a particular time and place. Whatever else the conception may imply, it involves a power of choice between alternatives, a choice which is real, not merely nominal, between alternatives which exist in fact, not only on paper . . . It means the ability to do, or to refrain from doing, definite things, at a definite moment, in definite circumstances.
> The right to education is obviously impaired, if poverty arrests its use in mid-career; the right to the free choice of an occupation, if the expenses of entering a profession are prohibitive; the right to earn a living, if enforced unemployment is recurrent; the right to justice, if few men of small means can afford the cost of litigation; the right to "life, liberty and the pursuit of happiness," if the environment is such as to assure that, as in a not distant past, a considerable proportion of the heirs to these blessings die within twelve months, and that the happiness investments of the remainder are a gambling stock (24, pp. 260, 267).

Two consequences flow from this definition. First, as the quotation from Tawney clearly shows, a variety of causes and circumstances have the capacity to abridge freedom. Compulsion is not seen to arise mainly in the political sphere. Economic factors, particularly, are no less coercive even though they present themselves as impersonal and anonymous. Second, because freedoms are concrete, discrete, and multiple, there arises the possibility of exchanges, or "trade-offs," among them. One freedom may be sacrificed to gain another that is more highly regarded. Similarly, a freedom enjoyed by one group may be sacrificed for the same freedom in another group, or a different freedom for all. For example, it may be expedient to submit to taxation during the working years in order to have during old age the capacity to receive or reject medical care, and to enjoy the other freedoms that the availability of medical care bestows. As Barker puts it: ''To enjoy the rights of social security is to be liberated from fears and dangers; to be more of a freeman, and to have more freedom for the development of personal capacity'' (25, p. 271). It is the sum total of all the freedoms enjoyed by all men in a society that determines whether one society is more free than another. In estimating this total sum, as we shall see in the next section, the welfare of each person is equal to that of any other.

A redefinition of the nature of freedom and of the threats to it is allied to a redefinition of the nature and role of government. This is no longer seen as the only, or even the major, threat to freedom. Nor is it seen to possess an inherent, almost uncontrollable, propensity to progressively encroach upon freedom. It is at once less foreign, more manageable and more benign. It is, in fact, in many situations, the major instrument that can assure for most people the liberties that they so devoutly desire.

It is still often assumed by privileged classes that, when the State refrains from intervening, the condition which remains, as a result of its inaction, is liberty. In reality, what not infrequently remains is, not liberty, but tyranny   (24, p. 261).

Government is not external: it is in us, or springs from us; and we regard political liberty as positive in its nature. It is a liberty not of curbing government, but of constituting and controlling it; constituting it by a general act of choice or election, in which we all freely share on the basis of universal suffrage; controlling it by a general and continuous process of discussion, in which we all freely share according to our capacities   (25, p. 147).

The state of government is not inherently hostile . . . public policy can reflect public opinion as determined by "the give and take and learn" of the democratic process. The state is no longer "them" but "us" as much as anyone. (5, p. 192).

A liberty that is protected by law is a right . . . Since important liberties are contested violently as they are born, they are transformed as quickly as possible into rights, so that they may be protected and nurtured (26, p. 342).

Finally, the concept of a natural, harmonious order of things that is brought about by a minimum of planned intervention, does not recommend itself to those who hold Viewpoint B. They are more prone to intervene and more apt to use the political process as an instrument for intervention. Centralized health planning is less feared; it is even encouraged. An expansion of the role of government in the provison of health services is regarded not necessarily as an evil, nor is compulsory insurance ruled out simply because it involves the abridgment of certain freedoms. The issue is whether the sum total of freedoms for the sum total of people is thereby enhanced.

Equality

VIEWPOINT A. Under this viewpoint, the concept of equality is rather narrowly defined to comprise, mainly, equality before the law. It covers only specifically defined constitutional and legal rights that cannot be extended to cover anything else to which one might want to lay claim. Furthermore, the emphasis appears to be on the potential for legally defined equality rather than on the equal realization, in practice, of this potential. In other words, the many factors that render constitutional and legal rights less operative for significant segments of the population do not appear to be so disturbing. It is held, in fact, that our system does not intend to provide equality of rewards, but only a legally defined framework within which competition can proceed and the resultant inequality in status achieved and maintained.

Another characteristic of Viewpoint A is emphasis on a seemingly irreconcilable conflict between freedom on the one hand and equality on the other, so that increases in one occur only at the expense of reductions in the other. Faced with this contradiction, the adherents of Viewpoint A would give precedence to freedom.

VIEWPOINT B. Those who adhere to Viewpoint B define equality more broadly as the equal opportunity for achievement through maximum development of the capacities within each person. It is held that the only moral justification for using personal achievement as a criterion for the distribution of rewards is the condition that all contestants start on some footing of equality. In a broader sense, one cannot use the prerequisites for achievement as rewards for achievement. The prerequisites must be made available to all.

Among these prerequisities, by general consent, is a certain level of preparatory education. More recently, health has been recognized as a similar prerequisite, and therefore a "right" to medical care is more generally asserted. It is interesting, for that reason, to note how similar are the arguments for and against the extension of public responsibility for medical care today, to the arguments for and against public education not much more than a hundred years ago (7). What is happening is a process by which equality is being constantly redefined as more and more goods are removed from the individual reward system and become part of the collective treasure available to all. Those who hold Viewpoint

A fear that this will so weaken the reward system that it will lose its efficacy as a spur to individual achievement. Those who hold Viewpoint B assert, on the contrary, that unless individual competition is placed on a more just footing, the whole system will fall into disrepute, placing it in jeopardy of total rejection.

Thus, the adherents to Viewpoint B see no contradiction between their emphasis on equality, as they define it, and the value of personal responsibility for achievement. Similarly, they do not see the contradiction between equality and freedom that is so salient for those who hold Viewpoint A. On the contrary, equality seems merely to be the extension, to a larger group of people, of freedoms now enjoyed by the relatively few. We shall return to this point when we discuss, in a subsequent section of this chapter, the reconciliation of seemingly dichotomous positions.

Summary of the Two Viewpoints

Simply as a device for demonstrating the relevance of social values to medical care policy, and for pointing out some of the intricate relationships among social values, we have constructed two archetypal viewpoints, designated, in order to postpone the thought-disturbing influence of labels, simply as Viewpoints A and B. Viewpoint A places major emphasis on personal achievement and the freedom of the individual from political compulsion. For this reason it may be most accurately called "libertarian." Viewpoint B places major emphasis on equality of opportunity and redefines liberty in terms of equalizing the opportunities for choice. For this reason it may be most accurately called "egalitarian."

Certain features of the analysis of values presented above require special mention. First, the more extreme ideological positions to either side of Viewpoints A and B (with the possible exception of Social Darwinism) have been purposely excluded. Although the more extreme positions are of major interest to political theory, they do not represent a significant force in our society. It is believed that the range of views presented here, though fairly narrow, embraces the large majority of the population. Second, it is clear that the value positions presented are highly interactive. Both Viewpoints A and B appeal to the same basic values and differ mainly in the way in which the values are defined and in the priorities given to the several values. In fact, it would not be uncommon for an individual, seemingly without inner discomfort, to hold a position composed of a mosaic of components taken from both sides of the model described. Perhaps, because the position each person takes may differ with the specific problem at issue, a kaleidoscope rather than a mosaic may be the more appropriate description. Third, some readers may feel that some of the more extreme libertarian views presented are mere straw men set up only to be demolished. This is not the case, as a reading of the medical care literature and an even superficial acquaintance with the practices (if not the theory) of public welfare medical care will quickly demonstrate.

A question of great interest is what accounts for individual preferences for certain value positions over others. A treatment of this question is beyond the scope of this book. It would seem, however, that the libertarian viewpoint is more frequently held by segments in the population who already possess a considerable fund of freedoms which they wish to exercise with a minimum of interference. There is, apparently, a willingness to accept devaluation of what is seen as a relatively small and rather marginal group of people, who are regarded not useful to society, in order to maintain what is seen to be the higher good of those who remain. By contrast, the egalitarian viewpoint appears to be more congenial to those who regard themselves as underprivileged, and who aspire to share in the freedoms which the more privileged already enjoy.

Reconciliation of Conflict

In the preceding section we emphasized the kinship between the two viewpoints presented in our model. One must also point out the differences and the potential for seemingly irreconcilable conflict. Such conflict arises especially when the situation to be faced is presented starkly as a choice between two totally disparate alternatives, for example: equality versus freedom, individualism versus collectivism, free enterprise versus socialism. Allied to this doctrine of dichotomies is another which Sidney Hook has called "the slippery slope" argument: "Once you begin, where will you stop?" (5) The allegation is that once one compromises in the smallest degree either of the two polar positions, total abandonment is the inevitable outcome. The following quotations are offered as illustrations of these points of view:

Let it be understood that we cannot go outside of this alternative; liberty, inequality, survival of the fittest; not-liberty, equality, survival of the unfittest. The former carries society forward and favors its best members; the latter carries society downwards and favors its worst members (William Graham Sumner quoted in ref. 18, p. 51).

The egalitarian . . . will defend taking from some to give to others, not as a more effective means whereby the "some" can achieve an objective they want to achieve, but on grounds of "justice." At this point equality comes sharply into conflict with freedom; one must choose. One cannot be both an egalitarian, in this sense, and a liberal (27, p. 195).

There are only two basic ways of organizing the activities of large numbers of people and, therefore, only two basic ways of organizing to satisfy people's desires for medical care . . . The choice is between (1) compelling and coercing people to provide that kind and quality of medical service desired by centralized authority, direction and control; and (2) inducing people to provide that care voluntarily by offering them, in exchange for their resources or services, generalised claims—usually in the form of money—against other goods and services. The first method requires coercion to some extent . . . The second alternative is . . . a medical care system organized through the market mechanism and voluntary exchange—a free, private-enterprise competitive exchange system . . . Are the proponents of a massive, State-owned and operated medical care system willing to draw the line at that point? If everybody's life must be run in terms of medical choices, what other aspects of people's lives must also be controlled? Where do they draw the line? (4, pp. 244, 243).

Fortunately, there are ways out of the impasse created by rigid positions such as the above. Two types of reconciliation are possible: one conceptual and the other pragmatic or operational. The conceptual solution rests upon emphasizing the points of kinship among the seemingly irreconcilable values. For example, we have already pointed out that the egalitarian viewpoint, far from rejecting the values of personal responsibility, social concern and liberty, merely recasts them into a new mold. By redefining equality and freedom, it postulates that the institution of equality with respect to certain fundamental requisites strengthens the validity of personal responsibility for the acquisition of other commodities and enhances the measure and distribution of freedom throughout society. As Tawney says in concluding his brilliant dissertation on Equality:

Insofar as the opportunity to lead a life worthy of human beings is needlessly confined to a minority, not a few of the conditions applauded as freedom would more properly be denounced as privilege. Action which causes such opportunities to be more widely shared is, therefore, twice blessed. It not only subtracts from inequality, but adds to freedom" (24, p. 268).

The pragmatic or operational reconciliation recognizes the relative meaninglessness of grand alternatives phrased in abstract and absolute terms. The emphasis is on the discrete, limited objectives that need to be attained and on the variety of means that are available to attain them. As Dahl and Lindblom so persuasively point out:

It has become increasingly difficult for thoughtful men to find meaningful alternatives posed in the traditional choice between socialism and capitalism, planning and the free market, regulation and laissez faire, for they find their actual choices neither so simple nor so grand . . . Capitalism is now hardly more than a name stretched to cover a large family of economies . . . Socialism has lost its unique character . . . Both socialism and capitalism are dead" (28, pp. 3ff).

Dahl and Lindblom go on to show that what social policy has to deal with are not choices between opposites, but the selection, or invention, of mechanisms situated at some point on a continuum between the traditional polar positions: private versus governmental and voluntary versus compulsory. In any one society, a variety of mechanisms or social institutions, dispersed so that they fall at different points along the entire continuum, can coexist. This is certainly true for medical care in the United States. At one extreme there are examples of state medicine typified by the government-owned and operated system of hospital care for veterans, and at the other extreme, private, solo medical practice in which physicians are paid out-of-pocket for each service rendered. The forms that are ranged in between include: (i) proprietary, voluntary, and public (local, state, and federal) hospitals; (ii) group practice sponsored by physicians, consumers, industry, or labor; (iii) individually purchased commercial health insurance; (iv) commercial and quasi-public, non-profit, health insurance provided under quasi-voluntary collective bargaining arrangements; (v) government-subsidized voluntary health insurance (Medicare, part B); (vi) compulsory health insurance, both state (Workmen's Compensation) and federal (Medicare, part A); and (vii) a variety of governmental programs, using mostly the charity approach, that make possible the purchase of medical care for private individuals from private sources. It is clear that one is not constrained to choose between one polar position or another. On the contrary, the emphasis should be on defining specific social tasks and using those social instruments that are most efficacious in performing these tasks at lowest cost. Part of the cost is monetary, or can be expressed in monetary terms. Another part may be some loss with respect to some deeply held value or general principle of conduct. The administrator's responsibility is to balance the losses and the gains and to make certain that society comes ahead in the balance.

There is always a price to be paid for rights. That price . . . is partly financial, or a matter of payment in money; partly spiritual, or a matter of payment in the acceptance of control. We need not pause to discuss the nature and implications of the financial price. That is a matter of economics: of national finance and the balancing of national income and national expenditure. It is the spiritual price which matters most: and the crucial balance to be struck is the balance between the spiritual profit gained in the increased enjoyment of rights and the spiritual loss incurred or involved in the increased acceptance of control. When we seek to strike this balance, we have two calculations to make. The first is a calculation of the gain and loss in the private account of each individual: it is a matter, as it were, of the private bankbook of each; it is a business of reckoning individual gain of liberty against individual loss. The second is a calculation of the gain and loss in what may be called the common account of the whole community; it is a business of computing the gain of one class or section, in liberty and personal rights, against the loss of another (25, p. 270).

As to the "slippery slope" argument, that once one begins moving in a certain direction, who knows where the movement will stop, one can respond with the refreshing rejoinder that "You stop where your intelligence tells you to stop, and an intelligent decision proceeds from case to case, from problem to problem" (5, p. 181).

A Personal Position

Since personal beliefs and biases strongly color recommendations for action in the medical care field, as in any other field of social policy, the reader should know where the author stands so that he may make the necessary allowances in evaluating the view of the medical care system which the author will proceed to present. It has, perhaps, become fairly clear that the author subscribes to Viewpoint B, the egalitarian orientation. Moreover, he finds particularly congenial the processes of conceptual and pragmatic reconciliation presented above. He believes that these processes call for careful analysis of all the factors, pertaining to values as well as to techniques, relevant to each problem and are, therefore, conducive to technically appropriate, politically feasible, and ethically defensible action.

DISTINCTIVE CHARACTERISTICS OF MEDICAL CARE

We have already referred to the argument whether medical care should remain within the reward system or be exempted, in the main, from the rule that rewards should be commensurate with the effort to earn them. The fundamental moral argument for withdrawing medical care from the reward system is that health is a prerequisite for successful achievement, and that competition, to be fair, must assure a reasonably equal level of health to all competitors. In addition, a number of more specific characteristics of illness, of medical care services, and of the medical care market, reduce the level of responsibility that the individual might be expected to exercise and provide justification for collective action, private or governmental, to assure a socially preferred distribution of health services. This section will deal with these specific characteristics. The discussion will be restricted to factors of general applicability. Excluded is consideration of services provided by government as an integral part of a broader function assigned to government (health services for the armed forces, for example) or provided to special groups for whom government has accepted particular responsibility: veterans, merchant seamen, Indians on reservations, and the like.

It may be useful to begin by pointing out the importance of medical care as part of the reward system. Certainly its capacity to safeguard life itself places it potentially among the supreme rewards a society can offer. The tendency to use it as such is clearly seen in most societies. In the United States, this intent is explicit in the system of medical care services for veterans, and implicit in the vast growth of health insurance under collective bargaining. In countries where medical care is more centralized and controlled, the same tendency may be exhibited in two ways. First, there may remain a sector of more sophisticated private medical care for the well-to-do. Second, especially liberal provision may be made in a public system for certain highly valued segments in the population, such as industrial employees or the military, who, by virtue of this, constitute "medically privileged groups" (29). Russia is an interesting case in point. By making medical care available to all, the Russian scheme removed medical care from the system of incentives. However, medical care is reintroduced into the incentive system by creating segments of higher level care which are reserved for elites whom it is the intention to reward. This is done in part by assigning private physicians to particularly prominent individuals or small groups of individuals, and partly by instituting a closed system of clinics, hospitals, and convalescent resorts reserved for the elite (30).

The characteristics of medical care as an economic good have been discussed by several authors, among them Lees (12), Mushkin (13), Weisbrod (14), and Klarman (15). Lees has contended that medical care differs little in any of its characteristics from other goods and services that are successfully rationed by a reasonably free market. Mushkin, Weisbrod, and Klarman have emphasized those characteristics of public health and medical services that set them apart from commodities more likely to be rationed successfully by the market. The following summary will draw on these sources without holding any of them responsible for the particular formulation to be presented.

Like all models, the classical economic model of the free market is an abstraction based on certain assumptions. The extent to which these assumptions do not hold for medical care services may be taken as evidence of the inapplicability, at least without modification, of the model to this particular commodity. The assumptions will be examined under the following headings: (i) limits on rationality, (ii) limits on consumer choice and control, (iii) other constraints in the medical market, (iv) external benefits and the public interest, and (v) health services as a public good.

Limits on Rationality

The success of the market in satisfying not only the individual's whims and desires but also, to a reasonable extent, his own welfare and the welfare of society at large, depends on choices by a reasonably well-informed and rational consumer. The ability of the consumer to act in this manner with regard to medical care is severely hampered by (a) limitations in knowledge, (b) the deferred consequences of present choices, and (c) the nonpleasurable nature of most medical care services.

There are severe limitations on the knowledge of the average consumer of what are his true needs for medical care, of where the best care is to be found, and of the technical quality of care which he receives. Furthermore, knowledge concerning these aspects is highly class-linked, so that persons in the lower socioeconomic groups are at a particular disadvantage in this respect.

The postulation that there are "true needs" for medical care distinct from the immediate wishes and desires of the individual, is a matter of critical importance to the argument under consideration. It is a well-established fact that professional estimates of need for medical care generally differ significantly from subjective estimates, and that there is a large reservoir of unmet need for medical care in the population (31).* What is at issue is whether this is a matter that calls for social intervention. To the libertarian, such social concern or intervention is contemptuously labeled as "paternalism." Others would contend that neither the medical care administrator, nor society at large, can be satisfied if there is a very large gap between professionally defined medical care needs and those needs as subjectively defined by the potential client. The disparity between the client's estimate of the quality of care and professional judgments of the quality of the same care should also be a matter of deep concern. This disparity is, of course, greatest in the technical domain. With respect to the amenities of care, the consumer may be the best judge. For this reason, the market should be more successful in assuring these amenities than it is in assuring technical quality.

With respect to most goods and services, the consequences of satisfy-

* For a more detailed discussion of need and unmet need see Chapter 3 in this book.

ing, or denying satisfaction, to the consumer's needs and wants are fairly immediate and readily discernible by him. This is also true for many situations in medical care: deprivation has immediate painful consequences, and receipt of service leads to fairly prompt satisfaction or relief. For such services, the market is a more adequate rationing mechanism. There are, on the other hand, many services, generally of a preventive nature, where the nonsatisfaction of needs, assuming that these are perceived, does not lead to any immediate injury. The long term effects could, however, be serious. There is evidence that the market mechanism of rationing by price selectively depresses the use of preventive services, health supervision, and the early diagnosis of illness (32).

Finally, receipt of medical care services, unlike consumption of other goods and services, is not pleasurable. On the contrary, it is fraught with anxiety and may even be painful. In consequence, there is greater need for knowledge, even conviction, to surmount the reluctance most people have to seek medical care.

Limits on Consumer Choice and Control

The model of the free market postulates a ''sovereign'' consumer who, by deciding whether to buy or not, what to buy, when and where, calls the tune to economic activity and, ultimately, bends the entire economy to his will. With respect to medical care, these assumptions are so wide of the mark as to be ludicrous. This is because (a) illness is involuntary and unpredictable, (b) medical care services are often necessary and unpostponable, (c) medical care services tend to be indivisible, (d) the need for services often coincides with reduction in earning power, (e) the physician decides what services are needed on behalf of his patient, (f) there are limits on the availability of alternative sources of care at variable price, and (g) ''shopping around'' is discouraged.

The ability of the client to control and manipulate his demands on the market is clearly diminished by the great extent to which illness is involuntary and unpredictable. These characteristics are what justifies health insurance and makes it actuarially feasible. The fact that, in most cases, medical care is a necessary and urgent need, imposes additional constraints on the capacity of the consumer to manipulate demand. This conjunction of unpredictability and necessity is particularly significant since medical care is one of the few necessities the need for which is also unpredictable. There is, of course, a discretionary element of undetermined (perhaps undeterminable) magnitude in medical care. Apologists for the status quo have tended to emphasize the discretionary component. For example, a spokesman for the Economic Research Department of the A.M.A. has the following to say:

The greater demand for physicians in higher income areas probably reflects the discretionary character of some medical care more than anything else. Not all medical care is urgent. Some of it is for the treatment of so-called self-limiting ailments, functional matters, symptoms, and complaints. Possibly as much as one-fifth of all the physicians' home and office visits belong in these categories. In short much of a physician's work consists of eliminating the pain and discomfort associated with an illness as well as accelerating a recovery which would occur anyway" (33, p. 797).

By arguing in this way, medicine is put in the strange position of saying that a great deal of what medicine has to offer is not that important after all! But there is another, and more important, aspect to the argument: namely, that it is impossible, in any given instance, to determine what is necessary or unnecessary *before* the event. The layman must act on a presumption of need and must place himself under medical observation before a definitive determination of need can be made. This means that in order to encompass necessary care, one has to provide access to competent and thorough medical evaluation.

In addition to the often urgent and necessary nature of medical care services, such services, to be effective, very often have to be taken whole. A visit or two to the physician or a few doses of a life-saving drug, may not suffice. Nor is there such a thing as a partial appendectomy or a heart operation tailored to the consumer's purse. Medical services, to a significant degree, are indivisible, or should be. The financial impact of these fairly large bundles of care is the more disturbing because the need for service often coincides with reduction in earning power brought about by illness. This is especially true when the illness is severe and prolonged, and care, in consequence, particularly costly. Furthermore, the decision concerning what services are to be received, when and, frequently from what source, is made not by the client, but, on his behalf, by the physician. The client is usually responsible for initiating care. From there on, the attending physician calls the tune, to the extent of determining what brand-name drug the client may buy, even when much less expensive equivalents are available.

Additional limits on the exercise of consumer sovereignty arise out of certain peculiarities of the medical care market. First, although firm information is not available, one has the impression that alternative sources of care at variable price are less a feature of this market than of others. However, some variability does exist. In the hospital, the ward, semiprivate and private services, though varying in price, are presumed to offer equally effective, though not identical, care.* A relatively small proportion of prescribed drugs is available in generic form at considerably lower cost than the brand name equivalents. One may also choose to receive care from a chiropractor, a general practitioner, or a distinguished specialist at some differential in price. In this instance, however, it is not likely that the effectiveness of care, in satisfying technical health needs, is equivalent.

Second, "shopping around" by the patient is considered reprehensible by the medical profession, assuming the client has the time or knowledge to engage in this practice. As already described, the patient is expected to place himself trustingly in the hands of his physician, who undertakes to pilot him through the intricacies of the medical care system. But the decisions of the physician are seldom made on the basis of how and where the patient may obtain the most benefit at the least expense. The route the patient takes is determined more directly by the network of professional and institutional relationships that constitute the "professional referral system" (36).

Other Constraints in the Medical Care Market

There are a number of features of the medical care market and of the production of health services that make these less susceptible of response to consumer preferences and to more broadly defined social needs.

First, the medical profession is believed to exercise a considerable degree of control on the recruitment and training of personnel. While this may be necessary to safeguard the quality of the product, it also has had the effect of creating distinct shortages. We shall return to these points in subsequent sections of this book. There are also professionally supported restraints on alternative, and probably more efficient, modes of organizing physician services. For example, many states place severe restrictions on the organization of prepaid group practice (37).

Second, there are certain aspects of the production of services that may justify some centralized form of planning and organization. Klarman has pointed out that it takes a very long time to prepare a person to assume the role of a physician and that short-term adjustments to

* Duff and Hollingshead have demonstrated differences in care between patients in the ward and those in the private service of a teaching hospital (34). Weisbrod has pointed out that the price differential between private and semiprivate services in a hospital is too large to encourage use of private services by persons who have health insurance that covers semiprivate care (35).

increased demand may, for that reason, be difficult to make. He also points out that a minimum mass of health personnel and facilities is needed to provide a reasonable range of medical care services, and that some geographic areas may be unable to assemble this minimum without public intervention (15). Another aspect of the organization of medical care services is the relationship between scale and unit cost of product. Some services, such as medical care, are expensive to produce on a small scale. Unit cost of service decreases as the hospital increases in size, provided the quality of the product is held constant. Similar economies may also accrue from the organization of medical practice into larger groups (see Chapter 4 of this book). Weisbrod has contended that this characteristic of at least some public health activities justifies public responsibility for bringing about, or helping to encourage the development of, the necessary scale of organization (14).

External Benefits and the Public Interest

Imperfections in the market mechanism for producing and distributing medical care would be more readily tolerated if the benefits of using, and the losses from not using, service were confined to individuals who have made the decision to use or not to use service. So far as medical care is concerned, it is clear that the benefits and losses go beyond the individual and involve others. One example of this is the propagation of infectious disease in a community due to the presence of unrecognized or untreated cases of individual illness. A recent experience, on a small scale, can serve as an illustration :

During the week that ended May 9, 1964, "4 cases (of diphtheria) occurred in the vicinity of Canby in Yellow Medicine County (Minnesota), which has reported 9 of the State's 10 cases this year. Six of the 9 cases have occurred in one family, which refused immunization and medical care, until late in the course of the disease. The cases involved children, age 4 to 17 . . . Two cases were fatal; a 4 year old died of respiratory failure despite a tracheotomy and administration of antitoxin late in the course of his illness, and an 11 year old died of myocardial failure. Three additional cases occurred in members of 3 other families which had school or community contact with this family of objectors (38, p. 1).

In another outbreak of diptheria, in Northern Texas, epidemiological analysis suggested that the occurrence of several cases among unimmunized migrant workers was responsible, probably through school contacts, for the spread of infection to broader segments of the permanent population who had become susceptible by virtue of the low prevalence of immunization (39). In a reverse direction, when a fairly large proportion of persons in a community are immunized, there is a level of "herd immunity" which prevents the spread of epidemics even though the community may still harbor many unimmunized persons. These characteristics of infections have traditionally served as justification for public action, including compulsion, to prevent and treat the more threatening infectious diseases (10). In some instances the state has gone even further by instituting compulsory procedures that are designed to protect the health of the newborn and of school children even when no threat to others exists (11).

Another aspect of the public interest in whether the individual receives medical care is the notion that the individual is a national resource. For one, he is a factor of production in economic activity. This aspect of the value of man, and its relationship to priorities in medical care, will be discussed in Chapter 3. The individual is also an important resource in national defense. The latter feature explains the resurgence of governmental interest in health during a national emergency. Furthermore, war conditions often make visible both the deplorable health of many recruits and the state of incoordination and disrepair in a nation's medical establishment. In Britain, first the Boer War, and then the Second World War, are credited with playing a part in bringing about National Health Insurance and the National Health Service respectively (21, pp. 84–98; 41). In the United States, the findings of health examinations of military recruits have also helped focus public attention on the large amount of unmet need for medical care among young men (42, 43). The concept of the individual as a national resource may also contribute to the interest in services for children and youth who must depend on parents, or others, to arrange for their care. Klarman refers to Pigou, who points out that investment in the welfare of future generations may not safely be left entirely to private personal initiative (15).

Finally, Klarman has pointed out that medical care services are often joint products with medical education and research, which benefit persons other than the immediate recipient of care, although the latter is also benefited by the higher level of care generally associated with research and teaching. It has been traditional for most medical teaching and research to use ward patients who, in return for free care or care at reduced prices, became available, sometimes without their knowledge, for teaching and research. The wide application of voluntary and compulsory insurance, and of public assistance medical care, has greatly reduced the reservoir of nonpaying or part-paying patients, and encouraged the use of paying patients for teaching as well as for research, provided "informed consent" has been obtained (44, 45).

For all these reasons, society, in its own interests, may feel compelled to assure that the individual receives adequate medical care. Society's interest in the health of the individual may, under certain circumstances, be greater than that of the individual himself. In a democratic system, this interest expresses itself by making care available. Compulsion is reserved for situations in which there is a clear threat to others. A totalitarian regime may be less punctilious, and insist that, in the national interest, to receive care is a legally enforceable obligation.

Health Services as a Public Good

The concern of this book is with personal health services rather than with manipulations of the environment for healthful purposes. Personal health services are consumed by individuals, so that the use of service by some leaves less to be used by others. Other activities in the health field are of a different nature. They produce benefits which can be used by one individual without thereby diminishing the potential for use by another. Such benefits constitute what economists call public, collective, or social goods. Examples are air pollution control, the provision of a safe public water system, the fluoridation of this system, and mosquito control through swamp drainage and the widespread use of insecticide. Economists contend that a commodity or service that has the characteristics of a "public good" calls for collective provision because individuals will invest insufficiently in the production of services of which they are not the exclusive beneficiaries. They would rather conceal their wishes and wait for someone else to put in the necessary money so that they themselves may enjoy the benefits. Under such circumstances, collective action may be private, governmental, or both, depending on the nature and scope of the action required.

Summary of Distinctive Characteristics

Medical care is perhaps not peculiar in *any one* of the properties mentioned above. It is therefore easy to take them one by one and show that medical care need receive no special consideration. This has been done very effectively by Lees (12). The peculiarity, perhaps even uniqueness, of medical care lies in the combination of properties that characterize it.

Briefly, medical care is a service, both necessary and unpredictable, which must compete with other necessities for which the need is more constantly pressing or with non-necessities the satisfaction of which is more pleasurable. It must be purchased by a relatively ignorant consumer in a market in which the free operation of consumer choice and the price mechanism are hampered by a variety of restrictive devices. It is, moreover, a service the receipt or nonreceipt of which by individuals affects society as a whole.

SUMMARY OF MAJOR ARGUMENTS

Social values	"Libertarian" viewpoint	"Egalitarian" viewpoint
Personal responsibility for achievement	1. Personal responsibility for achievement is stressed	1. General agreement with value of personal responsibility for achievement and the system of rewards that support it

	2. Nothing unearned should be given lest there be:
	   a. injury to recipient
	   b. injury to others
		2. Less emphasis on economic failure as moral failure

	3. Types of injury:
	   a. moral
	   b. economic
		3. Medical care should not be part of reward system (or should merit special consideration). Reasons are:

	4. Positive relationship between personal effort and moral excellence	a. Limits on rationality
		   (1) imperfect knowledge of need
		   (2) delayed consequences of nonsatisfaction of wants
		   (3) nonpleasurable use

	5. Medical care should remain part of reward system:
	   a. a highly valued reward
	   b. there is little that is essentially different about it	

	6. Confluence of:
	   a. "Protestant Ethic"
	   b. Laissez-faire economics
	   c. Social Darwinism: biological support for moral position
		b. Limits on consumer choice and control
		   (1) illness involuntary and unpredictable
		   (2) service necessary
		   (3) service indivisible
		   (4) reduction in earning power
		   (5) physician control of use

SUMMARY OF MAJOR ARGUMENTS

Social values	"Libertarian" viewpoint	"Egalitarian" viewpoint

		(6) limits on alternative sources with variable price
		(7) shopping around discouraged
		
		c. Other constraints in medical care market
		  (1) professional monopoly
		  (2) time lag in production of trained personnel
		  (3) relationships between scale of organization and production
		
		d. External benefits
		  (1) benefits accrue to non-users
		  (2) the individual as a national resource
		  (3) service, education and research as joint products
		
		e. Health services as a "public good." Applies mainly to environmental health services

Social concern and social responsibility	1. Recognition of partially antithetical nature of personal responsibility for achievement and of social concern for others 2. Reconciliation through limited exercise of social concern. This is made	1. Charity accepted as the least desirable expression of social concern a. demeaning to the recipient and corrupting to the institutions and individuals charged with its execution

SUMMARY OF MAJOR ARGUMENTS

Social values	"Libertarian" viewpoint	"Egalitarian" viewpoint

	easier by recognition that involuntary nature of disease partly removes blame for failure to achieve
	
	3. Charity is appropriate expression of social concern:
	  a. It is less likely to create entitlement to service.
	  b. Can be provided under conditions that do least violence to personal responsibility: needs not fully met (lesser eligibility), service under difficult conditions, etc.
	  c. Charity useful to giver provided it is voluntary and entails personal involvement. Can be expression of social elitism
	
	4. Strict Social Darwinism rejects social concern because it interferes with natural selection
		b. rather than being rehabilitative, leads to dependency, with atrophy in the capacity to exercise personal responsibility
		
		2. True expression of social concern is to reduce need for charity to a minimum, thus fostering personal responsibility and initiative

Freedom	1. Maintain maximum freedom 2. Emphasis on political freedom and coercion 3. Government seen tending to encroach on individual freedom unless curbed 4. Collective action is "paternalism"	1. Maintain maximum freedom 2. Redefinition of freedom as possibility of alternative choices 3. Compulsion not only political but also economic 4. The notion of trade-offs among freedoms a. group to group

SUMMARY OF MAJOR ARGUMENTS

Social values	"Libertarian" viewpoint	"Egalitarian" viewpoint
	5. Compulsion attenuates personal responsibility as well as individualistic and voluntary expressions of social concern	b. one type to another in any one person
		5. Government as a liberator
	6. A self-balancing state results if freedom is maintained: "natural harmony" a. "invisible hand" of economist b. the Social Darwinian tenet	6. Government as expression of public will or its agent 7. Much less fear of disturbing "natural harmony"
	7. Perils of disturbing this natural harmony	
Equality	1. Conceived mainly as equality before the law. Covers specifically defined constitutional and legal rights	1. Equality is broadly defined as equal opportunity to achieve
	2. Emphasis on potential for equality rather than its actual realization	2. Medical care as precondition of achievement; therefore it cannot be used as a reward for achievement. Similar to education, a social right
	3. Less concern about injustices suffered by the few if liberties of majority thereby maintained	3. Equality of opportunity foundation for morally acceptable contest to achieve
	4. Perceived conflict between equality and competitive personal achievement	4. Equality as dissemination of liberty
	5. Perceived conflict between equality and liberty; precedence to freedom	

READINGS AND REFERENCES

Social Responsibility for Medical Care

1. Roemer, M. I., ''Government's Role in American Medicine: A Brief Historical Survey.'' *Bulletin of the History of Medicine* 18:146–168 (July 1945).
2. Berge, W., ''Justice and the Future of Medicine,'' *Public Health Reports* 60:1–16, January 5, 1945. A shortened version appears in *Readings in Medical Care*, edited by Committee on Medical Care Teaching of the Association of Teachers of Preventive Medicine (Chapel Hill: University of North Carolina Press, 1958), pp. 666–676.
3. Titmuss, R. M., ''Ethics and Economics of Medical Care,'' *Medical Care* 1:16–22 (January-March 1963).
4. Kemp, A., ''Ethics and Economics of Medical Care.'' *Medical Care* 1:241–244 (October-December 1963). (A reply to professor Titmuss. See also responses by J. Jewkes and by D. S. Lees in the same issue, especially p. 236, on ''the question of quality'' and pp. 235–239 on the ''issues of method.'')
5. Hook, S., ''A Statement of Meaning—Summary of the Symposium,'' in The *Health Care Issues of the 1960's* (New York: Group Health Insurance, Inc. 1963), pp. 179–199.
6. Cohen, W. J., *Hospital Insurance Benefits for Social Security Beneficiaries.* An Examination of Some of the Main Features and Issues of a Proposed Plan (Ann Arbor: The Author, June, 1959), 57pp. (mimeographed). See especially ''Major Arguments in Favor of Providing Hospital Benefits under OASDI,'' pp. 21–25; ''Major Arguments Made Against Providing Hospital Benefits under OASDI,'' pp. 26–30; and ''The Issue of Compulsory Contributions,'' pp. 31–33.
7. Basch, S., ''The Pains of a New Idea.'' *Survey Graphic* 84:78–79 (February 1948).
8. Burns, E. M., ''Social Policy and Health Services: The Choices Ahead.'' *American Journal of Public Health* 57:199–212, (February 1967).
9. Cohen, W. J., ''Social Policy for the Nineteen Seventies,'' H.E.W. Indicators, May 1960, pp. 8–19.
10. Jackson, C. L., ''State Compulsory Immunization in the United States,'' *Public Health Reports* 84:787–795 (September 1969).
11. Hershey, N., ''Compulsory Personal Health Measure Legislation.'' *Public Health Reports* 84:341–352 (April, 1969).

Distinctive Characteristics of Health Services

12. Lees, D. S., *Health Through Choice* (London: Institute of Economic Affairs, 1961), 64pp.
13. Mushkin, S. J., ''Toward a Definition of Health Economics.'' *Public Health Reports* 73:785–793 (September 1958).
14. Weisbrod, B. A., *Economics of Public Health* (Philadelphia: University of Pennsylvania Press, 1961), 127pp.
15. Klarman, H. E., *The Economics of Health* (New York: Columbia University Press, 1965), 200pp. See ''Distinctive Economic Characteristics,'' pp. 10–19, and ''The Case for Intervention,'' pp. 47–56. These sections have also appeared respectively in *Journal of Health and Human Behavior* 4:44–49 (Spring 1963), and in *Medical Care* 3:59–62 (January-March 1965).

Other References in the Text

16. Tawney, R. H., *Religion and the Rise of Capitalism*. Paperback edition (New York: Mentor Book, The New American Library of World Literature, Inc., 1954), 280pp.

17. Weber, M., *The Protestant Ethic and the Spirit of Capitalism*. Paperback edition (New York: Charles Scribner's Sons, 1958), 292pp.

18. Hofstadter, R., *Social Darwinism in American Thought*. Paperback edition (Boston: The Beacon Press, 1960), 248pp.

19. Garnett, A. C., ''Charity and Natural Law.'' *Ethics* 66:117–122 (January 1956).

20. de Schweinitz, K., *England's Road to Social Security* (Philadelphia: University of Pennsylvania Press, 1943), 281pp.

21. Eckstein, H., *The English Health Service* (Cambridge: Harvard University Press, 1958), 289pp.

22. Phelps, E. S. (ed.), *Private Wants and Public Needs* (New York: W. W. Norton and Company, Inc. 1962), 148pp.

23. Cohen, W. J., ''Hospital Insurance for the Aged—The Conservative Approach'' (Washington, D.C.: The Author, January 5, 1965), 23pp. (mimeographed)

24. Tawney, R. H., *Equality*. Paperback edition (New York: Capricorn Books, G. P. Putnam's Sons, 1961), 285pp.

25. Barker, E., *Principles of Social and Political Theory*. Paperback edition (New York: Oxford University Press, 1961), 284pp.

26. De Grazia, A., *Politics and Government, Volume I: Political Behavior*. Paperback edition (New York: Collier Books, 1962), 388pp.

27. Friedman, M., *Capitalism and Freedom*. Paperback edition, (Chicago: University of Chicago Press, 1963), 202pp.

28. Dahl, R. A., and Lindblom, C. E., *Politics, Economics, and Welfare*. Paperback edition (Harper Torchbooks, New York: Harper and Row, 1963), 556pp.

29. Roemer, M. I., ''Medical Care and Social Class in Latin America,'' *Milbank Memorial Fund Quarterly* 42:54–64 (July 1964).

30. Field, M. G., *Doctor and Patient in Soviet Russia* (Cambridge: Harvard University Press, 1957), 266pp. See especially ''Social Position and 'Medical Category','' pp. 183–190.

31. Rosenfeld, L. S., Donabedian, A., and Katz, J., ''Unmet Need for Medical Care,'' *New England Journal of Medicine* 258:369–376 (February 20, 1958).

32. Donabedian, A., ''The Nature and Magnitude of Unmet Need in Medical Care.'' Pages 1–21 in *Institute on Planning and Administration of Nursing Service in Medical Care Programs—Selected Papers* (Ann Arbor: Continuing Education Service, School of Public Health, The University of Michigan, Ann Arbor, 1968), 230pp.

33. Meerman, J. B., ''Some Comments on the Predicted Future Shortage of Physicians.'' AMA Economic Research Bulletin 110. *Journal of the American Medical Association* 177:793–799 (September 16, 1961).

34. Duff, R. S., and Hollingshead, A. B., *Sickness and Society*. (New York: Harper and Row, 1968), 390pp.

35. Weisbrod, B. A., ''Some Problems of Pricing and Resource Allocation in a Non-Profit Industry—The Hospitals.'' *The Journal of Business* 38:18–28 (January 1965).

36. Freidson, E., *Patients' View of Medical Practice* (New York: Russell Sage Foundation, 1961), 268pp. See especially ''Professional Controls on Laymen,'' pp. 202–204.

37. Hansen, H. R., *Legal Rights of Group Health Plans, A Survey of State Laws through 1963* (Washington, D.C.: Group Health Association of America, 1964), 61pp.

38. U.S. Department of Health, Education, and Welfare, Public Health Service, *Morbidity and Mortality, Weekly Report* vol. 13, no. 9, May 15, 1964. 8pp.

39. Doege, T. C., Levy, P. S. and Heath, C. W. Jr., ''A Diphtheria Epidemic Related to Community Immunization Levels and the Health Problems of Migrant Workers.'' *Public Health Reports* 78:151–159, February, 1963.

40. Roemer, M. I., ''History of the Effects of War on Medicine.'' *Annals of Medical History* 4:189–198 (May 1942).

41. Titmuss, R. M., ''War and Social Policy,'' chap. 4, pp. 75–87, in Titmuss, *Essays on 'the Welfare State'* (New Haven: Yale University Press, 1959), 232pp.

42. Karpinos, B. D., ''Fitness of American Youth for Military Service,'' *Milbank Memorial Fund Quarterly* 38:213–247 (July 1960).

43. The President's Task Force on Manpower Conservation, *One-Third of a Nation. A Report on Young Men Found Unqualified for Military Service* (Washington, D.C.: U.S. Government Printing Office, July 1, 1964), 35pp. and appendices. (For a critique of this report see ''One Third of a Nation?'' *Journal of the American Medical Association* 188:1142–1144, June 29, 1964.)

44. Child, G. C., ''Residents, Physicians and Universities under Medicare.'' *The Journal of Medical Education* 42:392–403 (May 1967).

45. Perkins, W., ''Effects of Medicare and Title XIX on House-Staff Training Programs,'' *Journal of the American Medical Association* 201:94–97 (July 31, 1967).

I I

Program Objectives

THE NATURE OF OBJECTIVES

Almost intuitively, one arrives at the notion that organizations are set up to achieve certain objectives. Hence, a study of objectives, and of the means by which they are attained, appears to offer an excellent avenue to organizational analysis. A closer examination, however, reveals unexpected conceptual and operational difficulties in pursuing this approach.

At the very outset one is faced with the problem of distinguishing objectives from the means used to attain them. Simon, among others, has pointed out that the problem arises from the partially ordered nature of the underlying phenomenon (2, pp. 62–66). There is, according to this formulation, a hierarchy of states or events so that each item in a chain is partly or wholly dependent on the one that precedes it and contributes, in varying degrees, to the one that follows. The distinction between means and ends is thus effaced, so that each level in a chain can be viewed either as a means or as an end, depending on which is more relevant to the purposes at hand.

That there is a "hierarchy of ends" (2) is recognized in the health literature by repeated attempts, none entirely successful, to distinguish, and formalize by convention, the use of terms such as "mission," "purpose," "goal," "subgoal," "objective," "sub-objective," "intermediate objective," and "operational objective." Perhaps the most rigorously developed model is one that Deniston et al. have offered as a framework for evaluating the effectiveness of health programs (21). This model proposes a progression of objectives that begins with an "initial sub-objective" and proceeds to one or more "intervening sub-objectives," a "program objective" and an "ultimate objective." Any one program may comprise one or more chains of this kind, each with one or more branches. The most significant characteristic of the terminology proposed is the insistence that objectives, at any level in the progression, be stated only in terms of "a situation or condition of people or of the environment which responsible program personnel consider desirable to attain." This means that, by definition, work leading to these "desired situations or conditions" may not be recognized as an objective, but must be separately classified as an "activity" that is related to one or more sub-objectives that it serves. By distinguishing the category of "activities" from that of "objectives," Deniston et al. depart significantly from the model advanced by Simon.

A second, and perhaps more fundamental, conceptual obstacle to the study of organizational objectives is the validity of the concept itself: that there are identifiable, overriding objectives toward which the organization, as a collectivity, may be said to strive. Organizations are complex things. Each individual member in them has his own values, hopes, aspirations, and goals. In addition, each member has an assigned role and position to which are attached goals defined by professional training as well as by function and responsibility within the organization. Furthermore, the organization is divided into units and subunits constituted according to a variety of criteria: for example, purpose, process, and clientele. It is reasonable to assume that the objectives of these different components would vary in priorities if not in kind. In view of the multiplicity of purposes operative within the organization at all these levels, how can one postulate the emergence of a set of objectives that one might attribute to the organization as a collectivity? Cyert and March (3, 4) and Simon (5), among others, have addressed themselves to this question. The elements of the answer include, first, a recognition that the objectives of an organization (or objectives within an organization) are indeed complex, vaguely defined, in constant flux, and often internally inconsistent. It is also recognized that objectives formulated at one level in an organization may be modified at another level and further modified, even subverted, in actual execution. The diversity of goals has to be recognized. Equally true, however, is the observation that organizations act in ways that permit "the meaningful imputation of purpose to the total system" (2). It is this phenomenon that requires explanation.

Cyert and March (3, 4) take as a point of departure the fact that organizations must make decisions. The making of decisions in a group involves the formation of "viable coalitions" which are brought about by a process of bargaining. Part of the bargaining revolves around modifications in policy calculated to create and maintain a particular coalition. In this way there comes about at least partial agreement on objectives. Agreement sufficient for coalition formation and decision-making is made easier by a variety of features: (a) that at any given time only a limited number of actions are under consideration, (b) that a relatively small subset of participants in the organization are active with respect to a given problem, (c) that at any given time each person attends to only a small subset of his demands, and (d) that objectives are presented in forms that accommodate a range of positions. Whatever agreement is achieved tends to become stabilized by several mechanisms, which include (a) incorporation into the budget, (b) partitioning of functions and responsibilities through division of labor and specialization, and (c) the accretion to precedent which tends to severely constrain future action.

Simon (5) also begins with the need to make decisions, but appears to emphasize the more "rational" aspects of the process of problem-solving. According to Simon, the process of solving a problem consists in searching for alternative solutions and testing each alternative to see whether it satisfies a set of constraints or conditions. To the extent that each of the constraints has to be satisfied, it may be conceived as an objective or goal of the action envisaged by the solution to the problem. It is usual, however, for one of the constraints to take precedence over others in that it is used for the initial search for alternatives before these are tested to see whether the other constraints are also satisfied. The constraint used in this way—to generate alternatives—may be singled out and, more properly, designated as the goal or objective. This is because it possesses greater power to motivate the search and influences more profoundly the solution finally adopted. According to Simon, problem-solving by a group within an organization is likely to reveal considerable agreement on what constraints are relevant to a given problem, but also major differences on which of these constraints is used by each member of the group to generate alternatives for further testing. It can be said, therefore, that goals are shared and disparate at one and the same time, depending on whether all constraints are seen as goals or the designation of "goal" is restricted to the constraint used to generate alternatives. The communality of goals arises, according to Simon, from the relative precedence of role-related goals over personal goals in an organization and from the recognition that solutions, to be successful, have to be broadly acceptable. Differences arise from the fact that role incumbents, by virtue of professional training and expertise in specific techniques, view problems from their particular perspectives and that differences in personal goals and preferences are never fully submerged by the organizational role.

Models of how organizational goals are formulated must account not only for contemporaneous disparity and communality, but also for stability as well as change over time. Cyert and March discuss the effect on organizational objectives of both favorable and unfavorable experience, the emergence of specific problems, and the discovery of specific solutions to heretofore ignored problems (3, 4). Thompson and McEwen (6) emphasize the fact that most organizations are called upon constantly to reappraise their objectives in the light of changes in needs, demands, and other aspects of the environment within which they operate. The degree and nature of reappraisal depend on (a) the nature and pace of change in the environment, (b) the nature of the product of the organization, (c) the degree of control that the organization has over its environment, and (d) the strategies that the organization adopts to deal with the environment. Obviously, reappraisal must be more frequent, and perhaps more fundamental, when the environment is unstable or is undergoing rapid change. To the extent that the product of the organization is concrete and easily measurable, its unsuitability to environmental demands is more readily identified by the environment as well as by the organization. This means that the organization is subject to earlier challenge, but also is in a better position to anticipate and meet such challenge. When the product is less tangible (education or medical care, for example) environmental challenge may be delayed, but so is the capacity of the organization to anticipate, and adapt to, changing conditions. With respect to control over the environment, organizations vary over a continuum from virtually complete control (through monopoly, for example) to virtually complete powerlessness. With respect to strategies to deal with the environment, the agency has an option between competition and one of three cooperative strategies: "bargaining," "co-optation," and "coalition." All are likely to involve adjustments in organizational objectives. Competition means that the environment will not support organizational goals that society finds unacceptable. Through bargaining, adjustments in some goals may have to be made in exchange for enhancement in others. Through cooptation the organization absorbs potentially hostile elements into its own leadership in order to avert threats to its own existence; but thereby it also allows these elements to modify its own objectives. An example might be the incorporation of medical staff members on the board of a voluntary hospital or consumer-sponsored prepaid group practice. Through coalition with one or more other organizations, there results a greater ability to control the environment but also loss of ability to alter goals unilaterally.

A third difficulty in the analysis of organizational objectives arises from the discrepancy between the official or stated goals of an organization and its operative or real goals.* The models offered by Cyert and March and by Simon present objectives as arising from the constant give

---

* Etzioni uses the terms "stated" and "real" (1). Perrow uses the terms "official" and "operative" (7).

and take within the organization. This is part of the picture. In a larger sense, objectives also derive from the society which makes legitimate the organization and its activities, formally and informally. This is especially true for medical care organizations which are charged, in the public mind, with a duty to serve the public. This expectation is often incorporated in legal instruments that govern public and quasi-public programs and institutions as well as the health professions that participate in them. The organization is expected, therefore, to act within these broader legal and social guidelines, so that more specific objectives and actions conform to the broader purposes of the organization. As might be expected, this does not always happen. The real or operative goals, as inferred from what the organization actually does, can be different in many respects from the official or stated goals as found in enabling legislation, articles of incorporation, or official pronouncements of organizational intent, verbal or written. The tendency for organizations to deviate from their legitimate and avowed purposes is a general tendency referred to as "goal displacement." The inference is that the legitimate and avowed purposes are thereby less well served. A frequent form of goal displacement is when concern for the survival and welfare of the organization itself takes precedence over the broader objectives which the organization ostensibly exists to serve. Another is undue emphasis on procedures as if they were ends in themselves rather than means to a larger service objective. Procedures may also be subverted to serve unintended objectives. For example, Scheff describes how, in a mental hospital, staff-patient conferences and tranquilizing drugs were used to control patients rather than to further their rehabilitation as originally intended by the professional staff (18).*

It is clear from the foregoing discussion that organizational objectives, far from being immutable, are subject to change. In some situations it is possible to see distinct stages in the development of an organization, each stage characterized by a distinct shift in goals. This phenomenon is referred to as "goal succession." In rare instances it occurs when an organization has fulfilled the purpose for which it was originally formed and must look for new things to do if it is to survive. An excellent example, described by Sills, is the reorientation of the Foundation for Infantile Paralysis following the virtual conquest of poliomyelitis (23). More often, changes in the environment render the original objectives no

---

* Warner and Havens propose a more specific terminology than has been used in this text when they speak of "goal change" as comprising two subcategories: "(1) goal diversion, where the original objectives are supplanted by alternative ones, and (2) goal displacement, or what is here called means-ends inversion, the neglect of the claimed goals in favor of means as ends in themselves" (8, p. 541).

longer relevant, so new ones must be sought. Sills cites the Young Men's Christian Association (YMCA) as an example of successful adaptation through a shift in goals from predominantly religious to predominantly recreational activities. He cites the Women's Christian Temperance Union as an example of a failure to adapt to changing environmental conditions with consequent loss in power and prestige (23).

Perrow has described a phenomenon, akin to that of goal succession, whereby the operative goals of an organization are adapted to the tasks most appropriate to successive stages in its development (7). During its earliest stages an organization's greatest needs are to secure acceptance and obtain financial support. This is a responsibility which is assumed by directors or trustees who, during this stage, are the dominant force in setting organizational objectives. Subsequently, primary emphasis shifts to the most skillful performance of whatever tasks the organization exists to perform. During this stage, experts who have the relevant skills (engineers or physicians, for example) become the dominant force, and most influential in setting objectives. This is especially true if the needed skills are scarce and are based in a complex and rapidly growing technology—in medicine, for example. Finally, as the organization grows to become increasingly complex, perhaps embracing a large variety of skills and interacting wth many other organizations in its environment, there is paramount need for skillful management and coordination. During this stage, professional managers or administrators become dominant in setting objectives. Needless to say, all three groups (trustees, experts, and administrators) have some influence at all stages. What is postulated are differences in relative emphasis. Furthermore, the model includes the possibility of joint or multiple leadership with varying degrees of mutuality and conflict.

Perrow has shown that the three stages he describes may be discerned in the development of a single hospital. He also suggests that hospitals, as a whole, have historically gone through the first two stages and are entering their managerial phase. However, any given hospital today may be located in any one of the stages portrayed. In describing the goals likely to be pursued by the various dominant groups within the hospital, Perrow gives examples of socially desirable goals as well as of goal displacement in the service of more narrow interests. These examples are of particular interest because of their bearing on subsequent sections in this presentation.

Trustee Domination . . . Because of their responsibility to the sponsoring community, trustees may favor conservative financial policies, opposing large financial outlays for equipment, research, and education so necessary for high medical standards. High standards also require more delegation of authority to the medical staff than trustee domination can easily allow. As representatives drawn from distinct social groups in the community, they may be oriented towards service for a religious, ethnic, economic, or age group in the community. Such an orientation may conflict with selection procedures favored by the medical staff or administration. Trustees may also promote policies which demonstrate a contribution to community welfare on the part of an elite group, perhaps seeking to maintain a position of prominence and power within the community. The hospital may be used as a vehicle for furthering a social philosophy of philanthropy and good works; social class values regarding personal worth, economic independence and responsibility; the assimilation of a minority group; or even to further resistance to government control and socialized medicine . . .

Medical Domination . . . The operative goals of such a hospital are likely to be defined in strictly medical terms and the organization may achieve high technical standards of care, promote exemplary research, and provide sound training. However, there is a danger that resources will be used primarily for private (paying) patients with little attention to other community needs such as caring for the medically indigent (unless they happen to be good teaching cases), developing preventive medicine, or pioneering new organizational forms of care. Furthermore, high technical standards increasingly require efficient coordination of services and doctors may be unwilling to delegate authority to qualified administrators.

Various unofficial goals may be achieved at the expense of medical ones, or, in some cases, in conjunction with them. There are many cases of personal aggrandizement on the part of departmental chiefs and the chief of staff. The informal referral and consultation system in conjunction with promotions, bed quotas, and 'privileges' to operate or treat certain types of cases, affords many occasions for the misuse of power. Interns and residents are particularly vulnerable to exploitation at the expense of teaching goals. Furthermore, as a professional, the doctor has undergone intensive socialization in his training and is called upon to exercise extraordinary judgment and skill with drastic consequences for good or ill. Thus he demands unusual deference and obedience and is invested with "charismatic" authority. He may extend this authority to the entrepreneurial aspects of his role, with the result that his "service" orientation, so taken for granted in much of the literature, sometimes means service to the doctor at the expense of personnel, other patients, or even his own patient.

Administrative Dominance . . . If administrative dominance is based primarily on the complexity of basic hospital activities, rather than the organization's medical-social role in the community, the operative orientation may be toward financial solvency, careful budget controls, efficiency, and minimal development of services. For example, preventive medicine, research, and training may be minimized; a cautious approach may prevail towards new forms of care such as intensive therapy units or home care programs. Such orientations could be especially true of hospitals dominated by administrators whose background and training were as bookkeepers, comptrollers, business managers, purchasing agents, and the like. This is probably the most common form of administrative dominance.

However, increasing professionalization of hospital administrators has, on the one hand, equipped them to handle narrower administrative matters easily, and, on the other hand, alerted them to the broader medical-social role of hospitals involving organizational and financial innovations in the forms of care. Even medical standards can come under administrative control . . .

There is, of course, a possibility of less "progressive" consequences. Interference with medical practices in the name of either high standards or treating the "whole" person may be misguided or have latent consequences which impair therapy. Publicity-seeking innovations may be at the expense of more humdrum but crucial services such as the out-patient department, or may alienate doctors or other personnel, or may deflect administrative efforts from essential but unglamorous administrative tasks . . . Like trustees they may favor a distinctive and medically irrelevant community relations policy, perhaps with a view towards moving upward in the community power structure. Regardless of these dangers, the number of administration dominated hospitals oriented towards broad medical-social goals will probably grow" (7, pp. 858, 859, 860. References to the literature have been omitted).

CLASSIFICATION OF OBJECTIVES

From a consideration of the nature of objectives, and how they are formulated and modified, it is possible to derive a classification of objectives that the administrator may find useful in ordering his thinking. The classification offered has multiple axes that reflect various aspects of the phenomenon under consideration.

1. Hierarchical Aspects
   a. Causality
   b. Inclusivity
   c. Time sequence
   d. Value preference
2. Manifestational Aspects
3. Orientational Aspects
   a. Client-oriented
   b. Provider-oriented
   c. Organization-oriented
   d. Collectivity-oriented
   e. Multi-oriented

Hierarchical Aspects

These refer to relationships in which objectives are arranged according to some order. We have already presented the notion of a chain of events or states each of which is a means to a subsequent end and an end of a preceding means. Hence one speaks of "goals" and "subgoals" or of "objectives" and "subobjectives." This formulation implies that each link is totally, or in part, the cause of the one that follows. The causal relationship may be well established or merely presumptive. In some situations it is recognized that certain categories are included in others because they are parts of a more general concept. Here the relationship is one of inclusivity without postulation of a causal link. Under this heading we speak of "general" and "specific" goals or objectives. Objectives may also be ordered in a time sequence. This is certainly part of the concept of causality; but time sequence may also be relevant when there are no causal relationships. Hence one speaks of "proximate" versus "ultimate" goals or of "short-term" versus "long-term" objectives. Finally, there is a hierarchy of preference or priority according to which certain objectives are more valued or are regarded to be more important. Accordingly, objectives may be classified as "primary" or "secondary." In all of this, awareness of the precise nature of the ordering is more important than the terminology used. Since the terminology has not been standardized, it is necessary to define the words that one employs to designate the different types of ordering in this classification.

Manifestational Aspects

These refer to the degree to which objectives are manifest or concealed. We have already referred to the notion that the "official," "formal," or "stated" goals may differ in varying degree from the goals that are "operative," "informal," or "real."

Orientational Aspects

These refer to the groups whose interests the objectives are meant to serve primarily. These could be the clients, the providers of care, the organization or society as a whole. Any one objective may, of course, serve more than one of these groups. In fact, because service to clients, or the collectivity of clients, is what gives legitimacy to most activities in medical care, all objectives are ostensibly in the service of the client. What we have termed the orientation of an objective is usually best discerned by noting which party (client, provider, or organization) gives it relatively greater weight in the give-and-take of medical care organization.

SOME OBJECTIVES OF MEDICAL CARE ORGANIZATION

At the end of this chapter there are a number of references which deal with goals in a variety of medical care programs (9–14). A reading of these sources will give a notion of what issues have been of major concern in medical care policy. Since this will be the subject of much of this book, all that will be attempted here is to introduce some of the objectives and, at the same time, test the usefulness of the orientational classification.

Client-oriented objectives are the most distinctive feature of medical care institutions which represent a humanitarian tradition of service. Hence it is expected that in medical care programs primary attention be given to client welfare and adaptation to client wishes and desires. There is, however, a serious question about whether medical care organizations primarily serve the interests and wishes of the clients as seen by the clients themselves or those interests as interpreted by the professional and other elites who determine medical care policy. Increasingly, clients are insistent that the professional perspective on patient need be broadened to include the patient's own viewpoint.

Client-oriented objectives include: (a) access to service, (b) use of service, (c) quality of care, (d) maintenance of client autonomy and dignity, (e) responsiveness to client needs, wishes and convenience, and (f) freedom of choice. Among these objectives, ensuring or facilitating access to care has been the most pressing. This accounts for the multiplicity of schemes for financing health services through voluntary insurance, compulsory insurance, or some form of governmental service. Access to care is a preliminary to actual use of service. But it is actual use of service which demonstrates whether equality of access has become operational or remains a potential yet to be realized. In spite of this, attention to actual use has been limited. Partly this has arisen from the preoccupation with the financial barriers to care and insufficient attention to the many barriers, other than cost of care, that inhibit the use of service. Moreover, many financing schemes, especially those that operate on a voluntary basis, have no centralized responsibility or authority to supervise the total care of a specified population group. Even when such responsibility and authority exist, it is difficult to assemble and evaluate data on use of service, especially since the objective is not merely to equalize levels of use but to adjust use to need. These difficulties notwithstanding, perhaps the most important objective of a program to provide medical care is to achieve not merely equality of access to care, but also equal use for equal need. This would appear to be a reasonable application of the egalitarian point of view as presented in the preceding chapter. However, when need is professionally defined, the question arises whether persons should be compelled to receive care in pursuit of the egalitarian objective. The answer in our society has been in the negative, except in the most unusual circumstances. The objective then is to achieve equal service for equal need through the removal of barriers in addition to those of cost.

Another objective, often more honored in the breach than in the observance, is the intent to maintain and to promote quality. Certain dimensions of care subsumed by the concept of quality may be of greater relevance to client wishes and desires than are others. Insufficient attention to these may mean patient dissatisfaction in spite of technically superior care.

The objective to maintain client autonomy and dignity derives partly from more general norms and values that specify individual prerogatives and what are acceptable modes of social interaction. The interaction between a professional and a client needs particular protection since the client is often in a position of relative helplessness, open to exploitation. Hence, the additional legal, ethical, and administrative safeguards that surround the patient-physician relationship. Freedom of choice is believed to be one such safeguard, in addition to representing a deeply rooted libertarian tradition.

Provider-oriented objectives are meant to serve the interests of those who provide care, among whom the physician is paramount. However, since physicians and other health professionals maintain that their primary motivation is to serve patients, provider-oriented objectives are ostensibly advocated because they are necessary conditions for the maintenance of professional commitment and the proper provision of care. If one accepts this interpretation, provider-oriented objectives may be redefined as those to which providers tend to give greater importance in the planning and organization of care. Such objectives include: (a) freedom of professional judgment and activities, (b) maintenance of professional proficiency and the quality of care, (c) adequate compensation, (d) control over the conditions and terms of practice with special emphasis on control over remuneration, and (e) in general, maintenance of professional norms, usually as defined by each profession for itself.

Organization-oriented objectives may be similarly defined either as those that primarily serve the organization or as those which the organization regards as particularly salient. These include: (a) cost control, including prevention of abuse by client and provider, (b) control of the quality of care, (c) efficiency, (d) maintenance of the ability to attract clients, and (e) maintenance of the ability to recruit and keep employees, professional and other, and (f) mobilization of community support. In general, these and similar objectives are meant to assure the integrity of the organization and to increase its power over its environment. To the extent that the client is thereby served, these goals are considered legitimate. But we have already noted, under the rubric of "goal displacement," the tendency for such goals to take precedence over client-oriented objectives.

Collectivity-oriented objectives are postulated with the notion that some objectives are directed at preserving the social system and its values rather than serving merely the organization, the client, or the provider.* Thus, they are seen as more universalistic. Such objectives may be expressed in terms of values such as those discussed in the preceding chapter: personal responsibility, social concern, freedom and equality. They may, alternatively, be expressed in terms of a more concrete goal, such as contribution to higher levels of economic productivity. Finally, they may be expressed in terms of desired relationships to other institutions within the larger society. Examples are (a) the proper allocation of resources among competing needs, (b) nonpartisanship, (c) political representation, (d) representation of important interests involved in, or affected by, the program, and (e) coordination with other agencies, public or private, that perform similar or related functions. The notion of collectivity oriented goals includes the adjustment of the rival claims of clients, providers and the organization, and also the idea that what may be good for any group of clients, providers, or organizations, may not necessarily coincide with the public good more broadly construed.

Multi-oriented objectives are those that fit under more than one of the orientational categories. An excellent example is the maintenance of quality; another is maintenance of the patient-physician relationship. Both "quality" and the "patient-physician relationship" are rather vague concepts, which may be partly responsible for the handy use to which they are put in the polemics of medical care organization. This is not to say that they are without force or meaning. On the contrary, Eckstein points out that a general agreement over the need to maintain the traditional patient-physician relationship had important consequences to the way in which the British National Health Service was organized (15, pp. 172–173).

A major function of multi-oriented objectives is that they serve an integrative function, creating bonds that unite client, provider and organization in a common pursuit. In fact, most client-oriented goals have an integrative function, since patient welfare is recognized to be the

* Perrow suggests that organizations may have "social system goals, which refers to those contributions an organization makes to the functioning of a social system in which it is nested" (7, p. 855n).

ultimate objective of the medical care transaction. But the basis for cohesion within the medical care system is not only ideological, though the importance of ideological integration should not be minimized. There is also a functional interrelationship at the operational level. Conditions that honor professional norms and expectations do in fact contribute to better care. Similarly, a sound and flourishing organization can best serve both clients and providers. It is on the foundation of such mutualities that stable social structures stand.

ORGANIZATIONAL RESPONSIBILITIES

The medical care administrator has certain responsibilities with regard to the objectives of his program. These include (a) specification of objectives, (b) the choice of objectives, (c) resolution of conflict among objectives, (d) rendering objectives operational, and (e) keeping them current by adaptation to changing needs and conditions. This does not mean that all these responsibilities rest on the administrator alone, but that he is a major participant in discharging them. Issues relevant to each of these responsibilities will be discussed below.

Specification of Objectives

It is difficult to see how any purposive action can occur without the presence of objectives. The issue, therefore, is not whether to have objectives, but to consider the ways in which the more precise identification of objectives is relevant to program structure and operations. In this section we shall discuss (a) the uses and possible dangers of specifying objectives, and (b) the form in which objectives are to be stated. We shall also raise the question whether the specification of objectives may, under certain circumstances, have dangerous consequences.

The specification of objectives has several uses.* First, objectives constitute the moral and legal basis of a program. They give it legitimacy. Governmental programs generally rest on statutory provisions that give the general intent of the program and the rough outlines of its structure and function. A more detailed specification of all these features, including objectives, is a task for administrative, and sometimes judiciary, interpretation, not to say surmise (24). For this purpose the

---

* According to Etzioni, the goals of an organization serve the following functions: "provide orientation . . . set down guide lines for organizational activity . . . constitute a source of legitimacy . . . serve as standards [to] assess the success of the organization [and] as measuring rods for the student of organizations." (1, p. 5.)

language of the bill itself may not be enough. Increasingly, administrators, their legal advisers, and the courts have turned for guidance to ''committee hearings and reports, congressional debates, legislative journals, as well as executive messages, the long-standing interpretation of the laws by administrative officials responsible for their enforcement, and public acquiescence in such administrative construction'' (25, pp. 467–468). However, because of the nature of the legislative process, there are doubts not only about the validity of these sources in revealing legislative intent but, in a more fundamental way, about the validity of the notion of legislative intent itself. ''For Congress is so heterogeneous, its procedural machinery is so ill-adapted for rational decision-making, and the motives of its members so unrelated to their verbal professions that it may be completely unreasonable to inquire after its intent'' (26, p. 384). While this may be true, the important thing is that the ambiguities of legislation often leave a legitimate area of discretion within which the administrator can shape the objectives and operations of his program, subject, of course, to a variety of budgetary, administrative, political, and social pressures. The courts themselves, although they retain the full authority to reverse administrative interpretation, are increasingly deferential to established interpretations of statutes by the administrative agencies entrusted with their execution (24, p. 402).

A staff report to the Committee on Finance of the United States Senate, concerning problems in the implementation of Medicare and Medicaid, illustrates how administrative decisions of arguable conformity with congressional intent can profoundly shape program operations (27). For example, the authors of the Report contend that it was the intent of Congress to place as an upper limit on the ''reasonable charges'' of physicians, the scheduled fees paid by insurance carriers under comparable circumstances. The Social Security Administration was equally emphatic that the yardsticks intended by Congress were not the scheduled fees used by the carriers, but the customary charges of the physicians and the prevailing charges in the locality. According to the authors of the Report:

The Social Security Administration took an explicit statutory limitation on the maximum physician's charge which could be recognized as 'reasonable' for purposes of medicare payment and through fallacious logic turned it into a complex nullity. The 'comparable circumstances' phrase in the statute was interpreted as constituting a limitation *only* if a carrier had a policy or contract which paid benefits on a so-called 'customary and prevailing' basis. As has been pointed out, virtually none of the Blue Shield plans had such contracts generally available during the years of debate on medicare or at the time of medicare's consideration and enactment, or on the effective date of medicare. Thus, Social Security called for the application of a phantom yardstick (27, p. 64).

Without passing judgment on which of the two contending interpretations truly represents congressional intent, it is clear how important has been the impact of the administrative decision. The consequences are starkly visible in the unprecedented inflation of medical care prices that has accompanied the institution and implementation of Medicare and Medicaid (28).

The Report to the Senate Finance Committee illustrates still another way in which statutory intent can be frustrated, namely, through administrative adaptation to the imperatives of the real world. Under Medicare legislation, Congress recognized extended care to be a substitute for prior hospital care and to be provided by institutions certified for the purpose. The "conditions of participation" embodied in regulations contained reasonably high standards in conformity with the law. However, in the application of these standards the Social Security Administration required that the institutions be in substantial compliance and in progress toward full compliance. Under this interpretation of substantial compliance it was possible to certify relatively large numbers of homes only 30 percent of which were in full compliance with standards even two years after the institution of the program. As the Report notes: "Only about one-eighth of the 3,120 facilities not in full compliance in July 1967 were able to achieve full compliance within the next two years. The vast majority remain in the 'substantial compliance' category" (227, p. 94).

Related to the first function of objectives is a second, namely, that they serve as a basis for articulation with a broader value system or larger social or organizational units. We have already referred to the articulation with the value orientations which were discussed in Chapter 1. The need is obvious for mutually reinforcing linkages between medical care agencies and larger social institutions which include a medical care function among others. Later in this chapter we shall refer to the problems that arise when certain values and objectives of a larger social institution are inappropriate to the medical care function which they also purvey.

Third, congruence, or at least compatability, of objectives is the basis upon which planning for joint action can take place. Systematic and explicit exploration of objectives during the planning phase should reveal to what extent cooperative effort is possible and upon what grounds.

Fourth, objectives are the basis for the structure and operations of a program. Given specific objectives, one can progressively eliminate a variety of alternative ways of implementing a more general intent. Contrariwise, given a particular way of doing things, one can infer at least the operative, if not the official, objectives of a program. Taylor has pursued this type of reasoning in attempting to show how different objectives seem to result in different administrative structures and operating policies in three types of health insurance: "limited indemnity," "comprehensive service," and "prepayment-through-group-practice" (16, pp. 16–29). He makes clear that if the objective of health insurance is merely to offer financial help to meet large, unexpected bills, it is sufficient to enter into a direct agreement with the client under the terms of which the client receives specified sums of money after he gets hospital care. If the objective is to devise a method of financing that will promote health through the appropriate use of service, it becomes necessary to offer a broader range of services, including preventive procedures and office care; to offer benefits in the form of assured services rather than cash; and to give attention to appropriateness of the services received and to quality of care. To accomplish these objectives, it becomes necessary to enter into direct agreements with hospitals and physicians which involve, among other things, the acceptance of varying degrees of organizational control on hospital costs and on physician activities and fees. Taylor makes a good case for the general consonance between objectives and administrative structure and procedures in the several forms of health insurance. However, since the analysis is mostly after the fact, one cannot vouch for the objectives having preceded the organizational features. There is, in fact, good reason to assert that the reverse is partly true. Commercial insurance on the one hand, and medical societies and hospital associations on the other, developed different forms of health insurance partly because of differences in the values and objectives to which these two types of institutions were already committed and partly because the medical and hospital organizations had access to, and leverage over, providers which commercial insurance did not. The prepaid group practice movement, possibly because it is a reaction to inadequacies in the other forms of insurance, does demonstrate more clearly the precedence of objectives over organizational form.

The precedence of objectives, and the manner in which they shape organizational structure, is clearly visible in the deliberations that led to the establishment of the Saskatchewan Medical Plan (17, pp. 42–49). These discussions also demonstrate convincingly the relevance to health planning of the more general values presented in the first chapter of this book. Given the objectives of universality of entitlement, comprehensiveness, uniformity of benefits, financial stability, and administrative simplicity, coupled with maximum administrative control, it becomes clear why the choice was to institute a system based on compulsory contributions (taxes), under direct government control, that offers equal benefits to all residents in the Province. Similarly, Eckstein has shown that although the general objective of the British National Health Service was to provide to all patients, free of charge, all the medical and related services they may require, the structure and operations of the health care system that ensued can be only understood in terms of somewhat more specific objectives. According to Eckstein, these include adequate and rational public financing of services; rational control over the distribution of services; rationalization in the sense of the elimination of waste, the most efficient use of resources, and coordination; maintenance of an effective doctor-patient relationship, which was interpreted to mean perpetuation of the traditional form of this relationship; and democratic organization which, in the light of British tradition, included a large element of syndicalism, or the governance of professional affairs by the professions themselves (15, pp. 167–176).

Goss has studied the relationship between objectives and the medical care product by examining what is known about the quality of hospital care from the perspective of the objectives of categories of hospitals (20). She categorizes hospitals according to objectives as "teaching," "research as well as teaching," "profit making," "non profit," those with a "specialized medical-care goal," those with a "general care goal" and those with "configurations or combinations of hospital goals." A review of reported studies reveals the generally known relationships between the quality of care and characteristics of hospitals. What is distinctive about the analysis by Goss is that these relationships are translated into postulates about the operational relevance of organizational goals. Unfortunately, such postulates take us a very short way toward understanding how quality is attained. As Goss clearly recognizes: "Organizational goals can affect quality of performance only indirectly . . . through the specific types of organizational structures and procedural norms to which they give rise" (20, p. 256). Obviously, the identification of goals and their relevance to outcomes is only the beginning of the more definitive analysis that, as we shall see, Etzioni advocates under his "systems model" for the evaluation of organizational effectiveness (30, 31).

Fifth, an ordering of objectives should serve as the basis for setting priorities within a program and the allocation of effort among competing needs.

Sixth, objectives serve as the basis for solidarity and stability. We have already pointed out the integrative function of certain shared objectives. Agreement over objectives unites the activities of individuals and groups within an organization. Disagreement over objectives, or inconsistency and conflict among objectives, results in strain, conflict, and instability, possibly even dissolution. These expectations are supported by a study of the viability of ''entrepreneurial medical groups'' reported by DuBois. Viability was defined in terms of duration of the group association, rate of growth and current number of full-time medical staff, and duration of association of physicians with the group. A comparison of five groups which had discontinued operations with groups which rated higher than the median in viability scores, suggested that the presence of clear organizational goals and agreement over such goals serve as points around which conflict can be resolved. Furthermore, certain objectives which embody the professional ethic, including patient service and the practice of ''good'' medicine, were most useful in this respect.

> Successful groups were found to have had clearly formulated objectives. These objectives were expressed to recruits in the recruitment process and tended to help in the selection of recruits willing to serve the stated organizational objectives. In the establishment of group policies and the resolution of management problems, organizational objectives served as a basis for judgment. The nature of the objectives served by the highly viable medical groups was distinctly professional. Financial success for physician participants, leisure, professional advancement and relative status all were important aspirations implicit in the group structure, but professional excellence, patient service, the practice of "good" medicine, were the *principal* objectives and the ultimate criteria for decision making . . . Diminished viability or non-viability can result from organizational objectives which lead to organizational policies in conflict with the professional role or from failure to define or support organizational objectives as a central theme around which the organization is operated (19, pp. 8 and 9 of reprint).

A more recent account of the difficulties surrounding the Community Action Programs established under Title II of the Economic Opportunity Act supports the thesis that a common understanding about objectives is a necessary base for organizational stability (29). Moynihan has asserted that among the proponents and originators of these programs, as well as among those who staffed the federal agency, there were at least four different views of what the programs were supposed to accomplish. Some expected the local programs to coordinate disparate efforts in the interests of efficient operations. Others saw the programs as vehicles to bring much-needed services to localities where these were lacking. Still others were more concerned with the potential for political patronage and the mobilization of potential support for the local party establishment. For some others, however, the major object was to fuel discontent and foment conflict, and, through conflict, to create political awareness, self-respect, and power for the hitherto downtrodden. No wonder, seeing the obvious conflicts among these different purposes, that the programs were soon surrounded by controversy leading to disillusionment, bitterness, and, in the end, the scaling down or withdrawal of local and federal support. Moynihan concludes that the public interest requires "clarity and candor in the definition of objectives, and the means for obtaining them."

If there is a lesson here, it is somewhat as follows: government intervention in social processes is risky, uncertain—and necessary. It requires enthusiasm, but also intellect, and above all it needs an appreciation of how difficult it is to change things and people. Persons responsible for such programs who do not insist on clarity and candor in the definition of objectives, and the means for obtaining them, or who will settle for a short and happy life in office, do not much serve the public interest (29, p. 8).

Seventh, the specification of objectives may serve to prevent or minimize the displacement of organizational goals. Warner and Havens contend that the more intangible the goals of an organization, the more likely they are to be replaced by more concrete objectives that focus on means rather than ends (8). These means may or may not serve the intangible objectives that should be central to the organization. In medical care programs, intangible goals such as "the attainment of optimum health" need to be resolved into their more specific components. As we shall see, this is necessary for rendering the more intangible objectives operational and attainable, as well as for their use in evaluating organizational performance.

Finally, objectives serve as a basis for the evaluation of organizational effort. The specification of objectives will first permit a judgment to be made as to whether these objectives are "appropriate" or "adequate," given an external frame of reference. Second, it is possible to determine the extent to which the objectives which an organization sets for itself have been attained. Accordingly, some authors have defined "organizational effectiveness" in terms of the degree to which the organization, through its own efforts, realizes its objectives as specified by itself (1, 21). While, for some purposes, this is a useful approach to evaluation, it must be realized that a judgment still needs to be made as to whether the appropriate or relevant objectives have been pursued. An organization may appear to be highly effective by choosing easily attainable objectives. Consequently, what might be called "self-defined effectiveness" needs to be distinguished from "socially defined effectiveness."

Etzioni has pointed out some more general drawbacks of using, in the study of organizations, a "goal-model," based on the extent to which goals have been attained. Since goals are ideals which are seldom attained, attention is focused on the generally low effectiveness of organizations to the neglect of more penetrating analysis directed at exploring the relationships between specified organizational features and meaningful measures of performance. As an alternative to the "goal-model," in which each organization is compared to an ideal, Etzioni proposes a "systems-model" in which organizations are compared to one another with respect to specified organizational features that include, but are not restricted to, goals. The determination of what these additional features might be, which are chosen as variables in the comparative analysis, is a task that requires an intimate knowledge of each particular organization as well as much further development in organizational theory (30, 31).

The foregoing is a brief discussion of the usefulness of specifying, and making explicit, objectives in planning and administration. The case is made largely on the basis of what appears to be a rational approach to the analysis and resolution of administrative problems rather than on empirical observation and evaluation of actual administrative behavior. One may raise the question, therefore, about there being possible dangers in the explicit specification of objectives. Warner and Havens, while they emphasize the extent to which intangible goals are subject to erosion and displacement, also point out certain possible advantages to intangibility. These include the greater emotional appeal or motivating power of certain intangible goals, their contribution to the ability of the organization to accommodate diverse, and even inconsistent, subgoals, the greater ease with which adaptations can be made to changing conditions, and a greater immunity from critical evaluation (8). In some situations, participants in a cooperative enterprise, either in the planning stage or in actual operation, may have different and, to some extent, conflicting objectives. There is, however, a sufficient base for cooperation provided the areas of divergence and conflict, present or future, are not forced upon the attention of the participants. There may therefore be a danger that the explicit analysis of objectives and of their implications will reveal irreconcilable conflicts of values and interests either not previously perceived or intentionally ignored. Even here, however, one can make a case for the necessity to understand which objectives are shared, which are compatible though not shared, and which are in conflict either immediately or, through their implications or consequences, in the long run. It is then possible to use whatever strengths there are in the situation and to avoid moving into quicksand.

So much for the uses and possible dangers in the specification of objectives. A second consideration under the rubric of the specification of objectives is the form in which objectives are stated. The influence of educationalists is seen in the exhortation that objectives should be stated preferably in terms of behavior: what the subject (whether student or patient) is expected to be able to do as a result of professional effort on his behalf. Deniston et al. insist that, for purposes of program evaluation, a clear distinction be made between activities and objectives, and that objectives be stated in terms of "a situation or condition of people or of the environment" (21). It is perhaps more reasonable to adopt the viewpoint that objectives may be stated in a variety of forms, including (a) program activities, (b) behaviors of persons exposed to the program, or (c) states or conditions of people or of the environment that might be attributed to program activities. In each situation it is important to select the form of statement of objectives that is judged to be most appropriate. It is also essential that one be aware of what assumptions are made, or hypotheses advanced, when objectives are stated in one form or another. These assumptions or hypotheses are generally postulates that certain causal relationships exist between specified program activities and corresponding behaviors and states of clients.

Choice of Objectives

There are no specific guidelines to the choice of appropriate objectives for medical care programs. In general, it is necessary to have a clear understanding of the social mission of the program and make certain that subsidiary objectives do not frustrate or subvert that mission. As we have pointed out, and will discuss again in subsequent sections, it has become apparent that the mere reduction of financial obstacles to care is an insufficient measure. Responsibility has to be assumed for actual use of service and the quality of care received. Further discussion relevant to the choice of objectives will occur throughout this book, including the section on priorities.

Resolution of Conflict Among Objectives

Conflict among objectives is frequent in medical care programs, as it is in other organizations. Such conflict may be seen among objectives *within* any one of the "orientational" categories previously described as well as *among* such categories. As an example of conflict within the collectivity-oriented category, we have already discussed, in Chapter 1, the apparent conflict between the general principles of freedom and equality. More concretely, in the discussions leading to the institution of the Saskatchewan Medical Plan, the reader can see the conflict between the wish to achieve universal and uniform coverage on the one hand, and the desire to avoid compulsion on the other (17). Within the client-oriented category of objectives, conflict not infrequently arises between the objective of assuring quality, as professionally defined, and the objective of assuring responsiveness to the wishes of clients who may value free choice, prefer to be served by physicians of similar ethnic origin, or demand services which professionals regard as unnecessary or possibly injurious. There are also many examples of conflict between categories. Client-oriented and provider-oriented goals come into conflict when providers insist on controlling the terms of their own remuneration while clients need protection against unforeseen expenditures. Similarly, there is often conflict between the organization-oriented goal of control over costs and quality, and the provider-oriented goal of maintaining maximum professional autonomy. Conflict may even arise between collectivity oriented and client-oriented goals. For example, Mark Field has pointed out that the physician in Russia is unhappily caught between two sometimes conflicting demands: the desire to protect individual patients against hardship and the social necessity to keep the maximum number at work (32).

Some particularly significant types of conflict arise when medical care programs are part of a larger program, organization, or social institution. In such situations the goals of the larger unit may hinder the attainment of medical care objectives. Workmen's compensation and welfare medical care programs offer excellent examples. In workmen's compensation, the medical care component is part of a larger juridical institution which enshrines the adversary system for the resolution of conflicting claims. Cheit comments as follows on the consequences of this emphasis:

> It is sometimes argued that effective supervision of medical care is impossible so long as workmen's compensation is administered through an adversary system which permits, even encourages, conflict. The history of American workmen's compensation demonstrates clearly that an adversary system, due process and the right of appeal are valued more highly than is ease of administration. This makes complex the administration of workmen's compensation, and it is, therefore, inevitable that the special problems caused by the unique medical-legal relationship will continue (33, p. 89).

One might contend that the problems of workmen's compensation arise from the misapplication to medical care organization of values and objectives that may be fully appropriate and desirable in other contexts. These misapplied values and objectives include: (a) emphasis on the adversary system and due legal process; (b) belief that out of contending self-interests arises the maximum common good (in this case the contest of worker, union, employer, insurer and perhaps even physician); (c) restriction of governmental control and emphasis on the use of voluntary agencies as agents of government (in this case a multiplicity of good, bad, and indifferent carriers of insurance); (d) a variety of values related to professional prerogatives, free enterprise, and the like; and (e) states' rights, which leads to the development of multiple programs, one for each state, with little uniformity of practice.

Medical care under public welfare provisions is similarly hampered by the traditional values that permeate the institution of public welfare. The principle of lesser eligibility and the traditionally reluctant, miserly, even punitive approach to "helping" the poor are not in keeping with a program that would seek, aggressively, to bring persons who have suffered from long-standing medical neglect under care, and to provide the necessary range and intensity of service that would assure their medical rehabilitation. Even more enlightened approaches to welfare may pose unexpected problems. For example the principle, embodied in the Social Security Act of 1935, that persons on public assistance have their dignity and autonomy safeguarded by receipt of benefits in cash rather than in kind, was found, through experience, to be inapplicable to medical care. Amendments were made to allow direct payment, on behalf of welfare clients, to providers of care. In much the same vein, the notion that welfare clients would receive "mainstream medicine" by instituting a system of payment for care that welfare recipients seek on their own, runs counter to what is known about the type of care available in poverty-stricken areas.

The identification and resolution of conflict in objectives, as in other areas, is an ever-present task for the administrator. Fortunately for him, organizations appear to be able to tolerate a considerable degree of diversity in goals. According to Cyert and March (3) this is because (a) unifying objectives tend to be vague and ambiguous; (b) some objectives are stated in "nonoperational forms" which are "consistent with virtually any set of objectives"; (c) there is compartmentalization, by function or otherwise, within the organization; (d) only a small set of goals is at issue at any given time, so that conflicting objectives do not often present themselves simultaneously; and (e) participants in a cooperative endeavor ("coalition") are willing to exchange some degree of attainment in some objectives to a higher degree of attainment in others. The place that ambiguity and lack of simultaneity occupy in this model suggests, as we have already mentioned, that the explicit specification of objectives may exacerbate conflict. It is hoped, however, that in most instances such specification (at least by the administrator for himself) will lead to avoidance of conflict or its satisfactory resolution or containment. One mechanism of conflict resolution, implicit in the Cyert-

March model, is compromise, brought about through bargaining or otherwise. A good example is the compromise between medical needs and the objectives of legal adjudication achieved in the Ontario Workmen's Compensation program through vesting judiciary powers in a Board whose decisions take account of all relevant facts, but are final and cannot be appealed to the courts (34). Bargaining or compromise usually implies a system of priorities by value or attainability, or both. Hence, such a system of priorities can be considered an important mechanism for conflict resolution. What is less important may be sacrificed for what is perceived as more important, and what is immediately attainable for what can be scheduled for later development. Sometimes, conflict may be resolved by a separation of functions. The problem of whether welfare medical care should be part of a larger welfare function or a larger health function has been handled in some cases by assigning to the welfare agency the task of determining eligibility for aid and to a health agency the task of determining need for care and providing what is needed. For an approach to conflict resolution at a more general level the reader is referred to the discussion, in Chapter 1, of the conceptual and pragmatic reconciliation of the values of equality and freedom.

Implicit in our discussion of conflict resolution is the notion that conflict represents a threat to the organization which must always be avoided or allayed. Coser has argued that while this may be true under some conditions, which he specifies, it is not true in all cases (35). According to Coser, the thing to be most feared is the suppression of conflict, which only leads to its more intense eventual expression. By contrast, conflict can be useful if its expression is accepted and institutionalized, if it does not involve the basic assumptions upon which social or organizational relationships are founded, and if a multiplicity of conflicts exist over a multiplicity of issues, so that persons are only partially involved in any one conflict. Under such conditions the expression of conflict promotes responsiveness of the social system to changed conditions, enables the maintenance of a balance of power, or its readjustment, and reduces isolation and apathy by encouraging associations and coalitions of individuals around the differences at issue. Under this formulation the task of the administrator is not simply the reconciliation of conflicting objectives but the more general management of conflict so it can be put to constructive uses.

Rendering Objectives Operational

This involves the translation of general objectives into families of progressively more specific sub-objectives subservient to them and, eventually, to policies, organizational forms, standards, procedures and other activities that correspond to the objectives. Since this is, in large measure, the subject of this book, no further need be said at this point.

Keeping Objectives Current

We have already referred to the constant interchange between the organization and its environment, to the concept of "goal succession," and to the notion that a different constellation of goals may be operative at different stages in the development of an organization. The vigor—perhaps survival—and the social usefulness of the organization depends on its ability to keep its objectives current through adaptation to changing needs and conditions.

READINGS AND REFERENCES

General

1. Etzioni, A., *Modern Organizations* (Englewood Cliffs, N.J.: Prentice-Hall, 1964), chap. II, pp. 5–19.
2. Simon, H. A., *Administrative Behavior* (New York: Macmillan, 1961), 259pp.
3. Cyert, R. M., and March, J. G., "A Behavioral Theory of Organizational Objectives," chap. III, pp. 76–90, in M. Haire, ed., *Modern Organization Theory* (New York: John Wiley, 1959).
4. Cyert, R. M., and March, J. G., "Organizational Goals," chap. III, pp. 26–43, in *A Behavioral Theory of the Firm* (Englewood Cliffs, N.J.: Prentice-Hall, 1963).
5. Simon, H. A., "On the Concept of Organizational Goal," *Administrative Science Quarterly* 9:1–22 (June 1964).
6. Thompson, J. D., and McEwen, W. J., "Organizational Goals and Environment: Goal-Setting as an Interaction Process," *American Sociological Review* 23:23–31 (February 1958).
7. Perrow, C., "The Analysis of Goals in Complex Organizations," *American Sociological Review*, 26:854–866 (December 1961).
8. Warner, W. K., and Havens, A. E., "Goal Displacement and Intangibility of Organizational Goals," *Administrative Science Quarterly* 12:539–555 (March 1968).

Some Statements of Objectives in Medical Care Programs

9. Miscellaneous Authors, "Principles and Proposals," chap. XII, pp. 665–694, in Committee on Medical Care Teaching of the Association of Teachers of Preventive Medicine (eds.), *Readings in Medical Care* (Chapel Hill: University of North Carolina Press, 1958), 708pp. (See especially section on "Varying Approaches," pp. 676–693).
10. Health Program Conference, *Principles of a Nation-Wide Health Program: Report of the Health Program Conference* (New York: 1944), 34pp. (See especially section on "Objectives of a Nation-Wide Health Program, pp. 5–9.)

11. American Public Health Association, Subcommittee on Medical Care, ''The Quality of Care in a National Health Program,'' *American Journal of Public Health* 39:898–924 (July 1949). *Reprinted in Medical Care in Transition,* vol. I, pp. 17–43. (See especially section on ''Scope and Content of an Adequate Medical Care Program,'' pp. 898–899, in the *Journal* or pp. 17–18 in *Medical Care in Transition.*)

12. Davis, M. M., ''Moving Forces in Medical Care.'' *American Journal of Public Health* 47:525–538 (May 1957). Reprinted in *Medical Care in Transition,* vol. I, pp. 391–404. (See especially section on ''The Goal Ahead,'' pp. 530–532, in the *Journal,* or pp. 396–398 in *Medical Care in Transition.*)

13. New York Academy of Medicine, ''A Policy Statement on the Role of Government Tax Funds in Problems of Health Care,'' *Bulletin of the New York Academy of Medicine* 41:795–796 (July 1965).

14. Myers, B. A., ''Essential Elements of Good Medical Care,'' in *A Guide to Medical Care Administration,* vol. I: *Concepts and Principles,* pp. 23–39 in (New York: American Public Health Association, 1965 [Revised 1969].

Program Objectives and Their Relation to Structure and Function

15. Eckstein, H., ''Objectives,'' in *The English Health Service,* pp. 167–176 (Cambridge: Harvard University Press, 1958).

16. Taylor, M. G., ''Goals of Prepaid Medical Care'' and ''Relation of Goals to Administration,'' in *The Administration of Health Insurance in Canada,* pp. 16–29 (Toronto: Oxford University Press, 1956).

17. Advisory Planning Committee on Medical Care to the Government of Saskatchewan, ''Medical Care Insurance—Problems, Issues and Proposals,'' in *Interim Report of the Advisory Planning Committee on Medical Care to the Government of Saskatchewan,* pp. 42–59 (Regina: Queen's Printers, September 1961).

Some Studies of Goals in Medical Care Programs

18. Scheff, T. J., ''Differential Displacement of Treatment Goals in a Mental Hospital,'' *Administrative Science Quarterly* 7:208–217 (September 1962).

19. DuBois, D. M., ''Organizational Viability of Group Practice,'' *Group Practice* 16:261–270 (April 1967).

20. Goss, M. E. W., ''Organizational Goals and Quality of Medical Care: Evidence from Comparative Research on Hospitals.'' *Journal of Health and Social Behavior* 11:255–268 (December 1970).

Program Objectives in Program Planning and Evaluation

21. Deniston, O. L., Rosenstock, I. M., and Getting, V. A., ''Evaluation of Program Effectiveness,'' *Public Health Reports* 83:323–335 (April 1968).

22. Deniston, O. L., Rosenstock, I. M., Welch, W., and Getting, V. A., ''Evaluation of Program Efficiency,'' *Public Health Reports* 83:603–610 (July 1968).

Other References in the Text

23. Sills, D. L., *The Volunteers: Means and Ends in a National Organization* (Glencoe, Ill.: The Free Press, 1957), 320pp.

24. Murphey, W. F., and Pritchett, C. H., ''Statutory Interpretation,'' chap. XI, pp. 399–406, in *Courts, Judges and Politics* (New York: Random House, 1961).

25. Galloway, G. B., *The Legislative Process* (New York: Thomas Y. Crowell Company, 1953), 689pp.

26. Berman, D. M., *In Congress Assembled* (New York: Macmillan, 1964), 432pp.

27. Staff to the Committee on Finance, United States Senate, *Medicare and Medicaid: Problems, Issues and Alternatives*. Committee Print, 91st Congress, 1st sess. (Washington, D.C.: U.S. Government Printing Office, 1970), 323pp.

28. Horowitz, L. A., ''Medical Care Price Changes: Medicare's First Three Years.'' Social Security Administration, Division of Research and Statistics, Note no. 19 (Washington, D.C.: August 14, 1969), 6pp.

29. Moynihan, D. P., ''What is 'Community Action'?'' *The Public Interest* 5:3–8 (Fall 1966).

30. Etzioni, A., ''Two Approaches to Organizational Analysis: A Critique and a Suggestion,'' *Administrative Science Quarterly* 5:257–278 (September 1960).

31. Etzioni, A., *A Comparative Analysis of Complex Organizations* (Glencoe, Ill.: The Free Press, 1961), 366pp.

32. Field, M. G., *Doctor and Patient in Soviet Russia* (Cambridge: Harvard University Press, 1957), 266pp.

33. Cheit, E. F., *Medical Care under Workmen's Compensation*. Bulletin 244 (Washington, D.C.: U.S. Government Printing Office, 1962), 113pp.

34. Steele, E. C., ''Rehabilitation Program in Ontario for Occupational Injuries,'' *Journal of the American Medical Association* 172:163–167 (January 9, 1960).

35. Coser, L. A., *The Functions of Social Conflict*. New York: The Free Press 1956. (Paperback edition, 1964), 157pp.

III

The Assessment of Need

GENERAL FRAMEWORK

The medical care system, like all other stable institutions, exists to meet some need. The definition of what this need might be, the measurement of need, and the appraisal of the extent to which need has been met or neutralized become, therefore, central concerns of the medical care administrator. This chapter, and several that follow, will pursue this theme and its derivatives. But it is necessary, first, to present a general framework of ideas that will structure and guide this exploration.

The Medical Care Process and Its Environment

The author has found it useful in the study of medical care phenomena to abstract from the whole a set of rather intimate interactions involving health professionals and their clients which may be designated as the "medical care process." The medical care process, in turn, is seen to be surrounded by a host of influences which constitute its environment. The major phenomena of medical care, including use of service, quality of care, and the neutralization of need result from the behavior of participants in the medical care process and the manner in which such behavior is influenced by surrounding factors.

Fig. III.1 is a schematic presentation of the major components of the medical care process. The process is visualized primarily as two chains of activities and events that involve, in parallel but related fashion, the provider of care (most centrally the physician) on the one hand, and his client on the other. The activities that constitute the medical care process arise in response to some need, generally perceived as some disturbance in health or well-being. In some instances need may be first perceived by the health professional, who may take steps to set into action the process

Fig. III.1.   A model of the medical care process

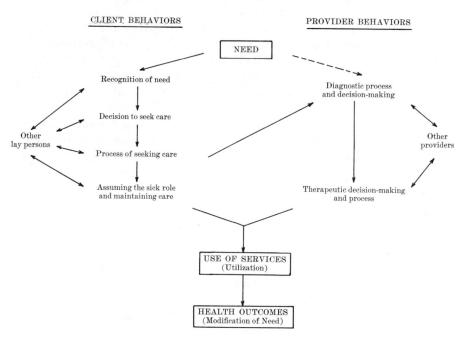

that may lead to care. More often it is the client who must recognize
need, decide to seek care, take appropriate action to seek it, and place
himself under care through adopting those behaviors that are considered
appropriate for persons who are ill. The process of seeking care often
leads directly to contact with a "primary" physician. In some instances
the route to the physician is circuitous and involves the intervention of
family members and friends, who constitute, in Freidson's terminology,
the "lay referral system" (261). In other instances there may be variable attempts at self-medication or resort to practices and practitioners
outside the pale of orthodox medicine. Assuming contact with the physician is ultimately made (which is not always the case), a train of activities is set up, within and by the physician, which constitute the second
chain in the model. First, there are the processes of investigation,
evaluation, and inference that constitute the diagnostic process and
which eventuate in a diagnosis, provisional or firm. These activities,
though much more elaborate and formalized, are analogous to recognition of need by the client and may therefore be seen to constitute
recognition and specification of need by the health professional. Then

follow the professional decision on appropriate therapy and the institution and execution of such therapy. The processes of diagnosis and therapy may require, in addition to the unaided activities of the primary physician, a complex set of interactions with other health professionals, including referral and consultation. Thus, the presence of a ''professional referral system'' (261) is a counterpart to the interactions between the primary client and his associates, and contributes to symmetry in the model.

The processes of diagnosis and therapy appear under the professional axis in the model because they are fundamental components of the professional role and are largely controlled by the professional. It is recognized, of course, that both diagnosis and therapy involve physician and client in intimate interactions which are governed by powerful professional and social norms. The termination of care is usually also a joint decision, although it may in some instances be brought about independently either by the physician or by the client.

Two fairly readily identifiable and measurable phenomena of central importance to medical care organization may be seen to result from antecedent client behaviors, provider behaviors, and their interaction. These are, first, use of service (utilization) and, then, some outcome expressed in terms of client health, well-being, or satisfaction. The two major axes of the medical care process (client behavior and professional behavior) converge, as it were, in use of service which, in turn, should bring about some alleviation of the need which first set the process into motion. The medical care process, therefore, may be seen to have this additional property of being circular. It begins in need and ends in some modification of need, whether partial alleviation or more complete neutralization (see Fig. III.2). There may also be failure to alleviate need and, if therapy is misapplied, the intensification of need or the creation of new need.

Another property of the model needs re-emphasis. The medical care process takes place not within a vacuum but within a context that we have referred to as its environment (Fig. III.2). While this environment is too complex to permit easy categorization, it is useful for the administrator to perceive it in two categories. First, there are the structures and processes that constitute medical care organization and which intimately surround and influence the medical care process. These in turn are surrounded and penetrated by the more pervasive societal and cultural features which also influence need and the perception of need, as well as client and provider behaviors in response to need. The separation of certain organizational features from all other social factors recognizes

Fig. III.2.   The medical care process and its environment

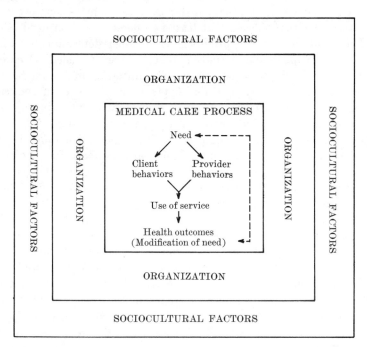

that the administrator has greater control over the former and that by manipulating these he may bring about desirable modifications in the medical care process and its outcomes.

The foregoing constitutes the briefest exposition of the medical care process. Client behaviors in response to need and the provider-client interaction constitute major concerns of the burgeoning field of medical sociology (262, 263). A brief but comprehensive review of client behavior in response to need may be found in a recent paper by Kasl and Cobb (264). By contrast, systematic exploration of the processes of diagnostic and therapeutic decision-making is still in its infancy. However, the prospect of using the computer as an aid in diagnosis and therapy has recently drawn increasing attention to the logical bases of clinical decision-making (265, 268).

The Concept of Need

To make things simpler at the start, the model of the medical care process that we have presented postulated a seemingly unitary concept of need, briefly defined as "some disturbance in health and well-being." Implicit in, and central to, the model, however, is a more complex view of need. It is clear that there are at least two perspectives on need: that of the client and that of the provider. Each must determine for himself whether in any particular situation there is need for medical care and the types of care likely to be needed. The initiation of the medical care process and its successful operation depend on the degree of congruence between the two assessments. To the extent that there is incongruence, the process may become inoperative or fraught with strain.

The physician's definition of need derives from the manner in which medical science defines health and illness and what medical technology has to offer as treatment or prevention. Characteristically, the concept of health receives relatively little attention in medical education. The central preoccupation is with the genesis and progression of disease states, their detectable manifestations, and the manner in which the disease process may be prevented, arrested, or reversed. Furthermore, the major preoccupation, even now, is with somatic disease rather than wth emotional illness and the disturbance in behavior that may be related to such illness (29). Consequently, disease is generally defined and understood in terms of microscopic or gross changes in the structure of cells and tissues, in terms of changes in the chemical composition of body fluids and cells, and in terms of the physiological function of organs and body systems. To the extent possible, the sensations and observations that patients report and the changes in behavior that they manifest are related to such changes in structure, composition or function. Whenever these relationships cannot be established, the physician may fall back on the conclusion, often arrived at after a lengthy and costly process of first excluding somatic disease (29, 30), that there is mental or emotional illness, psychosomatic disease, a "functional disorder," or, perhaps, malingering. Not infrequently the physician arrives at no definite conclusion and remains unsure of what may be wrong, if anything. Scheff has suggested that in such situations of uncertainty, physicians are prone to diagnose disease and thus to "create" it, because overlooking the existence of disease (false negative or Type-1 error) is more to be feared than diagnosing illness when it is not there (false positive or Type-2 error). Thus, generally, but not always, physicians appear to be guided by the rule: "When in doubt, continue to suspect illness (29)." On the other hand, Bogen, in an amusing but revealing paper, has shown how vague is the concept of "functional disease" in the minds of many medical students and, perhaps, in the minds of their instructors (270).

If one were to attempt a composite definition of "functional disease" based on Bogen's tabulation, it would run something as follows. Functional disease is idiopathic, psychogenic, due to multiple causation, and may be only a normal variation; it is sometimes, always and never organic, and it is usually harmless, although it may result in death" (12, p. 595).

In contrast to the ambiguity of the physician's assessment at one end of the spectrum, is the sensitivity, precision, and comprehensiveness of his grasp of illness at the other. Here the physician may be able to suspect (on the basis of familial history or personal constitution and habits) a propensity to certain diseases before disease may be said to have begun; to detect disease before the client is aware of its early inroads; and to assess the present significance of disease in terms of the injury it has already caused to vital body functions and of its capacity to cause progressive injury in the future.

The client's view of need is likely to differ from that of the physician in a number of ways (3–9). First, there is a less complete commitment to the "scientific" view of disease: its causation, evolution, and treatment. Residual folk beliefs color the client's view. Second, although the scientific view may be accepted in principle, there is imperfect knowledge of the characteristics of particular diseases as they are scientifically defined. Third, the time horizon of the client tends to be narrower, with emphasis on current manifestations rather than ultimate consequences. This is in marked contrast to the physician's view that, as Scheff puts it, "Disease is usually an inevitably unfolding process, which, if undetected and untreated, will grow to a point where it endangers the life or limb of the individual, and in the case of contagious diseases, the lives of others" (29, p. 168). Finally, the client is relatively more concerned with the impact of illness in terms of physical discomfort and interference with the activities of successful living as he defines them, and as they are defined for him by his place in society. Thus, physician and client are likely to define health in terms of different dimensions (9).

The upshot of all this is that the definitions of need by client and physician are, on the whole, only partly congruent. The degree of congruence varies from one client-physician pairing to another. Incongruence is likely to be greatest when the client belongs to a group with a distinctive subculture or one largely alienated from the larger society, and when the physician has a predominantly "somatic" view of health and illness.

Little is known about the quantitative relationships between physician estimates and client estimates of need. Some of the literature dealing with comparisons between clinically discovered morbidity and that reported by clients will be reviewed in a subsequent section. So far, the tendency in medical care planning has been to accept the professional estimate of need as the more definitive. From this perspective two phenomena are salient. First, there is in almost all populations, but especially among the underprivileged, a large reservoir of latent, unrecognized, and unmet need. Second, clients report needs ,that professionals cannot substantiate and make demands that professionals regard as inappropriate or excessive. Thus arises the notion of "abuse" of medical services by clients. Unfortunately, the notion of "abuse" has received little careful analysis. So-called abuse may well represent legitimate needs that the medical care system is either unwilling to meet or unable to meet because it was not designed, by professionals, to do so. There is reason to believe that need as viewed by clients, especially those who belong to alienated and less privileged groups, is less differentiated and categorized and, accordingly, the medical care system is seen as more multipotent than in fact it is. It is sobering to think that some clients may have a more "holistic" view of health than many professionals.

It is clear that the analysis of "abuse" is not complete unless one sees it from the differing vantage points of all the participants in the medical care transaction. The client may contribute to it by making inappropriate demands. The health professional may also make a contribution either by not responding to legitimate client needs or demands, or by prescribing inappropriate or excessive care. Congruence in the definitions of need should increase as clients learn more about the professional viewpoint through formal education and through personal experience of medical care, and as professionals broaden their own viewpoints to embrace nonsomatic disease and to acquire greater sensitivity to the interrelationship between social and health needs.

Need Equivalents

So far, we have defined need in terms of states of health or illness viewed by the client, or the physician, or both, as likely to make demands on the medical care system. Need is defined, therefore, in terms of phenomena that require medical care services. It is important to emphasize that these phenomena are broader than illness and include situations in which there is need for prevention or health promotion. For example, a pregnant woman or a well child represents definable needs.

Unfortunately, the word "need" is not always used in the medical care literature in this restricted sense. It is also used to denote the services needed in any particular situation or the resources required to

Fig. III.3. "Need" and its "equivalents"

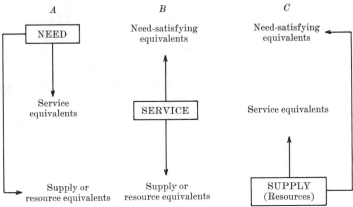

produce these services. The concept of need, then, has been applied to (a) states of health or ill health, (b) use of service, and (c) levels of supply. Influenced by Pennell, the author proposes the concept of "need equivalents" as one solution to this semantic problem. Under this proposal the word "need" would be reserved to describe states of the client that create a requirement for care and therefore represent a "service-requiring potential." Need so viewed can be translated into its "equivalents" in terms of service or of supply (resources) needed to provide the services required. Similarly, a particular bundle of services can be translated either into its capacity to satisfy need or into the resources required to produce that bundle of services. Finally, a given set of resources has its equivalents in the services that they can produce and the needs that they can satisfy. These relationships are shown schematically in Fig. III.3, columns A, B, and C respectively.

The significance of this model is not only, or primarily, in its contribution to classification. It dramatizes the fact that "need" may be conceived and assessed in terms of three different, though related, phenomena. It also emphasizes that, for purposes of planning, it is usually necessary to deal with all three sets of phenomena and with their known or presumed equivalences.

A Model for the Assessment of Need

We are now ready to consider a model for the assessment of need that assembles the elements discussed so far and prepares us for the discus-

Fig. III.4. A classificatory basis for determining need and unmet need

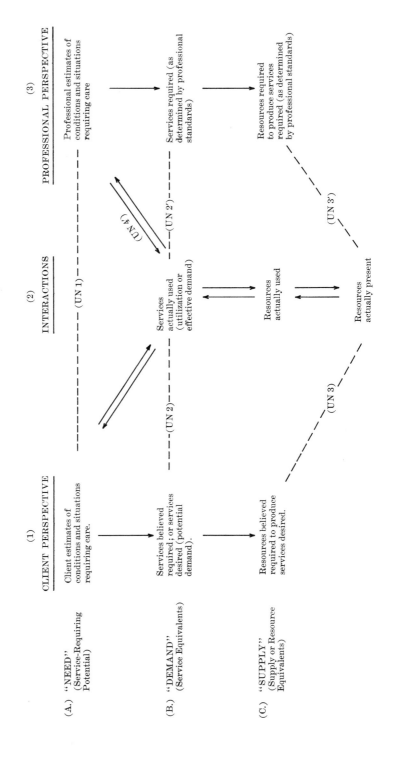

sion of "unmet need" that is to follow. This model is shown in Fig.
III.4. The reader will recognize that it represents a melding of the
medical care process and the notion of need equivalents. For purposes of
description, the model may be seen as a matrix composed of three
columns (1, 2, and 3) and three rows (A, B, and C). The rows represent
the three sets of phenomena that are used for measuring "need." The
designation "demand" (Row B) has been substituted for the category
of "service" in Figure III.3 to emphasize that this category is the
analogue, though not the *equivalent,* of the notion of demand as it is
ordinarily used.

Column 1 represents the client's perspective on need and its equivalents; Column 3 represents the professional perspective (whether of the
provider of care or of the administrator of health services) and Column 2
represents the interactions between the two perspectives and the phenomena that result from such interactions. Actual use of service (referred to
as "utilization," "effective demand," or simply "demand") is one such
resultant. It, in turn, determines, and is determined by, the resources
that are present and the extent to which these resources are employed in
the production of service. The double arrows, here and elsewhere in the
diagram, portray this reciprocal property in the relationship (to be discussed more fully in a later section) between the provision of resources
and their use. The arrows leading from the category of use of service
(Row B, Column 2) to client and professional estimates of conditions
and situations requiring care are intended to indicate how the latter are
altered, as discussed in the preceding section on the medical care process.
Under Column 1, we are already familiar with the notion that the client
has his own estimate of his own health and of his needs for medical care,
and appreciate how important a determinant this is likely to be of the
demand for care that the planner may want to assess and to meet. The
client may also express his needs in terms of resources (Column 1, Row
C), as when he demands a physician in his own neighborhood or a hospital in his town (269). The entries in Column 3 represent the professional
definitions of need and its equivalents. It is customary to accord these
definitions and estimates validity and authority much superior to those
of the client. This is especially true in arriving at estimates of supply or
resource equivalents. However, it is useful to remember, and the model
helps us do so, that each of the professional estimates has an analogous
element in the client's perspective. It is also important to subject to
critical analysis not only the client's viewpoint, but also the bases upon
which professional estimates are made.

Unrecognized and Unmet Need

The concept of unmet need can be readily defined in terms of the model in Fig. III.4. Unrecognized and unmet needs are incongruities between pairs of elements within the model which are viewed as deficits either by the client or the professional, or both. The concept of incongruity includes, of course, in addition to deficits, the complementary phenomenon of superfluity. In the interests of symmetry one might, therefore, add the notion of superfluously or excessively met ("over-met") need. We have already alluded to this problem in our referral to "abuse." We shall no doubt return to it repeatedly in later chapters. Insofar as deficits are concerned, some of these are indicated on the model by the entries (UN). These are:

—UN 1 : States of health or ill-health that are thought to require care by the physician but not by the client, or vice versa.
—UN 2 : Services desired by the client but not received.
—UN 2′: Services required by professional standards but not received by the client.
—UN 3 : Resources desired by the client but not present or available.
—UN 3′: Resources required by professional standards but not present or available.
—UN 4′: This is a variant of UN 1 but sufficiently different, and useful as a measurement device, to merit special mention. It denotes the presence of diseases or disabilities that the proper use of services should have prevented, eliminated, or ameliorated to a significant degree. For example, the prevalence of rheumatic heart disease and middle ear deafness, or the incidence of diabetic coma in a given population, might serve as indicators of insufficient or inappropriate prior care, even though it is recognized that these conditions are not fully preventable. The incongruity proposed in this category of the classification of unmet need is between the ability of services to modify need and the degree of such modification observed within the population. Since this is a purely professional determination, the analogue (UN 4) has not been entered in the diagram. However, the reader may wish, in the interests of symmetry, to add this element to the model and to speculate on what its precise meaning might be. The utility of models such as this is that they identify incompleteness in a conceptual framework and prompt its re-examination.

Another, and much more important, deficiency has been the omission of the dimension of quality from our discussions of the medical care process, of need and of unmet need. For now, it is sufficient to say that quality may be defined as an evaluative judgment about any component of the models so far present. For example, the presence of unprevented or unameliorated health problems in the community (UN 4′) may result not merely from deficiencies in the quantity of care, but also from inappropriate or poor care. Similarly, one can postulate a qualitative dimension to the other deficits indentified in the model. Briefly, the quantity of services and resources may be adequate, but their quality inadequate. The judgment of quality may be made either by the client or by the professional. The concept of the dual perspective, which has been a feature the models presented so far, applies with equal force to the dimension of quality.

ASSESSMENT OF NEED DEFINED AS HEALTH STATUS OR SERVICE-REQUIRING POTENTIAL

Reasons for Assessment

It is useful to distinguish three separate uses to which the assessment of need may be put. First, need defined as states of health and illness may be considered to constitute the outcome or end product of medical care. Hence, it can be used to indicate, in part, the success or failure of the medical care system in any given population. It reflects how effective has been the delivery of care both in quantity and quality. The relationship, however, is partial, since the prevalence of health and illness is also influenced by a host of social, biological, and physical factors additional to medical care. The first use to which estimates of need may be put is therefore evaluational. A second use is in the formulation of priorities for health action. The reasoning here is that a major consideration in the determination of priorities is the impact of specified states of ill-health on the population. A third use is for the purpose of translation into equivalent units of services and resources necessary to satisfy the varieties and levels of need prevalent in a given population. Such translation is an indispensable step in planning for the provision of care.

In this chapter we shall consider the measurement of need and the uses of the data for evaluation and for the setting of priorities. The discussion of the equivalents of need will be deferred to a separate chapter.

What to Measure

A number of categories or phenomena may be measured to give an indication of health status and of service-requiring potential. These include: (1) people, (2) mortality or survival, (3) morbidity, (4) situations that require care, but which cannot be classified as morbidity or mortality, and (5) health. There are, in addition, certain composite indices of health and illness.

The size of the population characterized, where possible, by demographic, socioeconomic, and geographic attributes, is perhaps the crudest, and yet most frequently used, measure of service-requiring potential for the purpose of planning. This is partly because accurate information on population size, by a number of attributes, is readily available in the decennial census reports. Estimates for intercensal years are less valid, but acceptable for most purposes. Data obtained for the 1970 census will be even more useful because they will include more detail on counties, census tracts, and other small areas which may be used for local planning or which may be combined to provide regional data. Other information relevant to health planning will include the presence and duration of disability that interferes with work, occupational history and income by source (137). A rough translation of population data to service needs is possible because of known or assumed relationships between population size and characteristics on the one hand, and the prevalence of conditions requiring care and the likelihood of use of service on the other.

Data on mortality are also readily available and, in most highly developed countries, virtually complete, with the exception of stillbirths. However, as chronic disease becomes a more prominent feature of morbidity and disability, mortality rates become a less accurate indicator of the burden of morbidity, and hence of the need for care. Methods for the measurement of morbidity, of health, and of morbidity and mortality combined will be discussed in subsequent sections of this chapter. We have already emphasized that the concept of need includes situations that cannot be classified as morbidity or mortality but which require care. For example, data on births and/or pregnancies can fairly readily be translated to service equivalents for prenatal, obstetrical, and well-child care, using reasonably agreed upon standards.

Measuring Morbidity

BASIC CONCEPTS. There are two properties of disease that profoundly influence its assessment: (1) its time-intensity gradient, and (2) the intensity-frequency relationship. The notion of a *time-intensity* gradient arises from the view of disease as a process in the individual that begins in subtle changes in the microscopic structure, chemical composition, and function of body cells, tissues, fluids, and organs. From these imperceptible beginnings, the disease process pursues its course to bring about progressively more severe derangement and correspondingly more obvious manifestations. The unfolding of the disease process and of its manifestations may take a variety of courses. In some instances it may progress rapidly or slowly, until death. Frequently, after reaching a peak, the disease process subsides, leading either to complete resolution or to varying degrees of permanent, but nonprogressive, damage which may be severe enough to be shown as disability. In other instances, the disease process and its manifestations follow a long-drawn-out course consisting of exacerbations and remissions, progressively severe damage, corresponding disability, and eventually death. More than one disease may coexist, usually, but not always, with reciprocally adverse effects (272). In fact, death in a chronic illness is often caused or aided by a superimposed acute illness, not infrequently an infection. The variations that result from the combinations of the several types of regression and progression can produce a bewildering variety of configurations in the time-intensity gradients.

The course of any given disease may vary greatly from person to person. On the average, however, and under a given set of circumstances, any given disease follows an expected course that may be designated as its "natural history" (16). The natural history of a disease may be modified to varying degrees, and in roughly predictable ways, by the institution of therapy. Sartwell and Merrell offer a classification of chronic disease based on nature of their evolution over time, and they point out some of the problems of measurement that are produced by the prolonged and variable course of chronic illness (49, p. 580ff).

An important part of the concept of the time-intensity gradient is that, as the disease process develops, its presence becomes increasingly evident. In its earliest beginnings, disease may be undetectable even to the best-equipped physician. It then becomes detectable through the application of particularly sensitive tests, but only when the body or its components are subjected to stress. For example, changes in the electro-cardiogram become evident after exercise, liver malfunction is revealed when it is incapable of removing speedily a dye injected into the blood stream, or damage to the kidney is demonstrated if it cannot function properly when the patient is either deprived of water, or given large amounts of water which the kidney is called upon to excrete. At a further stage of development, disease becomes evident through laboratory tests applied in the absence of stress and, still later, through the use of the ordinary clinical procedures of inspection, palpation, and auscultation. Either at this stage, or at a stage somewhat more advanced, the patient begins to feel unwell, to experience symptoms and to exhibit signs of illness. The disease has now emerged from the depths into the open, as it were. From here on it acquires significance not only to the individual but also to society, because it limits or prevents the discharge of social obligations. First, there may be interference with the performance of social roles, whether at work, in the family, or elsewhere. Then, there may be inability to perform simple tasks, including the activities of daily living. Finally, there is interference with mobility, total loss of mobility, and ultimately death.

Some aspects of the time-intensity gradients, as described in the text, are illustrated in Figs. III.5 and III.6. Certain features of these figures, and of the model as a whole, require further comment. First, as shown by hypothetical disease E in Fig. III.5, a disease may run its entire course without its presence ever becoming evident to the individual, or even to the physician unless he uses special tests to detect it. This is particularly likely to occur in infectious disease (subclinical infection). Second, it is obvious that each stage in the time-intensity gradient is included in the ones above it in Fig. III.6. Third, the stages that intervene between maximum health and death are never as neatly delimited, nor as orderly in their progression as Fig. III.6 shows. There may be considerable irregularity in sequence and overlap between stages. Nevertheless, the overall pattern remains valid and meaningful. For example, this model is meaningful because it has obvious implications for the measurement of illness. It also demonstrates the interrelationships between the medical, personal, and social definitions of illness. The relation to the recognition of need by the client is also evident. There may be, however, a gray period between the appearance of signs and symptoms that the client notices and feels and his recognition of these manifestations as ''illness''

Fig. III.5.   Some hypothetical time-intensity relationships in disease

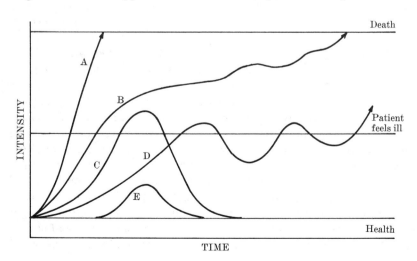

Fig. III.6.   The time-intensity gradient in one hypothetical disease[a]

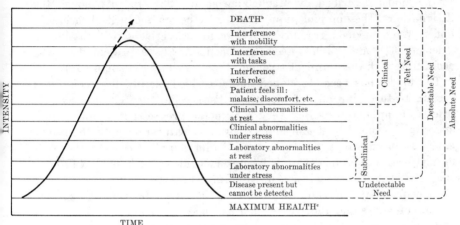

[a] The duration of each of the stages is almost never equal, but is determined by the range of intensities in each stage and, perhaps to a much greater extent, by the rate of change in the disease process at each stage. The impact or significance of each stage is determined by the area under the corresponding section of the curve.

[b] Mainly for convenience in presentation, death is shown as a zone rather than an end point.

[c] It is assumed that the individual has this one hypothetical disease. It is also assumed that there are degrees of health even in the absence of disease, so that "maximum health" is the limiting rather than the average state in this zone.

which requires some form of action. Little is known about this critical transition from feelings to recognition.

The model we have presented is coordinate with the work of others. Indeed, this view of disease derives mainly from the teaching of John E. Gordon at the Harvard School of Public Health (17–21). The model also fits in well with a classification of need offered by Winter and Metzner (273, p. 13, and personal communication). They designate as "undetectable need" that stage of illness during which disease exists, but is not detectable by the application of current medical technology. The inference is that as technology advances it may be possible to detect disease at an earlier stage and thus to broaden the definition of need. "Detectable need" is that stage in the development of disease during which it may be detected either by laboratory tests and investigations or by the application of the more ordinary clinical procedures. "Felt need" occurs when the patient is aware of the presence of illness. "Absolute need" includes the entire spectrum of disease from its earliest beginnings, including that portion which, using present technology, it is not possible to detect.

This formulation is itself remarkably similar in concept and terminology to the model described by Magdelaine et al. (22). In this model, the designations "besoin biologique absolu," "besoin médical théorique," and "besoin médical ressenti" correspond respectively to "absolute," "detectable," and "felt" need. The model we have presented is also coordinate with the "clinical taxonomy" proposed by Feinstein (31).

The model has been developed and described mainly to account for certain features initially of infectious disease and then chronic somatic disease. It appears to apply very well to the progression of nutritional states as described by Dann and Darby: (1) saturation with the nutrient; (2) unsaturated but functionally unimpaired; (3) potential deficiency disease, in which there is laboratory evidence of breakdown under stress; (4) latent deficiency disease, in which there are vague and nonspecific symptoms, and (5) clinically manifest disease with specific symptoms and signs and which, in turn, may be classified as (a) mild and (b) severe (274). The application of the model to mental illness and emotional disorder is somewhat more problematic, but appears to be possible, at least in part (19).

A corollary to the time-intensity relationships in disease is the *inten-*

Fig. III.7.   The intensity-frequency distribution of three hypothetical diseases during a relatively brief time-period[a]

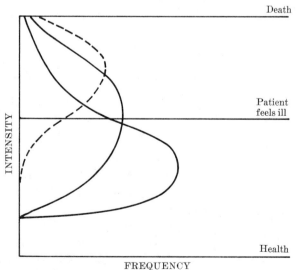

 a These are persons who have the disease in clinical or subclinical form. Persons who do not have the disease are not included.

sity-frequency relationship. This relationship is determined by the incidence of a disease in a given population, the natural history of the disease, and the degree of individual variability in its course. The intensity-frequency relationship is therefore a cross-sectional view of the impact of disease in a given population at a given moment, or during a short period, in time. Just as there is, under specified conditions, an average or typical course for each illness that is designated its "natural history," there is also a characteristic frequency distribution for each illness by stage of severity. Gordon has referred to this characteristic distribution as the "biological gradient" of disease. Figure III.7 shows the distribution for three hypothetical diseases. An important feature of this distribution is that a great share of it may be subclinical or "submerged." Hence it has been called, by Gordon and by others, the "iceberg phenomenon." Its relevance to the assessment of need has been recently re-emphasized by Last (23) and by Israel and Teeling-Smith (190).

The significance of the iceberg phenomenon (or of its absence) to the epidemiology of infectious diseases may be appreciated from the rough estimates shown in Table III.1.

Table III.1. Approximate relative frequency of subclinical to clinical forms of specified diseases

	Relative frequencies	
Disease	Clinical	Subclinical
Rabies	1	0
Measles	1	0.01
Pertussis	1	0.25
Diphtheria	1	5
Viral encephalitis	1	500
Poliomyelitis	1	5000

Table III.2 gives estimates of clinically recognized and unrecognized disease in an "average general practice" in England and Wales. The estimates were computed by Last based on methods for "completing the clinical picture" as discussed by Morris (217), and probabilities of the occurrence of illness derived from "surveys of whole communities for a particular condition" (23). There is, obviously, a large reservoir of undetected, but detectable, need made up of both infectious and noninfectious diseases. References to other studies of undetected and unmet

Table III.2.   Relative magnitude of detected and undetected, but detectable, illness during one year in a hypothetical average general practice, England and Wales, c. 1960

Diseases by Age and Sex Categories	Detected as Percent of Expected[a] (Percent)	Ratio of Detected to Undetected
Hypertension: males 45+	27	1:2.6
females 45+	18	1:4.4
Urinary infection: females 15+	51	1:2.0
Glaucoma: persons 45+	18	1:5.7
Epilepsy: all persons	57	1:1.8
Rheumatoid arthritis: all persons	44	1:2.3
Psychiatric disorders: males 15+	61	1:2.1
females 15+	47	1:1.6
Diabetes mellitus: all persons	48	1:2.1
Bronchitis: males 45–64	51	1:2.0
females 45–64	78	1:1.3

SOURCE: References: 23, Table II, p. 28; 190, Table 1, p. 44.

[a] Based on surveys of whole communities for a particular condition. The methods for detection used in the surveys are cited in the source reference.

need have been cited in a previous section. Discussion of the findings of health examination surveys occurs later in this chapter.

Implications for Medical Care Administration

The view of disease that we have expounded has a variety of implications for (1) the measurement of disease, (2) the interpretation of such measurements, (3) planning for health services, and (4) understanding the causation and distribution of disease.

With respect to measurement, it is clear that whether disease is present or absent depends on how sensitive is the instrument for the discovery of disease and, consequently, what portion of the spectrum of intensities is subsumed under the operational definition of what is "a case." The degree of variability in severity also emphasizes the limited utility of distinguishing merely the presence of disease and highlights the need for greater attention to measures of severity and impact. Certain problems of interpretation follow from the long-drawn-out course of chronic illness. This means that the discovery of new cases does not necessarily reflect the rate of inception. The present prevalence of chronic illness may well reflect infection rates in several generations, as in tuberculosis, or the operation of noxious influences over a lifetime, as in cancer of the lung.

There are many implications for planning health services. First, the natural history of disease influences the nature of services it requires. In particular, a disease that cannot be cured, but which pursues a variably progressive and disabling course, requires a degree of coordination, continuity and personal involvement in care, quite unlike the demands made by acute illness, even if severe or fatal. Second, a number of consequences flow from the submerged presence of a large portion of disease. This calls for the institution of special measures to detect early disease and to influence its course. Obviously, the interest in the detection of early disease depends to a large extent on the ability to do something about its presence. However, even if the disease is not amenable to interruption or retardation, the detection of early disease, and knowledge concerning its probable progression and consequences, may be important in predicting the future burden of disease and disability that the medical care establishment must handle when the disease becomes manifest.

A thorough grasp of these features is essential to understanding the epidemiology of disease. Inferences about the causation of disease cannot be made with confidence unless the entire spectrum of intensities has been mapped out and the course elucidated. The presence of subclinical infection is particularly important because such infection may be transmissible and because it may confer immunity and so influence the manner in which the disease spreads in a given population or its segments.

Measures of Morbidity

The presence of morbidity and its nature can be measured by one or more of the many manifestations that constitute the intensity gradient. These include:

    Fatal morbidities
        Data on deaths by cause of death
    Disability
        Limitation in mobility
        Task interference
        Role interference

Morbidity
>   Diagnosis
>   Signs
>   Symptoms
>   Clinical abnormalities
>   Laboratory abnormalities
>   Reactions to stress
>>   Clinical
>>   Laboratory

Nonmorbidity
>   The absence of morbidity
>   "Positive health"

In this section we are concerned with morbidities and disabilities. The measurement of nonmorbidity, or "health," will be discussed in a subsequent section.

There are at least three aspects to the measurement of morbidity for purposes of health planning: (1) the conceptual and operational definition of the phenomena to be measured, (2) the measurement of intensity, and (3) localization in time, person, and place. The discussion so far has provided a conceptual base for the *definition* of the phenomena to be measured. But for the actual measurement to take place, further specificity in the conceptual definition may be necessary and, equally important, the definition has to be made operational in terms of the data collected and the manner in which they are to be obtained, assembled, analyzed, and interpreted. Examples of what this may entail will be given when the household interview portion of the National Health Survey is briefly described in a subsequent section.

The framework we have presented also incorporates at least a partial *order of intensities* comprising a progression from subclinical to clinical, to symptomatic, to disabling, and finally to fatal disease. In clinical and epidemiological studies, where a great deal of detailed information may be available, it is possible to construct rather elaborate measures of the intensity or progression of the disease process. These are based on constellations of laboratory abnormalities, structural changes, signs, symptoms, subtle or gross disturbances in function or performance, response to therapy, and the like. Examples are certain schemes for staging cancer (36–38), heart disease (39), chronic respiratory disease (40), and arthritis (41). Similarly refined scales have been developed for the assessment of disability in handicapped patients (42–46). Walker et al. have proposed a scale for measuring social restoration of the mentally handicapped (47). A discussion of the rationale, uses and limitations of such measures exceeds the scope of this book and is beyond the competence of its author. It is a subject, however, that deserves thorough review and that constitutes one portion of the spectrum of methods available for the assessment of need.

For purposes of health planning and evaluation cruder measures of intensity suffice. These include (a) subjective measures such as whether the condition is painful, causes discomfort, or is "bothersome"; (b) the degree of interference with activity or mobility; (c) whether the condition called for medical care or hospitalization; and (d) the frequency and duration of the morbid phenomena in question. The household interview portion of the National Health Survey provides examples of the use of all these indicators. Consultation with a physician is, indeed, part of the definition of an acute illness, as we shall see. There is also considerable elaboration of the concept of disability for which three measures are used: interference with "usual activity," with "major activity," and with "mobility." The concept of "usual activity" is used to calibrate the impact of both acute and chronic illness. What constitutes usual activities is defined by what a person would have done ordinarily on the day, or the days, for which a morbid condition is reported. Hence, "usual activity" varies by individual as well as by age, sex, occupation, day of the week, or season. Scales of limitation in "major activity" and in "mobility" are used for the assessment of chronic conditions only. "Major activity" is defined, where preschool children are concerned, to mean "ordinary play with other children"; for school children, to mean going to school; for housewives, to mean housework; and for all other persons, to mean "work at a job or business." In tabular form, the three scales of disability are as follows:

Interference with usual activity
    Restricted activity day
    School-loss day
    Work-loss day
    Bed disability day
Limitation in major activity
    No limitation in activity
    No limitation in major activity, but otherwise limited
    Limitation in the amount or kind of major activity
    Inability to carry on major activity
Limitation in mobility
    Not limited in mobility

> Has trouble getting around alone
> Cannot get around alone
> Confined to the house

The several categories of disability specified by the National Health Survey are partially overlapping. Sullivan has proposed a mutually exclusive, graded categorization of morbidity in terms of disability, using some of the definitions of the National Health Survey, as follows (203, p. 12) :

1. Confined to resident institutions and unable to leave because of illness.
2. Not classified in 1 above, but confined to the house or cannot get around alone.
3. Not classified in either of the above, but unable to carry on the major activity for their group or limited in the amount or kind of major activity performed.
4. Not in any of the above categories but restricted in the performance of usual activities.

More recently, Sullivan has proposed alternative ways of combining the basic information contained in the household interview and resident institution survey components of the National Health Survey to arrive at an approximation of a mutually exclusive categorization of the total spectrum of disability.

One classification would categorize disability as follows (205) :
1. Bed disability :
   a) Confined to a long-stay institution.
   b) Is in a short-stay institution or is confined to bed at home for more than half the daylight hours.
2. Non-bed disability :
   Not classified in (1) but unable to carry on major or usual activity or restricted in the performance of these.
Another classification proposed by Sullivan is as follows (204) :
1. Long-term institutional disability :
   Confined to a long-stay institution.
2. Long-term noninstitutional disability :
   Not classified as (1) but has a chronic condition or impairment and is unable to carry on the major activity designated for his age-sex group.

3. Short-term disability:
   Not classified as (1) or (2) but is unable to carry on major or usual activities, or is restricted in the performance of these.

There would seem to be no a priori compelling reasons for selecting any one of these classifications over the others, but the first seems to be the most satisfactory. In the second classification, one might question the equating of institutionalization with bed disability and the fact that the category of non-bed disability includes bed disability for less than half the daylight hours. In the third classification, long-term disability that involves anything less than inability to carry on one's major activity would seem to be assigned to the category of short-term disability, which is, in fact, a residual class. Thus one sees a certain degree of confounding of two attributes of the seriousness or significance of a disability: its intensity and its duration. Furthermore, it should be noted that all the above are classifications of the status of any given person on any given day. For longer periods of time the days are summated to provide a cumulative picture of disability. Sullivan believes that "summing disability days in these four categories automatically weights each episode according to its duration and provides a measure of the burden of disability days during the year" (203, p. 13). It is clear, however, that the several categories cannot be collapsed into a single index of disability unless each category can be expressed in terms of a common unit (for example, dollars or man-hours of care, or whatever) and weighted appropriately before all the units are summed. We shall return to this problem later in this chapter.

In addition to the use of medical care and scales of disability, the National Health Survey uses *duration* and *frequency* as measures of intensity. The product of duration and frequency constitutes one measure of cumulative impact. The usual form of expression is the "person-days" of any one of the grades of disability. The "person-day" concept is a summary statement that does not distinguish the occurrence of disabilities of short duration in many persons from the occurrence of disabilities of long duration in fewer persons. Since such distinctions are important for medical care planning, person-day data must be supplemented with additional information: for example, the proportion of persons having experienced any disability during a given period, the average duration of disability for those who have experienced disability, the frequency distribution of persons by number of episodes of disability and of episodes of length of disability, and so on. Sheps has examined critically the application of the person-day concept to epidemiological studies and clinical trials, pointing out its serious shortcomings for this purpose (53).

The Commission on Chronic Illness used findings in a household survey to classify individuals into one of three groups using two types of criteria: disability and diagnosis (50). This approach was further developed by Katz and his colleagues to eventuate into an elaborate categorization of patients for clinical and epidemiological studies. For each person in a group, a profile is established which consists of (a) the established principal diagnosis, (b) additional chronic disease abnormalities revealed by standardized multiple screening, and (c) physical disability status. The entire population is categorized by each of three dimensions and their combinations (51).

More recently, Fanshel and Bush have extended the simple intensity scales of the National Health Survey, and their reformulation by Sullivan, into an eleven-point scale of mutually exclusive categories each of which represents a point or state on what they regard to be a "continuum of function/dysfunction" (206). These categories are designated: Well-being; Dissatisfaction; Discomfort; Disability, minor; Disability, major; Disabled; Confined; Confined, bed-ridden; Isolated; Coma; Death (206, pp. 1029–1030). As we shall see in a future section, they have also proposed a set of corresponding weights ranging from 1 for "well-being" to 0 for "Death," so that the several states can be aggregated into one measure of function/dysfunction. But position on the intensity scale is only one of two determinants of the "severity of illness"; the other is prognosis, which is expressed as the probability that a homogeneous group of persons who are in a given state at the beginning of a time period will be in the same or another specified state, or set of states, at the end of that time period. By applying these probabilities to the intensity categories over a succession of time periods, it is possible to describe the health of a population as an unfolding process in time. In this way, the model proposed by Fanshel and Bush provides mathematical expression to the "time-intensity" and the "intensity frequency" gradients as we have described them.

Moore has pointed out the inadequacies of the usual diagnostic categorizations of disease for purposes of health planning because these categories are not easily translatable into attributes such as urgency, degree of departure from health, requirements for care and probable outcome, all matters of primary concern to the planner (52). He refers to several attempts to develop alternative classifications, including one by the Department of the Army. In this study 100 common diagnoses were characterized according to urgency, survival, and extent of care required. Using similarity with respect to these attributes as the criterion for classification, it was possible to reduce the original 100 diagnoses into 11 classes of "good commonality." Moore himself offers an alternative scheme for classification which uses two dimensions—duration of care and intensity of care—to arrive at a partially ordered set of categories, as follows (52, pp. 43–44).

Class 1. Those patients who are considered to have a transitory condition and are expected to recover with outpatient care.
Class 2. Those patients who are expected to recover with short-term general hospital care.
Class 3. Those patients who have a chronic condition but are not disabled and are expected to be contained through outpatient care.
Class 4. Those patients who have a chronic condition and are expected to be contained by hospitalization.
Class 5. Those patients who are impaired but can be contained without hospitalization.
Class 7. Those persons who become patients for correction of impairments.

This classification is seen to incorporate a definition of severity partly in terms of impairment or disability, partly in terms of duration of impairment or of care, and partly in terms of duration of care and amenability to recovery. The problems and potentials of representing morbidity states in terms of their medical care equivalents will be dealt with at some length in the final chapter of this book.

To conclude this section, it may be useful to return to the need to categorize the impact of illness in terms of *episodes of illness* and their parallel, though not completely congruent expression, in episodes of care. The concept of episode flows naturally from the view of disease as a finite process with a beginning, unfolding, decline, and termination. We have found that while this picture is true for acute disease, and applies with some modification to the exacerbations of chronic disease, there are situations in which the disease remains active for long periods of time and the boundaries of its periodic fluctuations are not easy to determine. In other instances it may be difficult to fix the precise onset of disease or its termination. Further problems come about because of the concurrent presence of more than one disease process. Nevertheless, the delineation of episodes of illness and of episodes of care might be operationally possible, and would constitute an important tool for analysis. It should be easier to delineate episodes of care than of illness. Solon et al. have discussed the concept of an episode of care, have advanced some rules for the operational delineation of episodes, and have reported on the actual application of such rules (54, 55).

The *location of disease* in "person," "time," and "place" is a fundamental feature of classical epidemiology as it seeks clues to the causation of disease and the manner in which it is propagated (17–21, 56–58). The concern in medical administration is for the localization of need and the corresponding marshaling of resources. Although the priority of concerns is somewhat different, the basic concepts and methods are the same and constitute a major area of congruence between epidemiology and medical care administration (213). *Localization in person* refers to the distribution of disease by demographic and socioeconomic categories of the population. *Distribution in time* refers to trends in the incidence and prevalence of disease as well as its fluctuations around this trend. Fluctuations in the incidence of disease may represent random variation, especially where the population is small. In addition, many diseases exhibit a remarkable regularity in their periodocity, whether seasonal or with peaks spaced two or more years apart (58). The combinations of secular trend, seasonal and longer periodic rhythms, and random fluctuations often combine to produce a complex, but characteristic, pattern for each disease entity. An ''epidemic'' may be said to occur if the incidence of disease is unusually high. It is a moot point whether this term should be used to describe expected peaks in a periodic disease or be reserved for situations in which such expectations are significantly exceeded. The temporal variations in disease incidence are most marked, and have received most attention, in infectious disease. They do, however, occur in certain noninfectious diseases as well. In recent years, the upward trend in cancer of the lung has been so marked that some have spoken of an ''epidemic.'' It appears that this upsurge has run parallel, but with some decades of lag, to the spread of a social innovation—smoking. Certain features of the organization of place of work, place of residence, and leisure may interact with environmental features to produce seasonal, periodic, and even diurnal variations in motor vehicle accidents. Certain emotional phenomena, which appear to have some of the contagiousness of infection, have been described to occur in ''epidemics'' (20). The implications of the irregular occurrence of disease to the need for standby capacity of hospitals and other medical care resources will be discussed in a subsequent section.

Location in *place* is an especially important requirement for medical care planning because certain features of social organization conspire to concentrate particularly vulnerable populations in certain areas, notably the urban ghetto and some rural sections of the country. The association is often so close that mere residence in certain areas may constitute presumptive evidence of unmet need (64–72). Hence, an important tool for planning and for social research is the mapping out of disease, disability, and other indicators of need by small areas with relatively homogeneous populations (60–63). Such areas include city blocks, census tracts, postal zones, school districts, wards, towns and counties. A "block face" is the smallest areal unit used by the Census Bureau. Each block has an average of five block faces. The next larger unit is the "block grouping," which corresponds to the "enumeration district" in previous censuses. It contains approximately 10 blocks comprising about 200 to 600 households, or a population of between 500 and 1,600 persons. A block grouping is always a subdivision of a census tract. The census tracts themselves are "small, relatively permanent areas into which large cities and adjacent areas have been divided for the purpose of showing comparable small-area statistics. They are designed to be relatively homogeneous in population characteristics, economic status, and living conditions, and have an average population of 4000" (78, pp. 28–29; 79, p. 1). The decennial census has provided a fair amount of information concerning residents of blocks, census tracts, counties, and other small places. It promises to provide even more small area detail in the future (137). This is important because information concerning the population base is necessary for the computation of rates. In addition, there may be sufficient information in the census reports on educational, occupational, and income characteristics for each area, to permit the construction of simple or composite scores by which the areas are ordered so as to study correlations between such characteristics and the incidence or prevalence of indicators of need in each area or group of areas (59; 68, pp. 962–963; and 65, pp. 98–99). Such correlations depict accurately the associations between area characteristics but reflect none of the variation within areas (273, p. 107). Very frequently, the presence of associations between area-characteristics has led to the inference that similar associations exist between the same characteristics as they pertain to individuals. For example, if it is found that census tracts with higher average income also have a higher proportion of women who have received adequate care, the inference is made that individuals with higher income are more likely to receive adequate prenatal care. Robinson has warned that although the correlation between two attributes of a set of areas can be theoretically the same as that between the same attributes of individuals within the areas combined, this is not usually the case (63). The correlation is generally larger for the areas than for the individuals, and becomes larger as the number of areas is decreased as a result of grouping into larger subunits. In addition to changes in magnitude, area correlations may be different, sometimes showing associations in a reverse direction from those obtained when individuals are used as the unit of analysis.

An excellent example of such an occurrence is the admittedly absurd negative correlation between age and hospital use found by Rosenthal in a study in which states were the unit of analysis (275, p. 36). In spite of these dangers, correlations between attributes of areas continue to be used, at least as first approximations of their relationship in individuals (64–68). This is because socioeconomic data that are available for census tracts, for example, are often not available for the individuals in those census tracts who are the objects of study. Hence, the average character- istics of each census tract in a set are attributed to each of residents in that tract who also happens to be included in the particular study. Robinson has shown how and why large errors may ensue from this procedure (63). Generally, the nature and magnitude of the error remain undetermined. In a study in which both census tract and family data were available, Rosenfeld and Donabedian found roughly similar rela- tionships between the adequacy of prenatal care and income, when individuals were grouped first by family income and then by income of census tract of residence. However, the family data were more discrimi- nating in revealing the effect of particularly high incomes which could not be separated out in the census tract data because of averaging. For example, the highest group of individuals had a family income of $10,000–15,000, whereas the highest group of census tracts had a median income of $4,660 (66, pp. 1121–1122). The consequences to prenatal care of this large disparity in incomes may, however, have been somewhat reduced if, as Hochstim et al. suggest, residents in an area are more similar in some respects than would be indicated by differences in income or race (72).

An important corollary to locating need by geographic area is its degree of congruence with the spatial distribution of the service and supply equivalents of that need. As we shall see in a subsequent section, it is not sufficient to map the presence or absence of resources in a given area. The factors of travel distance, travel time, and other aspects of access and availability need to be taken into account.

Attempts to locate health-related events in person and in place are seriously hampered by the dispersed nature of the relevant information in a fragmented system of health care. One evidence of this is the large number of disparate sources of information which we shall describe in the following section. Generally, this information allows study only of the frequency and distribution of events. Often, even the several aspects of a given event cannot be assembled. For example, for any given episode of illness, care within the hospital cannot easily be related to that re- ceived either before or after the hospital experience. Similarly, it is seldom possible to study the many events experienced by the same person or family, or that occur in a given location. Studies that require information for many years of experience, perhaps a lifetime, are particularly difficult. Hence the need for methods that combine information from a variety of sources and over a long period of time.

The term "record linkage" was introduced by Dunn to designate such a method, originally in order to compile what he saw as a "book of life" for each individual (73). He later extended the notion to include the compilation of data for entire families (74). Newcombe and his associates have capitalized on the unusually complete information available in Canadian Vital Records to develop elegant methods of record linkage which they have used successfully in genetic studies (75). A clear account of past developments and current uses may be found in the book by Acheson (76).

The organization of information from disparate sources around a particular location requires that current information about place of residence be included in the sources in question. The more detailed this information, the more precise can be the localization of the events. Linkage is achieved by consulting a listing that translates addresses into the unit of aggregation used for statistical analysis, such as a block, block grouping, or census tract. The Bureau of the Census has developed methods for performing such translation by computer. In this way it is possible to link information that characterizes the geographic unit in question and to compare geographic units in terms of such characteristics (77–79). Computer mapping methods are also available (62, 77). These can produce either actual plots, in which each mark represents an event, such as perinatal death, or a visual display of frequencies represented by shadings of different intensity.

The linkage of records around individuals or families is a more difficult task. This is because each individual must be uniquely identified and his relationship to other members of a family specified. In theory, the simplest method for accomplishing individual linkage is to develop a system of numbers which are assigned to every person at birth and which characterize him throughout his lifetime. In the United States the Social Security number might serve this purpose. Lacking this, it is possible to select a number of basic attributes of which any individual configuration is sufficiently unusual to distinguish one person from another with a high degree of assurance. Such attributes might include surname, given names or initials, and place and date of birth. For married females, the maiden name must also be given. In order to accomplish family linkage, parents must be identified on at least one of the records of their children.

One major problem in achieving linkage is that this minimum required information does not always appear on every record. Furthermore, errors are made either in the reporting or the transcribing of one or more items of information. Names are particularly subject to variations in spelling and in order. To get around these difficulties procedures have been developed for the phonetic coding of names. Furthermore, where the identifying information on two or more records is only in partial agreement, known probabilities of the occurrence of the identifying characteristics are used to indicate the most probable match within specified limits of tolerance.

Given the necessary information and rules of procedure, linkage can be accomplished by manual processing of records. However, it is the remarkable advance in computer methods that brings with it the promise, as well as the possible dangers, of comprehensive record linkage on a national scale. The advantages are fairly obvious. The objections have been directed at possible breaches of the confidentiality of medical information and, more fundamentally, at the possible misuse of the information by government as an instrument for control. The assigning of unique, individual numbers, in particular, raises the specter of totalitarian rule. However, as Acheson persuasively contends, it should be possible in a democratic society to devise a system that provides the advantages of record linkage with adequate safeguards against abuse (76, pp. 98–106; 170–184).

SOURCES OF MORBIDITY INFORMATION

Having considered the phenomena that might be measured, it is necessary to turn to the sources from which information concerning these phenomena might be obtained. In this section, there will be a listing of sources, a description of their general characteristics, and a brief discussion of the interrelationship between the nature of the source and the nature of the phenomenon to be measured. More detailed description and evaluation of specific sources of information will follow in separate sections.

The following is a partial list of sources of morbidity information. The categories are not mutually exclusive.

1. Surveys
   a. Household interview survey
   b. Continuous local survey
   c. Surveys of institutional populations
   d. The symptom survey
   e. Self-administered questionnaires

2. Records
    a. Vital records
    b. Notifications
    c. Registers
    d. Records of special population groups
    e. Records of medical practice in institutions
    f. Records of office practice
3. Medical examination
    a. Clinical examination
    b. Laboratory and other tests
    c. Screening
4. Pathological examinations
5. Combinations of the above

It is notable that the National Health Survey combines elements from several of the categories listed above by including in its program: (a) a Health Interview Survey based on data collected in a continuing national sample of households; (b) Institutional Population Surveys based on national samples of establishments providing medical, nursing, and personal care services and samples of residents or patients; (c) a Hospital Discharge Survey based on a sample of patient records in a national sample of hospitals; and (d) a Health Examination Survey based on direct examination, testing, and measurement of national samples of the population (84).

The different sources of information listed above may be grouped into two major categories: those that embody the results of professional estimations of morbidity and those methods that tap nonprofessional or client views and valuations. The methods are coordinate, therefore, with the models of need that we have already presented, and raise similar questions concerning the validity and relevance of the two perspectives: of the professional and of the client. Our model would lead us to expect that the findings of the two kinds of methods would be different, but partly congruent. As a summary of experience, that will be discussed in greater detail in a subsequent section, it may be said that (a) a very low proportion of conditions found clinically, or recorded, is actually reported by clients; (b) many conditions are reported that cannot be substantiated in the record; (c) sometimes the "false positives" and the "true positives" reported by clients add up to a proportion of the population equal to the proportion of clinically substantiated ("true") positives, but this is an entirely spurious coincidence; and (d) the proportion of "false positives" and "false negatives" varies from condition to condition, and possibly in response to other influences, so that the

Fig. III.8.   A schematic representation of the relationship between morbidity phenomena and methods of obtaining information concerning these phenomena[a]

Phenomena to be measured	Client-oriented methods		Provider-oriented methods					
	Interview surveys	Self-administered questionnaires	Public health records	Clinical records	Clinical examinations	Screening tests	Comprehensive clinical and laboratory assessments	Comprehensive clinical, laboratory, and pathological assessment
Fatal morbidities								
Limitations in mobility								
Task interference								
Role interference								
Diagnoses								
Signs								
Symptoms								
Clinical abnormalities								
Laboratory abnormalities								
Reaction to stress: clinical								
Reaction to stress: laboratory								
Absence of morbidity								
"Positive health"								

[a] The list of methods presented in the text has been collapsed to a smaller number of more sharply differentiated categories.

result of client reports is not simply an underestimate or overestimate, but a distortion of the clinical diagnostic picture.

Because the biological gradient of morbidity itself is roughly divided into component spectra of professionally detectable, but unfelt, need, and felt need, there is a rough correspondence between the methods of obtaining information and the stage or zone in the spectrum of intensities and manifestations that the method can tap into. It is useful, therefore, to conceive of the relationship between the intensity-frequency gradient and the range of methods as a matrix (see Fig. III.8). Examination of such a matrix dramatizes the conclusion that the issue is not the superiority of one class of methods over another, but the particular suitability of the method to the type of information sought. If the objective is to assess the impact of morbidity on individuals and their behavior, client-oriented methods are indicated. If the objective is to arrive at the most valid and complete diagnostic categorization, a progression of increasingly valid methods has been proposed by Feldman as follows: (1) reports by respondents on behalf of other family members; (2) report by the respondent for himself; (3) diagnosis by the individual's regular physician in the course of routine medical care; (4) diagnoses which would be made on the basis of an extremely thorough examination in a clinical setting; and (5) diagnoses which would be made on the basis of an autopsy or exploratory operation (92). Possibly the most valid diagnostic categorization is based on the use of all the sources of information, including pathological tissue examination, rather than on the latter alone.

Finally, the reader should be warned that a whole science and "technology" has developed around methods for obtaining and analyzing population data which includes sampling and survey methodology. Not only are particular methods suited to eliciting certain kinds of information, but seemingly small variations in method or procedure bring about significant differences in the nature and quantity of information obtained. Kosa et al., for example, used three different instruments to obtain information about the health of a sample of families who used a medical emergency clinic for children: a questionnaire on utilization of service, a child health index similar to the Cornell Medical Index (which will be discussed in a subsequent section of this chapter), and a family "health calendar," or log. They found that measurements of morbidity within each instrument tend to be related, but that there was no significant relationship among instruments—each measures something different (102). Further examples will be cited when the individual methods are more fully assessed. The medical care administrator should know enough about the various methods so that he can exercise the necessary caution in the interpretation of the data they yield. Furthermore, he should be the expert in the particular medical care phenomena that the surveys set out to measure. As such, he should participate actively in the selection of the method most appropriate to the use to which the data are to be put.

Household Interview Survey. In this section there will be a discussion of the interview survey, its features, uses, and limitations, with special reference to the National Health Survey, both because it serves as a model and is the most important single source of current health data. Feldman (92) gives the following as the strengths of the household interview approach to measuring morbidity: (a) cost advantages over alternatives such as clinical examinations, (b) breadth of population coverage, (c) wide range of classifying data that can be obtained, including demographic, social, economic, and other variables, (d) availability of a population base for the construction of rates, and comparability of numerator and denominator data that are obtained at the same time and can be related to each other with greater confidence, and (e) quality of the sample. Often one obtains completion rates well over 90 percent. This is in contrast to medical examination surveys in which participation is generally low. However, the health examination component of the National Health Survey, by dint of considerable, carefully planned and staged effort, was able to obtain a response rate of 86.5 percent (194, p. 14). By contrast, the noninterview rate in the household survey component is about 5 percent, including 1 percent from refusals (84, p. 9).

On the debit side of the ledger are limitations of the household interview survey in the completeness and validity of the data obtained and considerable ambiguity about what precisely the data mean. Accordingly, the interpretation of interview survey data must take into account (1) the definitions of morbidity and the manner in which such definitions are made operational, (2) the nature of the sample, (3) problems of reporting, and (4) the validity of the information reported. These aspects of the household interview survey are dealt with in greater detail below.

An essential element in the interpretation of survey data, as well as any other type of statistical material, is a precise understanding of the *definitions* used to identify the phenomena being measured (88). This is particularly important if information from several surveys is to be compared. Terms that appear clear and unequivocal at first blush, are seen on closer scrutiny to be vague and subject to many interpretations. The basic health phenomenon measured in the household interview component of the National Health Survey is "a morbidity condition."

This is defined as "a departure from a state of physical or mental well-being resulting from disease or injury." As reported in the Survey, the concept of a morbidity "condition" includes three additional modifiers: awareness, impact, and action. Awareness is obviously a necessary pre-condition to reporting. Impact denotes some degree of disability and its duration; and action some effort to seek and receive care. Impact and action criteria are included in the definition to assure that the morbid condition reported exceeds a threshold of intensity below which its significance would be in doubt and reporting known to be much less reliable.

Operationally, the information which leads to the identification of reportable morbid conditions is derived from a series of questions that ask whether during the two weeks previous to the week of the survey the survey respondent, or the person on whose behalf the response is being made (a) has been "sick" or has experienced "ailments," "conditions," or "problems with health"; (b) has had "accidents or injuries"; (c) has experienced ill-effects from an accident or injury sustained prior to the two-week period, or (d) has "talked to a doctor" for any condition or has taken "treatment or medicine." In addition, information is sought on whether during the prior 12 months there has been (a) any one of 28 entries on a Check List of Chronic Conditions that include items such as asthma, heart trouble, stroke, stomach ulcer, allergy, epilepsy, hernia, and the like; (b) any one of 11 items on a Check List of Selected Impairments that includes conditions like deafness, having trouble seeing, cleft palate, club foot, and "any other condition present since birth" (88, p. 26); and (c) whether there has been admission to hospital or to "nursing home, rest home, or any similar place." Information is also obtained about the duration of each morbid condition and about the occurrence and impact of disability. The manner in which disability is defined and graded as to severity or impact has been described in a previous section. When a physician has been consulted for a "morbidity condition," the respondent is asked, "What did the doctor say it was?—did he give it a medical name?" Diagnostic categorization is based on the answers to these questions and to the check lists of chronic diseases and impairments.

The manner in which various attributes derived from the information cited above are combined to provide operational (22) definitions is illustrated in the following. A "chronic condition" is said to exist if (a) the condition is one of the items on the check lists of chronic conditions or impairments, or (b) the condition was first noted more than three months before the week of the interview. An "acute condition" must simultaneously satisfy three criteria: (1) not be an item on either check list of chronic conditions or impairments; (2) have lasted less than three months; and (3) either have received medical attention or caused re-stricted activity during at least one day (88, pp. 43–44). The incorporation of medical care as part of the definition of acute illness may introduce a bias because the propensity to seek care is not uniformly distributed in the population. For example, women and persons in higher income groups are believed to be more likely to consult physicians when illness oc-curs. The tendency to restrict activity or limit work is also likely to be in-fluenced by whether a person is employed, type of employment, and social class. Hence, the definitions of illness and disability in the National Health Survey include a significant but unmeasured social component. As we shall see, this and related factors raise questions about what the Survey data signify.

The *nature of the sample,* including the response rate, determines the degree to which it is possible to generalize from the findings of any survey. The response rate of the household interview portion of the National Health Survey is very high, about 95 percent. Adjustments for nonresponse are made in the published data. The sample has a highly stratified, multistage probability design (85) which eventuates in the weekly selection of clusters of 9 households in each of 357 primary sam-pling units which collectively represent the nation, but with some exclu-sions. Each weekly sample is independent of the others, so that weekly samples can be cumulated indefinitely into larger and larger samples while maintaining their representative nature. Needless to say, all the counts and measurements obtained are subject to a calculable sampling error which is cited in the Survey publications. Since the sample is designed primarily as a national sample with acceptable tolerances in sampling error, its findings cannot be applied, without considerable reservations, to the smaller units which are often the locus and concern of health planning. The Survey reports do, however, have considerable detail by age, sex, race, education, income, and urban-rural residence. With appropriate adjustments to local characteristics and the exercise of judgment, survey data may serve as a guide to local planning.

In addition to national estimates, the Health Interview Survey pro-vides some estimates for smaller geographic areas as follows: four major regions, three residence categories (standard metropolitan statistical areas, and farm and nonfarm classes outside these areas), and each of 22 metropolitan areas with population of 1,000,000 persons or more in 1960. In order to meet the demand for data at the state level, the National Center for Health Statistics has proposed a method that uses information from the national estimates in order to construct what are called "synthetic estimates'' for each of the states (86). The basic notion is that the occurrence of phenomena such as illness, disability, use of service, and possibly others as well, is determined by a number of specifiable population characteristics. The effect of such characteristics, singly and in combinations, on the occurrence of any specified phenomenon, can be determined from the national sample. If population size and characteristics for any given state are known, then the occurrence of a given phenomenon (illness, disability, use of service, etc.) in the state could be predicted by applying to the population of the state the relationships (between phenomenon and population characteristics) that have been determined from the national sample. Seven population characteristics are identified from the national sample and the scale of subclasses somewhat collapsed as follows: color (2 categories), sex (2), age (4), residence (3), family income (2), family size (2) and industry of head of family (2 categories). The seven characteristics and their subclasses produce 384 cross-classifications which are further collapsed into 84 cells. The national population and the occurrence of the phenomenon in each of these cells is obtained from the national sample data. Next, estimates need to be made of the state population for each of these 84 cells. In most cases such information becomes directly available only at each decennial census. For intercensal years an estimate can be made assuming that the population in each of the 84 cells has grown since the census at the same rate as the total population of the state has grown. (Estimates for state population growth are readily available.) Having arrived at an estimate of the number of persons in each cell in a given state, the next step is to apply the rate of occurrence of the phenomenon in each cell of the national matrix to the corresponding cell in the state matrix. The sum of all the cells in the state matrix gives the occurrence of the phenomenon in the state's population. The uses and limitations of this method and other variants that were tested are described in the original publication (86). The national estimates are unbiased and have a specifiable sampling variation. The ''synthetic estimates'' are neither one nor the other. ''Yet the rationale behind the model is plausible. Further, several tests of consistency and comparisons of results obtained by alternative methods suggest that these state figures do have merit, even though they are but provisional approximations. Lacking superior evidence, they should be useful'' (86, p. 2). Tentative confirmation of this expectation comes from a study in a semirural county in central Virginia. Here, data on use of physicians' services obtained from a household interview survey were compared with synthetic estimates obtained from national data by adjusting for the age composition and the urban-rural characteristics of the population of the county. The figures obtained by the two methods appeared to be similar, though no precise test of comparability was used. Further studies of this kind are required before one is assured that the agreement in this instance was not the fortuitous result of similarities between the other characteristics of the county and national samples or of interactions among the characteristics of the county. In this context, one might reemphasize that synthetic estimates become possible and attractive only when the relevant characteristics of the target population are already known or can be estimated with reasonable accuracy. If it is necessary to conduct a survey in order to find out what these characteristics are, one might decide to invest the additional effort needed to obtain directly the morbidity and use data which are being sought. Further, it is interesting to note that the characteristics of the national sample that are used to construct the synthetic estimates do not include the supply of personnel and health resources which are known to influence use of service, if not levels of disability. It is likely, however, that residence and family income, which are included, are so highly related to resource supply that they can be used as a substitute for the latter.

Omissions from the sampling frame also introduce significant limitations in the National Health Survey. The sample (1) is confined to the civilian population; (2) excludes persons in institutions, such as hospitals and nursing homes; and (3) excludes persons who have died since the survey period. The exclusion of the noncivilian population may be justified on the grounds that medical care services for them are provided by an autonomous and "closed" system that has little relevance to the general provision of medical care. On the other hand, the exclusion of persons in institutions and of the deceased results in significant underreporting, since such persons are more often ill and use more service. The degree of underreporting is not equal for all population subgroups, since death and institutionalization are significantly related to age, sex, and socioeconomic class. For example, inclusion of decedents has brought about 9 percent increase in reported discharges and about 14 percent increase in nights of care in general hospitals. The age bias is shown in Table III.3. Increments for males were higher than those for females in each age group, reflecting the higher mortality rate of the former (90). In addition to studies such as the above, which attempt to determine the degree and direction of error in Survey reports, the National Health Survey has introduced two components that supplement the picture obtained from the household interview. These are the surveys of institutions and the survey of hospital discharges.

Having considered the manner in which definitions and sampling

Table III.3.   Percent increase in hospital care, by age group, reported to the U.S. Household Interview Survey, brought about by including household members who have died since the period covered by the survey. Middle Atlantic States, 1957

Age	Percent Increase in Reported Nights of Care
0–44	3
45–64	15
65 plus	42

SOURCE: Reference 90.

influence the meaning and relevance of the household interview survey, we continue with the additional issues of *reporting* and *"validity."* The issue of "validity" arises largely from the dual perspectives of the client and the professional, and the obvious dependence of the interview survey on the first of the two. Since the term "validity" implies that the professional findings are always superior to the respondent's reports, it might be preferable, and certainly more neutral, to speak of "comparability." The ability and willingness to report depends to a large extent on the respondent's view of the phenomena in question; hence the two issues of reporting and of comparability will be considered together. First, we shall present some findings of comparisons between interview findings and other, more provider-oriented, methods of obtaining information. Then we shall briefly present some of what is known about the factors that influence reporting and consequently comparability. Finally, we shall speculate about the relevance of interview data to health planning in the light of what has been presented concerning their congruence or incongruence with the professional view of morbidity.

A number of studies provide comparisons between the *findings* of interview surveys on the one hand, and clinical examinations, physician reports, or clinical records on the other. The following brief review is intended to be illustrative rather than exhaustive.

Perhaps the most complete comparisons have been made in studies sponsored by the Commission on Chronic Illness. In the sample of an urban population, drawn in Baltimore, a case-by-case comparison was made between interview reports and conditions found on clinical examination. Of conditions found at clinical examination, and which were considered to have been also present at the time of the household interview, only 30 percent were reported by household respondents (95, p.

306). In the rural component of the studies sponsored by the Commission, carried out in Huntington County, N.J., Trussell et al. compared a wider set of alternative methods for collecting morbidity information. These included self-administered questionnaires, household interviews, reporting by the respondent's physician, findings on special clinical examination, and multiple screening (96). Comparisons of household interview reports and clinical findings were as follows: Of conditions reported by the respondents, 47 percent were matched by the clinical examination. Of conditions found by clinical examination, 22 percent were matched by household interview. The comparison included only conditions that the doctors felt were present at the time of the interview and should have been reported. An interesting, if somewhat comical, instance of the discrepancy between the report of a respondent and the findings of a physician is quoted by Sanders (93). It concerns self-reports of circumcised status and the findings of a physician as shown in

Table III.4. Percent distribution of males by circumcision status as reported and as found by an examining physician. Roswell Park Memorial Institute, Buffalo, New York, 1958

Report by Respondent	Finding by Physician		Total
	Yes	No	
Yes	19%	10%	29%
No	25%	46%	71%
TOTAL	44%	56%	100%

SOURCE: Reference 93.

Table III.4. There was agreement in only 65 percent of cases. Such ignorance about an object of considerable solicitude is difficult to believe!

It is clear from the above that the levels of agreement between household interview reports and clinical examination findings is very low. Trussell et al. (96) also tested the relationship between household interview findings and reports by the family physician. In one half of the cases the physician was informed by the researchers of what the household interview had shown, and in the other half he was not. The degree of agreement was as shown in Table III.5. Table III.6 shows the relationships for mutually exclusive categories for comparisons in which the physician was not informed of what the patient had reported.

In addition to the comparisons described above (interview versus clinical findings, and interview versus physician's report) several studies

Table III.5.   Proportion of conditions reported in a household interview survey which were also reported by the respondents' family physicians, according to whether the physicians were or were not informed of the interview report. Hunterdon County, New Jersey, 1951–1952

Extent of Agreement Between Physician and Household Interview Reports	M.D. Informed of Interview Diagnosis (percent)	M.D. Not Informed of Interview Diagnosis (percent)
Perfect agreement	56	46
Some agreement (including "perfect," "close," "general," "vague," or "remote")	92	75
Reported by patient only	8	25
New conditions reported by physician only	22/100 conditions reported by the patient	48/100 conditions reported by the patient

SOURCE: Reference 96.

have been done comparing clinical records and interview reports. Two such studies have been conducted under the auspices of the National Center for Health Statistics. One was conducted at the Health Insurance Plan of Greater New York (HIP) and involved a comparison between

Table III.6.   Number and percent distribution of conditions as reported by respondents and by their family physicians. Hunterdon County, New Jersey, 1951–1952

Patient Report	Physician Report		Total
	Yes	No	
Yes	441 (50%)	145 (17%)	586
No	292 (33%)	—	292
TOTAL	733	145	878 (100%)

SOURCE: Reference 96.

the regular, routine reports of the HIP physicians and the findings of the usual type of NHS interview survey (97). The second was done at Kaiser-Permanente (K-P) and involved comparisons of physician entries on a specially designed form with reports using several variants or modifications of the National Health Survey interview forms (98). For selected conditions, only 32 percent of conditions on the record were matched by interview reports in the HIP study. In the K-P study only 37 percent of conditions in the record were accurately matched by reported conditions, but some degree of matching was obtained for 55 percent of recorded conditions. The effect of a variety of factors on the degree of matching obtained in both the HIP and the K-P studies will be described below.

A constant finding in studies such as the above is that the extent of agreement between respondent reports and clinical sources varies strikingly by diagnosis or type of condition. This is clearly shown in Fig. III.9, which is based on data compiled by Sanders from the findings of the Commission on Chronic Illness. Assuming the clinical findings to be the criterion of validity, the figure shows, for each diagnosis, the relative magnitudes of "false positives" and "false negatives." The "true" prevalence of each condition (not shown in the figure) is the sum of the conditions found on clinical examination only (open columns) and those found or reported in both clinical examination and interview survey (striped columns). In the study by Trussell et al., the ratio "number found by clinical examination"/"number reported by respondent"

Fig. III.9.   Prevalence of selected chronic conditions determined by clinical evaluation and by household survey (Baltimore, 1953–1955)

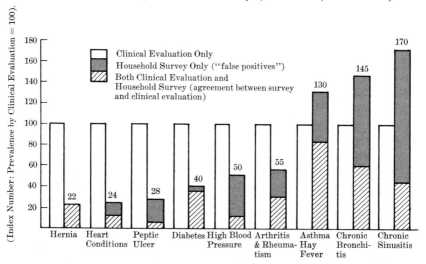

SOURCE: Data from the study by the Commission on Chronic Illness, assembled and analyzed by Barkev Sanders in reference 93.

ranged from 98–13 percent, by condition. The ratio "number reported by respondent" / "number found by clinical examination" ranged from 4–64 percent. Table III.7 shows the findings derived from a comparison

Table III.7.   Proportion of chronic conditions and services inferred from reports of physicians that were also reported by respondents in a household interview, according to specific diagnosis or diagnostic category and type of service. Subscribers of the Health Insurance Plan of Greater New York (New York, 1957)

Type of Condition or Service	Percent of Condition or Services Reported in Interview
Hay fever	79
Asthma[a]	71
Diseases of the gall bladder[a]	67
Bronchitis[b]	65
Diabetes[a]	62
Heart disease[a]	60
Ulcer of stomach and duodenum[a]	60
Back conditions[b]	56
Diseases of the kidney and ureter[a]	54
Hernia[b]	54
Sinusitis[b]	48
Hypertension without heart involvement[a]	46
Impaired hearing[b]	41
Diseases of the prostate[a]	38
Impaired vision[b]	33
Arthritis and rheumatism[a]	33
Malignant neoplasm[a]	33
Congenital malformations[a]	28
Mental illness[a]	26
Menstrual disorders	25
Benign and unspecified neoplasms[a]	21
Anemia	18
Obesity	10
Physician contacts during previous 2 weeks	64
Hospitalization during the previous year	87

SOURCE: Reference 97.

[a] Conditions specifically mentioned in the check lists used for interviewing.

[b] Conditions specifically mentioned in check list but with modifying qualifications (such as "chronic," "repeated," "serious," which the respondent must evaluate).

of interviews with Health Insurance Plan records. There is no completely satisfactory explanation for these differences. Sanders suggests that "medically diagnosed" conditions such as heart disease, hypertension, diabetes, and hernia, are under-reported in the health interview survey; whereas conditions based on self-diagnosis, such as sinusitis, hay fever, asthma, and chronic bronchitis, are more likely to be over-reported (93). The impact of the condition on the respondent and the social or psychological threat associated with it may also be factors. But these speculations lead to a more general discussion of the factors that influence reporting and comparability.

The following is a classification and listing of the *factors* that are thought to influence reporting and comparability. The classification incorporates the notion of ''saliency'' proposed as an analytic category perhaps most unambiguously by Mechanic and Newton (101).

1. Saliency of the morbid condition
    a. Self-response versus other-response
    b. Time elapsed since event
    c. Pain and discomfort
    d. Interference with activities or life style
    e. Receipt of medicine
    f. Medical care, number of visits to physician, length of hospital stay
    g. Communication with physician
2. Social or physical threat of the morbid condition
3. Respondent characteristics
    a. Demographic
    b. Socioeconomic
    c. Other
4. Interviewer characteristics
    a. Demographic
    b. Socioeconomic
    c. Other
5. Questionnaire design and interview techniques

Mechanic and Newton have suggested that several factors known to influence the completeness of interview data may be grouped under the heading of *saliency*. It is generally observed, for example, that respondents report more conditions for themselves than they do for other adults (see, for example, Table III.8). This may be largely a matter of knowing more about oneself than about others, especially where health matters are concerned. That there may be other factors as well, is suggested by the observation that respondents in the first phase of the Health Examination Survey were more likely to commit themselves to such an examination than they were to commit others (195, p. 4). For these reasons, the Health Interview Survey requires that each adult at home at the time of the interview be interviewed for himself. If a particular adult is not at home information may be supplied by spouse, parent, or adult children. Information about younger children is to be supplied by a parent unless some other adult is usually responsible for the care of the child (88, p. 10). Since most respondents are likely to be housewives and unemployed or retired males, one might speculate about bias introduced into household surveys because of this response factor.

That reporting is dependent upon recall is self-evident. The longer the *interval* between the time of interview and the occurrence of an illness or the use of service, the less likely is the event to be reported. Findings concerning the reporting of hospital use will be reported below. Table III.8 gives data on the comparison between records and interview reports

Table III.8. Percent of chronic conditions inferred from the reports of physicians that were also reported by respondents in a household interview, according to method of eliciting information and various respondent characteristics. Subscribers of the Health Insurance Plan of Greater New York, N.Y. 1957[a]

	Type of Chronic Condition[b]		
	Class I (Percent)	Class II (Percent)	Class III (Percent)
All services	44	28	20
By number of services per condition			
1 service	27	20	14
10+ services	88	56	56
By interval between last service and interview			
Two weeks or less	68	51	42
Four months or more	34	21	16
By identity of respondent			
Self respondent	48	36	21
Relatives	41	20	20
By age of person with the condition			
Under 15 years	36	17	18
65+ years	53	32	26

SOURCE: Reference 97.

[a] In this study the reporting of conditions was not related in a regular fashion to race, family income, education of the head of the household, or the number of conditions per person reported by the physician.

[b] "Type of Condition" refers to the manner in which the household interview elicits information about illness from the respondent. Both general questions and a checklist of specific conditions are used:

Class I: Specific condition in check list.
Class II: Condition listed in check list but the respondent given leeway in evaluating it as "chronic," "repeated," "serious impairment," etc.
Class III: Condition not listed in check list but elicited in response to questions on illness in general.

in the Health Insurance Plan study. The Kaiser-Permanente study provides an elegant demonstration of the influence of the recall period (Fig. III.10). This suggests a rapid decline over the first 40 days followed by a slow but steady deterioration thereafter. Mechanic and Newton refer to a report by Mooney that one-day recall produced monthly rates of morbidity that were four times those obtained by monthly recall. Mechanic and Newton also report very high rates of the reporting of symptoms based on a daily log kept by the mother for 15 days (101).

Other determinants of saliency are *pain,* or *discomfort,* and *interference* with activity or life style. The influence of such factors is well illustrated in the Kaiser-Permanente comparisons between reported and recorded conditions. Table III.9 gives some of the findings (98, Tables 30–35).

Trussell et al. have also reported that conditions that were characterized by some degree of seriousness ("keeping person from ordinary activities," "leaving a handicap or defect," "still bothering," or requiring medical attention or hospitalization) were more likely to be substantiated

Fig. III.10.   Percentage of conditions reported in medical records that were reported in interviews[a] by type of match and number of days since last visit to the physician. Southern California Kaiser Permanente Medical Group, 1960

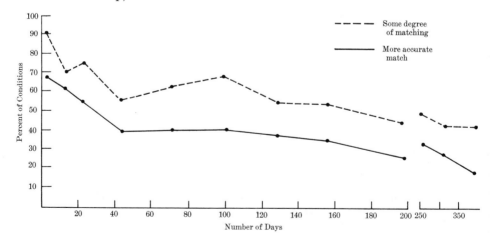

[a] Respondent reports for self only.
SOURCE: Reference 98.

Table III.9. Percent of conditions recorded by physicians which were matched, to specified degrees, by interview reports, according to specified behavioral consequences of the conditions. Southern California Kaiser-Permanente Medical Group, 1960

Consequences of Morbidity	Accurate Match (%)	Some Match (including accurate match) (%)
Has pain or discomfort		
Yes	47	66
No	32	48
Receiving medicine or treatment		
Yes	46	68
No	41	45
Ever had limitation of food or beverage		
Yes	43	61
No	31	44
Health problems source of worry		
Yes	51	71
No	35	51
Limitation of work or housework		
Yes	50	71
No	32	46

SOURCE: Reference 98.

by clinical examination if they had been previously reported on interview (96).

The receipt of *medical attention* and the intensity or duration of such care is another component of saliency. We have already noted that having received medicine or treatment appeared to improve comparability of reported and recorded conditions in the Kaiser-Permanente study. Conditions that require more visits to the physician are better reported. Analogously, hospitalization of longer duration is more likely to be reported. The relationship between number of visits to a physician and the degree and quality of reporting was noted in the HIP study (Table III.8), and also in the Kaiser-Permanente study as shown in Table III.10. Mechanic and Newton report the performance of surgery to be another factor in saliency under the general rubric of medical attention (101). The influence of medical attention is also postulated by Sanders,

Table III.10.   Percent of conditions recorded by physicians which were matched, to specified degrees, by interview reports, according to the number of visits to physicians made for each condition. Southern California Kaiser-Permanente Medical Group, 1960

Number of Visits	Accurate Match (Percent)	Some Match (including accurate match) (Percent)
1	27	44
2	39	53
3	45	65
4–5	56	74
6 and over	69	82

SOURCE: Reference 98.

who proposes that conditions likely to be self-diagnosed are more likely to be reported in excess of their prevalence as determined by clinical examination, and that conditions that are likely to be identified by physicians are under-reported in health interview surveys (93). A final factor in saliency that is also related to medical attention is the nature of the *communication* between physician and client. In addition to determining the nature of therapeutic regimen to be followed, and hence the potentially disruptive impact of that regimen, the physician may contribute to the impact and saliency of a condition by the manner in which he communicates with the patient. In the Kaiser-Permanente study, several questions dealt with the way in which the physician discussed the condition with the patient, and whether he stressed or played down the condition. "Analysis of responses to these questions in relation to the degree of under-reporting indicated that the greater the communication between patient and physician the smaller the percentage of conditions not reported" (98, p. 22).

A counterpart to saliency is the *social and psychological threat* posed by a disease, constituting, as it were, over-saliency. Such threat may actually inhibit reporting. One study of hospital admissions suggests that diagnoses such as syphilis, cancer of the breast, diseases of the male and female genital organs, and psychoneurotic disorders are considered to be threatening and less likely to be reported under certain circumstances (104). The study also showed that a set of factors, each of which has an adverse effect when present alone, can have an incrementally cumulative effect when present in combinations of two or three. Using short hospital stay, lengthy interval since discharge, and threatening illness as three factors adverse to reporting, it is possible to arrange them in such a manner as to demonstrate a reasonably scalar relationship to reporting, as shown in Table III.11.

Table III.11.   Percent of hospital stays that were not reported by respondents, according to number and nature of factors that characterize the hospital stay or the condition that caused it. U.S.A., 1958–1959

Number of Factors	Nature of Adverse Factors[a]	Percent Under-reporting
0	None	3
1	Threatening disease	0
	Short stay	7
	Long interval	17
2	Threatening plus short stay	7
	Threatening plus long interval	33
	Short stay plus long interval	27
3	Threatening plus short stay plus long interval	56

SOURCE: Reference 104, Table 4.

[a] Adverse factors are defined as length of hospital stay below 5 days, discharge from hospital 41–53 weeks prior to interview, and disease of a socially threatening or unacceptable nature.

Of the three factors, length of interval from discharge appears to be the most potent inhibitor of reporting. By contrast, the threatening property of disease alone, or in combination with short stay, has no or little effect. However, certain combinations, such as threatening illness with long interval, or all three factors present together, have a remarkably inhibiting effect on reporting.

The notions of saliency and threat are probably considerable over-simplifications of a complex process of selectivity in perception and reporting. Kosa et al., for example, describe the complicated manner in which mothers asked to keep a "calendar" of family health events, used judgment to report or not report ("censor") seemingly similar health events depending on their relevance or significance as viewed within particular contexts—season of the year or age of child, for example (102). Kahn and Cannell provide a more complete model, derived from social-psychological theory, of the variables related to the accuracy of reporting in interview surveys. The model regards the interview as an interaction between interviewer and respondent in which each influences the other and to which each participant brings his own attitudes, expectations, motives, and perceptions (107, p. 3; and 106). The similarity to the patient-physician relationship is striking. It is to be expected, therefore, that completeness and selectivity in reporting will be influenced by respondent characteristics, interviewer characteristics and the manner in which the interview situation is set up.

The findings concerning the influence of *respondent characteristics* are not consistent. Where demographic characteristics are concerned, the comparison of reported and recorded conditions in the Health Insurance Plan of New York showed that reporting was more complete for persons 65 and over than for persons under 15 years of age (Table III.8). On the other hand, a similar study at Kaiser-Permanente concluded that "generally speaking, the differences in reporting of chronic conditions by demographic characteristics were relatively small and seemed to be related to the seriousness of the condition" (98, p. 21). Since socioeconomic characteristics are an important determinant of need and unmet need, it is especially important to know whether bias in reporting illness and use of service is, or is not, associated with income, education, or employment. We have already referred to biases that may be introduced in health interview data, not due to reporting, but due to including in the definition of morbidity, components such as receipt of medical care or absence from work. We have also surmised that reporting by housewives for themselves and for employed adult family members will result in more complete reporting for the former and a relative underestimate for the latter. The findings of the Kaiser-Permanente study show no clear relationships between reporting and socioeconomic status. If anything, there may have been some tendency, with increasing education, to have fewer recorded conditions reported on interview. On the contrary, a study of underreporting of hospital episodes in the National Health Survey has shown that reporting becomes less complete as income decreases and as age increases, as shown in Tables III.12. and III.13. The

Table III.12.   Percent of hospital stays that were not reported by respondents to the U.S. Household Interview Survey, according to family income. 21 hospitals, April 1958 to March 1959

Income Group (in dollars)	Percent Underreporting
Under 2000	18
2000–3999	13
4000–6999	10
7000–9999	8
10,000 and over	8

SOURCE: Reference 105, Table 7, page 12.

study by Cannell et al. showed no significant correlation between education, family income, race or sex of the respondent and the amount of information obtained from the interview. Furthermore, "respondent feelings, level of information about the survey, motives, attitudes, and perceptions when measured the day after the interview are not directly related to health reporting behavior" (107, p. 5). In this study, however, there was no comparison of interview data with an external criterion. The index of performance was the number of chronic and acute conditions which the respondent reported for himself, corrected for the age of the respondent. One may conclude from all this that the precise relationships between respondent characteristics and reporting have not been established. In future studies it would be necessary to control for the factors of saliency and threat and also to look for the effects of definitional bias.

Table III.13.   Percent of hospital stays that were not reported by respondents to the U.S. Household Interview Survey, by age of person hospitalized. 21 hospitals, April 1958 to March 1959

Age	Percent Underreporting	
	All Episodes	Excluding Delivery
18–34	8	12
35–54	10	11
55–64	13	13
65–74	18	18
75 and over	14	14
All ages	10	12

SOURCE: Reference 105, Table 3, page 9.

That interviewers differ in performance, and that *interviewer characteristics* bias information elicited from respondents, has been known for a long time. Cannell et al. give a brief review (107, pp. 1–2). Consequently, a great deal of emphasis has been placed on the adequate training and supervision of interviewers and standardization of the interviewing schedules and procedures themselves. "There is no question but that better training of interviewers results in more accurate data, but even now not too much is known about factors underlying and leading to inaccurate reporting, although speculation abounds" (107, p. 2). Colombotos et al. (108) point out that the majority of interviewers in most surveys, including the National Health Survey, are women. They review opinions concerning possible effects of this factor, having in mind both the sex of the respondent (usually a housewife) and the nature of the information sought (whether regarded to be woman's province, such as health, or matters spoken of mainly among men, such as alcoholism, antisocial behavior, or sex). The study by Colombotos et al. showed that the sex of the interviewer did not influence significantly the amount of information about symptoms that have a psychiatric connotation.

A question that frequently comes up is whether, for certain kinds of data, including health, professional interviewers might not be more suitable. In considering this question, Sanders (93) refers to a study in which a comparison was made between conditions reported to lay interviewers and those reported to a physician, using the same check list of diseases during the examination of the same persons. Table III.14 shows

Table III.14.   Percent distribution of conditions by whether they were reported to a physician, lay interviewer or both, according to type of respondent. Nashville, Tennessee, 1959

| Condition Reported to | | Type of Respondent | | |
| | | All (Percent) | Woman Reporting for Self (Percent) | Mother Reporting for Child (Percent) |
Interviewer	Physician			
Yes	Yes	34	38	26
Yes	No	10	6	15
No	Yes	57	55	59
All conditions		100	100	100

SOURCE: Reference 93.

the percentage distribution of conditions by type of respondent and by person to whom the condition was reported. The conclusion is that very large amounts of information were simply not passed along to the lay interviewer. Contrary to the above, a study by the National Health Survey led to the conclusion that there was no advantage to using nurses in preference to lay interviewers. There was no indication that nurses, whether in or out of uniform, obtained higher frequencies in the four most frequent symptoms: joint stiffness, joint pain, joint swelling, and backaches. Similarly, when all symptoms were grouped into four categories, nurses again did not obtain more symptoms and may have obtained fewer. There was also no evidence that nurses elicited more reports of illness. In fact, nurses were more difficult to train and have accept the limited objectives of the study and to refrain from interpreting patient reports. The conclusion was that "for this type of interview, training in interviewing technique, particularly in probing for complete responses, is more important than medical training" (97, p. 19). The position of the National Health Survey has been summarized as follows:

In obtaining answers to certain questions specified by the questionnaire, the interviewer performs a function that is simply one of reporting what she hears. This function does not include any element of interpretation. For this reason, lay interviewers are generally preferred to medically trained interviewers, despite the nature of some of the information that is being handled. A person with a medical education is trained to interpret what the patient says, and this interpretation is difficult to standardize for statistical purposes (88, p. 11).

Cannell et al. broadened the scope of inquiry to include psychosocial characteristics that theory would predict to be relevant. Similar to the negative findings already reported for respondents, it was found that "interviewer attitudes, preferences, styles of interviewing, or expectations as measured here are not related to the reporting of conditions she obtained from her respondents" (107, p. 5). Only one factor appeared to influence the extent of reporting as measured in this study: the "amount of behavior" exhibited during the interview. Reporting was significantly better in those interviews during which both interviewer and respondent laughed and joked and talked a great deal, whether in pursuing the prescribed procedures of the interview or indulging in somewhat "unrelated" talk about the respondent and her family. This study may be of more general interest to the reader because the theoretical formulation, the methods used to observe and record interactions during the interview, the surprising findings and the new hypotheses that were prompted by these findings, all appear to be so germane to certain problematic aspects of the patient-physician relationship.

A final category of factors that influence reporting is subsumed under the heading of *questionnaire design and interview technique*. Considerable attention has been given to devising sets of questions that thoroughly explore each item concerning which information is sought, to the precise wording of questions so as to avoid misunderstanding or the introduction of bias, to the order of questions, and to the manner in which further probing is to be done. It is important to devise "a standard instrument to be applied in a standard manner" (107, p. 1). The formulation of questions, the construction of questionnaires, and the standardization of the procedures for obtaining information are, in fact, matters that require considerable expertise which the medical care administrator ordinarily does not possess. He would be advised, therefore, to seek proper help in anything beyond the simplest studies.

Several studies have examined the comparability of information obtained by variants of survey procedures. One such variant concerns the manner in which information about disease is elicited. In one comparison of interview reports with Health Insurance Plan records (97) three methods of eliciting disease information were used, each of which turned out to have a different level of comparability to the recorded information. The findings, which are summarized in Table III.15 may also reflect

Table III.15.　Percent of chronic conditions inferred from records of physicians that were reported to interviewers, according to the method used by the interviewer to obtain information from respondents. Subscribers of the Health Insurance Plan of Greater New York, 1957

Method of Obtaining Information	Percent of conditions on Record Reported by Interview
Specific condition in the check list	44
Condition listed in check list, but the respondent has leeway in evaluating it as "chronic," "repeated," "serious impairment," etc.	28
Condition not listed in check list but elicited in response to questions on illness in general	20

SOURCE: Reference 97.

differences in the conditions themselves, or the manner in which they are perceived.

In a similar study at Kaiser-Permanente, three versions of the questionnaire were tested. Here, "the main effect of differences among questionnaires seems to be not whether a condition in the medical records is reported in interview but where it is reported" (98, p. 21).

Other studies, conducted under the auspices of the National Health Survey, have attempted to compare the findings of self-administered questionnaires with those obtained using the usual Health Survey interview forms and specified modifications of these forms. In one study of the reporting of hospital episodes it was shown that there was underreporting by about 10 percent; in addition, about 7 percent of discharges were not reported because of the exclusion of decedents (105). Interestingly enough, a second interview with the same person was found to reduce underreporting to a mere 5 percent. This prompted the trial of three ways of obtaining information, with the results (109) shown in Table III.16.

Table III.16.   Percent of hospital stays that were not reported to interviewers, according to the procedure used to obtain information from respondents. Detroit, 1960–1961

Procedure	Percent Underreporting
The usual Health Interview Survey method	17
A revised interview schedule followed by a mail form in which any information about hospital stays that had been overlooked in the interview was to be recorded by the respondent and mailed in.	9
No questions about hospitalization in the interview; the requested information was to be entered on a self-administered form which was given to the respondent by the interviewer at the close of the interview.	16

SOURCE: Reference 109.

Still another study compared the information obtained by a "closed" interview form and that obtained using an "open" interview form; and between a "closed" interview form and a similar form used as a questionnaire to be filled by the respondent ("self-administered") (110). The distinction between open and closed questions is illustrated below:

Closed question: Did you have measles when you were a child? Yes_____,
        No_____.
Open question: What illnesses or diseases did you have when you were a child?
        (list)_____.

Comparing interviews using the open form with those using the closed form the findings were as follows: The open form yielded a considerably smaller volume of symptoms, but the symptoms reported were more bothersome. However, the more bothersome conditions—athlete's foot, for example—may not be as significant as some less bothersome conditions, such as early heart disease. Although the open form elicited fewer conditions, it had the advantage of reporting conditions not asked for in the closed form. The number of symptoms or illnesses reported in response to open questions was related to the respondent's self-perception as healthy or unhealthy. Those who regarded themselves as unhealthy reported more fully (using the yield from the closed form as the criterion). Comparing the yield from a closed form used for the interview with the same form used as a self-administered questionnaire, the findings were as follows. The volume of reporting appeared to be comparable. However, neither method could be considered to elicit a complete report, since items reported upon interview were sometimes not reported by self-questionnaire, and the reverse was also true. The interview was perhaps a little better in obtaining information on childhood conditions. Agreement between the two methods was better when the symptom was bothersome than when it was not. The conclusion is that the self-administered form can be used for eliciting adult symptoms and illness with accuracy equal to the interview.

Finally, we need to consider the *use of household interview data in medical care administration*, having regard to the many limitations which these data seem to have. We have already emphasized that the sampling scheme in the household interview portion of the National Health Survey by excluding decedents and institutional residents produces underestimates and introduces biases at least by age and sex. Furthermore the national scope of the survey makes it difficult to use the data without considerable uncertainty even after adjustments for local characteristics have been made. We have also discussed the biases that might be introduced by definitions which incorporate the receipt of medical care and staying away from work as components of the concept of reporting morbidity. Reporting may also be biased by a number of factors, including socioeconomic status and prior receipt of medical care. The prior receipt of medical care, which is related to socioeconomic status, is therefore not only part of the definition of "acute conditions" but also influences the amount and nature of information that the respondent has about his illness and how much of this he will report. Accordingly, Mechanic has suggested that health interview data are largely measures of the propensity to seek care (101). Since the absence of care, and poor communication between patient and physician, lead to underdefining and underreporting of morbidity, one may wonder to what extent the absence of care in itself may create a false picture of an absence of need for care.

It is clear, from all the evidence, that health interview data cannot show the diagnostic picture of illness in a population, nor should they be expected to do so. The interview survey presents disease as seen by the client, influenced, it is true, by prior experience of professional care. In terms of our model, it measures "felt need" rather than "detectable need." Feldman regards the essential distinction to be "phenotypical" as compared to "genotypical" reporting (92). There remains a question, nevertheless, about the scale along which the interview survey measures morbidity. Woolsey, speaking no doubt for the National Health Survey, has addressed himself to this question (89). The earlier notion was that morbidity was being measured along a "scale of awareness." Subsequent studies led to the view that what was being measured is a "scale of impact of the morbidity on the affected individual and his family."

It can be argued that in reflecting client views of morbidity, the health interview survey brings a unique and significant contribution to health planning. After all, health behavior is more likely to be influenced by subjective perceptions of health than by more "objective" criteria. For many purposes diagnostic categorization is not needed; an estimate in terms of symptoms and disabilities is sufficient, if not preferable.

Continuous Local, or Partial, Survey. Continuous local, or partial, surveys are simply one variant of national surveys, differing little in purpose or method. They do, however, permit adaptation to particular needs and, as breadth of coverage is restricted, make possible more intensive exploration of specific problems. Thus, local surveys may be indicated (a) in lieu of a national health survey, (b) as a supplement to such surveys, (c) for local community planning, and (d) for program planning and evaluation. Some aspects of these various uses will be discussed below.

Logan has discussed limitations in the usefulness of broadside national surveys for national health planning. He has pointed out that although many countries have initiated such surveys, only the United States has mounted such a survey on a continuing basis. In all other instances the survey has been discontinued. Logan favors, instead of a national survey, the use of repeated samplings of special population groups with a view to obtaining more detailed information for some particular purpose. This he considers more useful and less costly than the continuing accumulation of rather routine, and somewhat superficial, information. In any event, such special studies of subsamples adds to the usefulness of the routine national survey, if such a survey exists (210).

Some localities have found it necessary and useful to institute a local continuing survey, partly because the National Health Survey provides little useful information for units smaller than regions or major standard metropolitan areas. Tayback and Frazier have described such a survey in Baltimore. Each month a sample of about 100 households is drawn from a city directory. Information is obtained by public health nurses using a standard questionnaire to which are added special sections as dictated by the need for special information. The nursing workload is about one completed questionnaire per nurse per month. The cost is about $10,000 per year for 1,000 families ($10 per family). At the time of reporting, data collected included demographic and socioeconomic variables, inoculation status of children, the occurrence of respiratory diseases, and attitudes and practices relevant to health and health care. For medical care planning, other types of information could be added. This would include additional measures of need, unmet need, use of service, type and location of services used, etc. Data obtained from the household interview could be supplemented by data from hospital records, health insurance records, and other sources. The continuous monitoring of health and of health care activities on a local community basis is a feasible operation (128).

The continuous survey may be geared not to a geographic locality or community but to the beneficiaries of a specific program. Obviously, policy-making and administration in any program should rest on data concerning the operations and consequences of the program. For this purpose systems of reporting and data collection are set up. In certain situations, the formal data-reporting system is so cumbersome and slow that complete results are not available until a long time has elapsed. There may be need for faster feedback. Moreover, the reporting system may lack information on certain important items. A situation such as this prevailed in the Medicare program, leading to the institution of a continuous survey of Medicare beneficiaries (129). The sample is drawn from the 5 percent statistical sample of those enrolled in SMBI (Part B). It consists of 3,800 persons who will remain in the sample for 15 months (the period of time during which expenditures for covered services may be accrued to meet the $50 deductible), and of a small increment drawn to include persons "aging in" who are added to the sample each month. Personal interviews, utilizing a questionnaire and a diary form, are conducted by the Bureau of the Census for the Social Security Administration. The questionnaire and diary form are designed to obtain the following information: "name and address of respondent, date and place of doctor visits, type of physician, condition treated, and other medical services received, including covered medical services received in the hospital and nursing home, as well as X-rays, medical tests, ambulance services, and the like. Also included are questions relating to the total amount of the bill, the portion covered by the program, and the source of payment. Where no information on charges is available, an estimating procedure was established that is based on the assumption that charges will be the same for similar services rendered in the same area. Special efforts are made to obtain data for persons in the sample who died during the survey month.''

Symptom Survey. The "symptom" survey refers to a class of investigations in which the emphasis is on the occurrence and handling of specified indicators of need, which are usually symptoms experienced subjectively by the respondent, but may also be other concrete manifestations of illness which can be observed by others as well as by the respondents (technically designated as "signs" rather than "symptoms"). The symptom survey is usually a component or variant of the household interview survey. It has been executed and used in a number of ways. First, the incidence and prevalence of symptoms is elicited as some indicator of health status and need for care. Second, the respondent may be asked, for each symptom, whether care was received, how promptly care was sought, and what was the nature of the care received. From answers to these and similar questions inferences are drawn concerning the manner in which the respondent interprets symptoms, the degree of desire for health services and whether there are obstacles to the receipt of care and what these might be, and, ultimately, how much need for care remains unmet. A variant of the symptom survey is not to ask about symptoms actually experienced but to pose a hypothetical situation. The respondent is presented with a list of symptoms and asked, for each symptom, whether the respondent would seek care if that symptom were present. The object is to explore perceptions of illness rather than the actual operation of the medical care system, although, as we have said, the two are not unrelated.

It may be useful to review briefly the history of the symptom survey and some of what is known about its "validity" or comparability to clinically based estimates of need.

In their classic study on "The Fundamentals of Good Medical Care," Lee and Jones offer a list of symptoms for which, in their opinion medical attention should be sought. These are grouped into two categories: one of "sudden," and another of "chronic, persistent, or slowly developing departures from the normal of physical and mental well-being." Fourteen symptoms are listed under the first heading and 16 under the second (276, p. 28). Although this is the earliest such formulation known to the author, it does not appear to have influenced the development of the symptom list as a survey tool.

The symptom survey method appears to have been originated by

Schuler in the Bureau of Agricultural Economics during 1944 in response to the need for a simple technique to measure unmet need that could be used by lay interviewers. The questions were adapted from those used in a relatively standard clinical history (111). Each symptom was considered to be "a danger signal . . . which required the attention of a physician" (113). Lack of receipt of such care was considered to be unmet need. The symptoms selected included: running ears (watery, bloody, pus), unexplained nose bleeds (repeated), persistent pains in the chest, repeated vomiting, and hernia (rupture) or wearing of a truss. The list eventually included 22 items (113). Lay interviewers collected information relevant to the preceding six months. Housewives reported for themselves and for other members of the family. Two kinds of validation studies were done: first, comparison of the reports obtained by the lay interviewer with those obtained by a physician and, second, comparisons of determinations of unmet need based on the questionnaire survey with those based on clinical examination.

The first approach to validation was the comparison of the reports to the lay interviewer with the information elicited by a physician who also questioned each respondent. However, the physician did more than repeat the lay enumerator's approach. He actually used judgment in accepting or rejecting as "medically significant" the symptom elicited. Physician and lay interviewer findings were compared in two ways: (1) agreement on whether individuals were classified as those who had need or did not have need, and (2) agreement on the extent of unmet need. The degree of agreement on the present of need is shown in Table III.17. Agreement was obtained in 79 percent of respondents. However, the test was not a stringent one. Need was presumed to be present if the respondent reported one or more symptoms during any part of the study

Table III.17.   Distribution of persons by whether need for medical care was or was not present as judged by the presence of symptoms elicited by a lay interviewer and the presence and significance of symptoms as elicited by a physician. Warren County, North Carolina, 1945

Evaluation by Lay Interviewer	Evaluation by Physician Interviewer		Total
	Need Present	No Need	
Need Present	106	26	132
No Need	12	38	50
TOTAL	118	64	182

SOURCE: Reference 111.

period, and to be absent if none of the symptoms were reported. As the author understands it, there was not symptom-by-symptom matching in the lay interviewer–physician comparisons. In exploring the degree of agreement on unmet need, three categories of unmet need were set up (111) :

Medical needs met : all symptoms received medical care.

Medical needs partly met : some symptoms received care, others not.

Medical needs unmet : none of the symptoms received care.

The point to be made is that the mere receipt of care was judged to satisfy the need; appropriateness of care and quality of care were not considered. More detailed categories were evolved for later studies. The findings on the degree of agreement with respect to unmet need are summarized in Table III.18.

The comparison between the symptom survey report and the clinical evaluation, using medical examinations and laboratory and x-ray examinations, revolved around the decision whether there was need to consult a

Table III.18. Distribution of persons by specified judgments concerning presence of need for medical care based on information concerning presence of symptoms and care these have received as elicited by lay interviewers, and this same information as elicited and evaluated by physicians. Warren County, North Carolina, August, 1945

Lay Interviewer Reports	Physician Judgments				
	No Medical Needs	Medical Needs Unmet	Medical Needs Partly Met	Medical Needs Met	Total
No Medical needs	37	10	0	2	49
Medical needs unmet	16	38	6	7	67
Medical needs partly met	2	5	18	3	28
Medical needs met	9	3	6	20	38
Totals	64	56	30	32	182

SOURCE: Reference 113.

physician (112). The conclusion was that there was 80 percent agreement on the need to consult a physician using the two approaches. This, again, seems to be a non-specific kind of basis for agreement, and may have been unduly inflated by the large percentage of persons who need medical care in any event. This becomes evident when a symptom-by-symptom comparison is made. Reports by, and examination of, 153 persons revealed 138 symptoms of which 50 percent were true positive reports, 21 percent were false positive reports, 10 percent were unreported false negatives, and 19 percent were indeterminate, being neither confirmed nor denied by medical examination. In addition to revealing 14 symptoms (10 percent of 138) which were included in the questionnaire and should have been reported, the medical examination found, as might have been expected, an additional 53 symptoms (an increment of 38 percent to the 138 symptoms) which could not have been reported since they were not part of the questionnaire. In spite of these discrepancies the authors conclude that if the object is simply to classify persons into those who need medical attention and those who do not, the symptom survey is a "reasonably reliable" instrument (112).

A recent report from the National Health Survey adds some information concerning the relationship between reports of symptoms and the occurrence of hypertension as diagnosed by the physical examination survey. It was found that the occurrence of symptoms presumed to be related to hypertension, alone or in combination, were not related to the diagnosis of hypertension. The symptoms studied were headaches, nosebleeds, tinnitus, dizziness, and fainting. The conclusion was that "clearly if one wishes to obtain information about hypertension by use of a questionnaire . . . symptom information is totally noncontributory" (116). This study, however, addresses itself to the validity of using the symptom survey in a manner very different from the one originally envisaged. What is tested is partly the reporting of symptoms and partly the basic, medically postulated association between specific symptoms and a particular disease. The symptoms enumerated may not be related to the presence of hypertension; nevertheless, physicians might agree that such symptoms merit clinical investigation.

It may be of interest to conclude the discussion on the symptom survey by summarizing the findings using this approach to the delineation of need and unmet need. The studies of Hoffer et al., in three communities in Michigan (114) revealed unmet need (all symptoms untreated or treated by home remedies only) as follows: 5 to 27 percent of persons in the town and 18 to 37 percent of persons in the adjacent countryside. Unmet need, defined as above, was more common in lower income groups, in open country as compared to the town, in families where the wife or female head had lower educational levels, where there had been no medical examination during the previous year, and where there was no family doctor (38 percent as compared to 19 percent where there was a family doctor). Koos, in his classic study of health and medical care in a rural community, posed the hypothetical question of what the respondent would do if he had each of a list of symptoms. The responses showed that symptoms differed from one another in the frequency with which they were considered to require medical attention and, more important, persons in a lower occupational class would very frequently neglect symptoms that persons in a higher class would not (4). Mechanic and Volkart have also used the device of posing hypothetical situations to assess what they have come to call the "inclination" to seek care. They found that the self-perceived inclination to seek care is positively related to the actual seeking of care and that it is influenced by social characteristics, such as religion, and by personality traits, such as nervousness and anxiety (120). By contrast, Rosenfeld et al. obtained information on the actual occurrence of symptoms and the actual receipt of medical care for these symptoms in the Boston Metropolitan Area (65). The presence of considerable "unmet need" was again documented. "Of persons who had one or more symptoms believed to require medical attention, only 43 percent had received medical care. In the lowest socioeconomic group (as determined by census tract of residence), 50 percent of persons with symptoms had one or more untreated symptoms. In the highest socioeconomic group, the proportion with one or more untreated symptoms was 30 percent" (214, p. 373). The lists of symptoms used by Koos and by Rosenfeld et al. are shown in Table III.19, which also shows some of the findings by social class. Viewing these findings together, one is tempted to speculate about the differences between how people say they will behave, and how in fact thy do behave in response to symptoms. Cartwright was able to make such comparisons in a study of twelve areas in England and Wales. Persons who had actually experienced a given symptom or condition during the previous twelve months were less likely to have consulted a physician than would be expected from the responses to the hypothetical question by all persons in the sample (115, pp. 35–37).

More recently, White et al. used the symptom survey as one component in an international study of medical care need and use. A novel feature was the formulation of two "symptom-condition" lists, one for adults and another for children (91, pp. 7, 62, 70). Experience was compared in three specified areas—one each in the United States, the United King-

Table III.19.   Percent of respondents who recognized specified symptoms as requiring medical attention and percent of respondents who received medical treatment for specified symptoms, by social class or socioeconomic status of respondents, upstate New York, 1954 and Metropolitan Boston, 1956

Symptoms	Percent Recognizing Symptom as Requiring Medical Attention		Percent Receiving Medical Treatment for Symptom	
	Class I[a]	Class II	Groups IV & V[a]	Groups I & II
Loss of appetite	57	20	78	68
Persistent backache	53	19	90	46
Continued coughing	80	23	57	61
Persistent joint and muscle pains	80	19	72	53
Blood in stool	98	60	58	42
Blood in urine	100	69	100	80
Excessive vaginal bleeding	92	54	—	—
Swelling of ankles	77	23	—	—
Loss of Weight	80	21	100	45
Bleeding of gums	79	20	—	—
Chronic fatigue	80	19	65	52
Shortness of breath	77	21	74	54
Persistent headaches	80	22	56	60
Fainting spells	80	33	82	56
Pain in chest	80	31	80	83
Lump in breast	94	44	—	—
Lump in abdomen	92	34	—	—

SOURCES: (1) Data on the recognition of symptoms: Reference 4.
          (2) Data on treatment by symptom: Reference 65.
[a] The "higher" of the two social classes or socioeconomic groupings.

dom, and Yugoslavia. The study area in Yugoslavia differed from the other two in having a higher occurrence of symptoms-conditions and lower frequency of care for those conditions. Furthermore, the likelihood of receiving care for symptoms or conditions was no less in the United States, than it was in the United Kingdom. To the authors "this suggests that the presence of a financial barrier to the use of medical care, sometimes associated with the fee-for-service system, was not an important deterrent." However, since the study area in the United States had a rather prosperous, predominantly white population, it might not be safe to generalize from this finding. Perhaps more interesting than the differences among study areas, was the great frequency of medically unattended conditions in all areas. Of all adults with one condition or more, 40–70 percent had not consulted a doctor within the previous 12-month period, and of all conditions in adults that caused "great discomfort,'' 80–90 percent had not occasioned a consultation with a physician during a two-week period (91, Table M, p. 18).

White et al. wonder whether the differences in the reporting of symptoms and conditions that they observed are not a reflection of cross-cultural differences in the perception of morbidity rather than in the occurrence of morbidity as medically defined. There is good reason to believe that such cultural differences exist (119, 121, 123). Andersen et al. recently used the symptom survey to determine whether the much higher use of physicians' services in the United States as compared to Sweden could be attributed to a greater sensitivity to symptoms and a correspondingly greater propensity to seek care for such symptoms in the United States. The question was posed in terms of the perceptions of illness rather than illness itself, because it was assumed that illness levels, as clinically defined, would be the same in the two countries. A list of 15 ''symptoms'' (124, p. 19) was used in an interview survey to obtain information from representative samples of the population aged 16 and over. It was found that, contrary to expectation, most symptoms were somewhat more frequently reported in Sweden than in the United States, and that the patterns of response to symptoms were rather similar in the two countries. The large difference in the use of physician services cannot, therefore, be attributed to differences in the initiation of care in response to symptoms, but arises through differences in the way symptoms are medically managed after contact with the doctor has been established. In Sweden, where economic barriers to the receipt of physician care have been reduced to a greater extent than in the United States, there were no regular associations between socioeconomic status and response to symptoms. By contrast, ''in the U.S. the proportion of persons seeing a doctor tended to increase as family income, education and occupational rank increased.'' More important, however, was the weak nature of the association. It appears that at the national level (but not necessarily at other levels) the economic barrier has ceased to have a powerful differential effect by socioeconomic status. In addition to its findings, this study should be of interest to the reader because it provides a concrete example of the importance of several factors that we have already described as having a possible influence on the validity of survey findings.

In addition to the studies cited above, information on the prevalence of symptoms has been reported by Hammond for a large group of men and women followed prospectively in order to determine the relationship between smoking and disease (117); and by Mabry for a rural population in Vermont (118). Johnson et al. have reported the frequency of chief presenting complaints of patients who saw a sample of New York internists (277, pp. 917–918). More recently, the National Center for Health Statistics has provided data on the incidence of symptoms that have been used as indicators of "psychological distress" (126).

Self-Administered Questionnaires: The Cornell Medical Index. This is an instrument devised by physicians at the Cornell Medical Center for use in clinical management which can also serve as a survey device under appropriate conditions. The following brief account of the Cornell Medical Index is based on the excellent review by Abramson (131).

The Cornell Medical Index consists of 195 simply worded questions which the respondent answers "Yes" or "No." The detailed structure is shown in Table III.20. There is a form for males and another for females,

Table III.20.   Components of the Cornell Medical Index

Code	Number of Questions	Area
A	9	eyes and ears
B	18	respiratory system
C	13	cardiovascular system
D	23	digestive tract
E	8	musculoskeletal system
F	7	skin
G	18	nervous system
H	11	genitourinary system
I	7	fatiguability
J	9	frequency of illness
K	15	miscellaneous illnesses
L	6	habits
M	12	inadequacy
N	6	depression
O	9	anxiety
P	6	sensitivity
Q	9	anger
R	9	tension

SOURCE: Reference 131.

the latter differing in only six questions regarding the genitourinary system. The questionnaire, which can be self-administered, is usually completed in 10–30 minutes. When used for clinical purposes, there is further detailed elucidation of positive symptoms reported by the respondent. There is close correspondence between responses to the questionnaire and data given to physicians in oral interviews.

The Cornell Medical Index may be put to two kinds of uses: (1) to diagnose specific disease and (2) to arrive at a more global assessment of somatic, emotional, or general health. When interpreted by skilled physicians, the Cornell Index can be remarkably useful in identifying diagnostic categories and even specific medical conditions; hence its value as a tool in clinical management. In one study, interpretations made on the basis of the reports in the questionnaires predicted successfully 94 percent of diagnostic categories subsequently substantiated by hospitalization, and specific medical conditions "in 87 percent of these areas." Such successful interpretation appears to be based on the recognition of constellations of symptoms. A simple item-by-item comparison with findings on clinical assessment does not appear to be useful. The translation of patterns of symptoms latent within the questionnaire into diagnoses can be made with some success by a computer. In one study the computer was given the symptom combinations corresponding to the clinical diagnoses in 5,929 consecutive clinically substantiated cases. Subsequently, the computer was able to use this information to arrive at the correct diagnosis in 45 percent of male cases with the 60 most common diseases. But the proportion of success varied from 20 percent in 14 diagnoses to 70 percent in 6 diagnoses. Broadman and his coworkers, continuing their work with the Cornell Medical Index, have developed what they call a Medical Data Index-Health Questionnaire (MDI) consisting of 150 self-administering "medical questions" the answers to which can be translated to probable or "presumptive" diagnoses by using a computer. The computer does this by matching the symptoms reported by each respondent with the symptoms of persons, comparable by age and sex, who were diagnosed as having any of 100 common diseases during several years of experience in the outpatient departments of the New York Hospital-Cornell Medical Center. A precise estimate of the frequency of false positives and false negatives could not be made from the data given, but the authors claim that the instrument "performed this task with a large proportion of correct assignments and a low incidence of false-positive assignments" (133, p. 825). Collen et al. have reported on the use of Cornell-type questionnaires in conjunction with laboratory tests to obtain data for computer diagnosis of disease, and have discussed the mathematical bases for such diagnosis (191).

Global evaluations of health pose somewhat different objectives. It appears that scores constructed from total responses, or responses in specified segments of the questionnaire, or from the scatter of "yes" responses throughout all sections, are useful indicators of the degree of general emotional disability, but not of specific psychiatric disorder. By contrast, total or sectional scores do not appear to be useful specific indicators of the degree of "somatic health." However, in various studies, total scores have shown correlations with certain health behaviors and assessments of general health including: the number of sick calls among army inductees, absence from work among factory employees, over-all functional capacity among the aged, and appraisals of general health by physicians. These correlations may be due to the large emotional component in health, a component that the Cornell Index reflects well.

Finally, some studies suggest that there may be cross-cultural and subcultural variations in the response to the questionnaire. For example, in Okinawa, "yes" responses seemed to indicate the extent of courtesy rather than the presence of neurosis. A study of healthy inductees in New Jersey showed that those of Italian and Jewish origin had higher scores than those of British, Irish, or German origin.

Health Records. Under this heading we shall group several sources of information that assemble health data on a routine basis mainly for legal and administrative purposes. The purpose for which the data are obtained dictates the nature of the data and distinguishes the category of "health records" from that of "clinical records," which are primarily intended as a tool for the management of patients. Health records include vital statistics, records of notification of illness, and case registers. All these are general in scope and may be designated as "public health records." To them we shall add the category of records, often more detailed, that are available for special population groups. Since the subject of health records is well covered in standard textbooks of biostatistics and epidemiology, only the briefest description will be attempted here.

Vital statistics include data on population size and composition, births, deaths, and expectation of life. Needless to say, the population size and characteristics serve as the base to which all data on mortality, morbidity, use of service and supply or resources are to be related. In evaluating vital data, one must consider aspects of definition, completeness, and validity. Detailed consideration of these aspects is included in the standard texts on biostatistics, demography and epidemiology, and will not be attempted here. In the United States reporting tends to be quite complete, except for stillbirths. However, this may not be the case in some other countries. Moreover, the definitions adopted elsewhere may not be the same as those used in the United States. Such differences must be carefully considered in all international comparisons.

Reports of death are the main source of information on *fatal morbid-*

ities which, in turn, have long been the stage in the spectrum of disease concerning which most information has been available. This imbalance has been substantially corrected, first by the Health Interview Survey and, more recently, by the survey of hospital discharges and by some other components of the National Health Survey. Nevertheless, fatal morbidities remain a major source for the diagnostic categorization of morbidity and a major consideration in the evaluation of need. Unfortunately, the use of death reports has serious limitations from a number of causes: (1) the lack of correspondence between mortality and morbidity, (2) inaccuracies in the determination of the causes of death, (3) problems in the classification of disease, and (4) the conventions governing the reporting of the causes of death. Each of these will be discussed briefly below.

The lack of correspondence between mortality and morbidity arises from differences in the course and severity of disease. Deaths partly reflect the frequency of a given disease and partly the likelihood of that disease causing death. Hence, diseases that occur frequently but are seldom fatal are very decidedly underweighted in mortality statistics. Inaccuracies in the clinical determination of the causes of death are simply one aspect of a larger problem: the accuracy of clinical diagnosis in general, which is at a much lower level than most laymen would suspect. Sanders has published an excellent general review of the problem (176). More specifically, there have been several reports of comparisons between clinical certificates of death and autopsy findings (144–149). The recent study by Heasman and Lipworth from Britain show that, if one judges by certificates prepared prior to autopsy, there was an underestimate by 16 percent for lung cancer and 38 percent for pulmonary tuberculosis; by contrast, there was an overestimate by 110 percent for pulmonary embolism, 43 percent for cerebral hemorrhage, 57 percent for infectious hepatitis, and 14 percent for cancer of the colon (148). The clinical assessment is not merely an underestimate or an overestimate, but is a distortion of the diagnostic picture as revealed by autopsy. There is a question, however, whether cases that go to autopsy are a fair representation of all deaths and of their certification. Accordingly, Moriyama et al. examined a 10 percent sample of death certificates filed during a three-month period in 1956 in Pennsylvania. Questionnaires were sent to the attending physicians requesting information concerning each case. On the basis of a review of this information by a staff internist, the causes of death reported were judged to have been "solidly established" in 43 percent, "reasonable" in 36 percent, "in doubt" in 10 percent, and "probably wrong" in 8 percent. The ratings varied considerably by diagnostic category, by age (poorer above 65), by sex (poorer in females), and by residence (poorer for rural residence). Of course, several questions could be raised about the methods of this study, including reservations about the quality of physician reports and the reliability of the judgments of one internist (149).

Other difficulties in interpreting data on fatal morbidities arise from the problems of disease classification (32). Diseases may be classified by known or presumed causation, by the nature of the basic pathological process, by the more obvious manifestations of disease, by the organs, organ systems, or parts of the body affected, and even by the age and sex of the patient. For certain purposes some of these criteria are more meaningful than others, so that it is difficult to select one criterion uniformly in preference to all others. Furthermore, any one ''cause'' may produce a variety of manifestations in more than one organ system and, contrariwise, any one type of manifestation may be produced by a variety of causes. This produces considerable overlap among categories, however classified. Added to this are the severe imperfections in our knowledge of the causes of disease and the interrelationships among their manifestations. This means that as knowledge progresses, the assumptions underlying a given classification may require modification. The result is that current classifications of disease are somewhat untidy, if not confused, and tend to be, in some parts, distinctly provisional.

The classification most frequently used is the *International Classification of Diseases, Injuries and Causes of Death* which is published by the World Health Organization and is now in its eighth decennial revision (154–156). The classification, first introduced in 1948, is a descendent of the *International List of Causes of Death* adopted by international conference in 1893. It is intended primarily for the statistical compilation of morbidity and mortality data. However, an adaptation of it has been developed, and is now generally recommended, for the diagnostic coding of clinical hospital records (154). The classification consists of 17 sections with 612 categories of diseases and causes of death plus 182 categories for external causes of injury and 187 categories for the nature of injury. Except for the dual coding of injuries, each category is intended to provide a unique location for each diagnostic variant, which is identified by a three-digit code. Some categories are further subdivided into a four-digit designation. Gaps in the numbering system allow the insertion of additional categories. The Classification also provides standard ways for grouping diseases. In addition to the 17 sections, there is an ''Intermediate List'' of 150 causes suitable for reports of mortality and morbidity; an ''Abbreviated List'' of 50 causes for the tabulation of mortality; and a "Special List" of 50 causes for the reporting of morbidity in a manner suitable for social security purposes. Other groupings can be constructed which will be both reproducible by, and intelligible to, others, provided the component code numbers in each category are specified.

The Classification is revised approximately once every ten years to take account of changes in medical knowledge and opinion. One consequence of this is that morbidity experience coded using one revision will not correspond in significant ways with the same experience coded using the other versions of the Classification. For example, the coding of the same deaths occurring in 1966 by both the 7th and 8th revisions of the Classification reveals that the 8th revision brings about a 60 percent reduction in the category of hypertensive heart disease, a 68 percent reduction in syphilis and its sequelae, a 55 percent increase in "other diseases of arteries, arterioles, and capillaries," and a 67 percent reduction in birth injuries (139). Comparisons among the other revisions have also revealed similar changes brought about partly by changes in definition and partly by changes in the conventions for reporting the cause of death* (140–143). This means that trends in morbidity cannot be studied without appropriate adjustments. This has obvious applicability to projections of need based on past experience and to evaluations of the long term impact of changes in the organization of health services.

Finally, difficulties in the interpretation of fatal morbidities arise from the conventions governing the reporting of the "cause of death." Fundamental to these conventions has been the notion that each death must be counted only once and hence assigned only one cause (152). Since many patients have more than one disease, and most deaths are caused by a concatenation of circumstances, the notion of the single cause is a fiction that itself has been a long time dying. Earlier, the practice was to circumvent reality by applying a system of arbitrary rules that assigned relative priorities as cause of death to various diagnoses irrespective of which was most responsible for the death in any particular instance. Beginning with 1940 in Great Britain, and with 1949 in the United States and elsewhere, a new system was adopted which essentially left to the attending physician the designation of the relationship between the diagnoses present at the time of death and the event of dying. To accomplish this, the physician was asked to list the immediate cause of death (A), the antecedent cause of death (B), and the underlying cause of death (C), in a manner that indicated that C produced B which, in turn, produced A. Provision was also made for the listing of

* See below.

one or more significant conditions that contributed to the death but were not related to the immediate cause A. Several consequences flow from this procedure. The first is the degree of its dependence on the accuracy and completeness with which physicians determine the proper sequence of causes. In 1950 it was estimated that in about one-fourth of medical certificates the reported sequence was internally inconsistent, so that arbitrary rules had to be substituted to select the underlying "cause of death" (152). The second consequence is that the death certificate contains a great deal of information that is not used. The extent of this loss may be judged from a study of a national sample of death certificates for which multiple diagnoses were coded (153). For the data year 1955, about three-fifths of certificates reported more than one diagnosis, with an average of 1.9 diagnosis per certificate. The selection of one cause only, discarded about one-half of the diagnostic information. Finally, the selection of only one cause not only discarded valuable information, but also introduced serious distortion into perceptions of the relative importance of the contribution of various diseases to mortality. In the 1955 study, more than nine-tenths of the diagnoses included in the category, arthritis other than rheumatoid, were discarded. Of 28,213 deaths in which cancer of the lung was mentioned in the death certificate, 27,133 were ascribed to lung cancer as the underlying cause; but of 48,855 cases of chronic respiratory disease mentioned in the death certificate, only 13,609 were assigned to chronic respiratory disease as the underlying cause. Of particular interest to medical care administration is the gross underestimate of deaths in which therapeutic misadventure and operative intervention play a part. In such cases, deaths are assigned to the underlying disease which occasioned treatment or surgery, unless no such disease is mentioned. In 1955 there was mention of 3,261 therapeutic misadventures of which only 617 were coded as the underlying cause of death. The selection process was also found to introduce bias in comparisons among population groups. For example, "72 percent of the diagnosis of hypertensive heart disease entered on certificates for nonwhite persons were selected as the underlying cause of death; the corresponding percentage for the white population was 59" (153, p. 405).

Moriyama and Dorn propose a solution to the problems caused by the selection of a single cause of death (153). They suggest that there be virtually complete coding of the diagnostic information on death certificates. The 1955 study indicates that the coding of up to 5 diagnoses will include 99 percent of diagnoses reported. Routinely, the following information should be tabulated: (1) For each diagnosis, (a) the number of death certificates in which the diagnosis is mentioned, (b) the number in which it is the underlying cause, (c) the number in which it is the contributory cause, and (d) the percent of total mentions in which it is designated as the underlying cause; (2) A tabulation of deaths not by single causes of death but by composite diagnoses made up of combinations of diagnoses that are frequently associated in the causation of death. While the concept of underlying cause needs to be retained, the contribution of other concurrent diagnoses also needs to be documented. Furthermore, there is interest not only in fatal morbidities, but in a broader picture of morbidity at the time of death. A larger segment of morbidity will thus come into view. But even then, it will be only a partial and distinctly nonrepresentative view of morbidity in the total population.

Records of Notification are another form of health record. Certain diseases, notably those that are communicable, are notifiable, so that information concerning their occurrence can be obtained from official records. However, notification is notoriously incomplete. Moreover, only a few diseases are notifiable; and those that have been traditionally notifiable, the infectious diseases, are becoming less and less important as a consideration in planning health services in the more developed countries. This is not to say that infectious diseases are not still important in most countries, and predominant in some.

One form of notification and record-keeping involves the maintenance of what are called *Registers*. The register attempts to keep a current record of all known cases of a given disease in a given population. Examples are registers for tuberculosis, cancer (157–159), mental illness (160), neurological disease (161), blindness (162), congenital malformation and other chronic diseases of children and adults (163, 164). The maintenance of registers involves considerable effort to ensure reporting, comparability of definitions and quality of diagnostic categorization, avoidance of duplication, removing of decedents from the register, etc. A fundamental property of the register is that it records only known cases and consequently reflects more clearly the epidemiology of health care than it does the epidemiology of disease itself. It also reflects any special efforts for case-finding, as well as the kinds of institutionalized leverage that can be exerted on reporting. Reporting by private physicians, for example, is less likely to be complete than reporting by school authorities. While such influences can be very disturbing to the epidemiologist, they may provide useful information to the health administrator interested in the organization of care and its impact. The age at which congenital malformations are first reported or the stage in the progression of cancer when it first comes under notice, may indicate something about the effectiveness of the medical care system. Even more could be learned if, in addition to the standard demographic data, there were more information about socioeconomic characteristics of patients and the history of care. Logan suggests that if a national or regional register cannot be maintained, the register might be introduced on a sample basis or replaced by occasional surveys in depth. He also proposes that registers be expanded to include phenomena other than diseases. He lists the following as examples of diseases and conditions that might lend themselves to this approach (210) :

Diseases	Cancer
	Diabetes
	Chronic iron deficiency anemia
	Obesity
	Certain occupational diseases
Disabilities	Blindness
	Handicapping conditions
	Congenital malformations
	Certain pregnancies likely to result in malformation
Social Problems	Aged couple living alone (crisis if one dies)
	Attempted suicide
	Repeated accidents

Information on health status and use of service may be available more readily, more reliably, or in greater detail from the *records of special population groups* (165–174). Where the group selected is also the beneficiary of health services in a relatively closed system of medical care, clinical records as well as the more skimpy health records or health statistics may be available. Suitable population groups include the following :

> Armed services inductees
> Members of the armed services
> Veterans
> Industrial or employee groups
> School children
> College students
> Clients of insurance agencies
> Members of prepaid group practice plans
> Beneficiaries of social security systems
> Beneficiaries of other public programs of health care

In interpreting information from any one of these groups, special allowance must be made for the particular demographic, socioeconomic, and other factors of selection that characterize the population, as well as for the characteristics of the particular mode of financing and other aspects of the system of health care to which they are subject. Such peculiarities can constitute an advantage as well as a drawback. For example, when it is desired to examine what may be the effect of reducing the financial barrier to care, or of introducing coverage for office care in addition to hospital benefits, the experience of prepaid group practice plans becomes extremely valuable. Another advantage might be the availability of historical information for uninterrupted periods, as well as the opportunity for prospective studies with some special modifications in the information to be gathered.

Clinical Records. Clinical records may be obtained from hospitals and related institutions and from office practice. *Hospital records* provide an unusually reliable source of information on hospital use and on patient characteristics, including a great deal of detail concerning illness and its management. For institutions other than hospitals (as well as for many hospitals) the quality and completeness of the records may well be a question of serious concern. But even for the best hospitals, one must be certain that the information sought is reliably and validly represented in the record. In addition to the quality of recording, a major limiting factor in hospital data is the fact that they relate only to recognized illness of a certain spectrum of severity. As we have pointed out, it is only the physician's view of this segment of morbidity that is being presented; and only to the extent that the physician has made the correct diagnosis. Still another problem is that there is often no population base to which to relate use and morbidity data. In other words, one cannot construct rates, unless one is able to determine the population which feeds exclusively into the hospital or hospitals in question and the patients that derive from that population. Methods for determining the population served by a hospital will be discussed in a subsequent chapter. The determination of the population base is, of course, much less of a problem when one deals with a national sample, since few persons leave or enter the country for medical care.

In order to sample hospital discharges, the National Health Survey has developed a Master Facility Inventory which is used as the sampling frame (179). The Inventory is an unduplicated list of facilities classified according to uniform criteria. It includes all hospitals in the United States with 6 or more beds, as well as all resident institutions except for

Table III.21.   Master Facility Inventory, U.S.A., September 1963

A. Short-stay Hospitals

   1. General
   2. Special
      a. Maternity
      b. Eye, ear, nose, and throat
      c. Pediatric
      d. Other

B. Resident institutions

   1. Long-stay Hospitals
      a. General
      b. Psychiatric
      c. Mental retardation
      d. Geriatric
      e. Orthopedic
      f. Tuberculosis
      g. Chronic disease
      h. Other

   2. Nursing, Personal or Domiciliary Care Establishments
      a. Nursing care
      b. Personal care without nursing
      c. Domiciliary care

   3. Custodial Care Homes
      a. Homes for the deaf
      b. Homes for the blind
      c. Homes for unwed mothers
      d. Orphanages
      e. Other

   4. Correctional Institutions
      a. Prisons and reformatories
      b. Detention homes for juvenile delinquents

SOURCE: Reference 179.

nursing homes with less than 3 beds. Table III.21 gives the classification used and provides a picture of the scope of the inventory. The Master Facility Inventory provides the sampling frame for two components of the National Health Survey: The Institutional Population Surveys and the Hospital Discharge Survey. The former consists of a series of ad hoc surveys of the health status of residents in such institutions and of the factors relating to care. Examples are the studies of nursing home staffing patterns and patient characteristics. The Hospital Discharge

Survey proper is based on an approximately 10 percent sample of short-term hospitals listed in the Master Inventory. About 10 percent of discharges from the 10 percent sample are selected for review. Thus, about one in every 100 discharges in the United States is surveyed. For this purpose abstracts of the selected records are made, either by employees of the Bureau of the Census or of the hospital (180).

The Hospital Discharge Survey will provide more reliable information on hospital use (and possibly cost) than has been available until now from the Health Interview Survey. It will suffer from the drawback, also shared by the Health Interview Survey, of providing data only for the country and its larger subdivisions, so that its usefulness for local planning will be limited. Unlike the Health Interview Survey, the Hospital Discharge Survey will not provide data on persons hospitalized because the several hospitalizations by any one person are not linked. Hence, the data will refer to hospital episodes only. The unique contribution of the Discharge Survey will be the detailed and reasonably valid diagnostic information it will provide, for which the discharge diagnosis will be used. This is an important specification because the validity of admission diagnoses is known to be of a very low order (177). The Survey should also make possible examination of the way in which the hospital resources are employed to produce services, as distinct from the manner in which persons use hospitals. Special studies—of hospital service areas, for example—will also become possible.

The records of *office practice,* including that of general practitioners, might serve as an additional source of information. Here there are serious problems of completeness and validity, as well as of reporting. Access to such records is also difficult to obtain, unless the physicians are organized in group practice or in some other way. Finally, there would be problems of determining the population base for the construction of rates. In Britain the manner in which care is organized makes it possible to overcome some of these problems. The capitation system provides a fairly stable link between patient and physician, so that the physician's "list," provided it is reasonably well kept, constitutes the population base. Moreover, since access to specialists is generally through referral by the general practitioner, and the patient is almost always referred back to his family doctor, the general practitioner's records present a more complete picture of illness and care. As we pointed out in a previous section, the physician's record shows only known disease and leaves out a great part of the submerged "iceberg." In Britain a simple system has been developed that permits selected physicians to keep a running log of services and morbidities in their practices. This is based on the use of a

specially designed log called the "E"-Book (after Eimerl), and a simplified classification of illness developed by the College of General
Practitioners (181). In the United States and Canada records of general
practitioners (278, 279) and internists (280) have been used for some
special studies. Records of ambulatory care are more regularly available
for hospital outpatient departments and prepaid group practice. The
"Med 10," a simple form used by the Health Insurance Plan of Greater
New York to keep a running record of office, home, and hospital visits,
serves as the basis for statistical tabulations prepared by the Plan and
has also been used in several special studies. In prepaid group practice
plans, the membership provides the population base. However, approximately a third of all physician services may be obtained outside the plan.
Since the frequency with which this happens varies by type of condition
and type of patient, special adjustments for the deficit in plan records
will have to be made (281).

Measuring Health

THE CONCEPT OF HEALTH. So far we have concentrated on the measurement of morbidity. It is true that we have enlarged the concept of
morbidity both in scope and in depth: in scope to include the dual
perspectives of physician and client, and in depth to include a gradation
from early beginnings to total encroachment. But what of "health"? Is
there a view of health as something other than the absence of morbidity
and disability? Are there grades, levels, or intensities of health? Can one
distinguish mere "health" from "positive," abundant, or superabun-
dant health? If so, how can this phenomenon and its intensities be
measured and graded?

Almost all the definitions of health that the author has run across,
including the celebrated dictum by the World Health Organization, have
asserted that health is something other than the absence of disease. Here
are some examples:

Health is a state of complete physical, mental, and social well-being and not
merely the absence of disease or infirmity.—World Health Organization (282).

A healthy individual has been described as a well-integrated individual, both
as to his physical structure and as to his physiological and psychological functioning . . . Health is not a condition; it is an adjustment. It is not a state but
a process. That process adapts the individual not only to our physical but also
to our social environment (283, p. 13).

Positive health [is] a full sense of physical vigor and mental well-being and
maintaining a constructive and wholesome relation with others in a safe and
pleasant environment that promotes longevity and happiness (284).

The term "health" as affecting the individual, should embrace (in addition to those of sensory well-being and structural integrity) ideas of balance and adaptability; these in turn reflect the co-ordinated activity of component parts each functioning within its normal range (24).

Health is a relative term describing the degree of harmony which an individual is able to achieve in a particular, social, or cultural environment and in light of his own unique biological and physiological characteristics (5).

Health is a state of relative equilibrium of body form and function which results from its successful dynamic adjustment to forces tending to disturb it. It is not passive interplay between body substance and forces impinging upon it but an active response of body forces working toward readjustment (285).

Health is the perfect, *continuing,* adjustment of an organism to its environment (13).

The term normal or healthy can be defined in two ways. Firstly, from the standpoint of functioning society, one can call a person normal or healthy if he is able to fulfil the social role he is to take in that given society—if he is able to participate in the reproduction of society. Secondly (or alternatively), from the standpoint of the individual, we look upon health or normality as the optimum of growth and happiness of the individual—Erich Fromm (cited by Aubrey Lewis, 2, p. 110).

Health may be defined as the state of optimum *capacity* of an individual for the effective performance of the roles and tasks for which he has been socialized. It is thus defined with reference to the individual's participation in the social system. It is also defined as *relative* to his "status" in the society (1).

These definitions indicate that the notion of "health" differs from the "absence of disease" in at least two ways. First, the areas subject to evaluation have been broadened beyond physical and physiological functioning to include social, cultural, and mental or psychological aspects of performance. Second, certain criteria of successful functioning have been postulated which presumably apply to one or more of the aspects of performance previously enumerated. These criteria appear to belong under three categories. First, the notion of "health" embraces, possibly in ascending order, subjective feelings of contentment, "well-being," "vigor," and "happiness." Second, there is evidence, presumably in addition to self-estimates, of functional adaptation to external circumstances, including balance, harmony, and adjustment. Finally, there is the capacity to establish new adjustments should circumstances change, a property referred to as adjustment, adaptability, growth, and, perhaps, longevity. Thus, the determinants of health appear to be remarkably subjective and decidedly relative. They vary in stringency depending on the demands made upon the person in question: health for an accountant is different from health for a test pilot. Thus the criteria of health may be at once more stringent and less stringent than the absence of disease.

A person who "feels well" and is able to perform in a satisfactory manner what he usually demands of himself and what society ordinarily demands of him may be considered "healthy" even though he may have disease or significant disability. On the other hand, a person may show no detectable evidence of physical illness and yet be judged unhealthy because he feels unwell or cannot hold a job. The essential criterion appears to be successful adaptation. But perhaps the paradox of a judgment of "healthy" in the presence of disease is only apparent, and occurs because the third criterion of health, the capacity to adapt to changing circumstances, has been omitted. In other words, although at any given time a state of balance or harmony has been established, one must decide whether the precariousness of that condition, both over time and in the face of new stresses, is compatible with one's definition of "health." If one insists that the capacity for adaptation under changing stress is a necessary component of the definition of "health," the concepts of "health" and of "absence of disease" draw closer together. The concepts become still closer if one posits that (1) there are many aspects of human functioning; (2) for each function there are variations of encroachment on that function that range in continuous fashion from none to complete; and (3) any one person can be characterized by the position he holds on each continuum of encroachment of each function. This formulation recognizes the multidimensional nature of health and asserts that a profile of positions on several continua, rather than any single position, defines the degree of both "health" and "disease." Disease is a reflection of encroachment and health a reflection of non-encroachment, with the person's "health–disease" profile as the boundary between the two. This means that both disease and health are graded phenomena and that one is the complement to the other. By measuring any one aspect of one, we measure the same aspect of the other. However, measuring one aspect (say physical function) may not yield much information about another (emotional function, for example).

The formulation offered above appears to have at least two drawbacks. First, it leaves completely open the specification of what aspects of human functioning are relevant to the notion of "health." To that extent the formulation is inconclusive. But this openness has the advantage of recognizing the provisional nature of what the medical care system now considers to be within its scope. It also makes possible the conclusion that certain aspects of human functioning are of lower priority than others so far as the medical care system is concerned, and some altogether outside its purview. Another apparent drawback is that the emphasis on the disparate strands of functioning within the definition of health contradicts the general view of health as unitary, or reasonably so. But this contradiction is only apparent. The unitary aspects of health arise, in part, from the interrelatedness of the different aspects of human functioning. For example, encroachment on psychological function may influence physical performance, and the reverse is also true. Furthermore, subjective feelings, whether negative or positive, tend to be diffuse and nonspecific. It is difficult to be in constant pain but happy, or anxious and feel well. Encroachment on any one of several functions may result in rather similar states of feeling. In this way, feelings (an important determinant of the definition of health) unite the degrees of encroachment on disparate strands of functioning into one common expression.

OPERATIONAL MEASURES OF HEALTH. The conclusion to be drawn from the above is that when one measures encroachment on function, one measures both health and illness. The degree of encroachment, however, has to be viewed both subjectively and objectively, and its impact judged by the degree to which it interferes with the demands of living as defined by social obligations and personal preferences. This, in fact, has been fundamentally the approach to measurement of morbidity as we have presented it. What remains to be done is to consider greater emphasis on, and refinements in, measures of encroachment on social and psychological function. This, however, is a matter beyond the scope of this book and the competence of the author.

The concept of morbidity that we have used also placed emphasis on another component of the definition of health, adaptation to stress, as one measure of encroachment on function. In fact, in its earliest beginnings functional encroachment could be revealed only as a deficiency in adaptation measurable by the most sensitive devices. It is perhaps in this segment of the continuum of encroachment that "positive health" begins to have precise and measurable meaning. "Positive health" can perhaps be measured in terms of "functional reserve" in any given aspect of human functioning: physical, physiological, psychological, or social. It may be useful to elaborate on this notion as it applies to physical health.

The body, its organs and tissues, have inherent wide margins of safety in the form of redundancies of both function and structure. This means that ordinarily only part of the body's capacities are put to use, so that appreciable, sometimes considerable, structure and function can be destroyed before there is manifest impairment in ordinary function. Even in the absence of actual destruction, the habitual lack of use of functional reserve may itself result in defective response to stress. The amount of reserve function, or that part of it that can be mobilized, can be tested by performance under stress. Such measurements include tests of physical "fitness" which measure in physiological terms the capacity of the body to respond to the high metabolic demands of physical work and exercise with minimum evidence of stress as shown by the response of the circulatory and respiratory systems and changes in body chemistry (199, 200). The adjusting power of the body can also be tested under extremes of temperature, barometric pressure, water deprivation, and the like. The affinities of the notion of physiological homeostasis to the notions of social or psychological harmony or adaptation are quite obvious. In all such measurements, however, one must consider to what extent the results are relevant to the ordinary functioning or the longevity of the subject.

Another indicator of "positive health" may be derived from measurements of growth and development in the young or lack of evidence of senescence in the aging. However, it is not clear that rapid growth and early maturation are necessarily desirable, nor is it known what precisely constitutes senescence. Sullivan, after Gordon, has suggested that the degree of resistance to disease, to the extent that it is measurable, might be another approach to measuring "positive health" (203). All these proposals require further conceptual clarification and a great deal of investigation. But this should not give the medical care administrator undue concern. For a long time to come he will have his hands full measuring morbidity.

SUMMARY MEASURES OF HEALTH AND ILLNESS. There has been, for a long time, a search for a unitary measure of health and illness that would measure the impact of both morbidity and mortality and lend itself for use in the establishment of priorities and documenting the impact of care. No single satisfactory measure is now available, but there have been several proposals. They share in common the use of one unifying measure: the loss of function whatever the cause might be.

Sullivan has reviewed the conceptual and methodological problems in developing an "index of health," as he calls it, and has proposed mutually exclusive classifications of disability, which we have described in a previous section (203). The mere summation of the days of disability experienced in each of the four levels gives a total score of disability days. Sullivan recognizes that the days lost to disability, as he defines it, do not include losses due to death. He proposes, however, that "use of time units to measure morbidity may also facilitate the combination of morbidity and mortality measures into a single index. Although death and disability are not completely commensurable events, some life table values are also expressed in units of time'' (203, p. 13). We have pointed out two additional limitations to this index. While it is possible to add all days within each category, the summing of days across categories may be inappropriate without further weighting, since the degree of disability is graded by category. Furthermore, there are limitations in the person-day concept itself, since lengthy disability in a few persons may not mean the same thing, in terms of the uses of the index, as disability of short duration experienced by many persons.

Chiang has proposed an index that makes the assumption that Sullivan was somewhat hesitant to make—that days of life lost as a consequence of death are equivalent to days of activity or functioning lost due to illness (202). He also pays much less attention to defining precisely the nature of disability resulting from illness, than does Sullivan; but the two proposals are roughly congruent. One could readily use Sullivan's measure of disability in computing the Chiang index. According to Chiang, for any one person in the population, during one year:

$$1. \begin{pmatrix} \text{Average duration} \\ \text{of ill health} \end{pmatrix} = \begin{pmatrix} \text{Expected num-} \\ \text{ber of illnesses} \\ \text{during one} \\ \text{year} \end{pmatrix} \times \begin{pmatrix} \text{Expected} \\ \text{average} \\ \text{duration} \\ \text{of illness} \end{pmatrix} + \tfrac{1}{2} \begin{pmatrix} \text{Age-} \\ \text{specific} \\ \text{mortality} \\ \text{rate} \end{pmatrix}$$

2. (Average duration of health) $= 1 -$ (Average duration of ill health)

A weighted average, for example by number of persons in each age group, gives the measure for the entire population. When two populations of differing age-sex structure are to be compared, the usual techniques of standardization are used. The mathematics underlying the construction of the index are given by the author (202).

The reader should note that the last term in the first equation cited above states that each person who dies during a given year has suffered the loss of one-half year of life during that year. This is based on the assumption that persons die at a constant rate during a given year. Furthermore, since this term is stated in years, all the other durations are also stated in years. Conversion to days lost is, of course, easily done. A more fundamental characteristic of the formulation is that the accounting is limited to one year even though the effects of death extend beyond the year during which it occurs. Furthermore, it is clear that ''health'' is defined simply as the absence of ill-health. The objections we have raised about the Sullivan proposal also apply to the Chiang index.

Sanders has proposed a measure of ''functional adequacy'' which is similar to the two indices described above, but also has some essential differences (212). "Functional capacity" is defined as the ability to fulfil the requirements of the social role appropriate to an individual of specified age and sex. Losses in functional capacity due to death are added to losses due to illness. Unlike Sullivan, no operational definitions of "functional capacity" are offered. But the essential distinguishing characteristic of the Sanders proposal is that the horizon extends beyond the year during which death or disability occurs. It is proposed that if a cohort of births is exposed to the probabilities of losses in "functional capacity" that occur from illness and death as they are current for each age group in a population, a life table can be constructed of the remaining effective years of life at each age. This schedule (of effective life years remaining, by age) is the measure of health of that population. As we shall see in a subsequent section, the extension of the concept of loss to include the shortening of life brought about by death, produces important changes in how several diseases are ordered as to priority.

As a second step in his search for an index of mortality and morbidity, Sullivan has combined the life table method proposed by Sanders with his own notions about the classification and measurement of disability to arrive at summary and detailed quantitative representations of the health of a population, and of its subgroups, at any specified time (205). The principles and methods used are simple and conventional, but the measures that result should be remarkably useful. Given mortality rates by single years of age or by age group, as observed in a reference population during any specified period of time, it is not difficult, to construct a life table for that population. The life table tells us what would be the life experience of a cohort of births (say 100,000 persons) who would experience, at each age in its unfolding future history, the death rates observed in the reference population during the time period specified. From the life table one can tell how many persons will be alive at the beginning of each year of age or of each age interval, if ages are grouped. Similarly, one can tell how many years of further life remain at the beginning of each age interval to all the members of the cohort who survive to that age. Thus, one can compute the expectation of life for the average individual at birth or at any specified age. The average expectation of life is a summary measure of the net effect of the forces of longevity and mortality as they act upon the reference population during the specified period of time. It is not a true prediction or forecast of future life. It could be understood as a hypothetical prediction which says, in effect, "This would be the average remaining life span if the mortalities observed in the reference population during the specified period were unaltered in the future." Since this assumption of future constancy in mortality rates is often unrealistic, the life table is a method of representing in a summary measure (such as the life expectancy) or in full detail (as shown by the table in its entirety) the life experience of the reference population during the specified period. All this is fully conventional. Sullivan's accomplishment was to add to the mortality rates, the rates of specified levels of morbidity. Sanders had already proposed this in theory. Sullivan was able to use data from the National Health Survey to provide reasonably realistic estimates of bed disability and of non-bed disability, as he defined them. Thus, he was able to provide data on life expectancy with and without specified levels of disability. Table III.22, shows the estimates for subclasses of the

Table III.22.   Expectations at birth of years of specified types of disability and of life with and without specified disabilities, by color and sex, U.S.A., mid-1960's

	White		All Other	
	Female	Male	Female	Male
Total life	74.7	67.6	67.4	61.1
All disability	5.3	5.1	6.0	6.0
Bed disability	2.3	1.5	2.2	1.6
Nonbed disability	3.0	3.6	3.8	5.4
Life free of bed disability	72.4	66.1	65.2	59.5
Life free of all disability	69.4	62.5	61.4	55.1

SOURCE: Reference 205, Tables 1 and 2, pages 348 and 349.

population assuming these experience mortality and disability rates observed during the mid-1960's. One notes an orderly progression, so that life expectancy with and without disability is higher in females than males and higher for whites than nonwhites. In descending order of life expectancy are white females, white males, nonwhite females and nonwhite males. Including the disability estimates does not alter this ordering, but does change the relative magnitudes of the subparts. However, Sullivan warns that the comparisons by sex could be misleading because confinement to bed due to pregnancy and childbirth and restricted ability to do housework are disabilities that apply to females but not to males. A more detailed picture of longevity with and without disability is given by the life table as a whole. Figure III.11 is a visual representation of the lifetime experience of a cohort of males. With narrower age

Fig. III.11.   Years of life during each year of age[a] which are associated with disability and are free of disability. Cohort of 100,000 white males who experience sex- and age-specific death and disability rates as observed in the United States in the mid-1960's

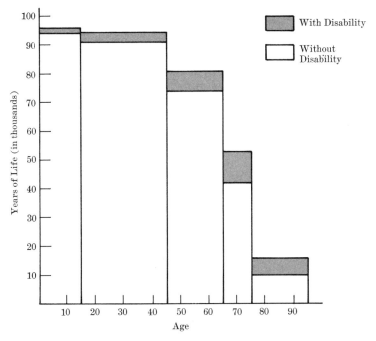

[a] The oldest age interval is arbitrarily closed at age 95.
SOURCE: Reference 205, Table 3, p. 351.

groups and further divisions in the disability classification, even greater detail would be possible. It should be noted, however, that the two classes of disability distinguished by Sullivan cannot be added without further weighting, since they differ in intensity and hence in the degree to which they interfere with functional integrity, physiological and social. A further characteristic of the Sullivan method is that each population subgroup is taken separately. Would it be possible to construct summary and detailed quantitative representations for the entire population that include adjustments for population characteristics and that permit the summation of different intensities of disability? One approach to such refinements is possibly based on the work of Fanshel and Bush (206) of Bush and his associates (207) and of Ortiz and Parker (208).

Fanshel and Bush begin, as did Sullivan, by classifying states of health into an ordinal scale of mutually exclusive categories ranging from "well-being" to death, and with 9 classes in between. This scale they regard as a continuum of "function/dysfunction," so that decreases in function are accompanied by corresponding increases in dysfunction, and the reverse. "Well-being" corresponds to the World Health Organization's "positive physical mental, and social well-being," and is assigned a value of 1. Death indicates "absolute dysfunction," or the total absence of health, and is given a value of zero. The problem is to weight, in some consistent and realistic manner, the 9 states in between. Fanshel and Bush discuss several alternatives for weighting but indicate preference for a method of paired comparisons which derives from prior work by Thurstone and is considered to be consistent with methods for scaling described by Tergerson. What is required is that informed people be asked to indicate at what point a certain quantity of one health state becomes so much the equal of another quantity of another health state that the choice between the two becomes a matter of indifference. Quantification is achieved using a variety of units such as dollars needed to achieve the two states, time periods of being subject to the two states or numbers of persons in each of the two states. For example, using time as the unit of exchange, one might ask how many years of life one would be willing to give up if one could be assured perfect well-being over a lifetime. Using the device of paired comparisons, in which all pairs of categories in the classification are compared to one another, it is possible to arrive at a set of weights that includes all categories and best approximates the paired choices. According to Fanshel and Bush, the most relevant group of judges whose choices would determine the weights, are the public officials who are charged with making the policy decisions that determine the national investment in health. One might, of course, question this contention on the grounds that it merely perpetuates existing bias and does not reflect the variety of perspectives on health, illness, and need for care that are bound to be present in any society. In any event, Fanshel and Bush have not had the opportunity to put their scheme to an empirical test. Instead, for purposes of illustration, they adopted an arbitrary set of weights on the assumption that each state in their scale has twice the quantity of function as the one preceding it and, by the same token, twice the quantity of dysfunction as the state preceding it. Table III.23 gives the ordinal scale of mutually exclusive categories proposed by Fanshel and Bush, their equivalents in terms of an arbitrary set of dysfunction weights, and a translation of the weights to a more concrete measure of loss of life. It is clear that the scale of categories is

Table III.23.   States of function/dysfunction, weights of dysfunction and equivalents in years of life lost during a lifetime in each state

Categories of Function/Dysfunction	Dysfunction Weights	Lifetime Equivalents (in years)
Well-being	0	0
Dissatisfaction	0.0039	0.33
Discomfort (not disabled)	0.0078	0.75
Disability, minor	0.0156	1.5
Disability, major	0.0313	2.8
Disabled (ambulatory)	0.0625	5.6
Confined (not bedridden)	0.125	11.1
Confined, bedridden	0.25	22.2
Isolated	0.5	45
Coma	1	90
Death	1	90

SOURCE: Reference 206, Table I, page 1046.

more complex and probably less easily amenable to operationalization than the scales proposed by Sullivan. For example, intrusion of the subjective terms "dissatisfaction" and "discomfort" into a scale largely, but not exclusively, based on physical and social disability, suggests multidimensionality and, therefore, problems in classification. As we have already remarked, the weights proposed are totally arbitrary, though plausible. In fact, Fanshel and Bush found it necessary to introduce small modifications in the weights in order to make them intuitively more satisfying to themselves. The lifetime equivalents that are cited embody an important feature of the method proposed by Fanshel and Bush: the decision to adopt the concept of "a standard life duration" (rather than the more usual life expectancy) in order to make losses from death commensurable to losses from other states. Coma and death are considered to represent equivalent disability during equivalent time periods (in this instance a lifetime). This feature aside, inspection of the weights, and of their more concrete equivalents, shows a bias toward illness rather than health, reflecting perhaps values inherent in our medical care system. For example, a lifetime of discomfort is considered to be so small a departure from perfect or "positive" health that it is equivalent to less than a year of loss from the standard life-span of 90. The configuration of weights is perhaps better appreciated from Fig. III.12. The curve D_1 in the figure shows the precipitous fall in function status attributed to the last few categories which are brought about by the successive doubling of the quantity of disability ascribed to each

Fig. III.12.   Proposed weights of function and dysfunction attached to a mutually exclusive ordered scale of health states.

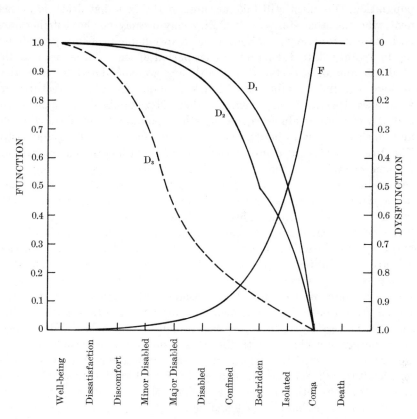

SOURCE: Reference 206, Tables I and II, pp. 1046 and 1047. (Curve D_3 added.)

successive state. The curve for function weights, shown as curve F, is, of course, a mirror image of the curve for dysfunction weights. This is because Function is mathematically defined as one minus Dysfunction. The curve D_2 shows the changes made in the original exponential progression of weights in order to achieve an intuitively more satisfying set. Note that the effect is to give greater weight to initial departures from perfect health. Curve D_3 is offered by the author simply to illustrate the consequences of a different set of values. Here, even greater attention is given to earlier departures from health, with greatest importance attached to the transition from minor disability to major.

The classification of health states and the weights attached to them is only a first step toward developing a measure of the health status of a population. One must still take account of the fact that death is permanent, whereas other states of disability may or may not be. Furthermore, each state of function/dysfunction has a specifiable probability of changing to another state during any given period of time. These peculiarities of death and of the states of health are accommodated by a method analogous to the life-table called Markov chain analysis. Its features are as follows. First, it is assumed that there is a standard life span at the end of which all or almost all persons in a population are dead. Fanshel and Bush took this to be 90 years, whereas Bush et al. used 100 years. This life-span is divided into periods of standard length. The population is then classified by function/dysfunction states, age, and any of a reasonable number of additional relevant characteristics such as diagnostic category, sex, and race. It is obvious that the result is a table which could be of considerable size. Each cell of the table contains a homogeneous segment of the population with specifiable characteristics and a specifiable weight of function/dysfunction. Also attached to each cell are probabilities of persons in that cell dying during the standard time period or of surviving to remain in the same state or to enter any of the other states of function/dysfunction by the beginning of the next period. The probabilities of transition from one state to another, including the irreversible state of death, are considered to be fixed for each cell; they do not change with the progression of time periods. In other words, it is assumed that whatever forces account for present mortality and health states will act unchanged in the relevant future. This is, of course, the conventional life-table assumption. It is also customarily assumed that the probability of transition of the population in one state to another state by the end of a time period is independent of the prior states of the population in that cell. When this cannot be assumed to be true, the analysis will have to be recast so that each cell contains people who have had the same antecedents (207). Thus it is possible to characterize the population by function/dysfunction states during each of a succession of periods until all its members are, theoretically, dead. A death during any period is credited with zero weight from that period to the end of the standard life span. All other states are represented by person-periods of full-function equivalents (state of well being). The sum of these values over cells and over periods gives the health index for that population. In this example a given population was carried forward, in theory, to the point where all its numbers were dead. The same method could be used to characterize the future hypothetical life experience of a cohort of births. This results in a life-table in which, instead of years of life, the unit of measurement is the full-function life equivalent derived from the function/dysfunction weights. In both instances one can characterize the population or cohort by the single aggregate index or by the area under the curve that results from plotting person-years of full-function equivalents against time.

The above description is meant to give only an approximate picture of the method. For a more precise and detailed view the reader is referred to the sources cited (206–208). The sources also offer examples of the application of the method, and of its variants, to situations that approximate real life problems. Precise applications are not now possible mainly because of a lack of data. For example, the weights proposed by Fanshel and Bush have not as yet been empirically derived. Further, it is not now possible to obtain information on morbidity and function/dysfunction states for target populations in the detail envisaged by the model. Most importantly, the prognoses, or the probabilities of transition from one state to another, are very imperfectly understood. However, as Fanshel and Bush emphasize, one reason for the paucity of requisite data is the absence of a prior conceptual framework that permits the use of the data for socially important ends. It is hoped that when the usefulness of certain kinds of data is established, the effort to obtain such data will be forthcoming.

Kisch et al. have taken a somewhat different approach to devising a unitary measure of health and illness (209). They argue that for many research purposes (as distinct from clinical management) it is sufficient to have a measure that is correlated with what a physician might find on clinical evaluation. Their "proxy measure" is a cumulative numerical score based on the reporting of four kinds of experiences during the previous year: (1) admission to hospital and duration of hospital stay, (2) the number of drugs or medications taken continuously for a month or more, (3) the number of acute conditions, of those on a check list, and (4) the number of chronic conditions, of those on a check list. The numerical score ranges from 0 to 146, with 0–20 designated as "good health," 21–60 as "medium health," and 61+ as "poor health." When these scores were compared to clinical judgments of "good," "medium," and "poor" health in 308 persons, there was complete agreement in 65 percent of cases. In 26 percent of cases, the proxy measure gave a higher rating of "health," and in 9 percent of cases a lower rating, than did the clinical evaluation. Because of the procedure used to trichotomize the numerical score of the proxy measure, these levels of agreement are probably the best that may be hoped for. Furthermore, the measure, by definition, is oriented to a professional determination of "health" as distinct from that of the client.

Evaluational Uses of Measures of Morbidity and Health

The reader will recall that three uses were postulated for measurements of need: (1) evaluation of the effectiveness of health services, (2) determination of priorities for health action, and (3) translation into service equivalents. In this section, the first of these uses will be briefly discussed. There will be further discussion of additional aspects later on in this chapter and in subsequent chapters.

Our model of the medical care process began with "need" defined by the client and by the provider in terms of conditions and situations that were judged to require care. The process terminated with some modification of need, usually the partial or complete satisfaction of need, but sometimes the creation of need, as when harm is done through excessive or ill-considered medical intervention. It follows that the prevalence and nature of need in a population should give some indication of the effectiveness of the medical care system which serves that population. In fact, "effectiveness" may be defined as the extent to which the existing potential of medical technology to preserve health and ameliorate disease has been achieved.

Pursuing this line of thought, Fanshel and Bush have shown how their index of health could be used to arrive at more precise operational expressions of the notion of "effectiveness" (206). Assume that it is possible to construct an index of the health status of a population. Further assume that it is possible to specify (1) what would be the value of the health index in the absence of medical care and (2) what would be the value of the health index if it were possible to apply fully our present knowledge about health care. It would then be possible to tell how far the present health care system has gone towards achieving the ideal. Using our own symbols, let:

H_0 = health index per unit population without the intervention of the health care system;

H_1 = health index per unit population at current levels of health care;

H_2 = health index per unit population at some "ideal" or "best practical" application of current knowledge about health care.

Then:

$$\text{Effectiveness} = \frac{H_1 - H_0}{H_2 - H_0}$$

Actually, the measure of effectiveness should also take account of changes in population size since the "health output" of the current system is $P (H_1 - H_0)$ where P is the current population. However, if P is the same for the numerator and denominator of the above ratio it can obviously be ignored.

The formulation described above is offered mainly in order to specify the manner in which health status could be used as a measure of the effectiveness of the medical care system and, consequently, a key tool in evaluation. Needless to say, present knowledge falls very far short of generating the necessary data in most situations. However, it is conceivable that the method could be applicable to measuring the observed incremental effects on health status of the introduction of a specific health program in a target population. Also, failing a total measure of health, it is customary to use partial measures, or "indices," of health status that presumably represent the totality of health, or at least that portion of it that is relevant to the program under evaluation. Whichever approach is followed, the use of health status as an evaluative tool is plagued by a number of difficulties to which we should now turn our attention.

A number of considerations govern the use of health status as an indicator of the effectiveness of the medical care system. First is the property of *exclusiveness,* signifying the extent to which health or ill health are attributable to the influence of medical care. This requirement is rarely met, but may be approximated. Deficiencies in health status reflect complex genetic and environmental factors, the latter including many features of the physical and biological environment and of social organization. By the same token, amelioration in health can be brought about by improvements in the conditions under which persons work and live quite independently of the effect of medical care. Medical care is only one among the many influences that determine health, often a relatively unimportant factor. Nevertheless, medical care does have an effect, and it is the task of the administrator to choose those circumstances under which the effect is most closely tied to antecedent medical care and least confounded by other influences. To some extent this depends on the second requisite property, that of *responsiveness,* which refers to the magnitude of the effect exerted by medical care on the phenomenon to be measured and the readiness with which such effects are exerted. These twin, and related, requirements have led to the choice of certain indices as particularly useful in the evaluation of health services. Logan has used the designation of "sensitive rates" to describe some of these indices (210). Where the purpose is not to make judgments concerning the medical care system alone, but to obtain some indicator of the conditions of life in general, responsiveness rather than exclusiveness becomes the prime criterion. The use of health indices for this purpose is certainly legitimate and, paradoxically, perhaps less open to criticism.

Among the indicators that rank reasonably high in exclusiveness and responsiveness are infant mortality, case fatality, and the occurrence or persistence of medically preventible mortalities, morbidities, and disabilities. Infant mortality and its components have served for a long time as an indicator both of medical care and of other factors in the physical and social environment. For more detailed analysis, where information is available, infant mortality may be subdivided into components: the first hour, the balance of the first day, the balance of the first week, the balance of the first month, and the balance of the first year, as well as sums of two or more adjacent segments. To the deaths during the first week or month of life, stillbirths may be added to obtain a measure of deaths that surround the event of birth (perinatal mortality). Since the factors that cause death during each of the segments of infant mortality differ to an appreciable degree, the responsiveness of the several mortalities differs, and their relative weights can give some insights into the nature of health and social problems in a population (230, 232, 233). For example, deaths during later infancy are generally caused by infectious disease and respond well to modern medical care or to general improvement in the conditions of life. Deaths during the first week of life are more often caused by imperfect development of the newborn or injury sustained during birth. Hence they are more purely medical in nature and, in part, less amenable to reduction by medical intervention or changes in the general social environment (232, 233). The device of segmental analysis of mortality can, of course, be extended to fetal mortality, on the one hand, and to broad age groups following the first year of life, on the other. The mortality of children and young mothers is often preventible, for example. One advantage of segmental mortality analysis is that, in the absence of a population base, one can construct ratios of the relative magnitude of one segment in relation to another. It is typical in underdeveloped countries to have a major share of mortality concentrated during infancy, exclusive of the first week of life, and during childhood. In more highly developed countries, infant mortality occurs predominantly during the first week of life, and general mortality predominantly in old age (230). Swaroop and Uemara have proposed as a measure of health status the number of deaths at age 50 and above expressed as a percent of deaths at all ages (236).

Case fatality rates have a closer relationship to medical care than does general mortality, and should be a more exclusive and sensitive reflection of the effectiveness of care, provided one chooses situations in which medical care is critically effective and one is able to correct for the effect of other variables, such as age, sex, the severity and stage of illness, and the presence of complicating conditions that might influence outcome. Case fatality rates, with some adjustments, have been used as an index of the effectiveness and quality of hospital care (221–223). Data on deaths in hospitals are easy to obtain. It is more difficult to obtain information concerning the mix of cases and particularly the severity of each case. Roemer et al. have described an attempt to use several variables as indicators of severity in order to adjust observed differences in fatality rates among hospitals (224). Of the several indicators considered, length of stay appeared to be the most satisfactory. However, since length of stay is also influenced by the level of hospital occupancy, a further adjustment for hospital occupancy was introduced. Serious a priori objections can be raised about the use of length of stay as a proxy for severity, and other aspects of the method used can be questioned. Nevertheless, the authors show that, after such adjustments were made, the observed hospital fatality rates were reordered to become concordant with other indicators of effectiveness, such as the number and variety of supportive services and accreditation status. Such reordering occurred because hospitals presumed to provide better care tend to be larger in size, to have a larger number of supportive sources, longer stays, and higher occupancy rates. The occurrence of preventible mortalities, morbidities, and disabilities in the population as a measure of unmet need has been discussed in the section on "unmet need." As may be expected, information concerning these more refined indices is more difficult to obtain.

Wallace et al. have examined the availability and "usefulness" of 29 indicators that might be used for characterizing census tracts in an urban area according to their need for medical or social services. To be "useful" an indicator had to be based on reliable data and be "associated with other high indexes in the same tract. It was assumed that the existence of several high indexes pointed to a need for medical or general services" (69). Of 29 indicators examined, the following were judged "useful":

Health Indexes:

Inadequate prenatal care: Live births with no prenatal care, or prenatal care only in the third trimester per 1,000 live births.
Fetal mortality: Infants over 400 grams born dead per 1,000 live births.
Incidence of prematurity: Infants born alive weighing 2,500 grams or less at birth per 1,000 live births.
Tuberculosis incidence: Reported new cases per 10,000 population.

Social Indexes:

> Unemployment: Unemployed males in civilian labor force per 1,000 males in civilian labor force.
>
> Low income: Families with annual incomes under $3,000 per 1,000 families.
>
> Inadequate education: Adults with 8th grade education or less, per 1,000 adult population.
>
> Overcrowding: Housing units with more than 1.0 persons per room per 1,000 housing units.
>
> Parental composition: Children under 18 not living with 2 parents, per 1,000 population under 18 years.
>
> School-age illegitimacy: Illegitimate live births to mothers aged 15–19 per 1,000 live births.
>
> Juvenile delinquency: Boys 8–17 charged with a non-traffic offense by police or juvenile court per 1,000 male population 8–17.

The work of Wallace et al. is a good example of the localization of need by geographic area and points out clearly the interrelationship of ill health and social pathology. It is interesting to note that several indexes, including neonatal and postneonatal mortality, that are reported by others to differentiate socioeconomic areas, were found not to be "useful" in this study.

We have already referred to the problems of exclusiveness and responsiveness in using health status to judge the effectiveness of medical care. Another problem referred to by several authors, but most emphasized by Sanders, is the occurrence of a "paradoxical effect" whereby better health services result in a greater prevalence of mortality and morbidity (212). Part of this effect is spurious, occurring because better medical care reveals hitherto unsuspected illness and, by establishing higher standards, makes greater calls for care. The possible biasing effect of medical care on morbidity reports was discussed in a previous section. Another component of the paradoxical effect is real. It arises in a number of ways. To the extent that medical care contributes to longevity, it permits the survival of persons who are subject to chronic illness and disability, and seemingly frustrates its own purposes by creating new needs. This points out the necessity to standardize for age and sex in estimates of health status as a measure of the effectiveness of medical care. There are, however, further paradoxical effects for which it is not so easy to correct. In certain instances, disease can be controlled but not cured. Hence the prevalence of such disease is increased in the population by virtue of effective medical care. Sartwell has surmised that the prevalence, though not the incidence, of diabetes has increased in the population for this reason (49). As Sanders has pointed out, higher standards of sanitation may so alter the natural history of certain diseases as to result in higher levels of manifest morbidity. Prior to the discovery of vaccine, poliomyelitis was an excellent example. In underdeveloped societies, infection with virus was almost universal early in infancy, when its effects were not noticeable or were mild. Where high levels of sanitation prevailed, infection occurred later in life, produced manifest disease more frequently, and had more serious consequences. Another paradoxically adverse effect of medical care has been advanced by some who speculate that persons of lower vigor or resistance to disease are permitted to survive only to suffer from unusually high morbidity throughout their life span. For example, Baumgartner has suggested that failure to bring about rapid reduction in neonatal mortality may be, in part, the result of better obstetrical care which permits children to be born alive, but only to die afterwards (286). Whether the survival and reproduction of persons with "inferior" genetic endowment will eventually create new problems for society is a question which the author is not competent to discuss.

A final problem in the evaluational use of health status is the question of standards. There are two ways in which standards may be derived: normatively and empirically. From a normative point of view, it is easy to postulate, in most situations, that the absence of disease and disability is the goal. What is lacking is a more precise estimate of what is reasonable to expect given a specified level of medical technology and medical care organization. Quantitative normative standards are difficult to specify. Williamson et al. have attempted to obtain such standards by asking physicians to predict the amount of disability following care for certain diagnoses. At least in the preliminary report they published, there was a remarkable degree of variability in these estimates (260). Further work, however, has led Williamson to conclude that in spite of "wide" variation among individual physicians, "group estimates proved specific and meaningful when compared to empirically measured follow-up findings" (287, p. 11). No evidence is cited to support this conclusion. In the absence of precise normative standards, most evaluational studies that use health status as the criterion rest on comparisons among population groups. Such comparisons should, of course, correct for extraneous variables that influence health status, so that differences in the organization of care are the remaining major variable that influences health. Needless to say, only the more obvious corrections can be made, and one is never certain that the differences in health that one observes are attributable to differences in medical care. Examples of such studies include comparisons of case fatalities in teaching and nonteaching hospitals (223) and the several investigations that have attempted to measure the impact of care under the Health Insurance Plan of Greater New York, a prepaid group practice, as compared to care organized along more traditional lines. The group practice studies have included comparisons of prematurity and perinatal mortality (219, 220), general mortality (218), and mortality among recipients of Old Age Assistance (225). Incidentally, the findings demonstrate the relative responsiveness to organizational change of infant mortality and the relative nonresponsiveness of general mortality, at least in the short run. Mortality in the aged did show a small but significant difference during a period of two years. One form of observational study is to compare health status before and after the introduction of some significant change in the organization of health services. However, since other changes may also occur in the interim, it is not possible to be certain what may have produced observed differences in health status. It would be useful, therefore, to have for comparison a population not exposed to the particular change in the organization of care. Less often it may be possible to introduce planned changes in medical care organization and allocate subjects in a controlled manner to one or more groups which are to be compared as to health status. These constitute "experimental," as distinct from "observational," studies, for which a variety of designs are available (217, 229). The controlled allocation of subjects involves some element of randomization which is meant to equalize the effects of variables, other than the particular aspect of medical care under study, on eventual health status. This adds greatly to confidence that the observed effects are due to the medical care variables. Horvits has described some simple experimental designs for evaluating health services (229). Shapiro has recently reviewed the evaluational uses of health status and cited a larger number of examples than we have been able to give (215).

Empirical studies, whether "observational" or "experimental," involve comparisons among populations subjected to different forms of medical care. One variant of observational studies that deserves special mention in the context of evaluation is the comparison of health status among socioeconomic groups. Socioeconomic status is an important determinant of access to medical care and of the quality of care received. Partly for this reason, and also for others, the lower the socioeconomic position, the greater the prevalence of ill health. If one accepts, in keeping with an egalitarian system of values, that medical care should be equally available to all, one can use changes in the socioeconomic distribution of need as one indicator of success in achieving this objective. Hence it might be postulated that a socially effective medical care system would (1) lower the levels of need for all socioeconomic groups

Fig. III.13.   Ratio of unmet need for five selected criteria, by socio-economic status, Metropolitan Boston, 1956, 1957

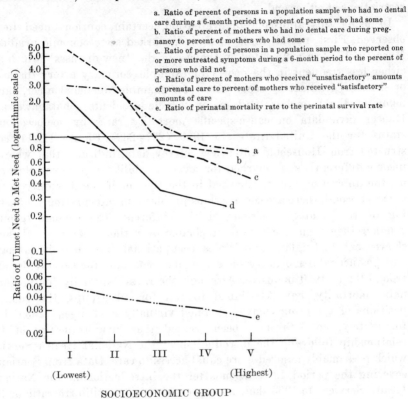

a. Ratio of percent of persons in a population sample who had no dental care during a 6-month period to percent of persons who had some
b. Ratio of percent of mothers who had no dental care during pregnancy to percent of mothers who had some
c. Ratio of percent of persons in a population sample who reported one or more untreated symptoms during a 6-month period to the percent of persons who did not
d. Ratio of percent of mothers who received "unsatisfactory" amounts of prenatal care to percent of mothers who received "satisfactory" amounts of care
e. Ratio of perinatal mortality rate to the perinatal survival rate

Ratio of Unmet Need to Met Need (logarithmic scale)

I (Lowest)   II   III   IV   V (Highest)

SOCIOECONOMIC GROUP

and (2) reduce the differences among groups. Figure III.13 offers one example of this approach as employed by Rosenfeld et al. (213, 214). It will be noted that several indicators of "unmet need" were used, including a partly preventible, undesirable outcome (perinatal mortality) and several measures of lack of receipt of adequate care (unsatisfactory prenatal care, nonreceipt of dental care during pregnancy and in the general population, and nonreceipt of care for significant symptoms). Following a recommendation by Professor Robert Reed, the ratio of unmet to met need was used to measure differences because this unit shows the same magnitude of differences between socioeconomic groups irrespective of whether the index is expressed in terms of met need or unmet need. To portray faithfully the proportionate differences between socioeconomic groups, the logarithm of the ratio of unmet need to met need has an additional advantage in that it may, theoretically, range from minus infinity to plus infinity, and offers a scale that is free of restrictions at either end.

In using this approach to evaluation, certain cautions need to be observed. First, not all diseases show a marked socioeconomic gradient. Morris (217) has commented on the rise of the "new diseases" which are either less frequent in the poor (for example, coronary artery disease), or show no gradient by social class (for example, duodenal ulcer, carcinoma of the bronchus, and motor vehicle accidents). Kitagawa and Hauser give data on cause-specific mortality rates by socioeconomic status for the United States in 1960 (237–239) Figure III.14, constructed from Household Interview Survey data, indicates that whereas income differentials are marked for severe disability in persons below age 65, the differences are less marked in the aged or if the disability is not severe. Second, there are some serious problems in interpreting the meaning of the relative positions of the different socioeconomic groups whether they remain constant or change over time. Morris et al. have shown that, in England and Wales, occupational differences in neonatal and postneonatal mortality have remained constant for several decades from 1911 to 1950 inclusive. Although the rates, especially for postneonatal mortality, have continued to fall for all groups, the relative positions of the groups have remained virtually unchanged (233). Unfortunately, no data have been located that give a picture of the relationship following the introduction of the National Health Service, which presumably assured more equal access to care. Data from Scotland, covering the period 1950 (soon after the introduction of the National Health Service) to 1963 show no convergence in the stillbirth ratio or the neonatal mortality rate (234). Data from the Netherlands also show an essentially invariant relationship between infant mortality and occupation of father between 1952–1954 and 1961–1962 (235). One explanation offered for these remarkably constant relationships is that even when medical care becomes more readily available to all, persons in higher social classes are better able to make effective use of such services (233).

Data from the U.S. confirm the British and Dutch experience, but only in part. In the United States, racial differences in neonatal and postneonatal mortality appear to have remained constant during the last 40 years, as shown by the data of Table III.24.

It is clear that the position of the nonwhite relative to the white has not improved, but may have deteriorated, especially in postneonatal mortality. On the other hand, the absolute difference in rates is smaller, especially for postneonatal mortality where the reduction is large. This

Fig. III.14.   Relative frequency of disability[a] by type of disability, age, and family income (White persons in families of two or more persons, U.S.A. July 1961–June 1963)

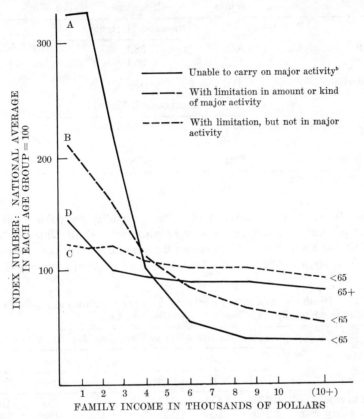

SOURCE: National Center for Health Statistics, *Selected Family Characteristics and Health Measures Reported in the Health Interview Survey.* P.H.S. Publication No. 1000, Series 3, No. 7, Washington, D.C., January 1967 (Table II, p. 25).
[a] The ratio of actual to expected events adjusted for age, sex and farm-nonfarm residence.
[b] Major activity refers to ability to work, keep house, or engage in school or preschool activities.

illustrates that different aspects of the situation are shown by relative positions and absolute differences, respectively. Kitagawa and Hauser have shown that in Chicago, between 1930 and 1950, there was considerable equalization in mortality rates for all ages by color, but much less

Table III.24.   Absolute and relative values of neonatal and postneonatal mortality rates, by race, U.S.A., 1915–1919 and 1963

	White	Nonwhite	Nonwhite as Percent of White
	Neonatal Mortality		
1915–1919	42.3	58.1	137
1963	16.7	26.1	156
Relative decline	61%	55%	
	Postneonatal Mortality		
1915–1919	49.6	89.5	180
1963	5.5	15.4	280
Relative decline	89%	83%	

SOURCE: Reference 231.

change in the relative magnitudes of infant mortality by color (Table III.25). Socioeconomic differentials were also reduced in Chicago between 1930 and 1950. Table III.26 shows the years by which the expectation of life at birth in the highest of 5 socioeconomic groups exceeds that

Table III.25.   Death rate and infant mortality rates for nonwhites as a percent of these rates in whites, by sex, Chicago, 1930, 1940 and 1950

	Rate for Nonwhite as Percent of Rate for White					
	Males			Females		
Rates	1930	1940	1950	1930	1940	1950
Crude death rate	175	154	104	174	151	110
Infant mortality rate	155	160	161	161	130	140

SOURCE: Reference 237, page 81.

in the lowest group; but for nonwhites the highest three groups had to be combined. The trend is similar, but with some aberrations, for infant mortality by socioeconomic status. Table III.27 shows mortality in the lowest economic group as percent of mortality in the highest group. As in Table III.26, the highest three groups for nonwhites had to be combined because of small numbers. The data on socioeconomic differentials cited by Kitagawa and Hauser are difficult to interpret because they are based on ecological analysis. "The five socioeconomic groups . . . were obtained by assigning residents of each of the 935 census tracts in Chicago

Table III.26.   Years of life by which expectation of
life at birth in highest socioeconomic group[a] exceeded
that in lowest group, by color and sex, Chicago, 1930,
1940 and 1950

Color and Sex	Years		
	1930	1940	1950
White males	11.8	7.5	8.0
White females	10.8	7.5	5.6
Nonwhite males	8.7	6.2	6.7
Nonwhite females	8.8	5.9	6.4

SOURCE: Reference 237, Table 17, page 80.
[a] For nonwhites, the three highest of five socioeconomic
groups were combined because numbers in each group
were small.

Table III.27.   Infant mortality in the lowest economic
group as a percent of infant mortality in the highest
group,[a] by color and sex, Chicago, 1930, 1940 and 1950

Color and Sex	1930 (%)	1940 (%)	1950 (%)
White male	230	180	147
White female	234	108	131
Non-white male	180	101	107
Non-white female	114	97	147

SOURCE: Reference 237, Table 18, page 80.
[a] For nonwhites, the three highest of five socioeconomic
groups were combined because numbers in each group
were small.

to a socioeconomic group on the basis of median rent (1920 to 1940) or
median family income (1950) of the tract. The underlying rationale was
to allocate the population of Chicago to the five socioeconomic groups in
approximately the same proportionate distribution on each date'' (237,
p. 70). The reader will recall that while such ecological correlations show
relationships between area characteristics, they may distort severely relationships between the corresponding characteristics of individuals. The
problems of interpretation are further increased, in this instance, by the
profound changes in the ecology of the metropolis that have occurred
during the years in question.

Whether differences in morbidity and mortality among classes have
increased, decreased or remained stable continues to be a matter for
controversy. Kadushin (240) has reviewed the findings of ten previous

investigations and has concluded that in western countries a progression has taken place. In the earliest studies there are clear differences among all classes. Later a difference is noted only between the lowest class and all the other, which are alike. Finally, in the most recent studies, one notes virtually no class differences, or only those that can be interpreted as differences in response to illness rather than in the occurrence of illness. Antonovsky has reviewed the evidence cited by Kadushin and concluded that it does not fully support the interpretation made by the latter. In addition to the conceptual difficulties of separating illness from the response to illness, it is doubtful that in the lower classes, response to illness is more marked or more readily reported (241). Antonovsky has himself reviewed thirty-odd studies from the United States and Western Europe covering a period from the middle of the 19th century to the period following World War II. He appears to agree with Kadushin in noting ''a blurring, if not a disappearance of a clear class gradient.'' Nevertheless, ''what seems beyond question is that, whatever the index used and whatever the number of classes considered, almost always a lowest class appears with a substantially higher mortality rate. Moreover, the differential between it and other classes evidently has not diminished over recent decades'' (242, pp. 66–67). Antonovsky offers the hypothesis that, historically, as mortality levels are reduced, class differentials will be most marked in the intermediate range and least marked at the extremes. Presumably, the means to avert death are at first available to no one, and eventually available to all.

There are severe problems of method in amassing and interpreting data such as those reviewed by Kadushin and by Antonovsky. Obviously, the validity of the data is at issue. The definition and classification of morbidity and the completeness of its reporting has changed markedly over time. The meaning of the socioeconomic classes and their comparability over time is also to be questioned. It may be very misleading to compare only the extremes in ill-health at both ends of the socioeconomic gradient. The diffusion of health within the population is better represented by comparing what proportion of the population accounts for what percentage of mortality or morbidity experience. The Lorenz graph is one convenient way of visually depicting this relationship. Briefly, the population is arranged in classes from low to high. The number of morbid or fatal events in each class is identified. If the distribution of these events is unrelated to socioeconomic class, plotting the cumulative percentage of the population against the cumulative percentage of events should yield a diagonal line. Figure III.15 shows one such graph in which the distribution of certain components of infant mortality are

Fig. III.15.   Percent of deaths in each of two specified age groups that occur among a specified percent of live births arranged by socioeconomic status.[a] A segment of Metropolitan Boston, 1950–1954

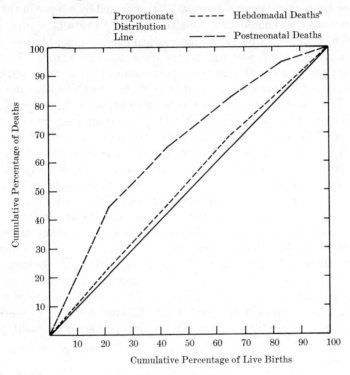

—————— Proportionate Distribution Line   – – – – Hebdomadal Deaths[b]

——— — Postneonatal Deaths

Cumulative Percentage of Deaths

Cumulative Percentage of Live Births

Arrayed from Low to High Socioeconomic Status

[a] Deaths and live births assigned to 5 groups of census tracts aggregated by a combined score of socioeconomic status using income, education and occupational characteristics of census tract residents.

[b] Hebdomadal deaths are those that occur during the first week of life. Postneonatal deaths occur during ages 28 days to 11 months.

SOURCE: Rosenfeld, L. S. and Donabedian, A., Unpublished data.

examined. It is clear that deaths during the first week of life are relatively indifferent to socioeconomic class, whereas deaths during the balance of the first month of life are markedly unequal in their distribution with respect to socioeconomic status. For example, inspection of the graph shows that a little over 20 percent of live births at the low end of the socioeconomic array account for 45 percent of all postneonatal deaths. Thus, the graph demonstrates differences in socioeconomic distribution of two segments of mortality within the same population. Needless to say, the same technique will reveal and measure differences between the socioeconomic distribution of the same event in two populations at any given time, as well as two populations separated by a lapse in time.

In conclusion, although the evaluative use of end results is surrounded by pitfalls, the responsibility for the medical care of a population carries with it responsibility for evaluating the impact of that care on the health and welfare of that population. The evaluation of health status reflects in part the impact of medical care and in part the effect of social and other factors. If it is desired to disentangle the effects of these two factors (medical care versus other), a great deal of attention needs to be given to the choice of measures of health and, even more important, to study design. The paucity of quantitative normative standards and the need for controls, dictate some kind of comparative study, usually observational, sometimes experimental. The study of socioeconomic differentials in health status and the manner in which such differentials change over time in response to changes in the organization of health services is an interesting evaluative tool which is also linked to basic policy issues and values. However, knowledge about what perpetuates or changes socioeconomic gradients in health status is incomplete at present. Socioeconomic gradients in the use of service, and the manner in which they change in response to medical care organization, would be easier to study and to interpret. There is evidence that such differences can be markedly reduced, but not abolished, through the institution of prepaid group practice (281, 288).

Health Status as a Determinant of Medical Care Priorities

Of the three uses for measurements of health status—translation into service and resource equivalents, evaluation of effectiveness, and the determination of priorities—this section will deal with the third. The question to which it addresses itself is the determination of what health problems are most "important" and, therefore, call for most attention in planning and in the allocation of resources. Here we shall deal mainly with technical considerations in the determination of priorities, although it will become clear that values permeate even these. Other, and perhaps more important, considerations in setting priorities—for example, political leverage and community support—will be excluded.

ELEMENTS IN THE DETERMINATION OF PRIORITIES. A simple notion underlies technical estimates of priority. Those health problems are most important which cause the greatest loss and are most amenable to prevention and amelioration. There are, however, a number of elements in the computation of loss, each of which derives from a somewhat different interpretation of value, brings its own contribution to the priority estimate, and modifies the relative contribution of other elements to the whole. As a prelude to more detailed discussion it may be useful to list these several components or alternatives in priority estimates, as follows:

A. Magnitude of loss
  1. Time lost due to death
  2. Time lost due to morbidity
  3. Single year losses versus lifetime losses
  4. The factor of productivity of time lost
  5. Losses due to the cost of care

B. Amenability to prevention or reduction

Magnitude of Loss. The elements that determine the magnitude of loss can be used singly or in combination to produce a variety of estimates each of which rests on different assumptions and may yield a different priority of health problems. The estimate of priority may rest on losses due to death or morbidity, or both combined. Each of these may be expressed in terms of time lost, productive time lost, or income foregone, and to each may be added the losses incurred due to the cost of care. Even when one considers that losses from morbidity are estimated for single years only, and that direct costs are only included when the measure of loss is income foregone, the number of possible combinations of elements is large. Fortunately, a description of a smaller set of these is sufficient to provide an understanding of the issues involved in the choice of estimate. The following discussion of the major determinants of priorities should, however, be read keeping in mind the more detailed presentation of morbidity and mortality in previous sections.

Loss of life due to mortality is an exceedingly imperfect indicator of the losses produced by a "health problem" or disease category. As the reader is well aware, this is because death constitutes only a small segment of the "biological gradient" of disease and because this segment varies markedly by disease. Nevertheless, the ready availability of mortality statistics, and the relative unavailability of alternative information, has made death the most frequently used determinant of the magnitude of loss from disease. The distortions that result from this are made worse by the inaccuracies in the reporting of the causes of death and the insistence that only one cause of death be tabulated. As Dorn and Moriyama point out, "the usual interpretation of (mortality) data is that they indicate the relative importance of the various causes of death. Yet this rank order is largely determined by the rules for selecting the underlying cause of death and by the way the causes are grouped" (152). A better estimate is obtained when losses from morbidity are added to those from mortality. This addition results in a rather significant rearrangement of priorities so that greater prominence is accorded the less fatal, but highly persistent and disabling diseases. Unfortunately, most representative population-wide morbidity information derives from household interview surveys and suffers from all the limitations of that method, including the fact that diagnostic categorization is highly invalid. Surveys of physician and hospital records linked with household interviews are needed to rectify this deficiency. In the meantime, rough estimates are possible on the basis of partial data. Another problem that has not been satisfactorily resolved is the concurrent presence of more than one illness which may be jointly responsible for disability. Since concurrent diseases are seldom equal in their contribution to disability, any system of partitioning must be highly arbitrary. Finally, one must determine what degree of disability constitutes a "loss" for purposes of counting. As we have seen, the degree of disability may vary over a wide spectrum, so that no one cut-off point is likely to be satisfactory. For all these reasons, current estimates of losses from specific disease categories are to be considered provisional, rough estimates.

The next issue is whether morbidity losses during any one year are to be combined with losses due to death during that year, or whether one must add the life-time losses from the deaths that occur during that year. We have already referred to this question in our discussion of summary measures of health and illness. When deaths are considered to produce a loss only during the year within which they occur (roughly an average of one-half year of loss per death) the effect is that deaths at any age are considered to be of equal value. However, if each death is considered to represent interruption of an expected average course of life, the earlier a death occurs, the greater is the loss attributed to it. Accordingly, deaths in the young are considered to have produced much greater loss than deaths among the aged. The effect is that a higher valuation is placed on the fatal diseases of infancy and childhood, whereas the survival of the aged is relatively devalued. The other effect is that the relative weights of mortality and morbidity are radically altered in favor of the first, since morbidity is considered to produce losses during a given year and mortality is considered to have produced losses over an expected lifetime.

So far, a year or day lost to mortality or morbidity has been considered equal to any other period of similar duration no matter when during the life span of an individual it occurs and no matter who is the individual affected. This method of priority estimation embodies a strongly egalitarian bias which some have challenged. The challengers have generally based their argument on the fact that some years of life, namely, the working years, are economically more productive than others. One might go further and say that some persons have a socially more highly valued product, so that the loss of some is more grievous than the loss of others. Interestingly enough, as far as we know, no one has yet gone so far as to explicitly place different values on different persons in computations of health priorities, even though the differential valuation of man is insisted upon in almost every other sphere. This may be due in part to the fact that the egalitarian argument is more applicable to health, as we have pointed out in our first chapter. To take a more cynical view, this may be mainly because the issue has been largely theoretical, with little practical impact on the allocation of resources to health in our society. Whatever the reason, the major application of differential values has been to the "economically productive" years. This definition does, however, raise questions about the value of those who are unemployed and, more important, the value of housewives whose product is not included in the national income accounts. These issues derive from the manner in which the factor of production enters the computation of losses from death and illness. This computation may be done in two ways: (1) the measurement of potential productive time lost, generally the years between 15 and 65, or (2) the estimation of the dollar value of the product lost. The money value of lost product is generally an estimate of the present value of future income lost due to death or illness. Since the value of money in hand is greater than the promise of money yet to be earned, the latter has to be reduced by a yearly "discount rate" so that the present value of future income is lowered in proportion to the remoteness of the actual possession of that income. Generally, some average value—for example, average wages—is applied to all time losses, so that all persons in the labor force are treated equally. There is, however, some difficulty in estimating the output of nonemployed housewives. Feminists have been dismayed by the decision in one series of studies to assign housewives the average earnings of a domestic worker!

(250). To summarize, then, the placing of a money value on life lost due to illness and death tends to devalue the young (who have no current earnings and whose future income is discounted over many years), the old, and perhaps many women, so that diseases that have a proportionately large impact on these persons are lowered in priority ranking. Another consequence of the emphasis on loss of product, whether expressed in time or dollars, is that some tangibles, and many intangibles, are omitted from the computation. The tangibles include the loss of productivity due to suboptimal performance brought about by levels of ill health that do not completely interrupt work (246). The intangibles include pain, suffering, grief, family disruption, and the like. Since some diseases and certain personal or family situations are more likely to be associated with unmeasured losses than are others, the priority rankings of "health problems" may be altered by these omissions. Finally, there are a large number of technical issues in the measurement of the money value of lost product which only an economist can competently discuss and which may have some effect on priority ranking (245–250). These include the magnitude of the discount rate to be used to estimate the present value of future income, how to handle the question of unemployment, whether taxes and transfer payments are to be included in the cost of illness, and whether the loss of the nonproductive (children and aged) is partly a gain because it reduces consumption, or is a loss for the same reason.

The losses of output due to illness and death represent the "indirect cost" of illness. There is also a "direct cost" which consists of expenditures for actual health services (consumption) as well as the current value of the investment in the production of health services as represented by research, training, and capital investment in facilities and equipment. The addition of direct costs to indirect might conceivably alter the priority rankings of disease by emphasizing those diseases that require a great deal of costly care and last a long time. In addition to the nature of disease, direct costs reflect current levels of medical technology and medical care organization. They also reflect the many complex factors that influence utilization of care by type of disease and by socioeconomic and geographic attributes of clients. Any element in the priority estimate that reflects levels of use of service introduces a curious circularity by which the priority estimate creates further priority. In other words, a disease on which we spend a great deal becomes one for which one ought to spend a great deal. A particular example of an analogous situation will be discussed later in this section.

Table III.28.   Specified estimates of the cost of mental illness, according to basis for the estimate, U.S.A., specified years

Source	Year	Basis of Estimate	Cost estimate (in billions)
Fein, R. (Ref. 247, pp. 57–58)	1952	Loss of earnings to persons institutionalized due to mental illness and cost of care for both institutionalized and noninstitutionalized persons.	$2.4 (2.6)[a]
Rice, D. (Ref. 250, p. 81)	1963	Added to the above is the loss of the product of the non-institutionalized mentally ill who are "unable to work" or who suffered "work loss."	$7 (6.6)[a]
Conley et al. (Ref. 253)	1966	Used a "broad definition" of mental illness and included, in addition to losses due to inability to work, the losses due to "reduction of productivity among the unemployed mentally ill," as well as the cost of a "wider range of treatment services."	$19.5 (17.2)[a]

[a] Adjusted for changes in consumer prices: 1957–1959 = 100. See Statistical Abstracts of the United States, 1969, Table 500.

A study by Conley et al. illustrates the effects of several factors on estimates of the cost of mental illness (253). A comparison of their own estimates with those made by others demonstrates how sensitive are such estimates to factors such as the definition of mental illness and the nature of the losses included in the estimates. A brief summary is given in Table III.28. Conley et al. point out that even their much higher estimate does not include the cost of "illegal and other undesirable behavior" or of the "intangible psychic loss that so often accompanies mental illness."

AMENABILITY TO PREVENTION OR REDUCTION. The second set of factors in estimates of priority relate to the readiness with which the disease may be prevented or its adverse effects minimized. Magnitude of loss and amenability are two essentially independent properties which jointly constitute decision rules or guides for health action. Assuming only two degrees of each, Table III.29 serves as an illustration of possible decision rules:

Table III.29.   Decisions concerning priority that correspond to levels of the magnitude of loss from hypothetical illnesses and to levels of the amenability of such illness to medical intervention.

Magnitude	Amenability	Decision
High	High	High priority for delivery of service
High	Low	High priority for research
Low	High	Second priority for delivery of service
Low	Low	Second priority for research Lowest priority for delivery of service

Amenability is, of course, a function of the state of medical science and technology as well as of the organization and delivery of health services. Although the two factors are interrelated, it is useful to think of the two separately. It is quite possible that a disease may be technically subject to ready control, but for a variety of reasons be resistant to control, because the technology cannot be implemented. Hence, it may be useful to distinguish technical amenability from social or operational amenability. It is operational amenability that is the more relevant to the setting of priorities for action.

Amenability is more accurately portrayed by a relationship between inputs and outputs. The inputs may be stated either as measures of work or of effort, or as expenditures. The outputs can be stated, in this context, either as states of health or ill health, or as the money value (positive or negative) of such states. Usually one uses the following pairings: (1) effort-effect relations, or (2) cost-benefit relations. The relationship between effort and effect, or between cost and benefit, is best represented by an equation or graph. In terms of this relationship, the following problems face the inclusion of sophisticated amenability estimates in the assessment of priorities: (1) the nature of the relationship for any one disease and any given input is very poorly understood. (2) The relationship is likely to be curvilinear, as shown in Fig. III.16. (3) The relationship is likely to differ by disease and by type of input, and perhaps for the same disease in different ecological (including social) settings. (4) Because of curvilinearity, the rate of change in response for any unit of change in input is different at various points on the curve. Hence, the yield differs depending on the magnitude of the health problem in the

Fig. III.16.   Hypothetical input-output relationships signifying the amenability of disease to prevention of amelioration

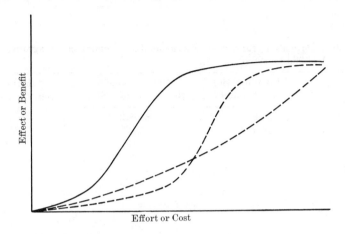

population at the time additional effort is implemented. By the same token, there is a level of prevalence below which a great deal of effort produces very little response. Also, effort below a certain range produces very little response. (5) Because of certain interrelationships among health problems, any one set of inputs may have effects on several categories of disease or health problem. It would be necessary to get an estimate of this total effect in arriving at estimates of priority. (6) For the same reason, the incremental effect of any input may depend, at least to some extent, on the type and level of inputs already present. (7) Any one health problem may be susceptible to amelioration through the effect of a variety of inputs. Hence one must search for the input that has the greatest effect (benefit) in relation to effort (cost). It may well be that this is not a medical care action, but something else—nutrition, for example, or housing, or education. Frequently, it is some form of environmental control procedure.

Several of the characteristics enumerated above are due to the fact that we are dealing with a delicately balanced but highly interactive system. Axnick et al. provide a rather elegant example of how a change in the ecology of disease brought about by a health-oriented action can itself influence, in this instance favorably, the effectiveness of further action. They show that expenditures on immunization for measles bring about progressively greater benefits relative to expenditures. This is because the effect of immunization persists beyond the year during which it is received. Furthermore as the density of immunized children increases, their very presence becomes an obstacle to the propagation of disease from one susceptible person to another. The data are shown in Table III.30.

Table III.30.   Estimated yearly costs and benefiits of immunization against measles, U.S.A., 1963 to 1968

Year	Cost of Immunization (thousands of dollars)	Dollar Benefits (thousands of dollars)	Ratio of Benefits to Cost
1963	$11,700	$5,842	0.5
1964	12,900	2,161	0.2
1965	18,900	55,189	2.9
1966	24,300	88,231	3.7
1967	19,500	160,040	8.2
1968	21,000	220,080	10.5

SOURCE: Reference 254 and personal communication.

Special considerations arise when one is confronted with a situation in which an infectious disease may be eradicated. We have, intuitively, postulated a relationship between effort and effect that will progressively yield diminishing returns after a certain intensity of effort has been exceeded. If one could envisage, however, that with still greater effort a disease could be eradicated, a benefit would accrue in perpetuity. In this instance, as in the one preceding, the time horizon becomes a critical element in the evaluation of inputs relative to outputs. Another example of change in basic relationships over time is the spread of infectious disease if efforts at control are relaxed or eliminated. Thus a disease of low-current priority will gain progressively in importance if it is not held in check by current expenditures of effort.

The complexity of the system is readily apparent. Equally great is our ignorance of anything approaching even a crude statement of the quantitative relationship between input and output. For this reason, only the crudest statements of amenability can usually be included in estimates of priority. Fortunately, in practice, it is rarely necessary to know the complete effort-effect curve. The realistic question faced is whether further expenditures on one program directed at disease A will yield more (in days of health or their money value) than similar additional expenditures on another program directed at disease A or disease B. For such purposes it is only necessary to have some estimate of the slope of the effort-effect curve over the relatively short, relevant stretch of the amenability function. Such estimates usually rest on informed guesses by experts. However, the Division of Indian Health has hit upon a rather brilliant statagem for arriving at an estimate of amenability for any given health problem (255–257). This is derived from a ratio of the magnitude of a health problem in the "target group" (the population for whom plans are to be made) to the magnitude of the same problem in a "reference group" (a standard population). The ratio

$$\frac{\text{magnitude of health problem in target population}}{\text{magnitude of health problem in reference population}}$$

measures what we have called the "operational amenability" of that problem to the influences of whatever incremental factors are operative in the standard population. In other words, the state of health in the standard population tells us what is possible given more favorable conditions, and directs our attention to those problems which show the greatest excess over the standard. This approach to the determination of amenability will be further discussed in a subsequent section.

In concluding the discussion on the elements which go into determining priorities, it is useful once again to emphasize the limitations in knowledge and data. Current estimates are at best crude and, of necessity, based on assumptions and computational methods that are not always fully justified. The medical care administrator ought to examine carefully the data and the manner in which they are used. In doing so he will be particularly impressed by the confidence with which persons from other disciplines walk in areas where he himself is reluctant to tread. This may be partly a matter of less knowledge on the part of the former of all the possibilities of error. It may, in part, be justified by the assertion, often heard, that even crude estimates are better than none. While this is often true, the administrator should also be aware of the dangers of misplaced concreteness. Etzioni has expressed very well the dangers of measuring only what is measurable in the process of evaluation and planning in organizations:

Most organizations under pressure to be rational are eager to measure their efficiency. Curiously, the very effort—the desire to establish how we are doing and to find ways of improving if we are not doing as well as we ought to—often has quite undesired effects from the point of view of the organizational goals. Frequent measuring can distort the organizational effort because, as a rule, some aspects of its output are more measurable than the others. Frequent measuring tends to encourage over-production of highly measurable items and neglect of the less measurable ones . . . The distortion consequences of over-measuring are larger when it is impossible or impractical to quantify the more central, substantive output of an organization, and when at the same time some exterior aspects of the product which are superficially related to its substance, are readily measurable (243, pp. 9–11).

ILLUSTRATIONS OF THE RELATIVE MAGNITUDE OF HEALTH PROBLEMS. In this section we shall present some examples of the relative importance of the several elements in determining the magnitude of loss due to illness and illustrate how the relationships between morbidity and mortality, as well as the rank ordering of selected diseases, is altered in consequence of selecting specified measures of loss in preference to others. It is hoped that this will lend greater concreteness to, and result in a firmer grasp of, the general considerations in the previous section. Almost all of the illustrations are derived from the work of Dorothy Rice at the Social Security Administration.

Fig. III.17 shows how the relative weights of morbidity and mortality from all diseases are altered as different elements are selected to compute loss. The major difference, as one would expect, is between single-year losses from mortality and lifetime losses from that cause. The introduction of the notion of productivity causes some reduction in the relative weight of mortality, especially when computed over a lifetime. This effect is evident when one compares Bars (3) and (4) of Fig. III.17, which use man-years as the unit of measurement, as well as Bars (5) and (2) which compare man-years to dollar value of output lost.

In order to illustrate effects by disease category, three such categories from the International Classification were selected. These were chosen to differ widely with respect to case fatality, chronicity, and age distribution, as follows: (A) "Diseases of the nervous system and sense organs" are heavily loaded with chronic and fatal diseases of older persons, including strokes; (B) "Diseases of bones and organs of movement" are largely represented by various forms of arthritis which involve mature and old persons, producing considerable disability, but which are not frequently reported as causes of death; and (C) "Certain diseases of early infancy and congenital malformations" obviously occur in the very young and, in addition, are often fatal. Fig. III.18 shows the absolute losses in man-years from annual (single-year) morbidity, annual (single-year) mortality, and the increment over single-year losses from mortality that occurs when one considers lifetime losses from mortality. It is clear that in Category A there is a great deal of morbidity and a fair amount of mortality during any one year, but that the effect of mortality is not well represented unless lifetime losses are computed, at which time it becomes the dominant element. In Category B we see clearly the extent to which mortality alone, even when computed to include lifetime losses, would greatly underestimate the impact of the disease group. The third Cate-

Fig. III.17.   Percent distribution of components of the costs of illness[a]
by type of cost, using specified methods of computation (U.S.A., 1963)

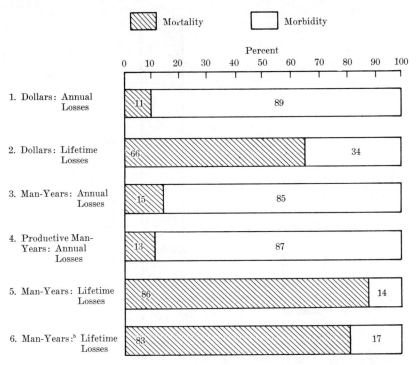

SOURCES: Reference 250, Tables on pp. 58, 66, 81, 94, and 110, and ref. 255.

[a] Only "indirect" economic losses arising from loss of output are included. Losses
due to morbidity are annual losses. To this are added losses due to mortality computed
either for one year ("annual losses") or for expected remaining years of life
("lifetime losses"). The basic method for computing economic value of lost output
was to apply prevailing average earnings to productive time lost which was defined as
time lost to work or housework. Lifetime earnings were discounted at 6 percent.

[b] Q Index, Division of Indian Health (see pp. 179 ff).

gory (C), shows how certain diseases of infancy that are rather infrequent, so that losses from morbidity do not show on the graph, cause
tremendous loss by interrupting life almost at its inception. These three
disease categories have, of course, been chosen to make a point and, to
that extent, are not representative. On the other hand, if one were able to
select single-disease entities, rather than categories of disease, differences
even more extreme would have been revealed.

Another way of seeing the effects of these same factors is to examine

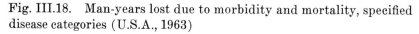

Fig. III.18.   Man-years lost due to morbidity and mortality, specified disease categories (U.S.A., 1963)

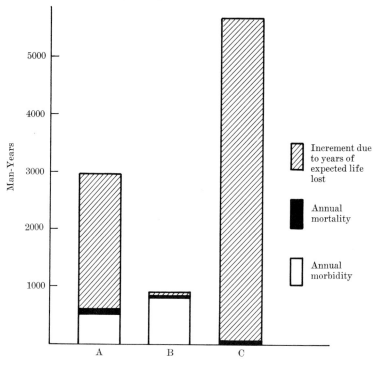

SOURCE: Reference 250, Tables on pp. 20, 66, and 99.
DISEASES: A. Diseases of the nervous system and sense organs. B. Diseases of bones and organs of movement. C. Certain diseases of early infancy and congenital malformations.

how the relative positions of the three disease categories are altered when one uses different elements in the assessment of the magnitude of loss expressed in man-years. The top half of Fig. III.19 shows the relative priorities expressed as percentages of total time loss attributed to the three disease categories combined. The radical changes in relative magnitude of loss attributed to each disease category, depending on the elements in the assessment, are very clear. In particular, Bars (1) and (2) show the effects of including morbidity in the computation; and Bars (3) and (4) show the effect of the change from single-year losses from mortality to lifetime losses. The effect of computations on the basis of using the economic cost of illness and death are shown in the bottom half of the same figure. Bars (4) and (5) in Fig. III.19 are analogous. However, Bar (5) shows the influence of the element of productivity. As a result of including this factor, diseases of the nervous system, which influence adults and interfere with current productivity, gain in relative weight over diseases of early infancy. Deaths from the latter cause prevent earning rather far in the future and therefore lose more in

Fig. III.19.   Relative significance of specified diseases using specified criteria (U.S.A., 1963)

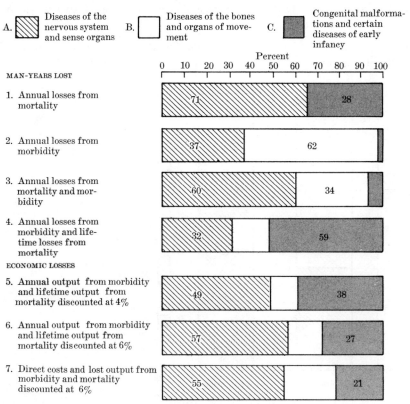

SOURCE: Reference 250, Tables on pp. 20, 66, 99, 109 and 110.
    The basic method for computing economic value of lost output was to apply prevailing average earnings to productive time lost which was defined as time lost to work or housework. Direct costs of illness comprise expenditures for prevention, detection, treatment, rehabilitation, research, training, and capital investment in medical facilities.

present value through discounting. Bar (6) shows that the rate of discount itself has an appreciable effect. Diseases of early infancy are further devalued in relation to the diseases that affect persons in their productive years when the rate of discount is increased from 4 percent (in Bar 5) to 6 percent. Finally, Bar (7) shows the effect of adding some direct costs to the computation. Such costs appear to be relatively high in diseases of bones and organs of movement, and relatively lower in diseases of early infancy. Accordingly, the relative priorities are still further altered.

The relationships of direct costs to indirect costs are shown in a more general way in Fig. III.20. The figure shows, for each of two ways of

Fig. III.20.　Percent distribution of components of the costs of illness[a] by type of cost, using two methods of computation (U.S.A., 1963)

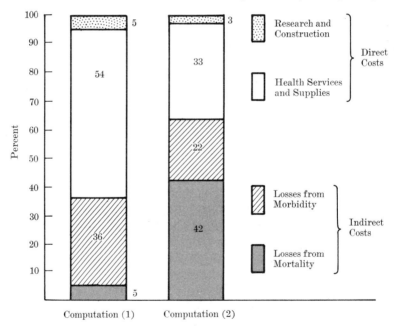

Computation 1: Yearly direct costs plus yearly losses from morbidity and mortality.
Computation 2: Yearly direct costs, yearly losses from morbidity and life-time losses from mortality.
[a] Economic value of lost output is computed by applying prevailing average earnings to productive time lost. Life-time earnings were discounted at 6%.
SOURCES: U.S. Department of Health, Education and Welfare, *Social Security Administration, Research and Statistics Note No. 10–1965.* Washington, D.C., May 3, 1965 and reference 250, Table 19, p. 77, and Table 32, p. 110.

computing mortality losses (single-year and lifetime losses), the relative weights of the indirect losses from morbidity and mortality as well as the direct costs of expenditures on health in two categories: research and construction (investment), and health services and supplies (consumption).

SOME SPECIFIC PROPOSALS. In this section we shall describe, and comment briefly on, some specific proposals for ranking health problems. These examples are offered partly as a consolation for the practitioner who has become discouraged by the preceding analysis; but mainly as illustrations of the application of the more general concepts already discussed, and some further elaboration of these concepts.

Indices of Health. Some of the indices of health that we have described in an earlier section could, theoretically, produce a measure of time lost due to illness and mortality, if the necessary data were available. The complement of the Chiang Index is a measure of time lost due to morbidity and mortality during a single year (202). The index proposed by Fanshel and Bush is expressed as function-years of life per person, assuming a life span of 90 years (206). Hence, 90 minus the function-years of life would be a measure of losses due to illness. As we have pointed out, the Chiang Index assumes that each death causes one-half year of loss of life during the year in which it occurs. The Fanshel and Bush index would, by contrast, yield life-time losses from morbidity and mortality combined. In addition, it would weight different levels of disability according to functional loss. This is an important feature that has been absent from the measures of losses from illness that we have described in this section, although one could argue that direct costs of care might be a proxy for severity of disability. Another feature of the measures of health and illness is that they do not explicitly include the factor of productivity. All days lost appear to be equal in worth irrespective of what part of the life span is abridged. But this may not be completely so, because the definition and weighting of disability does include in it the factor of inability to do gainful work for those whose "major activity" is to do so.

Needless to say, the factor of amenability would have to be added, if the measures of loss derived from the health index were to be used for the purpose of determining priorities for action.

The "Q-Index," Division of Indian Health. For some years the Division of Indian Health has been at work on a system for planning, resource allocation, and evaluation which has attracted considerable attention both within and outside government. An important feature of this system has been the "Q-Index," a method for determining the relative importance of disease categories to be used as a guide in the allocation of resources (255–257). Since the system is in process of development and testing, several variants of the Index have appeared. The version which we use is not necessarily the latest. It is presented here mainly as an illustration of the basic concepts involved in its construction. For any disease category, or for all diseases combined,

$$\text{Index } Q = M\,D\,P + \frac{C}{N}\,(274) + \frac{A}{N}\,(274) + \frac{B}{N}\,(91)$$

(1) M = Health Problem Ratio
   The ratio of the age adjusted death rate of the target population to the age adjusted death rate of the reference population. (The "target population" is the one for which plans are being made. The "reference population" is the one which serves as a desirable standard of achievement.)

(2) D = Crude mortality rate per 100,000 per year in the target population.

(3) P = Average years of life lost due to each death over a lifetime.

(4) C = Days of restricted activity during the year in the target population.

(5) A = Number of inpatient days during the year in the target population.

(6) B = Number of outpatient visits during the year in the target population.

(7) N = Number of persons in the target population.

(8) $274 = \dfrac{100,000}{365}$ = Conversion constant used to change restricted activity days or inpatient days to years (since mortality losses are expressed in years).

(9) $91 = \dfrac{100,000}{365} \times \frac{1}{3}$ = Conversion constant used to change days into years, assuming each outpatient visit equals the loss of $\frac{1}{3}$ day of activity.

The Index, then, has several major components:

   Estimate of amenability   M
   Estimate of magnitude of loss
      Lifetime losses due to mortality   D and P
      Single year losses due to morbidity   C, A, and B.

Each of these major components will be discussed briefly below. It seems reasonable to discuss first the elements that determine the magnitude of loss and then the factor of amenability.

The magnitude of loss is measured in man-years of life, with all years given equal weight. In some versions of the formula, the term "P" stands for "productive years," defined as those between the ages of 15 and 65. The substitution of productive years for all years would obviously exclude the effect of deaths above 65 and reduce appreciably the effect of deaths below 15. Maximum weight would be given deaths in young adults, of both sexes, since productivity, as defined here, would not depend on employment but simply on age. In none of the versions of the formula that the author has seen has there been an adjustment for productivity applied to the morbidity terms (C, A, or B). The three determinants of losses from morbidity should, of course be mutually exclusive so that no double counting occurs. But even with this precaution, a problem arises because of the inclusion of two terms—hospital stay and clinic visits—that are measures of use of service as well as measures of time lost. These terms reflect not only the occurrence of disability, but also the effects of all the many factors that influence the availability of service and the receipt of care. Hence, a disease which receives much care stakes a claim for high priority for further care. However, the magnitude of the morbidity losses in relation to the lifetime losses from mortality is so small that the distortion we refer to above may not be important. This also applies to omission of productivity adjustments to the morbidity terms. The Division of Indian Health, and later the Bureau of Health Services, has studiously avoided the placing of a money value on life, even though they have at times emphasized the productive time lost from mortality. Nor has there been an attempt to incorporate a measure of the direct cost of illness. The terms A and B do, of course, represent indirectly the costs of hospital and outpatient care, in addition to reflecting disability. Their contribution in this respect could perhaps be more equitably represented by some process of weighting. If the average cost per hospital day and per clinic visit were known, it would seem reasonable to add to each of the two terms (A and B) a number of work days equal in value to the cost of care received. The rationale is simple. For each day of time lost receiving care, there are also losses which can be represented as man-days of work that needs to be done to pay for the cost of care. This is output deflected from other uses to meet needs created by illness. This suggestion makes the general point that economic losses can be converted to a uniform measure of time lost using the same rationale which has been used to place a money value on time lost. The essential thing is to use the same unit (of time or money) to sum all the losses.

The rationale underlying the use of "health problem ratio" as a measure of amenability has already been mentioned. Briefly, the degree to which a health problem is of smaller magnitude in the reference population, as compared to the target population, indicates the ameliorating effects of certain conditions in the former. We do not know, however, what these helpful conditions might be, nor are we certain that they necessarily belong under the general rubric of "health actions." Furthermore, it is not clear what should be the standard population. Should this population be one that is similar in socioeconomic and other ecological circumstances to that of the target population? Or should the comparison be with experience in the "best" identifiable group in the nation? Obviously, the conclusions drawn might be different. Under ideal circumstances, the two populations would be similar in all respects except for the inputs whose effectiveness it is desired to test. This would argue for the comparison of populations that are roughly similar with respect to urban-rural residence, occupational characteristics, and the like. Needless to say, adjustments also need to be made for differences in age and sex. Also, because amenability varies by disease, adjustments for differences in disease mix should be made when a single representative (national or areawide) ratio is to be computed.

The version of the Q-Index that we have given includes an amenability factor for mortality only. This means that the factor of mortality is likely to be even further enhanced in relation to morbidity. Other versions have included terms that could be interpreted to signify that amenability of certain components of morbidity was also incorporated in the Index. For example, an amenability ratio could be attached to "days of restricted activity" (term C) under the same rationale applied to mortality. There are, however, certain serious reservations to doing so, partly because the occurrence of restricted activity in response to a given level of illness is much influenced by economic and social factors. Moreover, as we have seen, more effective treatment may reduce mortality but increase morbidity from the same cause. This last characteristic is not necessarily a limitation in this instance, because one might argue that a disease in which mortality can be reduced without increases in morbidity is more amenable than another in which mortality can be decreased but at the cost of increased morbidity. The remaining two terms in the Index are, as we have pointed out, qualitatively different because they are also measures of service. In computing a "health problem ratio" for these terms it would be necessary first to correct for differences in the composition, incidence, and prevalence of illness. In other words, for each homogeneous or comparable disease category, one needs to compare use of service per 1000 patient-days, rather than per 1000 persons, including the well. When this is done, it may well be that the use of service is higher in the standard population, signifying amenability to care, though not necessarily amenability to improvement in health status. Amenability to improvement and suitability for care are of course related. However, there are certain basic differences between them, when used as priority estimates, which will be emphasized when we discuss planning in terms of health status in the concluding paragraphs of this chapter. Finally, one must consider whether amenability should be combined with the measure of magnitude of loss (as is done in the Q-Index) or kept separate. As we have indicated, different decision rules flow from different combinations of levels of amenability and levels of loss. This would suggest that, at least at some point, the two measures should be examined separately.

The foregoing has been an attempt to analyze the characteristics of the Q-Index as a measure of priority. The space devoted to this subject does not necessarily indicate the value of the Index. It does indicate the need to understand thoroughly any index before it is put to use. Additional insights into the Q-Index, or any other, would occur when it is subjected to empirical testing so as to determine what are the contributions of each of its components to the total, and to see how the total compares with other, and perhaps simpler, measures of priority. As we have already pointed out, and as shown in Bar 6 of Fig. III.17, the Q-Index is overwhelmingly a measure of lifetime losses from mortality. Accordingly, one wonders how the rankings by disease category would differ from those that one would obtain using crude mortality alone. The Bureau of Health Services, Public Health Service, has provided computations from which may be derived priority rankings, in the United States as a whole, for selected disease categories by the Q-Index and by cause-specific mortality (255). These rankings and the difference between them are shown in Table III.31. The table also shows the contribution to the total Q-Index of its component elements. In this computation, because the U.S. population is itself the reference population usually employed, the amenability factor M is taken to equal 1. Hence, the effect of differences in amenability is, unfortunately, not demonstrated. For all disease, it is clear that losses from mortality are by far the dominant factor, with losses from restricted activity a poor second. Losses from hospital stay or ambulatory care are negligible by comparison. The relative contribution of the several elements does, however, vary markedly by disease category. In spite of this, the priority rankings are not drastically altered when the Q-Index is used in place of losses from mortality by cause. The Bureau of Health Services has also conducted studies in Maryland, with a view to

Table III.31. Contributions of specified elements of the total Q-Index, priority rankings by the Q-Index and by crude mortality rate, and differences in priority rankings using the foregoing two criteria, specified disease categories, U.S.A., 1963–1964

Causes of Death	Percent of Total Q Value Contributed by Each Element Specified Below[a]				Priority Ranks		
	DP	$\frac{C}{N}$ (274)	$\frac{A}{N}$ (274)	$\frac{B}{N}$ (91)	By Q-Index (1)	By Mortality (2)	Difference[b] (2)−(1)
ALL CAUSES	83	13	2	2	—	—	—
I. Infective and parasitic	40	52	1	6	6	8	+2
II. Neoplasms	97	1	1	0.4	3	2	−1
VI. Nervous system	92	4	1	3	5	3	−2
VII. Circulatory system	97	1	1	1	1	1	0
VIII. Respiratory system	42	52	5	5	4	5	+1
IX. Digestive system	78	13	8	3	6	6	0
X. Genitourinary system	70	19	18	3	8	7	−1
XI. Complications of pregnancy	20	53	4	8	9	11	+2
XII. Skin and cellular tissue	26	46	19	24	11	9	−2
XIII. Bone and organs of movement	16	49	1	15	10	10	0
XVII. Accidents, poisonings, etc.	82	16	1	1	2	4	+2

SOURCE: Reference 255.

a $M = 1$. For key to symbols see page 180.

b Plus sign means increase in priority brought about by Q-Index; minus sign means a reduction in priority brought about by using Q-Index as compared with mortality losses alone.

applying the Q-Index to the population of a state (256). However, the difficulties in obtaining data were so great, and so many compromises had to be made, that to report the findings would be only to mislead.

Health Problem Index, Pan American Health Organization. A publication on planning issued by the Pan American Health Organization proposes a method for ranking diseases using three elements: (1) "incidence," (2) "importance," and (3) "vulnerability" (258). *"Incidence"* is measured by the proportional mortality ratio, which is the ratio of the mortality from one disease to the total mortality from all diseases. A refinement in computing the ratio is offered so as to allow "for the existence of certain diseases typical of particular age groups" (258, p. 24). *"Importance"* alludes to the differences in the impact of death in different age groups. The considerations are analogous to those we have already discussed in connection with lifetime losses from mortality with and without corrections for "productivity" or for money value of lost output. The issues are not, however, explicitly or rigorously discussed. It is recognized that adult lives may be regarded as "more important than those of children and still more important than those of old people." On the other hand, the reverse position may be taken, so that the "coefficient of importance" is:

1   for each death below 15 years of age
0.75 for each death between 15 and 69 years
0.50 for each death at other ages

Assuming that the importance of death is inversely proportional to age at death (all years of equal value) an alternative, and more extended, scale is proposed which assigns the weight of 1 to children less than one year old and reduces this by one-hundredth for each subsequent year of age, as shown in Table III.32.

Table III.32.   Proposed coefficients of importance (weights) for deaths occurring at specified ages

Age	Coefficient of Importance	Age	Coefficient of Importance
below 1	1.00	50	0.50
1	0.99	60	0.40
2	0.98	65	0.35
5	0.95	70	0.30
10	0.90	80	0.20
20	0.80	90	0.10
30	0.70	100	0.00

SOURCE: Reference 258.

"Vulnerability" is analogous to, but not synonymous with, "amenability" as we have used it. It signifies the degree of response to health action. However, the Pan American Health Organization makes a distinction between the vulnerability of morbidity and the vulnerability of mortality, and confines its attention to the first. The concern, apparently, is with the ability to prevent illness rather than the fatal consequence once illness occurs. Using this limited definition of vulnerability, a four-point scale is proposed as shown in Table III.33.

Table III.33.   A proposed classification of disease according to vulnerability to control, corresponding coefficients (weights), and examples of diseases in each class

Vulnerability of Disease	Coefficient of Vulnerability	Examples
Eradicable	1.00	Smallpox
Reducible	0.66 or ⅔	"Majority of communicable diseases": dysentery, gastritis, duodenitis, pulmonary tuberculosis.
	0.33 or ⅓	Influenza, the pneumonias and bronchitis, transportation accidents.
Nonreducible	"Near zero" For example, 0.1	Cardiovascular diseases, tumors, accidents, excluding transportation.

SOURCE: Reference 258, page 25, and Table 3, page 28.

The determination of what diseases are "eradicable," "reducible," or "nonreducible" is primarily a matter of expert judgment. There is recognition, however, that estimates of vulnerability, at least for some diseases, might be obtained from comparisons of the trends of disease in different populations (258, p. 26n).

Under the foregoing assumptions, the health problem index is computed to equal:

$$\begin{pmatrix} \text{Proportionate} \\ \text{mortality} \\ \text{ratio} \end{pmatrix} \cdot \begin{pmatrix} \text{Coefficient} \\ \text{of} \\ \text{importance} \end{pmatrix} \cdot \begin{pmatrix} \text{Coefficient} \\ \text{of} \\ \text{vulnerability} \end{pmatrix}$$

In the above computations the proportionate mortality ratio is expressed as a percentage, whereas the other two terms are decimal fractions, as shown above. The incremental contributions of each of the terms to the

priority rating has been tested in an empirical application to the State of
Aragua, Venezuela, 1966 (258). Table III.34 gives the priority rankings

Table III.34.   Ranking of specified diseases from highest to lowest priority,
using specified factors in the determination of priority. State of Aragua,
Venezuela, 1966

Causes of Death	Factors Taken into Account in Priority		
	Proportionate Mortality	Proportionate Mortality, and Importance	Proportionate Mortality, Importance, and Vulnerability
Cardiovascular disease	1	1	4
Dysentery, gastritis, duodenitis, etc.	2	2	1
Premature births	3	3	2
Tumors	4	4	8
Accidents (excluding transportation)	5	6	9
Influenza, pneumonia, bronchitis	6	5	3
Transportation accidents	7	7	6
Pulmonary tuberculosis	8	9	5
Other diseases of early childhood	9	8	7

SOURCE: Reference 258, Tables 1–3, pages 27–28.

of certain disease categories when specified factors are taken into account. Examination of the table shows that the inclusion of a coefficient
of importance makes little difference in ranking over the use of mortality
alone. This, however, should be interpreted keeping in mind the considerable degree of grouping of diseases in the above categories. The
inclusion of a coefficient of vulnerability does appear to be critical. In
summary, the proposed index, though conceptually more primitive than
it needs to be, provides a rough-and-ready means for arriving at priorities. Perhaps its most important distinguishing characteristic is the
emphasis on the prevention of illness rather than care for illness. This
may be in part due to the rather restricted orientation in traditional
public health. More likely, it represents the belief that when resources are
limited, returns are greater when attention is focused on prevention.

Modified Pan American Health Organization Index. Stewart has described a modification of the index presented in the preceding section
(259). The major modification is the introduction of a term that represents the cost of caring for illness. There are also changes in detail, which
include the use of a mortality rate instead of a proportionate ratio as a
measure of incidence and a preference for 10-point scales for the other
coefficients. The index proposed is as follows:

$$\text{Priority Index} = \frac{M \; \cdot \; T \; \cdot \; V}{C}, \text{ where}$$

M is mortality per 100,000

T (for "trascendencia" in Spanish) is the coefficient of importance,
ranging from 0 (least importance) to 10 (greatest importance).
"The relative importance to be assigned in saving lives is closely
tied in with life years expected to be saved if successful treatment
is provided and the potential productive capacity of the patients
most affected."

V is "vulnerability of the disease to treatment . . . assessed arbitrarily and approximately on a scale running from 0 (not vulnerable to
treatment) to 10 (very vulnerable to treatment). This cannot be
assessed without considering the existing potential resources and
personnel likely to be available."

C is "Cost of personnel and resources required to treat an average
case of the disease" expressed as a point on a scale from 0 (negligible
cost) to 10 (highest cost).

The precise characteristics of the index are not easy to determine from
the brief account given by Stewart. It is not clear, for example, how the
vulnerability factor enters the term T. It appears, however, that the
index is oriented to determining priorities for treatment rather than
prevention. It is also important to note that vulnerability is stated in
operational and not technical terms. In other words, the issue is not how
effective treatment can be in the abstract, but how effective it can be
using the resources at hand. The effect of introducing the cost factor may
be conjectured. Theoretically, both V and C may range from 0 to 10.
Hence, the fraction V/C may vary from 0 to infinity. However, it is not
very often that C is zero or negligible. If C equals 1, the value of V
remains unchanged. If C is greater than 1, the value of V is reduced.
Hence, the introduction of the cost coefficient would appear to reduce the
impact of the vulnerability coefficient or the index as a whole.

Priorities for Hospitalized Illness, Williamson et al. This is an index developed for use in highly specific situations, but which has some very interesting general implications. Williamson et al (260) began with the notion that the medical staff in a hospital should give greatest emphasis in its educational and quality control programs to diseases that cause the largest volume of preventible disability. To arrive at measures of preventible disability it is necessary to estimate, first, how much disability each disease can cause (A) if it is not treated, (B) as currently treated, and (C) if treated optimally. Using the above notation, A − C equals the total preventible disability, and B − C represents the need for improvement over current methods of care in any particular situation. The magnitude of the term B − C is a measure of priority among diseases; it is also, and not incidentally, a measure of the quality of care for any given disease.

Williamson et al. used several approaches to make their basic idea operational. To begin with, they were able to obtain empirical information concerning the clinical impact, or "disability," produced by various diseases from data accumulated by the Commission on Professional and Hospital Activities in Ann Arbor, Michigan. A set of arbitrary weights was developed to take account of the notion that the degree of "social disruption" caused by disease varies with age. This concept is different from, but roughly analogous to, the more precisely defined concepts of lost product or lost output which we have already discussed. Williamson et al. also developed a set of arbitrary rules for partitioning the total impact of disease during any hospital episode, among the several diseases that might be present simultaneously in any one person. The several coefficients or weights are shown in Table III.35.

Based on the information given above,

$$\frac{\text{Total}}{\text{impairment}} = \frac{\text{Disability}}{\text{coefficient}} \cdot \frac{\text{Social disruption}}{\text{coefficient}}$$

Total impairment can then be partitioned among several diagnoses according to the percentages given in Table III.35.

Williamson et al. have encountered greater difficulty in estimating the term A, which is the amount of impairment that would be expected if no treatment were given, and term C, the amount of impairment that would be expected if care were optimal by current standards. Both of these terms could be derived empirically if it were possible to observe cases who have received no treatment and other cases (of comparable severity, etc.) who have received care at one or more near-perfect hospitals. The problems that might be encountered in attempting either of these will not be discussed. Williamson et al. have chosen to derive normative, rather than

Table III.35. Proposed weights to be used in the determination of priorities for diseases in order to account for the hospital experience of the patient, the patient's age, and number of coexisting diagnoses

Patient Experience (CPHA data)	"Disability Weights"
Hospital days	0.1 per day
Complications	1 per complication
Death	30

Patient Age (Years)	"Social Disruption Weights"
0–9	1
10–19	2
20–59	3
60–69	2
70 and over	1

Number of Diagnoses	Proportionate Priority Weight Assigned to:			
	Dx1[a] (%)	Dx2 (%)	Dx3 (%)	Dx4 (%)
1	100	—	—	—
2	60	40	—	—
3	50	30	20	—
4	40	30	20	10

SOURCE: Reference 260.

[a] "Dx = diagnosis. Diagnoses are in order of importance—Dx1 being primary, Dx2 secondary, etc."

empirical, expectations for both A and C. After a comparatively fruitless search of the literature that involved "searching nearly 11,000 citations and reading nearly 2,000 articles," they decided to construct normative standards by obtaining the opinions of experts concerning what the expectations of disability and of improvement might be. They found considerable differences of opinion among physicians, but also sufficient agreement, in their opinion, to warrant continuing work in this direction. If successful, the technique developed would provide measures of priority that include fairly well-authenticated factors of technical vulnerability, as well as a method for assessing the quality of care. Further work along these lines continues to be encouraging (289, 290).

PLANNING IN TERMS OF HEALTH OUTCOMES. In several preceding sections and some that will follow, the reader will find evidence of a duality of orientations: to the process of care, on the one hand, and to the outcomes of care, on the other. In the chapter on objectives, for example, we discussed whether objectives should be set only in terms of states of health, or whether activities themselves can serve as appropriate bench marks of achievement. In this chapter we have emphasized health outcomes as evaluators of care and determinants of priorities for care. Since it is the prime social function of the medical care system to bring about amelioration in health, it seems self-evident that program activities should be directly primarily, perhaps exclusively, toward the end results of care. And yet one encounters reservations, doubts, and even covert or overt opposition to the use of priority systems or evaluations based primarily on health outcomes. There is something more fundamental behind this reluctance than mere conservatism or inertia in individuals or organizations.

There is no doubt that at some level, or levels, there must be concern with overall health outcomes and the relationship of health services to health outcomes. But are these concerns appropriate at all levels? The answer could be "No." A program directly responsible for the health of a population, with virtually complete control over the range of environmental and personal services for that population, must obviously allocate scarce health resources in terms of contribution to health outcome. The situation described above is, unfortunately—some say fortunately—not often encountered in our society, although it may be more often approximated in restricted spheres of activity. Planning and evaluation in terms of health outcomes may become irrelevant, and insistence upon it frustrating, if the agency has no control over the range of activities that are necessary to influence outcome in all diseases or even in one specified disease. The agency finds it more reasonable and satisfying to plan in terms of its own mission, often restricted by legislation, which is the performance of a usually limited task as one component of a very loosely structured set of public and voluntary health activities. In our system, fortunately or unfortunately, these multifarious activities nowhere come to a single focus of overall direction and control. This does not mean that planning oriented to health outcomes cannot be done, but that it can only be done incompletely and in limited segments. At all times one must be oriented to health outcomes, but to insist that this become the only orientation and the exclusive framework for planning and evaluation is probably unrealistic.

There is another basic consideration of a philosophical nature. Health services have come to be regarded as a good in themselves. True, this derives ultimately from their perceived effect on health. Nevertheless, this effect only needs to be perceived and generally accepted for it to become a powerful social imperative. The purveyance of health services to all segments of the population in a manner proportionate to socially defined need becomes the objective. Public programs often influence more directly underprivileged segments of the population. To insist that for them, and for them alone, demonstrated effectiveness be the criterion in planning becomes heresy in an egalitarian society.

Opposition to exclusive reliance on health outcomes as determinants of planning also derives from current ignorance about the relationship between health services and health outcomes. That there is a relationship is sometimes not clearly established. More often, we do not know the precise quantitative relationships. The need to remedy this situation is universally recognized. In the meantime, it is easier to assume that present medical custom should serve as a guide for what one must do.

Perhaps the duality referred to could be reconciled if attention were sharply focused on the specification of what the relevant or desired outcomes are, irrespective of how readily these can be measured, and on elucidating beyond doubt the relationships between specific program activities and the end results that we have agreed to accomplish.

READINGS AND REFERENCES

Concepts of Health and Illness

1. Parsons, T., ''Definitions of Health and Illness in the Light of American Values and Social Structure,'' pp. 16–187, in E. G. Jaco (ed.), *Patients, Physicians and Illness.* (Glencoe, Ill.: The Free Press, 1958), 600pp.

2. Lewis, A., ''Health as A Social Concept,'' *The British Journal of Sociology* 4:102–124 (June 1953).

3. Saunders, L., *Cultural Differences in Medical Care: The Case of the Spanish-Speaking People of the Southwest* (New York: Russell Sage Foundation, 1954), pp. 141–173.

4. Koos, E. L., *The Health of Regionville* (New York: Columbia University Press, 1954), pp. 30–52, 93–111, and 138–158.

5. Strauss, R., ''Determinants of Health Beliefs and Behavior. II. Sociological Determinants,'' *American Journal of Public Health* 5:1547–1552 (October 1961).

6. Apple, D., ''How Laymen Define Illness,'' *Journal of Health and Human Behavior* 1:219–225 (Fall 1960).

7. Baumann, B., ''Diversities in Conception of Health and Physical Fitness,'' *Journal of Health and Human Behavior* 2:39–46 (Spring 1961).

8. Blum, R. H., ''The Patient's Definition of Illness,'' in *The Management of the Doctor-Patient Relationship*, pp. 1–28 (New York: McGraw-Hill, 1960).

9. Friedsam, H. J., and Martin, H. W., ''A Comparison of Self and Physicians' Health Ratings in an Older Population,'' *Journal of Health and Human Behavior* 4:179–183 (Fall 1963).

10. Riese, W., *Conception of Disease, Its History, Its Versions and Its Nature* (New York: Philosophical Library, 1953). 120pp.

11. Dubos, R., *Mirage of Health: Utopias, Progress and Biological Change* (New York: Harper, 1959). 236pp.

12. Hudson, R. P., ''The Concept of Disease,'' *Annals of Internal Medicine* 65:595–601 (September 1966).

13. Wylie, C. M., ''The Definition and Measurement of Health and Disease,'' *Public Health Reports* 85:100–104 (February 1970).

14. Kohn, R., *The Health of the Canadian People.* Royal Commission on Health Services (Ottawa: Queen's Printer, 1967). pp. 4–16.

15. Dunn, H. L., ''What High-Level Wellness Means,'' *Canadian Journal of Public Health* 50:447–457 (November 1959).

16. Leavell, H. R., and Clark, E. G., ''Health as a Relative State,'' ''Disease as a Process,'' and ''The Natural History of Disease and Multiple Causation,'' in *Preventive Medicine for the Doctor and His Community: An Epidemiologic Approach,* 3rd ed., pp. 14–19 (New York: McGraw-Hill, 1965).

17. Gordon, J. E., ''The Newer Epidemiology in Tomorrow's Horizon in Public Health'' (New York: Public Health Association of New York City, 1950).

18. Gordon, J. E., ''Evolution of an Epidemiology of Health, III. The World, the Flesh and the Devil as Environment, Host and Agent of Disease,'' in Iago, Galdston, ed., *The Epidemiology of Health,* pp. 60–73 (New York: Health Education Council, 1953).

19. Gordon, J. E., O'Rourke, E., Richardson, F. W., Jr. and Lindemann, E., ''The Biological and Social Services in an Epidemiology of Mental Disorder,'' *American Journal of the Medical Sciences* 223:316–343 (1952).

20. Knight, J. A., Friedman, T. I. and Sulianti, J., ''Epidemic Hysteria: A Field Study.'' *American Journal of Public Health* 55:858–865 (June 1965).

21. Gordon, J. E., and Ingalls, T. H., ''Medical Ecology and Public Health,'' *The American Journal of the Medical Sciences* 235:337–359 (March 1958).

22. Magdelaine, M., Pequignot, H., and Rosch, G., ''Un Modéle mathématique de la consommation des soins médicaux,'' *La Presse medicale* 73:1319–1321 (May 1, 1965).

23. Last, J. M., ''The Iceberg: 'Completing the Clinical Picture' in General Practice,'' *Lancet* 2:28–31 (July 6, 1963).

24. Ryle, J. A., ''The Measuring of Normal,'' *Lancet* 1:1–5 (January 4, 1947).

25. Pickering, G., ''The Quantitative Approach to Disease, Exemplified by Essential Hypertension,'' in *Ciba Foundation Symposium* (Boston: Little, Brown, 1959). 356pp.

26. Elvebak, L. R., Guillier, C. L., and Keating, F. R., ''Health, Normality, and the Ghost of Gauss,'' *Journal of the American Medical Association* 211:69–75 (January 5, 1970).

27. Crombie, D. L., ''Diagnostic Process,'' *Journal of the College of General Practitioners,* 6:579–589 (1963).

28. Starfield, B., and Borkowf, S., ''Physicians' Recognition of Complaints Made By Parents About Their Children's Health,'' *Pediatrics* 43:168–172 (February 1969).

29. Scheff, T. J., ''Preferred Errors in Diagnosis,'' *Medical Care* 2:166–172 (July-September 1964).

30. Goshen, C. E., ''The High Cost of Nonpsychiatric Care,'' *G.P.* 27:227–235 (April 1963).

31. Feinstein, A. R., ''Boolean Algebra and Clinical Taxonomy, I. Analytic Synthesis of the General Spectrum of a Human Disease,'' *New England Journal of Medicine* 269:929–938 (October 31, 1963).

32. Moriyama, I. M., ''The Classification of Disease—A Fundamental Problem,'' *Journal of Chronic Diseases* 11:462–470 (May 1960).

Measuring Morbidity: Frequency and Intensity

33. MacMahon, B., Pugh, T. F., and Ipsen, J., ''Measurements of Disease Frequency,'' in MacMahon et al., *Epidemiologic Methods,* pp. 51–71 (Boston: Little, Brown, 1960).

34. Dorn, H. F., ''A Classification System for Morbidity Concepts,'' *Public Health Reports* 72:1043–1048 (December 1957).

35. Dunn, J. E., ''The Use of Incidence and Prevalence in the Study of Disease Development in a Population,'' *American Journal of Public Health* 52:1107–1118 (July 1962).

36. Kottmeier, H. L., *Annual Report of the Results of Treatment in Carcinoma of the Uterus*, vol. 13 (Stockholm: P. A. Norstedt and Söner, 1964).

37. Anderson, W. A., *Pathology*, 5th ed. (St. Louis: Mosby, 1966). 1439pp. See section on cancer of the cervix, pp. 1152–1155.

38. Dukes, C. E., ''Cancer of the Rectum: An Analysis of 1000 Cases,'' *Journal of Pathology and Bacteriology* 50:527–539 (May 1940).

39. Criterion Committee of the New York Heart Association, *Nomenclature of Diseases of the Heart and Blood Vessels* (New York Heart Association, 1953), pp. 80–82.

40. Medical Research Council, Committee on the Aetiology of Chronic Bronchitis, ''Definition and Classification of Chronic Bronchitis for Clinical and Epidemiological Purposes,'' *Lancet* 1:775–779 (April 10, 1965).

41. Lansbury, J., ''Methods for Evaluating Rheumatoid Arthritis,'' in Hollander, J. L., ed., *Arthritis and Allied Conditions*, pp. 269–291 (Philadelphia: Lea and Febiger, 1966).

42. Sokolow, J., Silson, J. E., Taylor, E. J., Anderson, E. T., and Rusk, H. A., ''A New Approach to the Objective Evaluation of Physical Disability,'' *Journal of Chronic Diseases* 15:105–112 (January 1962).

43. Katz, S., Ford, A. B., Moskowitz, R. W., Jackson, B. A., and Jaffe, M. W., ''Studies of Illness in the Aged: The Index of ADL, A Standardized Measure of Biological and Psychosocial Function,'' *Journal of the American Medical Association* 185:914–919 (September 21, 1963).

44. Wylie, C. M., and White, B. K., ''A Measure of Disability,'' *Archives of Environmental Health* 8:834–839 (June 1964).

45. Schoening, H. A., Anderegg, L., Bergstrom, D., Fonda, M., Steinke, N., and Ulrich, P., ''Numerical Scoring of Self-Care Status of Patients,'' *Archives of Physical Medicine* 46:689–697 (October 1965).

46. Kelman, H. R., and Willner, A., ''Problems in Measurement and Evaluation of Rehabilitation,'' *Archives of Physical Medicine and Rehabilitation* 43:172–181 (April 1962).

47. Walker, R., and Frost, E. S., ''Measurement of Social Restoration of the Mentally Handicapped by the General Adjustment and Planning Scale (GAPS),'' *Health Services Research* 4:152–160 (Summer 1969).

48. Fisher, J. W., Bristow, M. E., and Henderson, L., ''An Actuarial Procedure for Assessing the Experience of Mental Hospital Patients,'' *Medical Care* 2:84–94 (April–June 1964).

49. Sartwell, P. E., and Merrell, M., ''Influence of the Dynamic Character of Chronic Disease on the Interpretation of Morbidity Rates,'' *American Journal of Public Health* 42:579–584 (May 1952).

50. Commission on Chronic Illness, *Chronic Illness in the United States. Vol. IV: Chronic Illness in a Large City* (Cambridge, Mass.: Harvard University Press, 1957), pp. 375–377.

51. Katz, S., Ford, A. B., Downs, T. D., and Adams, M., ''Chronic-disease Classification in Evaluation of Medical Care Programs,'' *Medical Care* 7:139–143 (March–April 1969).

52. Moore, W. S., ''Classifying Morbidity.'' *Inquiry* 7:41–45 (December 1970).

53. Sheps, M. C., ''On the Person Years Concept in Epidemiology and Demography,'' *Milbank Memorial Fund Quarterly* 44:69–91 (January 1966).

54. Solon, J. A., Feeney, J. J., Jones, S. H., Rigg, R. D., and Sheps, C. G., "Delineating Episodes of Medical Care," *American Journal of Public Health* 57:401–408 (March 1967).

55. Solon, J. A., Rigg, R. D., Jones, S. R., Feeney, J. J., Lingner, J. W., and Sheps, C. G., "Episodes of Medical Care: Nursing Students' Use of Medical Services," *American Journal of Public Health* 59:936–946 (June 1969).

Measuring Morbidity: Localization in Time, Person and Place

56. MacMahon, B., Pugh, T. F., and Ipsen, J., "Place" and "Time," in MacMahon et al., *Epidemiologic Methods*, pp. 141–186 (Boston: Little, Brown, 1960).

57. Taylor, I., and Knowlden, J., "Time" and "Place," in Taylor and Knowlden, *Principles of Epidemiology*, pp. 265–302 (Boston: Little, Brown, 1964).

58. Aycock, W. L., Lutman, G. E., and Folet, G. I., "Seasonal Prevalence as a Principle in Epidemiology," *American Journal of Medical Sciences* 209:395–411 (March 1945).

59. Shevky, E., and Bell, W., *Social Area Analysis* (Stanford University Press, 1955), 70pp.

60. Foley, D. L., "Census Tracts in Urban Research," *Journal of the American Statistical Association* 48:733–742 (December 1953).

61. Moore, F. J., "Defining Aggregations of the Poor for Community Health Center Location," *Health Services Research* 4:188–197 (Fall 1969).

62. U.S. Bureau of the Census, *Census Study: Computer Mapping.* Report No. 2 (Washington, D.C., 1969), 44pp.

63. Robinson, W., "Ecological Correlations and the Behavior of Individuals," *American Sociological Review* 15:351–357 (June 1950).

64. Altenderfer, M. D., and Crowther, B., "Relationships Between Infant Mortality and Socio-Economic Factors in Urban Areas," *Public Health Reports* 64: 331–339 (March 1949).

65. Rosenfeld, L. S., Katz, J., and Donabedian, A., *Medical Care Needs and Services in the Boston Metropolitan Area.* (Boston: United Community Services of Metropolitan Boston, 1957). 147pp.

66. Rosenfeld, L. S., and Donabedian, A., "Prenatal Care in Metropolitan Boston," *American Journal of Public Health* 48:1115–1124 (September 1958).

67. Anderson, U. M., Jenss, R., Mosher, W. E., Randall, C. L., and Marra, E., "High Risk Group—Definition and Identification," *New England Journal of Medicine* 273:308–313 (August 5, 1965).

68. Stockwell, E. G., "Use of Socioeconomic Status as a Demographic Variable," *Public Health Reports* 81:961–966 (November, 1966).

69. Wallace, H. M., Eisner, V., and Dooley, S., "Availability and Usefulness of Selected Health and Socioeconomic Data for Community Planning," *American Journal of Public Health* 57:762–771 (May 1967).

70. Hunt, E. P., "Infant Mortality and Poverty Areas," *Welfare in Review* 5:1–12 (August–September 1967). (Application of geographic area analysis.)

71. Fox, R. I., Goldman, J. J., and Brumfield, W. A., "Determining the Target Population for Prenatal and Postnatal Care," *Public Health Reports* 83:249–257 (March 1968).

72. Hochstim, J. R., Anthanasopoulos, D. A., and Larkins, J. H., "Poverty Area Under the Microscope," *American Journal of Public Health* 58:1815–1827 (October 1968).

73. Dunn, H. L., "Record Linkage," *American Journal of Public Health* 36:1412–1416 (December 1946).

74. Dunn, H. L., and Gilbert, M., ''Public Health Begins in the Family,'' *Public Health Reports* 71:1002–1010 (October 1956).

75. Newcombe, H. B., Kennedy, J. M., Axford, S. J., and James, A. P., ''Automatic Linkage of Vital Records,'' *Science* 130:954–959 (October 1959).

76. Acheson, E. D., *Medical Record Linkage* (London: Oxford University Press, 1967). 213pp.

77. Gabrielson, I. W., Siker, E., Sohler, K. B., and Stockwell, E. G., ''Relating Health and Census Information for Health Planning,'' *American Journal of Public Health* 59:1169–1176 (July 1969).

78. U.S. Bureau of the Census, *Census Use Study: Family Health Survey*. Report No. 6 (Washington, D.C., 1969). 41pp.

79. U.S. Bureau of the Census, *Census Use Study: Health Information System*. Report No. 7 (Washington, D.C., 1969), 67pp.

80. Chase, H. C., *The Study of Infant Mortality from Linked Records: Method of Study and Registration Aspects, United States*. National Center for Health Statistics, Public Health Service Publication, No. 1000—ser. 20, no. 7 (Washington, D.C., U.S. Government Printing Office, February 1970). 44pp.

Sources of Morbidity Information: General

81. MacMahon, B., Pugh, T. F., and Ipsen, J., ''Sources of Mortality and Morbidity Data,'' in MacMahon et al. *Epidemiologic Methods*, pp. 72–85 (Boston: Little, Brown, 1960).

82. National Center for Health Statistics, *Origin, Program, and Operation of the U.S. National Health Survey*. P.H.S. Publication No. 1000—ser. 1, no. 2 (Washington, D.C.: U.S. Government Printing Office, August 1963). 41pp.

83. Several Authors, *Trends in the Study of Morbidity and Mortality*. (Geneva: World Health Organization, 1965). 196pp.

The Household Interview Survey

84. National Center for Health Statistics, *Origin, Program, and Operation of the U.S. National Health Survey*. P.H.S. Publication No. 1000—ser. 1, no. 1 (Washington, D.C.: U.S. Government Printing Office, August 1963). 41pp.

85. U.S. National Health Survey, *Health Statistics from the U.S. National Health Survey: The Statistical Design of the Household-Interview Survey*. P.H.S. Publication No. 584–A2 (Washington, D.C.: U.S. Government Printing Office, July 1958). 40pp.

86. National Center for Health Statistics, *Synthetic State Estimates of Disability Derived from the National Health Survey*. P.H.S. Publication No. 1759 (Washington, D.C.: U.S. Government Printing Office, 1968) 16pp.

87. McCormack, R. C. and Miley, C. E., ''Health Service Utilization in Central Virginia: A Comparison of Estimated and Observed Rates.'' *American Journal of Public Health* 60:1733–1738 (September 1970).

88. National Center for Health Statistics, *Health Survey Procedure: Concepts, Questionnaire Development, and Definitions in the Health Interview Survey*. P.H.S. Publication No. 1000—ser. 1, no. 2 (Washington, D.C., May 1964). 66pp.

89. Woolsey, T. D., ''The Concept of Illness in the Household Interview of the U.S. National Health Survey,'' *American Journal of Public Health* 48:703–712 (June 1958).

90. National Center for Health Statistics, *Hospital Utilization in the Last Year of Life*. P.H.S. Publication, No. 1000—ser. 2, no. 10 (Washington, D.C.: U.S. Government Printing Office, July 1965). 30pp.

91. White, K. L., and Murnaghan, J. H., *International Comparisons of Medical Care Utilization.* P.H.S. Publication, No. 1000—ser. 2, no. 3 (Washington, D.C.: U.S. Government Printing Office, June 1969). 74pp.

92. Feldman, J. J., "The Household Interview Survey as a Technique for the Collection of Morbidity Data," *Journal of Chronic Diseases* 11:535–557 (May 1960).

93. Sanders, B. S., "Have Morbidity Surveys Been Oversold?" *American Journal of Public Health* 52:1648–1659 (October 1962).

94. Woolsey, T. D.; Lawrence, S. P., and Balamuth, E., "An Evaluation of Chronic Disease Prevalence Data from the Health Interview Survey," *American Journal of Public Health* 52:1631–1637 (October 1962).

95. Commission on Chronic Illness, "The Household Interview in Studies of Prevalence—An Evaluation," in *Chronic Illness in the United States, Volume IV, Chronic Illness in a Large City,* pp. 297–328 (Cambridge: Harvard University Press, 1957).

96. Trussell, R. E., Elinson, J., and Levin, M. L., "Comparison of Various Methods of Estimating the Prevalence of Chronic Disease in a Community—The Hunterdon County Study," *American Journal of Public Health* 46:173–182 (February 1956).

97. U.S. Department of Health, Education, and Welfare. Public Health Service. *Health Statistics from the U.S. National Health Survey: Health Interview Responses Compared with Medical Records* (Washington, D.C.: P.H.S. Publication No. 584—D5, June 1961).

98. National center for Health Statistics, *Interview Data on Chronic Condition Compared with Information Derived from Medical Records,* P.H.S. Publication, No. 1000—ser. 2, no. 23 (Washington, D.C.: U.S. Government Printing Office, May 1967). 84pp.

99. Gordon, R., *Three Views of Hypertension and Heart Disease.* (Washington D.C.: U.S. Government Printing Office, March 1967). P.H.S. Publication, No. 1000, ser. 2, no. 22 (Washington, D.C., U.S. Government Printing Office, March 1967).

100. Suchman, E. A., Phillips, S., and Streib, G. F., "An Analysis of the Validity of Health Questionnaires," *Social Forces* 36:223 (1958).

101. Mechanic, D., and Newton, M., "Some Problems in the Analysis of Morbidity Data," *Journal of Chronic Diseases* 18:569–580 (1966).

102. Kosa, J., Albert, J. J., and Haggerty, R. J., "On the Reliability of Family Health Information: A Comparative Study of Mother's Reports on Illness and Related Behavior," *Social Science and Medicine* 1:165–181 (July 1967).

103. Solon, J. A., et al., "Patterns of Medical Care: Validity of Interview Information on Use of Hospital Clinics," *Journal of Health and Human Behavior* 3:21–29 (Spring 1962).

104. Simmons, W. R., and Bryant, E. E., "An Evaluation of Hospitalization Data from the Health Interview Survey," *American Journal of Public Health* 52:1638–1647 (October 1962).

105. National Center for Health Statistics, *Reporting Hospitalization in the Health Interview Survey.* P.H.S. Publication No. 1000—ser. 2, no. 6 (Washington, D.C.: U.S. Government Printing Office, July 1965). 71pp.

106. Kahn, R. L., and Cannell, C. F., *The Dynamics of Interviewing.* (New York: John Wiley, 1957). 368pp.

107. Cannell, C. F., Fowler, F. J., and Marquis, K. H., *The Influence of Interviewer and Respondent Psychological and Behavioral Variables on the Reporting in Household Interviews.* P.H.S. Publication No. 1000—ser. 2, no. 26 (Washington, D.C.: U.S. Government Printing Office, March 1968). 65pp.

108. Colombotos, J., Elinson, J., and Loewenstein, R., "Effect of Interviewer's Sex on Interview Responses," *Public Health Reports* 83:685–690 (August, 1968).

109. National Center for Health Statistics, *Comparison of Hospitalization Report-*

ing in Three Survey Procedures. P.H.S. Publication, No. 1000—ser. 2, no. 8 (Washington, D.C.: U.S. Government Printing Office, July 1965). 48pp.

110. Cannell, C. F., and Axelrod, M., *Health Statistics from the U.S. National Health Survey: A Study of Special Purpose Medical-History Techniques.* P.H.S. Publication No. 584–D1 (Washington, D.C.: U.S. Government Printing Office, January 1960). 27pp.

Symptom Surveys and the Meaning of Symptoms

111. Schuler, E. A., Mayo, S. C., and Makona, H. B., "Measuring Unmet Needs for Medical Care: An Experiment in Method," *Rural Sociology* 11:152–158 (June 1946).

112. Hoffer, C. R., Schuler, E. A., Nelight, R., and Robinson, T., "Determination of Unmet Need for Medical Attention among Michigan Farm Families," *Journal of the Michigan State Medical Society* 46:443–446 (April 1947).

113. Hoffer, C. R., and Schuler, E. A., "Measurement of Health Needs and Health Care," *American Sociological Review* 13:719–724 (December 1948).

114. Hoffer, C. R., et al., " 'The Symptoms Approach' in Determining Unmet Needs," in *Health Needs and Health Care in Michigan*, pp. 13–15 (East Lansing: Michigan State College, June 1950). 94pp. Pages 15–18 give some findings.

115. Cartwright, A., *Patients and Their Doctors* (New York: Atherton Press, 1967). See pp. 35–37.

116. Gordon, T., "Symptoms as a Diagnostic Tool," in *Three Views of Hypertension and Heart Disease*, pp. 9–10. P.H.S. Publication, No. 1000—ser. 2, no. 22 (Washington, D.C.: U.S. Government Printing Office, March 1967).

117. Hammond, E. C., "Some Preliminary Findings on Physical Complaints from a Prospective Study of 1,064,004 Men and Women," *American Journal of Public Health* 54:11–23 (January 1964).

118. Mabry, J. H., "Lay Concepts of Etiology," *Journal of Chronic Diseases* 17: 371–386 (May 1964).

119. Zborowski, M., "Cultural Components in Response to Pain," *Journal of Social Issues* 8:16–30 (1952). (Reprinted in *Patients, Physicians and Illness*, ed. E. G. Jaco (Glencoe, Ill.: The Free Press, 1958), pp. 256–268.

120. Mechanic, D., and Volkart, E. H., "Stress, Illness Behavior and the Sick Role," *American Sociological Review* 26:51–58 (February 1961).

121. Hetherington, R. W., and Hopkins, C. E., "Symptom Sensitivity: Its Social and Cultural Correlates," *Health Services Research* 4:63–75 (Spring 1969).

122. Zola, I. K., "Culture and Symptoms—An Analysis of Patients Presenting Complaints," *American Sociological Review* 31:615–630 (October 1966).

123. Winsberg, B., and Greenlick, M., "Pain Response in Negro and White Patients," *Journal of Health and Social Behavior* 8:222–227 (September 1967).

124. Andersen, R., Anderson, O. W., and Smedby, B., "Perceptions and Responses to Symptoms of Illness in Sweden and the United States," *Medical Care* 6:18–30 (January–February 1968).

125. Haberman, P. W., "Ethnic Differences in Psychiatric Symptoms Reported in Community Surveys." *Public Health Reports* 85:495–502 (June 1970).

126. National Center for Health Statistics, *Selected Symptoms of Psychological Distress, United States.* Public Health Service Publications No. 1000—ser. 11, no. 37 (Washington, D.C.: U.S. Government Printing Office, August 1970). 44pp.

127. Elder, R. and Acheson, R. M., "New Haven Survey of Joint Diseases, XIV. Social Class and Behavior in Response to Symptoms of Osteoarthritis." *Milbank Memorial Fund Quarterly* 48:449–502 (October 1970), pt. 1.

Continuous Local or Partial Survey

128. Tayback, M., and Frazier, T. M., ''Continuous Health Surveys a Necessity for Health Administration,'' *Public Health Reports* 77:763–771 (September 1962).

129. Scharff, J., ''Current Medicare Survey: The Medical Insurance Sample,'' *Social Security Bulletin* 30:4–9 (April 1967).

Self-Administered Health Histories

130. Brodman, K., et al., ''The Cornell Medical Index: An Adjustment to Medical Interview,'' *Journal of the American Medical Association* 140:530–534 (June 11, 1949).

131. Abramson, J. H., ''The Cornell Medical Index as an Epidemiological Tool,'' *American Journal of Public Health* 56:287–298 (February 1966).

132. Brodman, K., et al., ''Interpretation of Symptoms with a Data-Processing Machine,'' *Archives of Internal Medicine* 103:776–782 (May 1959).

133. Brodman, K., and Goldstein, L. S., ''The Medical Data Screen: An Adjunct for the Diagnosis of 100 Common Diseases,'' *Archives of Environmental Health* 14:821–826 (June 1967).

134. VanWoerkom, A. J., and Brodman, K., ''Statistics for a Diagnostic Model,'' *Biometrics* 17:229–318 (June 1961).

135. Brodman, K., et al., ''The Cornell Medical Index—Health Questionnaire VI: The Relationship of Patients' Complaints to Age, Sex, Race and Education,'' *Journal of Gerontology* 8:339–342 (July 1953).

136. Alexious, N. G., Wiener, G., Silverman, M., and Milton, T., ''Validity Studies of a Self-Administered Health Questionnaire for Secondary School Students,'' *American Journal of Public Health* 59:1400–1411 (August 1969).

Vital and Health Statistics

137. National Center for Health Statistics, *The 1970 Census and Vital and Health Statistics: A Study Group Report of the Public Health Conference on Records and Statistics*. Public Health Service Publication No. 1000—ser. 4, no. 10 (Washington, D.C.: U.S. Government Printing Office, April 1969). 14pp.

138. Israel, R. A., and Klebba, A. J., ''A Preliminary Report on the Effect of Eighth Revision ICDA on Cause of Death Statistics,'' *American Journal of Public Health* 59:1651–1660 (September 1969).

139. National Center for Health Statistics, ''Provisional Estimate of Selected Comparability Ratios Based on Dual Coding of 1966 Death Certificates by the Seventh and Eighth Revisions of the International Classification of Diseases,'' *Monthly Vital Statistics Report,* vol. 17, no. 8, Supplement (October 25, 1968). 8pp.

140. National Center for Health Statistics, ''Comparability of Mortality Statistics for the Sixth and Seventh Revisions: United States, 1958,'' *Vital Statistics—Special Reports,* vol. 51, no. 4 (March 1965).

141. National Center for Health Statistics, ''Comparability of Mortality Statistics for the Fifth and Sixth Revisions: United States, 1950,'' *Vital Statistics—Special Reports,* vol. 51, no. 2 (December 1963). Also, vol. 51, no. 3 (February 1964).

142. World Health Organization, ''Comparability of Statistics of Causes of Death According to the Fifth and Sixth Revisions of the International List,'' *Bulletin of the World Health Organization,* Supplement 4 (1952). 59pp.

143. Dunn, H. L., and Shackley, W., ''Comparison of Cause-of-Death Assignments by the 1929 and 1938 Revisions of the International List: Deaths in the United States,

1940," *Vital Statistics—Special Reports,* vol. 19, no. 14, pp. 153–277 (June 14, 1944).

144. Emerson, H., "Reliability of Statements of Cause of Death from Clinical and Pathological Viewpoints," *American Journal of Public Health* 6:680–685 (July 1916).

145. Swartoot, H. O., and Webster, R. G., "To What Degree are Mortality Statistics Dependable?" *American Journal of Public Health* 30:811–815 (July 1940).

146. Pohlen, K., and Emerson, J., "Errors in Statements of Cause of Death," *American Journal of Public Health* 32:251–260 (March 1947).

147. James, G., Patton, R. E., and Heslin, A. S., "Accuracy of Cause of Death Statements on Death Certificates," *Public Health Reports* 70:39–51 (January 1955).

148. Heasman, M. A., and Lipworth, L., *Accuracy of Certification of Causes of Death.* General Register Office. Studies on Medical and Population Subjects, no. 20 (London: H. M. Stationary Office, 1966). 133pp.

149. Moriyama, I. M., Baum, W. S., Haenszel, W. M., and Mattison, B. F., "Inquiry into Diagnostic Evidence Supporting Medical Certification of Death," *American Journal of Public Health* 48:1376–1387 (October 1958).

150. Hewitt, D., Milner, J., and Csima, A., "Some Proposed 'Comparability Areas' for U.S. Statistics on Cause of Death," *Public Health Reports* 84:857–863 (October 1969).

151. Moriyama, I. M., Baum, W. S., Haenszel, W. M., and Mattison, B. F., "Inquiry into Diagnostic Evidence Supporting Medical Certification of Death," *American Journal of Public Health* 48:1376–1378 (October 1958).

152. Moriyama, I. M., "Development of the Present Concept of Cause of Death," *American Journal of Public Health* 46:436–441 (April 1956).

153. Moriyama, I. M., and Dorn, H. F., "Uses and Significance of Multiple Cause Tabulations for Mortality Statistics," *American Journal of Public Health* 54:400–407 (March 1964).

154. National Center for Health Statistics, *International Classification of Diseases, Adapted* (rev. ed., vols. I and II) P.H.S. Publication No. 719 (Washington, D.C.: U.S. Government Printing Office, 1962). Vol. I, 375pp.; vol. II, 417pp.

155. National Center for Health Statistics, *Eighth Revision International Classification of Diseases, Adapted for Use in the United States (ICDA).* Public Health Service Publication No. 1693 (Washington, D.C.: U.S. Government Printing Office, October 1967). Vol. I, 671pp.; vol. II, 685pp.

156. World Health Organization, *Manual of the International Classification of Diseases, Injuries and Causes of Death,* 8th ed. (Geneva: WHO, 1967). Vol. I, 478pp.; vol. II, 616pp.

Case Registers

157. Cutler, S. J., "The Role of Morbidity Reporting and Case Registers in Cancer Control," *Public Health Reports* 65:1084–1089 (1950).

158. Griswold, M. H., Wilder, C. S., Cutler, S. J., and Pollack, E. S., *Cancer in Connecticut 1935–1951.* (Hartford: Connecticut State Department of Health, 1955). 141pp.

159. Cancer Registry of Norway, *Cancer Registration in Norway* (Olso: The Norwegian Cancer Society, 1964).

160. Bahn, A. K., "Psychiatric Case Register Conference, 1965," *Public Health Reports* 81:748–754 (August 1966).

161. Task Force on Stroke Registries, "Feasibility and Value of Stroke Registries for Regional Medical Programs," *Public Health Reports* 83:537–550 (July 1968).

162. Goldstein, H., "Blindness Register as a Research Tool," *Public Health Reports* 79:289–295 (April 1964).

163. Miller, J. R., "The Use of Registers and Vital Statistics in the Study of Congenital Malformations," in *Second Scientific Conference on Congenital Malformations*, pp. 334–340 (New York: International Medical Corps, Ltd., July 1963).

164. Mott, G. A., "The Report of Handicapped Children and Adults in British Columbia," *Canadian Journal of Public Health* 54:239–245 (June 1963).

Data from Special Groups

165. Perrot, G. St.J., "Physical Status of Young Men, 1918 and 1941," *Milbank Memorial Fund Quarterly* 19:337–344 (October 1941).

166. Britten, R. H., and Perrot, G. St.J., "Summary of Physical Findings on Men Drafted in the World War," *Public Health Reports* 56:41–62 (January 10, 1941).

167. Goldstein, M. S., "Physical Status of Men Examined Through Selective Service in World War II," *Public Health Reports* 66:587–609 (May 11, 1951).

168. Karpinos, B. D., "Fitness of American Youth for Military Service," *Milbank Memorial Fund Quarterly* 38:213–247 (July 1960).

169. Taylor, H. L., et al., "Death Rates Among Physically Active and Sedentary Employees of the Railroad Industry," *American Journal of Public Health* 52:1697–1707 (October 1962).

170. DeBakey, M. E., and Beebe, G. W., "Medical Follow-Up Studies on Veterans," *Journal of the American Medical Association* 182:1103–1109 (December 15, 1962).

171. Compton, A. S., "Health Study of Adolescents Enrolled in the Neighborhood Youth Corps," *Public Health Reports* 84:585–596 (July 1969).

172. Metropolitan Life Insurance Company. *Statistical Bulletin.* A monthly publication that provides useful summaries of data from various sources including the experience of insured groups. (May be obtained from the Editor, *Statistical Bulletin*, Metropolitan Life Insurance Company, 1 Madison Avenue, New York 10, N.Y.).

173. Densen, P. M., Balamuth, E., and Deardorff, N. R., "Medical Care Plans as a Source of Morbidity Data: The Prevalence of Illness and Associated Volume of Service," *Milbank Memorial Fund Quarterly* 38:48–101 (January 1960).

174. Chamberlain, J., "Selected Data on Group Practice Prepayment Plan Services," *Group Health and Welfare News.* Special Supplement (June 1967). 8pp.

Clinical Records

175. Bachrach, C. A., "Patient Record as a Source of Useful Statistics," *Hospitals* 29:67–71 (October 1955).

176. Sanders, B. S., "Completeness and Reliability of Diagnosis in Therapeutic Practice," *Journal of Health and Human Behavior* 5:84–94 (Summer and Fall 1964).

177. Koen, M. H., "Discharge Diagnoses and Their Importance to Blue Cross," *Inquiry* 3:55–74 (February 1966).

178. Doyle, D. M., "Accuracy of Selected Items of Blue Cross Information," *Inquiry* 3:16–27 (September 1966).

179. National Center for Health Statistics. *Development and Maintenance of a National Inventory of Hospitals and Institutions.* P.H.S. Publication No. 1000—ser. 1, no. 3 (Washington, D.C.: U.S. Government Printing Office, February 1965). 25pp. (The findings are reported in ser. 12 of the Reports from the National Center for Health Statistics.)

180. Sirken, M. G., "The Hospital Discharge Survey," *Public Health Reports* 82:9–16 (January 1967).

181. Last, J. M., "Primary Medical Care: Record Keeping," *Milbank Memorial Fund Quarterly*, vol. 43, no. 2 (April 1965), pt. 2, pp. 266–276.

182. National Center for Health Statistics, *Use of Hospital Data for Epidemiologic and Medical Care Research.* A Report of the United States National Committee on Vital and Health Statistics. P.H.S. Publication No. 1000—ser. 4, no. 11 (Washington, D.C.: U.S. Government Printing Office, June 1969). 9pp.

183. Vacek, M., "Information on Morbidity from Medical Practice," in World Health Organization, *Trends in the Study of Morbidity and Mortality,* pp. 69–77 (Geneva: World Health Organization, 1965). 196pp.

184. Logan, W. P. D., and Cushion, A. A., *Morbidity Statistics from General Practice, Vol. 1: (General).* General Register Office Studies on Medical and Population Subjects, no. 14 (London: Her Majesty's Stationery Office, 1958). 174pp.

185. Patton, R. E., "The Sampling of Records," *Public Health Reports* 67:1013–1019 (October 1952).

Multiple Screening and Health Examination Surveys

186. Levin, M. L., "Screening for Asymptomatic Disease: Principles and Background," *Journal of Chronic Diseases* 2:367–374 (October 1955). This entire issue is devoted to multiple screening.

187. Thorner, R. M., and Remein, Q. R., *Principles and Procedures in the Evaluation of Screening for Disease.* P.H.S. Monograph no. 67 (Washington, D.C.: Government Printing Office, 1961). 24pp.

188. Wilson, J. M. G., and Jungner, G., *Principles and Practice of Screening for Disease.* Public Health Papers, no. 34 (Geneva: World Health Organization, 1968). 163pp.

189. Sharp, C. L. E. H., and Keen, H., eds., *Presymptomatic Detection and Early Diagnosis* (London: Pitman Publishing Company, 1968). 384pp.

190. Israel, S., and Teeling-Smith, G., "The Submerged Iceberg of Sickness in Society," *Social and Economic Administration* 1:43–56 (January 1967).

191. Collen, M. F., et al., "Automated Multiphasic Screening and Diagnosis," *American Journal of Public Health* 54:741–750 (May 1964).

192. National Center for Health Statistics. *Plan and Initial Program of the Health Examination Survey.* Public Health Service Publication No. 1000—ser. 1, no. 4 (Washington, D.C.: U.S. Government Printing Office, July 1965). The findings are reported in ser. 11 of the Reports from the National Center for Health Statistics.

193. McDowell, A., "U.S. National Health Examination Survey," *Public Health Reports* 80:941–948 (November 1965).

194. National Center for Health Statistics. *Cooperation in Health Examination Surveys.* P.H.S. Publication No. 1000—ser. 2, no. 9 (Washington, D.C., U.S. Government Printing Office, July 1965). 38pp.

195. National Center for Health Statistics, *Factors Related to Response in a Health Examination Survey,* United States, 1960–1962. P.H.S. Publication No. 1000—ser. 2, no. 36 (Washington, D.C.: U.S. Government Printing Office, August 1969). 48pp.

196. Kilpatrick, G. S., "Observer Error in Medicine," *Journal of Medical Education* 38:38–43 (January 1963).

197. "Bibliography on Observer Error and Variation," in Witts, L. J., ed. *Medical Surveys and Clinical Trials,* pp. 43–49 (London: Oxford University Press, 1964). 367pp.

Measuring Health

198. Dunn, H. L., "Points of Attack for Raising the Levels of Wellness," *Journal of the National Medical Association* 49:225–235 (July 1957).

199. Whittenberger, J. L., "Physiologic Aspects of Physical Fitness," *American Journal of Public Health* 53:792–795 (May 1963).

200. Fleishman, E. A., *The Structure and Measurement of Physical Fitness.* (Englewood Cliffs, N.J.: Prentice-Hall, 1964). 207pp.

201. Lawton, M. P., Ward, M., and Yaffe, S., "Indices of Health in an Aging Population," *Journal of Gerontology* 22:334–342 (July 1967).

Summary Measures of Health and Illness

202. Chiang, C. L., *An Index of Health: Mathematical Models.* Public Health Service Publication No. 1000—ser. 2, no. 5 (Washington, D.C.: U.S. Government Printing Office, May 1965). 19pp.

203. Sullivan, D. F., *Conceptual Problems in Developing an Index of Health.* National Center for Health Statistics—P.H.S. Publication No. 1000—ser. 2, no. 17 (Washington, D.C.: U.S. Government Printing Office, May 1966). 18pp.

204. Sullivan, D. F., *Disability Components for An Index of Health.* National Center for Health Statistics, P.H.S. Publication No. 1000—ser. 2, no. 42 (Washington, D.C.: U.S. Government Printing Office, July 1971). 35pp.

205. Sullivan, D. F., "A Single Index of Mortality and Morbidity." *HSMHA Health Reports* 86:347–354 (April 1971).

206. Fanshel, S. and Bush, J. W., "A Health-Status Index and Its Application to Health Services Outcomes," *Operations Research* 18:1021–1060 (November–December 1970).

207. Bush, J. W., and Zaremba, J., "Estimating Health Program Outcomes Using A Markov Equilibrium Analysis of Disease Development." *American Journal of Public Health* 61:2362–2375 (December 1971).

208. Ortiz, J. and Parker, R., "A Birth-Life-Death Model of Planning and Evaluation of Health Services Programs." *Health Services Research* 6:120–143 (Summer 1971).

209. Kisch, A. I., Kovner, J. W., Harris, L. J., and Kline, G., "A New Proxy Measure for Health Status," *Health Service Research* 4:223–230 (Fall 1969).

Evaluational Uses of Measures of Morbidity and Health

210. Logan, R. F. L., "Assessment of Sickness and Health in the Community: Needs and Methods," *Medical Care* 2:173–190 (July–September 1964) and 2:218–225 (October–December 1964).

211. World Health Organization, *Measurement of Levels of Health.* Technical Report Series, no. 137. (Geneva: W.H.O., 1957). 32pp.

212. Sanders, B. S., "Measuring Community Health Levels," *American Journal of Public Health* 54:1063–1070 (July 1964).

213. Rosenfeld, L. S.; Katz, J., and Donabedian, A., "Measuring the Need for Medical Care," in *Medical Care Needs and Services in the Boston Metropolitan Area* (United Community Services of Metropolitan Boston, 1957). pp. 1–6.

214. Rosenfeld, L. S., Donabedian, A., and Katz, J., "Unmet Need for Medical Care," *New England Journal of Medicine* 258:369–376 (February 20, 1958).

215. Shapiro, S., "End Result Measurement of Quality of Medical Care," Part 1, *Milbank Memorial Fund Quarterly* 45:70–80 (April 1967).

216. World Health Organization, *Trends in the Study of Morbidity and Mortality.* Public Health Papers, no. 27 (Geneva, 1965). 196pp.

217. Morris, J. N., *Uses of Epidemiology,* 2nd. ed. (Baltimore: Williams and Wilkins, 1964). 135pp.

218. Committee for the Special Research Project in the Health Insurance Plan of Greater New York, *Health and Medical Care in New York City* (Cambridge: Harvard University Press, 1957). 275pp.

219. Shapiro, S., Weiner, L., and Densen, P. M., ''Comparison of Prematurity and Perinatal Mortality in a General Population and in the Population of a Prepaid Group Practice Medical Care Plan,'' *American Journal of Public Health* 48:170–185 (February 1958).

220. Shapiro, S., Jacobziner, H., Densen, P. M., and Weiner, L., ''Further Observations in Prematurity and Perinatal Mortality in a General Population and in the Population of a Prepaid Group Practice Medical Care Plan,'' *American Journal of Public Health* 50:1304–1317 (September 1960).

221. Moses, L. E. and Mosteller, F., ''Institutional Differences in Postoperative Death Rates. Commentary on Some of the Findings of the National Halothane Study.'' *Journal of the American Medical Association* 203:492–494 (February 12, 1968).

222. Roemer, M. I., ''Is Surgery Safer in Larger Hospitals?'' *Hospital Management* 87:35–37, 50, 77, 101 (January 1959).

223. Lipworth, L., Lee, J. A. H., and Morris, J. N., ''Case Fatality in Teaching and Non-teaching Hospitals, 1956–1959,'' *Medical Care* 1:71–76 (April–June 1963).

224. Roemer, M. I., Moustafa, A. T., and Hokins, C. E., ''A Proposed Hospital Quality Index: Hospital Death Rates Adjusted for Case Severity,'' *Health Services Research* 3:95–118 (Summer 1968).

225. Shapiro, S., Williams, J. J., Yerby, A. S., Densen, P. M., and Rosner, H., ''Patterns of Medical Use by the Indigent Aged Under Two Systems of Medical Care,'' *American Journal of Public Health* 57:784–790 (May 1967).

226. Bakst, J. N., and Marra, E. F., ''Experience with Home Care for Cardiac Patients,'' *American Journal of Health* 45:444–450 (April 1955).

227. Katz, S., Vignos, P. J., Moskowitz, R. W., Thompson, H. M., Svec, K. H., Hurd, G. G, Rusby, D. I., and Walker, F. B., ''Comprehensive Outpatient Care in Rheumatoid Arthritis: A Controlled Study,'' *Journal of the American Medical Association* 206:1249–1254 (November 9, 1968).

228. Hanchett, E., and Torrens, P. R., ''A Public Health Home Nursing Program for Outpatients with Heart Diseases,'' *Public Health Reports* 82:683–688 (August 1967).

229. Horvitz, D. G., ''Methodological Considerations in Evaluating the Effectiveness of Programs and Benefits,'' *Inquiry* 2:96–104 (September 1965).

230. Behar, M., ''Death and Disease in Infants and Toddlers of Preindustrial Countries,'' *American Journal of Public Health* 54:1100–1105 (July 1964).

231. Chase, H. C., ''White-Nonwhite Mortality Differentials in the United States,'' *Health, Education, and Welfare Indicators* (June 1965), pp. 27–37.

232. Donabedian, A., Rosenfeld, L. S., and Southern, E. M., ''Infant Mortality and Socioeconomic Status in a Metropolitan Community,'' *Public Health Reports* 80:1083–1094 (December 1965).

233. Morris, J. N., and Heady, H. A., ''Social and Biological Factors in Infant Mortality in Relation to Father's Occupation, 1911–1950,'' *Lancet* 1:554–559 (March 12, 1955).

234. National Center for Health Statistics, *Infant and Perinatal Mortality in Scotland*. P.H.S. Publication, No. 1000—ser. 3, no. 5 (Washington, D.C.: U.S. Government Printing Office, November 1966). 44pp.

235. Posthuma, J. H., and de Haas, J. H., *Infant Loss in the Netherlands*. P.H.S. Publication, No. 1000—ser. 3, no. 11 (Washington, D.C.: U.S. Government Printing Office, August 1968). 63pp.

236. Swaroop, S., and Uemura, K., ''Proportional Mortality of 50 Years and Above,'' *Bulletin of the World Health Organization* 17:439–481 (1957).

237. Kitagawa, E. M., and Hauser, P. M., "Trends in Differential Fertility and Mortality in a Metropolis—Chicago," in E. W. Burgess and D. J. Bogue, eds., *Contributions to Urban Sociology* (Chicago: University of Chicago Press, 1964).

238. Kitagawa, E. M., "Social and Economic Differentials in Mortality in the United States, 1960." Paper prepared for session on socioeconomic differentials in mortality, General Assembly and Conference of International Union for Scientific Study of Population held in London, September 3–11, 1969 (Chicago: Population Research Center, University of Chicago, 1969). 24pp. Processed.

239. Kitagawa, E. M., and Hauser, P. M., "Education Differentials in Mortality by Cause of Death, United States, 1960," *Demography* 5:318–353 (1968).

240. Kadushin, C., "Social Class and the Experience of Ill Health." *Sociological Inquiry* 24:67–80 (Winter 1964).

241. Antonovsky, A., "Social Class and Illness: A Reconsideration." *Sociological Inquiry* 37:311–322 (Spring 1967).

242. Antonovsky, A., "Social Class, Life Expectancy and Overall Mortality." *Milbank Memorial Fund Quarterly* 45:31–67 (April 1967) part 1.

Health Status as a Determinant of Medical Care Priorities

243. Etzioni, A., "Effectiveness, Efficiency, and the Danger of 'Over-Measurement,'" in *Modern Organizations*, pp. 8–10 (Englewood Cliffs, N.J.: Prentice-Hall, 1964). 120pp.

244. Hickman, J. C., and Estell, R. J., "On the Use of Partial Life Expectancies in Setting Health Goals," *American Journal of Public Health* 59:2243–2250 (December 1969).

245. Mushkin, S. J., "Toward a Definition of Health Economics," *Public Health Reports* 73:785–793 (September 1958).

246. Mushkin, S. J., and Collings, F. d'A., "Economic Costs of Disease and Injury," *Public Health Reports* 74:795–809 (September 1959).

247. Fein, R., *Economics of Mental Illness* (New York: Basic Books, Inc., 1958). 164pp.

248. Weisbrod, B., *Economics of Public Health* (Philadelphia: University of Pennsylvania Press, 1961). 127pp.

249. Klarman, H. E., "Costs and Benefits of Health Programs," in *The Economics of Health*, pp. 162–176 (New York: Columbia University Press, 1965). 200pp. (See bibliography on pp. 190–192.)

250. Rice, D. P., *Estimating the Cost of Illness*. P.H.S. Publication No. 947–6 (Washington, D.C.: U.S. Government Printing Office, May 1966). 16pp.

251. Rice, D. P., "The Economic Value of Human Life," *American Journal of Public Health* 57:1954–1966 (November 1967).

252. Klarman, H. E., "Present Status of Cost-Benefit Analysis in the Health Field," *American Journal of Public Health* 57:1948–1953 (November 1967).

253. Conley, R. W., Conwell, M., and Arrill, M. B., "An Approach to Measuring the Cost of Mental Illness," *American Journal of Psychiatry* 124:63–79 (December 1967).

254. Axnick, N. W., Shavell, S. M., and Witte, J. J., "Benefits Due to Immunization Against Measles," *Public Health Reports* 84:673–680 (August 1969).

255. Bureau of Health Services, Public Health Service, "Health Planning: The Basic Information System," in *Training in Health Planning: Philosophy and Concepts of Planning: Programming and Budgeting Systems, Instruction Manual* (Washington, D.C.: The Bureau, 1967). 25pp. (Processed).

256. Bureau of Health Services, Public Health Service, "Study Summary: Utiliza-

tion of a Health Problem Index Formula at the State Level'' (Washington, D.C.: The Bureau, January 24, 1968). 26pp. and appendices. (Processed).

257. Michael, J. M., Spatafore, G., and Williams, E. R., ''A Basic Information System for Health Plannings,'' *Public Health Reports* 83:21–28 (January 1968).

258. Pan American Health Organization, *Health Planning, Problems of Concept and Method.* Scientific Publication No. 111 (Washington, D.C., April 1965). See pp. 24–29.

259. Stewart, D., ''Planning as an Integral and Essential Part of a National Health Program,'' *Medical Care* 6:439–453, (November–December 1968).

260. Williamson, J. W., Alexander, M., and Miller, G. E., ''Priorities in Patient-Care Research and Continuing Medical Education,'' *Journal of the American Medical Association* 204:303–308 (April 22, 1968).

Additional References Cited

261. Freidson, E., *Patients' Views of Medical Practice* (New York: Russell Sage Foundation, 1961). 268pp.

262. Freeman, H. E., Levine, S., and Reeder, L. G., *Handbook of Medical Sociology* (Englewood Cliffs, N.J., Prentice-Hall, 1972). 598pp.

263. Mechanic, D., *Medical Sociology* (New York: The Free Press, 1968). 504pp.

264. Kasl, S., and Cobb, S., ''Health Behavior, Illness Behavior and Sick Role Behavior,'' *Archives of Environmental Health* 12:246–266 (February 1966); 12:531–541 (April 1966).

265. Ledley, R. S., and Lusted, L. B., ''Reasoning Foundations of Medical Diagnosis,'' *Science* 130:9–21 (July 3, 1959).

266. Von Woerkom, A., and Brodman, K., ''Statistics for a Diagnostic Model,'' *Biometrics* 17:299–318 (June 1961).

267. Warner, H. R., Toronto, A. F., Veasey, G., and Stephenson, R., ''A Mathematical Approach to Medical Diagnosis: Application to Congenital Heart Disease,'' *Journal of the American Medical Association* 177:177–183 (July 22, 1961).

268. Lincoln, T. L., and Parker, R. D., ''Medical Diagnosis Using Bayes Theorem,'' *Health Services Research* 2:34–45 (Spring 1967).

269. Kane, R. L., ''Determination of Health Care Priorities and Expectations Among Rural Consumers,'' *Health Services Research* 4:142–151 (Summer 1969).

270. Bogen, J. E., ''Some Student Concepts of Functional Disease,'' *Journal of Medical Education* 31:740–745 (November 1956).

271. Pennell, E. H., ''Location and Movement of Physicians—Methods for Estimating Resources.'' *Public Health Reports* 59:281–305 (March 3, 1944).

272. Gordon, J. E., et al., ''Synergism and Antagonism in Mass Disease of Man,'' *American Journal of Medical Sciences* 225:320–344 (March 1953).

273. Winter, K. E., and Metzner, C. A., *Institutional Care for the Long-Term Patient* (Ann Arbor: The University of Michigan School of Public Health, Bureau of Public Health Economics, Research Series, no. 7, 1958). 137pp.

274. Dann, W. J., and Darby, W. J., ''Appraisal of Nutritional Status (Nutriture) in Humans, with Especial Reference to Vitamin Deficiency Diseases,'' *Physiological Reviews* 25:326–346 (April 1945).

275. Rosenthal, G. D., *The Demand for General Hospital Facilities.* (Chicago: American Hospital Association, Hospital Monograph Series, no. 14, 1964). 101pp.

276. Lee, R. I., and Jones, L. W., *The Fundamentals of Good Medical Care.* Number 22 of the Publications of the Committee on the Costs of Medical Care (Chicago: The University of Chicago Press, January 1933). 302pp.

277. Johnson, A. C., Kroeger, H. H., Altman, I., Clark, D. A., and Sheps, C. G.,

"The Office Practice of Internists. III: Characteristics of Patients," *Journal of the American Medical Association* 193:916–922 (September 13, 1965).

278. Peterson, O. L., Andrews, L. P., Spain, R. S., and Greenberg, B. G., "An Analytical Study of North Carolina General Practice: 1953–1954," *The Journal of Medical Education*, vol. 31, no. 12, pt. 2 (December 1965). 165pp.

279. Clute, K. F., *The General Practitioner: A Study of Medical Education and Practice in Ontario and Nova Scotia* (Toronto: University of Toronto Press, 1963). 566pp.

280. Kroeger, H. H., Altman, D. A., Clark, A. C., Johnson, A. C., and Sheps, C. G., "The Office Practice of Internists. I: The Feasibility of Evaluating the Quality of Care," *Journal of the American Medical Association* 193:371–376 (August 2, 1965).

281. Donabedian, A., *A Review of Some Experiences with Prepaid Group Practice* (Ann Arbor: The University of Michigan, School of Public Health, Bureau of Public Health Economics, Research Series no. 12, 1965). 74pp.

282. World Health Organization, "Constitution," In *The First Ten Years of the World Health Organization* (Geneva: W.H.O., 1958). 538pp.

283. President's Commission on the Health Needs of the Nation, *Building America's Health: A Report to the President*. Vol. 2: *America's Health Status, Needs, and Resources* (Washington, D.C.: U.S. Government Printing Office, 1952–1953). 320pp.

284. Kandle, R. P., "Report of the Chairman of the Technical Development Board to the Governing Council 1959–1960," *American Journal of Public Health* 51:287–296 (February 1961).

285. Perkins, W. H., *Cause and Prevention of Disease* (Philadelphia, Lea and Febiger, 1938). 713pp.

286. Baumgartner, L., "Public Health Aspects of Problems of Current Interest in Neonatal Pediatrics," *Pediatrics* 11:489–501 (May 1953).

287. Williamson, J. W., "ABCD Strategy of Patient Care Evaluation—Key to Continuing Education Planning," Johns Hopkins School of Hygiene and Public Health. Unpublished paper, undated. 12pp. plus 6pp. of figures.

288. Donabedian, A., "An Evaluation of Prepaid Group Practices," *Inquiry* 6:3–27 (September 1969).

289. Williamson, J. W., "Outcomes of Health Care: Key to Health Improvement." Pages 75–101 in Hopkins, C. E., (Editor) *Methodology of Identifying, Measuring and Evaluating Outcomes of Health Service Programs, Systems and Subsystems*. U.S. Department of Health, Education, and Welfare, National Center for Health Services Research and Development (Washington, D.C.: U.S. Government Printing Office, 1970). 274pp.

290. Williamson, J. W., "Evaluating Quality of Patient Care. A Strategy Relating Outcome and Process Assessment." *Journal of the American Medical Association* 218:564–569 (October 25, 1971).

I V

Assessment of Supply

GENERAL FRAMEWORK

In the preceding chapter we presented a model for the evaluation of need. With a few modifications and extensions, the same model can serve as a framework for the evaluation of the resources that provide care. To recapitulate briefly, our framework began with a model of the medical care process that included two components, contributed by client and professional respectively, and the interactions between the two components. Use of service and health outcomes was seen as the resultant of the antecedent behaviors and interactions of clients and professionals in response to certain events or situations that one, the other, or both interpret as relevant to health care. To adapt this model to the evaluation of "need" it was necessary to introduce the concept of "need equivalents" which means, simply, that "need" may be expressed in terms of (1) health states, (2) services believed to be required to care for these states of health or illness, or (3) resources believed necessary to provide the services believed required. It was pointed out that a major task of health planning was the determination of these equivalences. In this chapter we shall deal with the resources that generate services and with their equivalents. The examination of these equivalents will require the explicit introduction of one last additional element into the model. This is the notion that certain factors influence the extent to which specified units of supply can be converted into equivalent units of service or equivalent capacity to satisfy health needs. These factors are conceived as characteristics of service-producing resources, of their internal organization and of their external relationships. They might be called "conversion factors" except that this phrase might mislead by suggesting the availability of precise, quantitative terms that enable a conversion to be made from one need equivalent to another. The state of knowledge concerning such "conversion factors" will be discussed in a subsequent chapter. What we are concerned with here is more the exploration of those variables that intervene between resources and their service equivalents or between the latter and their equivalents in satisfaction of health needs. We will therefore refer to these as "intervening factors." To reiterate, we shall be concerned with only a limited set of intervening factors, namely, those that we can conceive of as characteristics of the resources and of their organization.

A schematic presentation of the model for assessing supply is shown in Fig. IV.1. The reader will immediately recognize the four columns labeled "Equivalences," "Interactions," "Client Estimates," and "Professional Estimates," as well as the three rows that roughly correspond to "supply," "demand," and "need." The major differences from the model for assessing need, as shown in Fig. III.4, is that the column for "Interactions" has been transposed and that the rows have been rearranged so that the attention focuses first on "supply" rather than "need." Also, to keep the diagram simple, only a few of the arrows, indicating interrelationships, have been drawn in. Finally, four major intervening factors are shown. These are briefly indicated as "productivity," "potency," "appropriateness," and "accessibility." The factors that determine "productivity" intervene between the units of supply (resources) and the services which these units are able to produce. They refer to those characteristics of supply which influence its ability to produce service. It is recognized that this is only one possible definition of "productivity." In a subsequent section we shall further develop the

Fig. IV.1. A model for evaluating supply

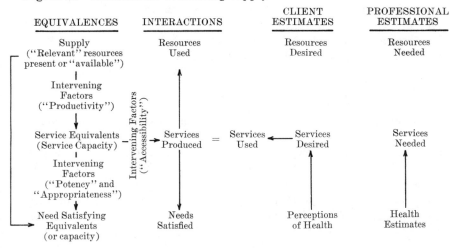

notion of productivity. The factors that determine "potency" and "appropriateness" intervene between service equivalents and need-satisfying equivalents because they determine the extent to which specified units of service are effective in actually influencing health status. "Potency" refers to the ability of medical science and technology, at any given time, to bring about changes in health status. "Appropriateness" refers to the extent to which available knowledge and techniques are used or misused in the management of illness and health. Thus, "appropriateness" is a major attribute, though not the whole, of "quality" (270, pp. 7–11). "Accessibility" intervenes between the capacity to provide service and the actual production of services, because it subsumes those characteristics of resources that make them more or less readily usable. There are, of course, many factors, other than "accessibility" that influence the use of service, but those other factors are conceived to be characteristics of professionals, of clients or of the medical care system as a whole. In this model, "accessibility" is distinguished from "availability," which is regarded as the mere presence of the resource and is therefore included under the heading of "supply."

The general notion of "equivalents" and the expressions "service equivalent" and "service capacity" are taken from a paper by Pennell (96). The observation had been made that of all physicians, those in the age group 35–44 made the most visits. This meant that if one was concerned with how many physicians were required to serve a given population, physicians could not be considered equal unless a correction had been made for age. This correction was "the decimal fraction obtained by dividing the average weekly number of patients seen by a physician of designated age by the corresponding number seen by a physician at the peak of his career" (96, p. 282n). This fraction was the "service capacity" or "service equivalent," terms which Pennell used interchangeably. The derivation of the "equivalent" was clearly empirical, based entirely on service load as it varied by age. Pennell was also aware, however, of the relevance of the question: How much *could* a physician produce, as visits, at any given age? He used the term "service potential" to signify possible, if not desirable, service load at each age.

In our formulation we have extended the notion of equivalents to include the ability to modify health states in addition to producing services. We differ somewhat from Pennell in placing much more emphasis on the normative determinations of equivalents. We are initially concerned with the question: How many visits or hospital days *should* a physician or hospital bed produce and what *should* the effect of these visits or days on health be? As a necessary second step, however, we shall be concerned with how many services are actually produced and what changes in health status are actually accomplished. One can then compare actual with potential as a measure of how the system performs and what prospect for better performance remains.

One concept not shown in the model, but which relates to important attributes of it, is that of "efficiency." The reader will recall the analogous omission of the concept of "quality" from the schematic presentation of the medical care process. This was because "quality" was conceived as an evaluative statement about any aspect of the process. Somewhat analogously, the concept of efficiency belongs in the model for assessing supply, though it cannot be shown graphically. This is because efficiency deals with a very different dimension of the model: the relationship between output and input usually expressed in terms of the money value of each. An omission from the model of an entirely different nature is that of "unmet" or "overmet" needs. The points in the model where such deficits or superfluities may arise can be readily identified by the reader. Their omission is merely in the interests of simplicity in visual presentation.

In subsequent sections of this chapter, there will be a discussion of (1) the specification and measurement of units of supply, (2) the factors that influence the capacity of these units to provide service, (3) the relationship between the capacity to provide service and the actual production of service, and (4) the relationship between the capacity to provide service and the need, as well as the demand, for service. In the process, the brief definitions of "productivity," "potency," "appropriateness," "efficiency," and "accessibility" that were given above will be considerably amplified and, hopefully, clarified.

SPECIFICATION OF UNITS OF SUPPLY

General Considerations

It is a truism that the first issue in assessment is a clear understanding of what is being assessed. Unfortunately, with respect to supply, this condition is not always satisfied. Misunderstanding may arise at the very outset because, as Klarman has pointed out, "supply" is used in the literature of medical care organization to mean something rather different from what it means in economics (1). In medical care usage, "supply" generally refers to a count of the *units that produce service* which are present at any given time in a given locality—for example, the number of physicians or of hospital beds. Almost always, the count of service-producing units is related, either explicitly or implicitly, to some rough measure of need or demand. The usual expression of "supply," therefore, is a ratio of the service-producing unit (physician, bed) to a unit of population. Hence there are the usual expressions of "supply" such as the physician : population ratio or the bed : population ratio. It might clarify things considerably if this usage of the word "supply" were abandoned and, borrowing from epidemiology, we were to speak of the "prevalence" of physicians, beds, or whatever service-producing resource is the object of concern.

A less frequent practice in medical care organization is to specify "supply" not in terms of service-producing resources, but in terms of *functions* that need to be performed : for example, nursing care in the home, prenatal care, rehabilitation services, and the like. The fundamental difference is that each of these functions includes the organized contribution of several categories of service-producing units. Each of the units may be present at a given level in each community, but the issue is whether the particular mode of organization that is necessary for the optimal performance of the function is present or absent. This book largely adheres to traditional, medical-care usage in quantitating "supply" primarily in terms of service-producing units, and secondarily in terms of the "service-equivalents" of those units. The organization of these units and services to perform certain functions, and the relationship between the presence of units and the satisfaction of need or demand, are the concerns of the evaluative process.

Having come to some agreement as to what one means by the word "supply," the next decision to be made is the choice of units to be enumerated or measured and the explicit definition of these units. The choice and definition of unit or units depends in turn, on two major considerations : (1) functional differentiation in the production of services, and (2) the relevance of such functional differentiation to the purposes of the assessment. The purpose, generally, is to determine the availability of service-producing resources to meet certain service needs. Personnel, facilities or equipment not relevant to the service needs in question, obviously, should not be enumerated. As an example, for physicians one needs to decide whether doctors of medicine and doctors of osteopathy are equivalent sources of service, and whether chiropractors can also qualify for the same purpose, or must be excluded. Similarly, one needs to determine whether all physicians qualify (including those in teaching, research, or administrative work) or whether one is concerned only with those who provide patient care. The specialization of health personnel raises further questions. For example, if one were interested in measuring the capacity to provide general patient care, one might want to exclude from consideration a large number of specialists, or to develop some method of rating certain specialties in terms of part-time equivalents of general patient care that they provide, or are capable of providing. Full-time equivalents of part-time practice may have to be developed. Similar considerations pertain to hospitals and other facilities. Hospitals, for example, are not homogeneous but are differentiated from one another in several ways, including major function and clientele. Within hospitals, beds are also often assigned to special uses. The characterization of the prevalence of hospitals must therefore take these categories into account.

An additional aspect of relevance that applies to both health personnel and hospitals is the operational or nonoperational nature of the supply. Obviously, hospital beds that are not fully staffed and equipped cannot be considered equivalent to those that have a full complement of staff and equipment; nor can physicians who are inactive or in semiretirement be considered part of the service-providing establishment. However, the concept of operationality is not completely distinct. On the one hand, it overlaps with that of functional differentiation and, on the other, with some of the factors that influence productivity, which are to be discussed in a subsequent section. Perhaps the clearest examples of nonoperational supply are the inactive health professional and the bed in the closed wing of a hospital. Professional inactivity is a particularly salient feature of certain occupations staffed largely by women. For example, at any given time, about one-third of nurses and about half of dental hygienists are reported to be inactive (33, Table 6, p. 13; 31, p. 193). Here, one purpose of the assessment may be to estimate the extent to which, given certain incentives, such nonoperational supply may be made operational.

An illustration of the relevance of some of these considerations may be found in the Report of the Surgeon General's Group on Medical Education (379). They assembled figures to show that although the number of physicians (MD) per unit population had increased between 1931 and 1957, a closer examination revealed certain adverse trends. Among these was a marked decline in "family physician potential" as represented by pediatricians, internists, and physicians in general practice or part-time specialty. Table IV.1, derived from data which the Group assembled, illustrates how different conclusions concerning the adequacy of supply may be drawn depending on what premises, explicit or implicit, the investigator has accepted. More recent information shows that certain of the trends shown in Table IV.1 continue to be observed. For example, between 1950 and 1965 physicians in private practice per 100,000 civil-

Table IV.1.   Physician-population ratios for 1931 and 1957 and percent change from 1931 to 1957, according to specified categories of physicians, U.S.A.

Categories of Physicians	Physicians per 100,000 Civilian Population			
	1931	1957	Absolute Change	Percent Change
All physicians (MD)	126	132	+14	+5
All physicians in active practice[a]	116	112	−4	−4
All physicians in private practice	108	109	−17	−16
"Family physician potential"	94	60	−34	−36

SOURCE: Reference 379, pages 10 and 83–84.

[a] Arrived at by the exclusion of the categories of "teaching, research, public health," "Federal government" and "retired."

ians were reduced from 103.0 to 92.0, an absolute decline of 11.0 per 100,000 and a relative decline of over 9 percent. During the same period, physicians in "family practice" were reduced from 75.8 to 50.0 per 100,000, an absolute decline of 25.8 and a relative decline of 34 percent (380, Appendix Table 5, p. 75). Recently, Overpeck has reexamined trends in the availability of physicians for family practice between 1931 and 1967 with due regard to the noncomparability of data over time (381).

Somewhat similar considerations have gone into the determination of pediatric manpower in the United States. If it is assumed that the general care of children below 15 years of age requires special competence possessed by general practitioners and pediatricians, but not by internists or physicians in other specialties, one can make estimates of what might be called "child care potential" as distinct from "family physician potential." The historical data and estimates in Table IV.2 are quoted by Bergman et al. based on work by Stewart and Pennell (25). The point made is that although the total physician:population ratio might remain unchanged, a particular subsection of it, relevant to some special need, may become ostensibly inadequate. The reader may, however, question the assumption implicit in the foregoing formulation.

A final precondition in the assessment of supply is knowledge of the sources of published, or otherwise available, information concerning service-providing units one has elected to enumerate or measure. One

Table IV.2.   "Child health physicians" per 100,000 children, U.S.A., at decennial intervals, 1930–1980

Year	Child Health Physicians per 100,000 Children
1930	314
1940	336
1950	242
1960	146
1970	106 (estimate)
1980	68 (estimate)

SOURCE: Reference 171, Table 7, page 262.

needs to know not only what information is available, but also the precise manner in which the units are defined, the data assembled, the completeness of the data, and their validity. The availability of information may indeed influence the choice of units and their classification for the purpose of assessment.

It follows from the preceding discussion, that the execution of the most meaningful characterization of supply requires a profound understanding of the structure and function of the service-producing apparatus and of the uses to which it may be put. It is, obviously, beyond the scope of this book to bring about this kind of understanding. Here, our attention will be confined to certain selected facets of the assessment, with emphasis on procedural, rather than substantive, aspects. We will identify the kinds of factors that need to be taken into account and furnish some illustrations as a guide to the administrator. Where possible, the examples will be chosen to show the applicability of the factors or approaches described to health personnel and to facilities. Physicians will generally be chosen to represent the category of health personnel, and hospitals to represent health facilities. This choice is made because of the key importance of these two resources, the greater availability of literature concerning them, and the greater familiarity of the author with this literature.

Data on Health Personnel

SOURCES OF INFORMATION. A brief description and evaluation of the major sources of information concerning the supply of health personnel is to be found in the introduction to the compendium on Health Resources published by the National Center for Health Statistics in 1968

(3). These sources include (1) the records of individual professional and vocational schools, and compilations of these records prepared by associations of such schools (for example, the Association of American Medical Colleges) and by the National Center for Educational Statistics; (2) licensure and registration data kept by the appropriate official agencies; (3) certification or registration by bodies established by the professions themselves; (4) association membership lists; (5) information from places of employment, including surveys of such establishments—for example, by the National Center for Health Statistics; and (6) a portion of the decennial census that is based on a 5 percent sample of the population. The bibliography to this chapter gives concrete references to publications that contain information from one or more of these sources (7–11).

The reliability of estimates of manpower varies by source and by occupation. In some instances, the best available estimates may be off by as much as 50 percent (3, p. 7). Information obtained from professional or vocational schools is meant to give a picture of entry into the health occupations. The accuracy and completeness of this information is best for the established professions that require highly formalized and distinctive educational preparation: medicine and dentistry, for example. The quality and completeness of information from educational institutions deteriorates progressively at the baccalaureate and sub-baccalaureate levels and is totally absent for those occupations, or segments of them, who are prepared by on-the-job training. The data are also incomplete, at any level of training, if a significant number of foreign graduates are recruited into the profession, as is true for medicine. Data from educational institutions are a particularly valuable, perhaps unique, source of information concerning certain aspects of the qualifications of health personnel. They can also provide information concerning an additional aspect of recruitment into the profession, namely, the number of qualifications of applicants for admission, as compared with those who are actually admitted (22). After corrections are made for multiple applications, these figures give a picture of the demand for professional education. When corrections are made for those unqualified by current standards, one obtains a picture of the pool of potential manpower, at least in the short run. Data from educational institutions cannot, of course, provide an estimate of the actual prevalence of manpower since they offer no information on depletion through inactivity, retirement, outmigration, or death.

Licensure statistics are fairly complete for some professions and incomplete or absent for others.

About 25 occupations in the health field are licensed in one or more States. All States and the District of Columbia require that the following health personnel have a license to practice: dental hygienists, dentists, environmental health engineers, optometrists, pharmacists, physicians (MD and D.O.), podiatrists, practical nurses, registered nurses, and veterinarians. All except a few States license chiropractors and physical therapists. About 20 to 30 States license midwives, opticians, psychologists, and sanitarians or sanitary inspectors. Fewer than one-third of the States license clinical laboratory directors, including bioanalysts, clinical laboratory personnel such as medical technologists or technicians, naturopaths and other drugless healers, and social workers. Ten States license nursing home administrators. Health department administrators, hospital administrators, and radiologic technologists (X-ray technicians) are licensed in one State each (10, p. 4).

At any level, licensure statistics have to be carefully scrutinized for licensure of the same person in several states, as well as for inactivity or death of the licensee. In some states, periodic renewal of licensure is not required, and where it is, active practice is not usually a requirement for licensure.

Professional associations may provide considerable information, additional to mere numbers, concerning members as well as nonmembers. For example, "A master file of physicians has been maintained by the American Medical Association since 1906. It has included information on every physician in the United States and on those graduates of American medical schools practicing overseas on a temporary basis. The file includes members and non-members of the Association. It also includes aliens residing in this country. Inclusion in the file starts during the medical school phase of a physician's career or upon entry into the country. The master file is divided into two sections: (1) current records of professional activities, and (2) historical records. "Historical data such as "previous professional addresses and licenses . . . facilitate studies of geographical mobility and specialization trends in medical practice" (19, p. 1). Beginning with 1966, the A.M.A. has also conducted a yearly mail-questionnaire survey of a national sample of physicians in "office-oriented" practice, which has included questions on aspects of the physician's practice, such as workload and income, concerning which reliable information has been very difficult to come by (20, 162).

Information from the master file of the American Medical Association has appeared in periodic issues of the *American Medical Directory* which, for decades, has been the major source of information concerning the characteristics of the corps of physicians in the United States (16). The *Directory* lists physicians by name and, for each, provides coded information on education, training, and aspects of practice. These include professional mailing address, year of birth, medical education (state, school, year of MD degree), year of license in present state, National Board (year), American Specialty Board, "primary specialty," "secondary specialty," and type of practice (intern, research, etc.). From 1906 to 1958, the *Directory* also included summary tabulations of the number and characteristics of physicians. Starting with the year 1963, a comparable series of tabulations has appeared in other annual publications of the American Medical Association (4, 18). The data in all these publications are compiled from responses to yearly questionnaires mailed to all physicians (MD) known to the AMA, irrespective of membership in the Association. The characterization obtained is therefore that described by the physician for himself. This feature influences, in particular, the reported specialization status of the physician. For this purpose, "primary specialty" used to be defined as the "Recognized Specialty Field to which the physician devotes his major interest," and "secondary specialty," the "Recognized Specialty Field in which the physician indicates that he has a limited interest." Since 1968, primary, secondary and tertiary specialty designations have been assigned according to the average number of hours during a typical week that are allocated to each specialty, as reported by each physician respondent. More detailed information about an altogether different subset of specialists, those who have achieved certification by a specialty Board, is available in the *Directory of Medical Specialists* (17). The author knows of almost no published studies of the completeness and validity of the information in either of these directories. It is known, however, that the A.M.A. goes to considerable lengths to keep its master file complete and current. The yearly mail questionnaires of the recent past (1968 and 1969) have achieved a usable response rate of around 87 percent after 5 mailings (19). For the future, there will be a complete census of the entire physician population every three years. In between, there will be a weekly updating system based on "indications" from physicians, hospitals, government agencies, medical schools, medical societies, specialty boards, and the like (19).

A partial test of reliability, if not validity, was obtained in 1966 as a by-product of a mailed questionnaire survey of a random sample of 3,544 physicians in "office-oriented practice" listed in the AMA master file (162). The response rate was almost 89 percent, but only 80 percent of questionnaires yielded responses that were used. The specialty reported in the survey was identical with that in the AMA Directory in 88 percent of cases and different in 12 percent. There were variations by specialty in the degree of correspondence, with the difference largest for the category of general practice, namely, 22 percent. The differences noted were attributed partly to the lapse of as much as one year for some of the respondents and partly to the different criterion used to judge specialty status in the survey: namely, the derivation of 50 percent or more of medical income from that specialty. Lists of certified specialists are probably very accurate, provided efforts are made to update them, to remove decedents, and to identify those who are no longer active. However, they provide information on a rather limited segment of the profession.

Additional problems arise, when time series are examined, because of changes in the definitions used or procedures employed in the assembling of information. Fein has pointed out that "at various times . . . osteopaths were included in the Bureau of the Census definition of physicians; at other times they were not. On occasion, the Bureau of the Census included only those physicians gainfully employed as physicians; at other times, physicians seeking work were also included" (289, p. 65). A major change occurred in the reporting of physicians as a consequence of a conference called in 1963 by the Federal Office of Emergency Planning. Table IV.3, derived from a report by Pennell, gives a brief descrip-

Table IV.3.   Conventions used in the reporting of the supply of physicians, U.S.A., before and after 1963

Characteristics of Data or Physicians	Previous to 1963	Recommended in 1963
Reporting date	Mid year. Excludes current year's graduates	December 31. Includes current year's graduates
Non-federal physicians with temporary foreign address	Included	Excluded
Non-federal physicians with address temporarily unknown to AMA	Included	Included; but dropped if no reply after three yearly requests
Foreign physicians in training programs in the U.S.	Excluded	Included
Unlicensed foreign physicians other than interns and residents	Excluded	Included
Physicians not in practice (retired, not in practice)	Included	Included
Doctors of Osteopathy	Excluded (by AMA)	Included (when labeled MD and DO)

SOURCE: Reference 24 and personal communication from author.

tion of the changes made and illustrates the kinds of questions that arise in the categorization of supply (24). The major changes are the inclusion of doctors of osteopathy in the aggregate number under the rubric of "physicians," the inclusion of the rather large number of foreign physicians in training programs who temporarily provide significant care to the U.S. population and the inclusion of the graduates from U.S. schools who qualify during the year of the report. The Conference also made recommendations concerning the manner in which the population base of the prevalence ratio should be constructed. For example, it was recommended that U.S. citizens overseas who are Government civilian employees, their dependents, and dependents of Armed Forces personnel be included, but that U.S. civilian citizens residing abroad be excluded. The net effect of all these revisions in the rules governing the reporting of physicians was a spurious increase in the reported prevalence. Apparent lack of awareness of the purely procedural basis for this change, resulted in two sets of figures and two conclusions concerning trends in the prevalence of physicians, one by some spokesmen for the AMA and another by representatives of the Public Health Service (371). The data were as shown in Table IV.4.

Table IV.4.   Physician population ratios in 1960 and 1963 and percent increase between the two dates, as reported by the American Medical Association and the Public Health Service, U.S.A.

Year	Physicians/100,000 as Reported by	
	A.M.A.	P.H.S.
1960	137.8	144.2
1963	146.7	145.9
Percent increase	6.5%	1.2%

SOURCE: Reference 371.

Further information concerning the sources of data on health manpower and the reliability of the data will be found in the publication referred to (3). Enough has been said to indicate the need to evaluate carefully the nature of the information before it is used in assessment. This does not mean that only perfect information can be used. On the contrary, in many instances rough information is quite adequate, and it would be both costly and inappropriate to seek unnecessary refinement. For other purposes, high degrees of refinement may be essential.

CLASSIFICATION. As we have already pointed out, the classification of units of service-producing resources and the choice of the appropriate unit or units are activities that require thorough understanding of health manpower resources in general, of the structure and functions of each component health occupation, and of the basic purposes of the assessment. The following, therefore, are merely illustrations of possible ways in which health occupations may be classified in order to display aspects of their structural and functional configuration.

The Census of Occupations by Industry identifies certain occupations as primarily engaged in the provision of health services. For these occupations, as well as for a larger listing of other occupations, it identifies how many are employed in health services, how many in all industries including health services, and the percent of all employees in each category who are employed in health service industries. This classification of occupations primarily engaged in the provision of health services is given in Table IV.5. The reader will note, first, that the listing is incomplete. Second, it contains peculiar anamolies, such as the inclusion of chiropractors and medical technicians in the same broad group with physicians. A much more complete listing of health occupations, with relatively homogeneous categories, has been prepared by the National Center for Health Statistics, and is used in the compilation of data reported by the Center. A condensed version of the classification is shown in Table IV.6. The full version contains 32 "fields" (categories) plus another designated as "miscellaneous." It identifies about 125 health occupations and "approximately 250 alternate titles such as synonyms or designations related for form of practice, type of specialty or place of practice." There are approximately 375 titles in all. Occupations essential, but not unique, to the health service industry are omitted from the list.

Attempts to group the health occupations into functionally meaningful families date at least back to the Committee on the Costs of Medical Care which proposed the following classification (12) :

1) Primary practitioners : physicians, dentists
2) Secondary practitioners : midwives, chiropodists, optometrists
3) Cultists or sectarian practitioners : osteopaths, chiropractors, Naturopaths (including herbalists), homeopaths, Christian Science practitioners, New Thought healers.

The classification cited above would evoke much argument today concerning the extent to which the several professions have a primary

Table IV.5.   Occupations primarily engaged in the provision of health services, as identified by the U.S. Census, 1970[a]

PROFESSIONAL TECHNICAL AND KINDRED WORKERS

Physicians, dentists, and related practitioners
   Chiropractors
   Dentists
   Optometrists
   Pharmacists
   Physicians, medical and osteopathic
   Podiatrists
   Veterinarians
   Health practitioners, n.e.c.

Nurses, dietitians, and therapists
   Dietitians
   Registered nurses
   Therapists

Health technologists and technicians
   Clinical laboratory technologists and technicians
   Dental hygienists
   Health record technologists and technicians
   Radiologic technologists and technicians
   Therapy assistants
   Health technologists and technicians, n.e.c.

Teachers, college and university
   Health specialties teachers

MANAGERS AND ADMINISTRATORS, EXCEPT FARM
Health administrators

CLERICAL AND KINDRED WORKERS
Secretaries
   Secretaries, medical

CRAFTSMEN AND KINDRED WORKERS
Dental laboratory technicians
Opticians, lens grinders and polishers

SERVICE WORKERS, EXCEPT PRIVATE HOUSEHOLD
Health service workers
   Dental assistants
   Health aides, except nursing
   Health trainees
   Lay midwives
   Nursing aides, orderlies and attendants
   Practical nurses

SOURCE: Information provided by Maryland Y. Pennell, Division of Allied Health Manpower, Public Health Service.

[a] Because of changes in classification which include the addition of some new categories and different assignments to some existing categories, 1970 and 1960 data cannot be compared without adjustment.

function or are merely secondary to, or auxiliary to, those identified in the classification as "primary." The classification of osteopathic physicians as sectarian practitioners is no longer justified, although most physicians would still relegate chiropractic to the status of a cult.

More recently, Weiss has examined critically the Census classification of health occupations and has proposed an alternative which he considers more meaningful for the study of developments in the health services industry. Using an approach developed by Scoville (13) he has identified a set of occupations that make up the "health care job family"; has further categorized these into subsets (also called "families") according to "technical focus" and, finally, has grouped the occupations by "level of job content" (14, 15). Two criteria were used to identify occupations that belonged in the health care job family:

(1) the job can be performed only by persons whose principal training has been oriented toward the provision of health services; (2) transfer of persons performing the job to a job not oriented toward the provision of health services would entail either a great deal of retraining or failure to utilize acquired skills (14, p. 55).

Using available information on the "technical focus of care," Weiss has distinguished the following categories ("families") of health occupations:

1. Health jobs . . . directly concerned with patient care.
   Patient care—mental
   Patient care—nursing
   Patient care—medical
   Patient care—dental

2. Health jobs . . . not oriented toward direct patient care.
   Technical and laboratory focus
   Administration and planning—health
   Data-processing—health
   Environmental health focus
   Health research

Perhaps the most interesting, and analytically most useful, of the classifications devised by Weiss is one that classifies health occupations by "level of job content." To do this, he used two surrogate measures of job content to each of which he gave equal weight in the final ranking. These were: (1) "the minimum number of years of formal education required—regardless of whether the education was geared or oriented toward a specific vocation—plus an estimate of on-the-job time required for training," and (2) "the median earnings of persons who worked in

Table IV.6.   Classification of health occupations, National Center for Health Statistics, 1970

1. ADMINISTRATION
   Health administrator
   Health administrative assistant
   Health program analyst
   Health program representative
   Health systems analyst

2. BIOMEDICAL ENGINEERING
   Biomedical engineer
   Biomedical engineering technician
   Biomedical engineering aide

3. CHIROPRACTIC AND NATUROPATHY
   Chiropractor
   Naturopath

4. CLINICAL LABORATORY SERVICES
   Clinical laboratory scientist
   Clinical laboratory technologist
   Clinical laboratory technician
   Clinical laboratory aide

5. DENTISTRY AND ALLIED SERVICES
   Dentist
   Dental hygienist
   Dental assistant
   Dental laboratory technician

6. DIETETIC AND NUTRITIONAL SERVICES
   Dietitian
   Nutritionist
   Dietary technician
   Dietary aide
   Food service supervisor

7. ENVIRONMENTAL CONTROL
   Environmental scientist
   Environmental engineer
   Environmental technologist
   Environmental technician
   Environmental aide

8. FOOD AND DRUG PROTECTIVE SERVICES
   Food technologist
   Food and drug inspector
   Food and drug analyst
   Food and drug technician

9. HEALTH EDUCATION
   Health educator
   Health education aide

10. INFORMATION AND COMMUNICATION
    Health information specialist
    Health science writer
    Health technical writer
    Medical illustrator

11. LIBRARY SERVICES
    Medical librarian
    Medical library assistant
    Hospital librarian

12. MATHEMATICAL SCIENCES
    Mathematician
    Statistician

13. MEDICAL RECORDS
    Medical record librarian
    Medical record technician
    Medical record clerk

14. MEDICINE AND OSTEOPATHY
    Physician
    Osteopathic physician
    M.D. or D.O.

15. MIDWIFERY
    Midwife

16. NATURAL SCIENCES
    Anatomist
    Botanist
    Chemist
    Ecologist
    Entomologist
    Epidemiologist
    Geneticist
    Hydrologist
    Immunologist
    Meteorologist
    Microbiologist
    Nutritionist
    Oceanographer
    Pathologist
    Pharmacologist
    Physicist
    Physiologist
    Sanitary sciences specialist
    Zoologist

17. NURSING AND RELATED SERVICES
    Nurse
    Practical nurse
    Nursing aide
    Orderly
    Attendant
    Home health aide
    Ward clerk

18. OCCUPATIONAL THERAPY
    Occupational therapist
    Occupational therapy assistant
    Occupational therapy aide

19. ORTHOTIC AND PROSTHETIC TECHNOLOGY
    Orthotist
    Orthotic aide
    Prosthetist
    Prosthetic aide
    Restoration technician

20. PHARMACY
    Pharmacist
    Pharmacy aide

21. PHYSICAL THERAPY
    Physical therapist
    Physical therapy assistant
    Physical therapy aide

22. PODIATRIC MEDICINE
    Podiatrist

23. RADIOLOGIC TECHNOLOGY
    Radiologic technologist
    Radiologic technician

24. SECRETARIAL AND OFFICE SERVICES
    Secretary
    Office assistant

25. SOCIAL SCIENCES
    Anthropologist
    Economist
    Psychologist
    Sociologist

26. SOCIAL WORK
    Clinical social worker
    Clinical social work assistant
    Clinical social work aide

27. SPECIALIZED REHABILITATION SERVICES
Corrective therapist
Corrective therapy aide
Educational therapist
Manual arts therapist
Music therapist
Recreation therapist
Recreation therapy aide
Homemaking rehabilitation consultant

28. SPEECH PATHOLOGY AND AUDIOLOGY
Audiologist
Speech pathologist

29. VETERINARY MEDICINE
Veterinarian
Veterinary technician

30. VISION CARE AND SERVICES
Ophthalmologist
Optometrist
Vision care technologist
Technician:
    Vision care technician
    Orthoptic technician
    Optician
Vision care aide

31. VOCATIONAL REHABILITATION COUNSELING
Vocational rehabilitation counselor

32. MISCELLANEOUS HEALTH SERVICES
Assistance for physicians:
    Physician's associate
    Physician's assistant
    Physician's aide
Emergency health service
    Medical emergency technician
    Ambulance attendant (aide)
Inhalation therapy
    Inhalation therapist
    Inhalation therapy aide
Medical machine technology
    Cardiopulmonary technician
    Electrocardiograph technician
    Electroencephalograph technician
    Other
Nuclear medicine
    Nuclear medical technologist
    Nuclear medical technician
Other health services
    Community health aide
    Extracorporeal circulation specialist
    Other

SOURCE: Reference 3 (1970), pp. 350–356.

that category for at least 50 weeks'' in a given year. In this way it was possible to classify health occupations into three levels: high, middle and low, as shown in Table IV.7. One might debate the degree to which the proxy measures chosen, and especially income, regularly reflect level of job content. For various reasons, nursing, for example, is likely to be underrated by the income criterion (294, 297). Nevertheless, the general

Table IV.7.   Health care jobs by level of job content

HIGH LEVEL

Psychiatrist and neurologist	Biochemist
Physician and surgeon (MD, DO)[a]	Administrator—hospital and
Dentist	other health institution
Veterinarian	Psychologist—clinical
Life scientist—health	Optometrist
Podiatrist	Pharmacist
Biophysicist	Health education specialist
	Sanitary engineer

MIDDLE LEVEL

Social worker, psychiatric	Medical laboratory technologist-
Social worker, medical	technician
Chiropractor	Dietitian and nutritionist
Rehabilitation counselor	Medical record librarian
Speech and hearing therapist	Medical X-ray technician
Sanitarian	Dental laboratory technician
Industrial hygienist	Optician and lens grinder and
Physical therapist	polisher
Occupational therapist	Nurse, professional
Other therapist	Dental hygienist
	Midwife

LOW LEVEL

Dental assistant, dental office	Practical nurse
Medical office assistant	Attendant, hospitals and other
Medical record technician	institutions

SOURCE: Reference 14, Table 6, page 61.
[a] Excludes psychiatrists and neurologists.

concept appears to be valid and useful as demonstrated by Weiss in his analysis of the changing structure of health manpower (15).

The National Center for Health Statistics has introduced a further refinement in terminology by suggesting the designations ''Technologist'' or ''Therapist'' be used for persons with educational preparation at the baccalaureate level or above, "Technician" or "Assistant" for those with two years of formal preparation beyond high school, and "Aide" for health personnel with less than two years of education beyond high school as well as those who have only received on-the-job training (3–1970, p. 349).

A categorization of health occupations is often only a prelude to more detailed classification of any particular occupation. For this purpose, one or more of the following axes of classification may be appropriate: legal status, education or training, post-graduate training, specialization, organization of practice, source of income, and employer, the latter politically or functionally defined. Legal status is, of course, germane to the availability of manpower for practice within a particular political jurisdiction. It may also distinguish a hierarchy of function within a given occupation or family of occupations. The legally permissible functions assigned to the "registered nurse" and the "licensed practical nurse" are an example. Educational distinctions are particularly important in occupations, such as nursing, where a very wide range of preparation is subsumed under the generic designation of the occupation; hence the compulsion to further distinguish nurses in the precise order of their hagiarchy as doctoral, masters, baccalaureate, associate degree or merely diplomaed! The American Nursing Association would like to see the first three positions in this order designated as "professional nurse practitioner," the last two as "technical nurse practitioner," and everything beneath it as "assistants to nurses" (372). By contrast, organized medicine has an aversion to invidious educational comparisons, other than its near obsession with the distinction between graduates of U.S. schools (which include, for this purpose, Canada) and all other schools, which are designated as "foreign." In justification, it may be pointed out that the few studies that have been published indicate that foreign graduates from large segments of the world, though not all, tend to be inferior in their performance in the United States (373–375). Students during the course of their education, and professionals during post-graduate training, may provide significant service. The Census, for example, has had a separate category for "nurses, student professional" (even though the use of nursing students for patient care is no longer significant outside the hospital-based schools, and much reduced in the latter), and the National Center for Health Statistics distinguishes physicians in training as "intern," "resident," or "fellow."

The classification of physicians by the American Medical Association indicates the significance for certain purposes, including availability for care to the civilian population, or classification by organization of practice and employer. For many years this classification was as follows (5; p. 102) :

Private practice
Other Practice
  Non-federal
  Federal
In training programs
Retired, not in practice or status not reported

In 1966, the A.M.A. adopted a new classification more oriented to care-providing potential than the merely political implications of the mode of employment. The new classification has been incorporated in recent tabulations of the National Center for Health Statistics (3, p. 124) :

A. Non-Federal

   1. Patient care
      a. Solo, partnership, group or other practice
         (1) General practice
         (2) Other full-time specialty
      b. Training programs
      c. Full-time hospital staff

   2. Other professional activity
      Includes teaching, administration and research

   3. Inactive

B. Federal

   1. Patient Care
      a. Training programs
      b. Full-time hospital staff

   2. Other professional activity
      Includes teaching, administration, and research

C. Address unknown

In 1968 the American Medical Association introduced still another classification which carried even further the emphasis on the locus and nature of professional activities as the basis for distinctions among categories and which, accordingly, required a major change in the

Table IV.8.   Percent distribution of physicians by each of two classifications, and percent change in numbers of physicians in each category when the new classification is compared with the old, U.S.A., December 31, 1968

Major Professional Activity	Percent Distribution		Percent Change
	Old Class.	New Class.	
Total physicians	100	100	0
Patient Care	89	83	− 8
Office-based practice	61	58	− 5
Hospital-based practice	28	24	− 14
Interns	3	4	+ 4
Residents	12	11	− 4
Full-time physician staff	13	9	− 27
Other professional activity	6	11	+ 77
Medical teaching	4	2	− 55
Administration	1	4	+199
Research	1	5	+251
Other	—	1	—
Inactive	4	6	+ 54
No classification	—	—	—
Address unknown	1	1	+ 2

SOURCE: Reference 19, Table C, page 18.

questionnaire used to obtain information from physicians (19). Table IV.8 shows the new classification, and gives the magnitude of the changes that occur in the relative importance of categories of physicians when the new classification is used, instead of its predecessor, to categorize the same population of physicians. Where the number of physicians in a category is large, the relative changes are small. However, for some of the smaller categories, the method of classification is shown to be a matter of decisive importance. For example, whereas the physicians assigned to the category of "patient care" are reduced by about 8 percent, those described as engaged in professional activities other than patient care are augmented by 77 percent. This is the resultant of a 55 percent decrease in physicians who are reported to be primarily involved in medical teaching, while those in research and administration are shown to have increased by 251 and 199 percent respectively. Thus, the use of one classification as compared to another may not change our general view of the population of physicians, but it can be critical when dealing with smaller subgroups. The same is true when one examines the percent distribution of physicians by specialty. The new procedures increase the number of diagnostic roentgenologists by 1700 percent, of therapeutic radiologists by 450 percent, of forensic pathologists by 286 percent, and of pediatric allergists by 229 percent! The numerically more important specialties are less influenced, in relative terms, though the shifts in numbers from one category to another can be large. For example, according to the new classification there are now 6000 fewer general practitioners, or a reduction of 9 percent in the total.

The changes that we have discussed occur not only because of differences in the categories in the two classifications, but also because of new definitions or rules of allocation. The most important of these is that the physicians are asked to report the average number of hours spent on specified activities during a typical week. Physicians are separated into active and inactive depending on whether they report 20 or more or less than 20 hours of work per week, without regard to how they describe their activity status (retired, semiretired, disabled, temporarily not in practice or not active for other reasons, being the categories specified in the classification). Similarly, assignment to practice and specialty categories depends on the number of hours allocated to each category by the physician. By this rule, a physician may claim as many as three specialties: "primary," "secondary," and "tertiary." When the hours of work allocated to two or more categories are equal, uniform procedures are used to break the tie. An important feature of the classification is that no physician shall be without his niche, even if it is only a residual category such as "no classification," for those who have not responded to current or past survey, or "address unknown," for those truly lost to the fold.

Perhaps the most significant attribute of the physician establishment, other than availability for patient care, is specialization status. The significance of functional differentiation to productive capacity will be discussed in a subsequent section of this chapter. Here we are concerned merely with classification. We have already referred to the fact that the A.M.A. *Directory* classified a physician as a specialist if he said he "devotes his major interest" to a specialty field recognized by the A.M.A. The *Directory* currently recognizes "primary" and "secondary" specialties. In former years prominence was given in the tabulations to a category of "part-time specialist" that does not figure in current reports (16). Prior to 1969 the American Medical Association "recognized," in addition to general practice, 20 "specialties," 7 "sub-specialties," and 7 "special fields." All these, excluding general practice, were grouped into 4 categories as follows: medical specialties, surgical specialties, psychiatry and neurology, and other specialties. (5, Table 75, p. 103; and 16). In 1969

"Family Practice" was accepted as a recognized specialty, replacing general practice in A.M.A. tabulations. In 1970 the list was radically expanded to comprise 63 entries, including "hypnosis," but not, as yet, acupuncture (19, pp. 28, 29). The Advisory Board for Medical Specialties, which is largely a creature of the A.M.A., recognizes certification by one of its member Boards, of which there are 20—some with subspecialties. A list of these is given in Table IV.9. A category, often recognized, but not included in the Directory of Specialists is that of "Board eligible" persons who have completed the requirements for certification, but have not attempted the examination or have failed in one or more attempts. In 1961, only 45 percent of full-time specialists were diplomates of the American Boards. Other criteria for designation as a specialist may be membership in specialist associations (such as the American College of Surgeons), academic rank, position on a hospital staff, or recognition by some governmental agency such as a state workmen's compensation board.

Data on Hospitals and Related Facilities

SOURCES OF INFORMATION. The *Directory of Health Resources Statistics,* 1968, of the National Center of Health Statistics, gives a brief account of the sources of information concerning inpatient facilities (3, pp. 215–219). Perhaps the most complete count of inpatient institutions in the United States is to be found in the Master Facility Inventory (MFl) of the National Center for Health Statistics (39). Provision has been made for keeping the Inventory current through additions and deletions. It is estimated that the Master Facility List for 1963 included about 90 percent of all inpatient facilities, coverage being most complete for hospitals, about 90 percent for nursing and personal-care-type homes, and about 80 percent for all other types of institutions (3, p. 219). The list is the sampling frame for the continuing survey of short-stay hospital discharges (See Chapter 3, pages 133–135) and for the periodic censuses of inpatient facilities to determine type of business and number and characteristics of employees and residents or patients. Thus, the Master Facility Census provides information concerning health manpower as well as the resources for inpatient care.

Other sources of data include annual publications by the American Hospital Association (42), the National Institute of Mental Health (54–55), and the Division of Hospitals and Medical Facilities of the Public Health Service, under provision of the Hill-Burton Hospital Survey and Construction Act (37). The Social Security Administration publishes

Table IV.9.   American Boards of Specialists, by Year of Incorporation, and subspecialties or subfields of specialization under each

AMERICAN BOARD OF:	AMERICAN BOARD OF:
Ophthalmology (1917)	Internal Medicine (1936)
	Internal Medicine
Otolaryngology (1924)	Allergy
Otolaryngology	Cardiovascular Disease
Limited branches	Gastroenterology
	Pulmonary Disease
Obstetrics and gynecology (1930)	
Obstetrics	Pathology (1936)
Gynecology	Anatomic Pathology
Obstetrics and gynecology	Anatomic Pathology and Clinical
	Microbiology
Dermatology (1932)	Anatomic Pathology and Clinical
	Pathology
Pediatrics (1933)	Anatomic Pathology and
Pediatrics	Neuropathology
Pediatric allergy	Clinical Chemistry
Pediatric cardiology	Clinical Microbiology
	Clinical Microbiology and
Orthopaedic Surgery (1934)	Clinical Chemistry
	Clinical Pathology
Colon and Rectal Surgery (1934)	Forensic Pathology
	Hematology
Psychiatry and Neurology (1934)	Neuropathology
Psychiatry	
Neurology	Anesthesiology (1937)
Psychiatry and Neurology	
Child Psychiatry	Plastic Surgery (1937)
Radiology (1934)	Surgery (1937)
Diagnostic Roentgenology	
Medical Nuclear Physics	Neurological Surgery (1940)
Radiological Physics	
Radiology	Physical Medicine and Rehabilitation
Radium Therapy	(1947)
Roentegen Ray and Radium Physics	
Roentgenology	Preventive Medicine (1948)
Therapeutic Radiology	General Preventive Medicine
Therapeutic Roentgenology	Aviation Medicine
	Occupational Medicine
Urology (1935)	Public Health
	Thoracic Surgery (1948)

SOURCE: Reference 17.

listings of certified providers (38, 43, 52, 58, 71). The Joint Commission on Accreditation of Hospitals reports on accreditation of hospitals, extended nursing and resident care facilities, and accredited rehabilitation facilities. Information may also be obtained from state licensing bodies and similar regulatory agencies of which there are an estimated 100. Associations, additional to the American Hospital Association, include The American Osteopathic Hospital Association, the American Nursing Home Association, and the American Association of Homes for the Aged. The 1960 Census of Population, also provided information on the number of institutions, by type and size, and the characteristics of persons under care or in custody, based on a 25 percent sample of the population (3).

The most readily accessible and the most widely used compendium of information concerning hospitals is published yearly in the *Guide Issue of Hospitals*, the journal of the American Hospital Association. To be eligible for listing, a hospital need not be a member of the association, but it must have at least 6 beds and should satisfy certain conditions which, collectively, define what qualifies as a "hospital" for this purpose (42, p. 17). Since these stipulations are very revealing of the minimum components of the concept of "hospital," they are quoted in full below:

1. The hospital shall have at least six beds for the care of patients who are nonrelated, who are sick, and who stay on the average in excess of 24 hours per admission.
2. The hospital shall be constructed, equipped, and maintained to insure the safety of the patients, and shall provide uncrowded and sanitary facilities for the treatment of individuals accepted for care.
3. Doctors of medicine, doctors of osteopathy, and doctors of dentistry may admit patients to hospitals registered by the American Hospital Association. (Patients admitted to the hospital by doctors of dentistry must have an admission history and physical examination done by a doctor of medicine or doctor of osteopathy on the staff of the hospital, and the doctor of medicine or osteopathy shall be responsible for the patient's medical care throughout his stay.)
4. There shall be an organized medical staff (which may include doctors of osteopathy and dentistry) governed by by-laws adopted by said staff and approved by the governing board of the hospital.
5. The hospital shall submit evidence of regular care of the patient by a doctor of medicine, doctor of osteopathy, or doctor of dentistry and of general supervision of the clinical work by doctors of medicine.
6. Records of clinical work shall be maintained by the hospital on all patients and shall be available for reference.
7. Registered nurse supervision and such other nursing service as is necessary to provide patient care round the clock shall be available at the hospital.
8. The hospital shall offer services more intensive than those required merely for room, board, personal services, and general nursing care.

9. Minimal surgical or obstetrical facilities (including operating or delivery room), or relatively complete diagnostic facilities and treatment facilities for all patients, shall be available at the hospital.

10. Diagnostic X-ray services shall be regularly and conveniently available.

11. Clinical laboratory services shall be regularly and conveniently available.

For each hospital listed, the *Guide Issue* gives the address, accreditation, approval for internship and residency, medical school affiliation, nurse training programs, participation in Blue Cross and in Medicare, facilities and services out of a list of 16, control, major function, length of stay, beds, admissions, births, census, occupancy, personnel, total expenses and payroll. In addition to the hospital by hospital listing, the *Guide Issue* provides extensive tabulations of hospital statistics, including staffing and fiscal data, and a narrative account of trends and major developments in the hospital establishment.

CLASSIFICATION. The classification of inpatient facilities is made particularly difficult because about two-thirds of these are composed of homes that provide nursing and personal services at a confusing variety of levels to an extremely heterogeneous population. The degree of uncertainty concerning how these institutions are to be categorized is evident by the number of classifications that have been offered for this type of facility, as shown in Table IV.10. Added to the categories listed in the table is that of "extended care facility" recognized for participation in the Medicare program (53). Table IV.11 shows the classification developed for the Master Facility Inventory for all inpatient institutions. Table IV.12 offers an alternative classification developed by a conference called by the American Hospital Association in 1966. The greater precision and quantitative orientation of the definitions of the Master Facility Inventory can be appreciated by comparing the roughly parallel definitions for the group of nursing and personal care institutions in the two classifications, as shown in Table IV.13.

Within the category of "hospitals," further classification is usually necessary. As shown in Tables IV.11 and IV.12, the Master Facility Inventory and the A.H.A. Conference both use major function as the primary axis of classification. The latter also uses control or ownership as a secondary classifier. The *Guide Issue* makes use of four main classifiers: "control," "service," length of stay and size (number of beds excluding bassinets for the newborn). The detailed categories, their groupings, and some combinations are shown in Table IV.14. Berry has used the A.H.A. classification by service and length of stay combined to distinguish four "hospital industries": (1) psychiatric hospitals, (2)

Table IV.10. Selected classifications of nursing homes and related institutions

Source	Type of Facility	Type of Care

National Inventory of Nursing Homes, Public Health Service, 1954(47)	1. Skilled nursing home
	2. Personal care home
	   a. with skilled nursing
	   b. without skilled nursing
	3. Personal care home
	4. Sheltered home
		a. Skilled nursing care
		b. Personal care
		
		c. Shelter

National Conference on Nursing Homes and Homes for the Aged, 1958(51)	1. Comprehensive services facility 2. Nursing care facility 3. Personal care facility 4. Residential facility	a. Comprehensive services b. Nursing care c. Personal care d. Residential services

Public Health Service Survey, 1961(48)	1. Nursing homes
	2. Homes for the aged
	3. Boarding homes
	4. Rest homes
		a. Skilled nursing care
		b. Personal care
		   (1) with skilled nursing
		   (2) without skilled nursing
		c. Residential care
		   (1) with skilled nursing
		   (2) without skilled nursing

National Center for Health Statistics Resident Places Survey(50)	1. Nursing care home 2. Personal-care-with-nursing home 3. Personal care home 4. Domiciliary care home 5. Boarding or rooming-house	

National Center for Health Statistics, Master Facility Inventory, 1963(39)	1. Nursing, personal or domiciliary care establishments
	   a. Nursing care
	   b. Personal care with nursing
	   c. Personal care
	   d. Domiciliary care
	2. Custodial care homes	

American Hospital Association, Classification of Health Care Institutions, 1966(41)	1. Extended care institutions
	   a. General
	   b. Special
	2. Health-related care institutions
	   a. Personal care institutions
	     (1) Resident care institutions
	     (2) Sheltered care institutions
	   b. Nonresident institutions	

Table IV.11.   Classification of facilities, Master Facility Inventory, National
Center for Health Statistics, 1963

A. Short-stay hospitals

    1. General
    2. Special
       a. Maternity
       b. Eye, ear, nose, and throat
       c. Pediatric
       d. Other

B. Resident institutions

    1. Long-stay hospitals
       a. General
       b. Psychiatric
       c. Mental retardation
       d. Geriatric
       e. Orthopedic
       f. Tuberculosis
       g. Chronic disease
       h. Other

    2. Nursing, personal or domiciliary care establishments
       a. Nursing care
       b. Personal care with nursing
       c. Personal care
       d. Domiciliary care

    3. Custodial care homes
       a. Homes for the deaf
       b. Homes for the blind
       c. Homes for unwed mothers
       d. Orphan Asylums
       e. Other

    4. Correctional institutions
       a. Prisons and reformatories
       b. Detention homes for juvenile delinquents

SOURCE: Reference 39.

tuberculosis hospitals, (3) short-term, general, and other special hospitals, and (4) long-term, general, and other special hospitals. He recognizes certain problems in this kind of categorization, including the fact that hospitals in one group may, currently or potentially, serve some functions of those in another; that the designation "other special" subsumes institutions with differing products; and that nursing and

Table IV.12.   Classification of health care institutions, Conference on Classification on Health Care Facilities, American Hospital Association, June 1966

CLASSIFICATION BY PRIMARY FUNCTION

I. Health care institutions

   A. Medical care institutions

      1. Inpatient care institutions
         a. Hospitals.
           i. General
           ii. Special
         b. Extended care institutions
           i. General
           ii. Special
      2. Outpatient care institutions
           i. General
           ii. Special
      3. Home care institutions
           i. General
           ii. Special

   B. Health-related care institutions

      1. Personal care institutions
         a. Resident care institutions
         b. Sheltered care institutions
      2. Nonresident institutions

II. Noninstitutional health services

CLASSIFICATION BY CONTROL

I. Governmental institutions

   A. Federal institutions

   B. Nonfederal governmental institutions

      1. State institutions
      2. Local governmental institutions
         a. District institutions
         b. County institutions
         c. City-county institutions
         d. City institutions

II. Nongovernmental institutions

   A. Voluntary nonprofit institutions

   B. Proprietary institutions

SOURCE: Reference 41, pp. 10 and 11.

Table IV.13.   Classifications and definitions of institutions that provide nursing and personal care services as developed by the National Center for Health Statistics, Master Facility Inventory and by the Conference on Classification of Health Care Facilities, American Hospital Association

Master Facility Inventory	A.H.A. Conference[a]
Nursing Care Home	*Extended Care Institution*
is defined as one in which 50 percent or more of the residents receive one or more nursing services and the facility has at least one registered nurse (RN) or licensed practical nurse (LPN) employed 35 or more hours per week. Nursing services include nasal feeding, catheterization, irrigation, oxygen therapy, full bed bath, enema, hypodermic injection, intravenous injection, temperature-pulse-respiration, blood pressure, application of dressing or bandage, or bowel and bladder retraining.	Establishments with permanent facilities that include inpatient beds; and with medical services, including continuous nursing services, to provide treatment for patients who require inpatient care but do not currently require continuous hospital services, and who have a variety of medical conditions (General Extended Care Institution) or who have special medical conditions (Special Extended Care Institution).
Personal-Care-with-Nursing-Home	
one in which either (a) some, but less than 50 percent, of the residents receive nursing care or (b) more than 50 percent of the residents receive nursing care, but no RN's or LPN's are employed full time on the staff.	
Personal Care Home	*Personal Care Institution*
one in which the facility routinely provides three or more personal services, but no nursing service. Personal services include rub or massage service or assistance with bathing, dressing, correspondence or shopping, walking or getting about or eating.	Establishments with permanent facilities that include resident beds, and with health-related services to provide continuous general supervision and direct personal care services to residents in their activities of daily living.
Domiciliary Care Home	*Sheltered Care Institution*
one in which the facility routinely provides less than three of the personal services specified in the definition above, and no nursing service. This type of facility provides a sheltered environment primarily to persons who are able to care for themselves.	Establishments with permanent facilities that include resident beds, and with health-related services to provide continuous general supervision and protection, with only occasional direct personal care services to residents who are in need of protective environment but who are otherwise able to manage the normal activities of daily living.

SOURCE: Reference 3, page 216, and Reference 41, pages 12–13.

[a] Further specification of terms is to be found in a Glossary included in the conference report.

Table IV.14.   Classification of hospitals, American Hospital Association, Guide
Issue of *Hospitals*

BY CONTROL

Governmental, non-federal (also referred to as state and local governmental)
    State
    County
    City
    City-county
    Hospital district

Nongovernmental nonprofit
    Church-related or -operated
    Other nonprofit

Nongovernmental for-profit
    Individual
    Partnership
    Corporation

Governmental, federal (also referred to as federal)
    Air Force
    Army
    Navy
    Public Health Service Indian Service
    Public Health Service, other than above
    Veterans Administration
    Department of Justice
    Other federal

BY SERVICE

General
Hospital unit of an institution (prison hospital, college infirmary, etc.)
Psychiatric
Tuberculosis
Maternity
Eye, ear, nose, and throat
Orthopedic
Chronic and/or convalescent
Other specialty
Children's
Institution for mental retardation
Epilepsy
Alcoholism and/or addictive diseases

BY LENGTH OF STAY

Short-term: over 50 percent of all patients admitted have a stay of less than 30
      days.
Long-term: over 50 percent of all patients admitted have a stay of 30 days or
      more.

Table IV.14.   (continued)

SERVICE AND LENGTH OF STAY COMBINED
Psychiatric
Tuberculosis
Short-term, general and other special (excludes psychiatric and tuberculosis)
Long-term, general and other special (excludes psychiatric and tuberculosis)

BY SIZE
Under 25
25–49
100–199
200–299
300–399
400–499
500 and over.

SOURCE: Reference 42.

personal care homes overlap in their functions with hospitals in all four categories. Nevertheless, Berry proceeds to show the validity and usefulness of viewing hospitals as differentiated into the four industries which he postulates (123, pp. 19–23). Hospitals may also be classified by a host of additional characteristics, including those for which the A.H.A. listing obtains information: accreditation, approval for residency and training, medical school affiliation, number and type of "facilities and services," and levels of staffing and cost. As we shall see, many of these characteristics have important implications for the nature and quality of the hospital product and are therefore important considerations in the assessment of the hospital establishment. Ways of characterizing hospitals in studies of productivity will be found in the work of Carr and Feldstein and of Berry (122, 124–126). Morrill and Earickson refer to an "index of specialization" which is "the sum of the number of facilities and the number of specialties with interns and/or residents" (45, p. 227, and Fig. 1, p. 226). Still other classifications derive from the growing interest in the ecology of hospital services. The notion of a regional organization of hospitals has resulted in the categorization of hospitals in a variety of functional hierarchies and the study of the actual and desired relationships between these and location in space and in relation to aggregations of people and of health personnel. Mountin et al., who did much of the original work in this regard, have visualized a hierarchy of "base hospital," "district hospital," "rural hospital," and "health center," as follows:

In the system the base hospital would have the most advanced equipment and specialized staff, associated, wherever practicable, with the teaching, research, and study opportunities of a medical school. This hospital would offer diagnosis and treatment to patients with conditions requiring services not available in most local hospitals. Large, well-equipped district hospitals would be strategically located within the area served by the base hospital and would provide general and specialty services beyond the resources of smaller local hospitals; thus only the more complex cases would have to be referred to the base hospital. Other hospitals, including those in the more built-up rural areas, should be prepared to meet the ordinary demands of a community and select for transfer to district and base hospitals those cases requiring highly specialized care. Finally, there would be health centers equipped for diagnosis and treatment of ambulatory patients, as well as the more traditional health department services. Probably a few of these located in sparsely populated areas would contain accommodations for limited hospital service" (360, p. 1).

However, the more recent maps issued by the state Hill-Burton agencies seem to distinguish only two main groupings of hospitals: (1) base, regional, or district and (2) rural or community. Weiss used a number of characteristics to classify counties in a hierarchy of "medical centers," depending on the medical care personnel and functions located in each, as shown in Table IV.15.

Table IV.15. Counties of the United States grouped and ranked according to the medical care resources found in each county, U.S.A., 1965

Type of Center	Characteristics	No. of Counties
4	Each county includes a medical school, interns, residents, and service staffs	56
3	Each county contains interns, residents, and service staffs	132
2	Each county contains residents and service staffs	49
1	Each county contains over twenty physicians in the service functions	8
0	Each county with fewer than twenty center personnel present	2818

SOURCE: Reference 344, pages 52–53.

Although the units of analysis were counties rather than institutions, it is clear that the classification reflects the nature of facilities present and the aggregation of physicians, in training and in practice, within and adjacent to such institutions. Morrill and Earickson refer to a study of Cincinnati hospitals by Schneider in which a three-level hierarchy was suggested, depending on hospital size and types of specialty services present. For example, very large hospitals had a "virtual monopoly" on a group of services constituted of dermatology, plastic surgery, psychiatry, neurology, and thoracic surgery; whereas "large and medium-size hospitals share a second level of specialties, absent in smaller hospitals" (45, p. 225). Morrill and Earickson have themselves offered the following a priori classification of the 123 hospitals in the Chicago Area:

Group A. Teaching and research hospitals
Group B. Regional and district hospitals, intermediate service level
Group C. Community hospitals
Group D. Very small hospitals (mean = 64 beds)
Group S. Long-term institutions

When hospitals in these groups are mapped out, a roughly concentric arrangement becomes evident, with a nucleus of Group A hospitals surrounded by hospitals in the B and C groups and finally a few outlying hospitals in the C and D categories (45, pp. 228–229, and Fig. 2, p. 230). As a second stage in their study of Chicago hospitals, Morrill and Earickson used 99 variables to characterize 123 hospitals. Factor analysis showed that two-thirds of the variance among all the 99 variables was accounted for by the following nine "dimensions": (1) amount and volume of service, (2) character of the service area and relative location, (3) length of stay and quantity and scope of service, (4) importance of obstetric and pediatric care, (5) recent dynamism (growth), (6) competitive position, (7) propensity to admit nonwhite patients, (8) personnel expenses per bed and proportion of patients on public aid, and (9) importance of elderly patients. Using these dimensions, Chicago hospitals were grouped into the following types:

Teaching and research
Medium competitive (inner city and suburban)
Satellite city
Medium suburban
New suburban
Small, inner city
Small, outer city
Small, far suburban
Negro
Veterans
Isolates (do not fit any of above categories)

Table IV.16.   Examples of types of
distinctive inpatient care facilities

---

1. By Patient age
     Geriatric
     Adult
     Pediatric
     Newborn

2. By patient sex

3. By patient religion

4. By patient race

5. By patient residence

6. By procedure or
   attending M.D. specialty
     Obstetric
     Medical
     Surgical
     Psychiatric
     Orthopedic
     Gynecologic

7. By Length of stay
     Short (overnight)
     Intermediate
     Long-term

8. By Size of patient room
     Private
     Semiprivate
     Ward

9. By level of nursing care required
     Intensive
     Intermediate
     Self-Help

10. By source of payment for care
     Patient (or his insurance)
     Closed prepayment plan
     Private charities
     Public welfare

11. By availability for teaching
     Teaching
     Nonteaching

SOURCE: Reference 213, Table 1,
page 76.

As a final element in hospital classification, units within each hospital may be classified by department or service; by sex, age, or even religion or race; by type of accommodation or source of payment; by availability for teaching; and by level of nursing care required. The internal subdivisions, to the extent that they influence substitutability among units or beds, have, as we shall see, an important influence on the capacity of the hospital establishment to respond to need or demand. Blumberg has proposed that the term "distinctive patient facility" be used to describe such administrative or functional subdivisions that restrict internal substitution (213). Table IV.16, derived from Blumberg, gives the most common internal categorizations. Needless to say, such internal divisions, though much less elaborate, can also be a feature of inpatient institutions other than hospitals.

THE CAPACITY TO PRODUCE SERVICE

Definition of Productivity and Efficiency

In the previous section of this chapter, we discussed some aspects of selecting and specifying the units of supply that are relevant to the purposes of assessment. The next step is to translate the count, or measurement, of such units into "service equivalents" or "service capacity," in the terminology of our model (Fig. IV.1). The methods of counting or measuring service capacity and of services produced will be discussed in the following section. Here, our attention will focus on the "intervening factors" that influence the capacity of a specified set of service-producing resources to produce service. These factors are subsumed under the rubric of "productivity," with the understanding that "productivity" is used in a rather restricted sense: that of a "partial productivity."

"Productivity" and "efficiency" both consider output-input relationships but in somewhat different, though related, ways. Productivity is a measure of the relationship between output and input when both are expressed in real physical volume terms:

$$\text{Productivity} = \frac{\text{Total output}}{\text{Total input}}$$

When only one output relates uniquely to only one input so that there is a one-to-one correspondence between them, the conceptual and operational problems of measurement are considerably simplified. But severe problems may arise when the outputs, the inputs, or both, are multiple.

These difficulties are further compounded when any one input is partly responsible for several outputs, each of which in turn is the product of several inputs. In such situations one is seldom certain that outputs and inputs have been compared in such a way as to include all the relevant outputs and inputs, and to exclude those that are irrelevant. In other words, a complete correspondence between the numerator and the denominator of the productivity ratio becomes very difficult to achieve. Further difficulties arise because measures of productivity are used in a comparative rather than an absolute sense. One is interested in changes in productivity over time, or in comparisons of productivity among several ways of organizing inputs. This means that the outputs and inputs must all be qualitatively similar and measured in standard ways. If, for example, the outputs of two firms, or of two time periods, are not similar, the outputs must be made comparable through some process of standardization, such as weighting. Finally, as we shall see, there may be some ambiguity about the distinction between inputs and outputs; and considerable disagreement may arise about what precisely is the nontangible output of a service such as medical care.

Let us consider a rather simple situation where it is possible to specify a single output (O) and several related inputs (I). In this instance, the total measure of productivity would be a ratio of output to all relevant inputs, thus:

$$\text{Total productivity} = \frac{O}{I_1 + I_2 + I_3 + \ldots \ldots I_n}$$

Under certain circumstances, it is expedient or appropriate to dispense with a measurement of all the relevant inputs and to measure a smaller set, or only one. What is obtained is a partial measure of productivity:

$$\text{Partial productivity} = \frac{O}{I_1}$$

This simplification is both expedient and appropriate when it is known that one major input (I_1) reasonably represents all other inputs either because other inputs are relatively negligible in magnitude, or because they have a fixed relationship to the major input so that changes in this input are a valid indicator of changes in all the others. To the extent that these assumptions are not true, the partial measure of productivity does not represent total productivity. Another reason for considering only one input, sufficiently different from the above to merit separate mention, is particular interest in one input which, for a variety of reasons, is considered to be critical. Such reasons include the functionally central role of this input, its relative scarcity, or the comparative difficulty of manipulating it in the interests of production. The distinction being made (though it is not always complete) is that in some instances partial measures of productivity appear to be a proxy for more complete measures. In other instances, they are used because of a substantive interest in the partial productivity itself. It appears to the author that in the analysis of medical care resources both uses obtain. A study of the productivity of the physician or dentist is predicated on the central role and relative unmanipulability of this resource as compared to associated inputs of other health manpower and capital. These resources are relatively scarcer than others are, they take longer to replenish or augment, and their contribution to the outcome of care is regarded as more critical as well as unique, to the extent that they can substitute for the inputs of allied health professionals but the latter cannot substitute for the former. On the other hand, when the productivity of the hospital is under study, the hospital bed is regarded as a rough proxy for all the inputs that the hospital is able to marshal.

When, for whatever reason, a partial measure of productivity is used, problems arise in the interpretation of observed differences between firms or of observed changes over time. Specifically, to what extent are the differences or changes observed due to differences in the input measured and to what extent, and in what ways, due to differences in associated (but unmeasured) inputs? For example, are increases in the productivity of physicians attributable to the physicians themselves or due to the use of auxiliary personnel and equipment? There are, of course, some ambiguities in the separation between "the physician himself" and all other associated inputs. To what extent, for example, may one separate the state of the technology, an external factor in productivity, from the internalized ability to use the technology? However, after such matters are disposed of, by convention if nothing else, it is possible by appropriate tehniques to identify the contribution of each of several inputs to the differences in productivity. Unexplained differences may be the contribution of the critical input (for example, the physician) or of other unidentified or unmeasured inputs.

In the presentation of our model for the assessment of supply we mentioned the reason for not showing "efficiency" graphically as an element of the model. This was because efficiency was seen as a different dimension of the relationship between output and input than that of productivity. Since productivity and efficiency are closely related concepts, it is necessary to consider in what ways they are similar as well as different. In studies of productivity, what is measured is the relationship between outputs and inputs expressed in real physical volume terms. "Economic efficiency," on the other hand, deals with the monetary value of the outputs and the cost of the inputs. This distinction is important because the relationship that is most productive need not be economically most efficient. For example, it may be possible to increase output significantly by the use of fewer but very highly trained employees. However, this is economically less efficient if it is more costly than the use of a larger number of less well-trained employees who produce the same product. Thus, the use of primitive technology may be economically more efficient where cheap labor is plentiful and machinery costly to acquire, maintain, and operate. In many situations, however, productivity and economic efficiency are closely related. When this is so, appropriate measures of partial productivity may also be used as approximate indicators of economic efficiency.

The example cited above illustrates another attribute of the concept of "efficiency"—that it applies to comparisons among methods of production. In studies of efficiency, the object is to identify the combination and quantities of inputs that result in the largest output under a given set of constraints. That is, the concern is with what inputs are selected from among alternatives, and in what amounts relative to each other. For example, a given number of patients can be "taken care of" by employing various combinations of physician time, nursing time, and medical equipment. The most efficient method is one that takes care of a given number of patients with the least input, or takes care of more patients when the inputs are the same. Obviously, judgments such as the above require that terms such as "similar input" or "least input" be defined and measured. This is done by identifying and summating the costs of these inputs. In the example given above, there was a single output identified as number of patients "taken care of." However, if there were differences in degrees of being "taken care of" and/or several outputs, comparisons among outputs could not be made without some way of adding them up. The monetary value of outputs is one device for doing this. Hence, comparisons among different production processes, which share certain elements in common, are made in terms of "economic efficiency."

Issues in the Measurement of Productivity

DEFINITION OF OUTPUT. The first issue in the measurement of productivity is the specification of the product. Generally, where the product is concrete, this is not a matter of great difficulty. In medical care, on the contrary, the nature of the product remains a matter for debate and disagreement. In examining the problem, one encounters once again the curious duality of process and outcome to which we have already referred and to which we shall have occasion to return repeatedly. Those who are oriented to process define the product of the medical care system as medical care. They are concerned, therefore, with identifying the specific contribution of the service-producing units (for example, the physician) to the medical care process. Those who are oriented to outcome are inclined to consider the process of medical care as an intermediate input, and to emphasize the end-results of care expressed as some state of health or well-being in the client. The preference of the author, as the model for the assessment of supply clearly shows, is for maintaining the separateness of process and outcome to the extent that this can be done without violence to reality. Reference to Fig. IV.1 shows "productivity" to be the "intervening factor" between resources and their service equivalents. The implicit assumption is that the product is to be measured in terms of the process of care. But assessment does not stop here. The services produced are themselves translatable to some expression of impact on health. Intervening between services and the satisfaction of need are factors that influence the "potency" and "appropriateness" of these services. It is possible, of course, as the model also shows, to translate resources directly into need-satisfying equivalents. This happens when the product is defined in terms of health and well-being. When this is done, there is no need to distinguish "potency" and "appropriateness" from "productivity," since the first two factors become part of the third. The preference for maintaining the separation between process and outcome (and hence between "productivity" and "potency-appropriateness" as here defined) rests on several considerations. First, medical care standards, quantitative as well as qualitative, are almost always formulated in terms of service. The socialization of health professionals centers on the provision of appropriate care rather than on the attainment of results that are often not precisely predictable. Second, services appear to be more readily definable and measurable, at least in approximate form, than are states of health or well-being. Third, the relationship between services and health may be very partial, even paradoxical. Some of the factors that account for this have already been discussed in a previous section on the evaluative uses of health status. It follows from these considerations that greater insight into the workings of the medical care system can be obtained if one measures the product of the system, successively, first as services and then as health and well-being.

There is a third approach to the definition of product which may be viewed as a synthesis of the two already discussed. This is a definition in terms of episodes of illness appropriately cared for. When this is done, "potency" and "appropriateness" become part of "productivity," because they enable the provider to satisfy need with fewer services or in a shorter time through the application of more intensive care, or both. A very similar approach has been used by Scitovsky in a study of medical care prices (78). Martin Feldstein has also argued for using the hospital "case" rather than the patient-day (or patient week) as the unit of output. The number of cases is measured by the number of discharges from hospital, dead or alive (2, pp. 24–25). Not as similar, but kin to some extent, is the proposal by Daniels that "another yardstick of productivity may be how many individuals and families are maintained in a state of adaptation, relatively free of physical or psychological discomfort. In such measurements, the absence of visits to a physician might be credited to his productivity if they were the results of his preventive efforts" (93, p. 71). The definition of the product in terms of episodes of illness that are appropriately cared for has the advantage of relating service to some health objective, a property that many find more satisfying than the measurement of activities which may represent, in part, misapplied or wasted effort. It does this without requiring a measurement of outcome. It also would seem to be unaffected by the imperfect or paradoxical nature of the relationship between health and medical care. There are, however, some new problems. Who is to say what is appropriate care? In general, the burden of this decision is left to the physician, and it is assumed that care is appropriately conducted and terminated in each instance. Then there are problems of delineating discrete episodes of illness and corresponding episodes of care, a matter which we have discussed in a previous section. Finally, the problems of comparability of morbidity states, which we shall discuss below, are not removed simply because end results are not measured. Martin Feldstein, in proposing the "case" as the measure of hospital output, is aware of precisely these limitations. He recognizes the need for correcting for differences in case mix if the "case" is to be used as the measure of output. He also recognizes that the use of the case as a measure of output contains the implicit assumption that the "doctor's decision to discharge a patient indicates that the patient's medical care is adequately completed"; and that, if this assumption is made, it must be recognized that patients may be discharged or transferred to other hospitals before the care is completed. These limitations notwithstanding, Feldstein believes that the "case" has a major advantage as a measure of output because it recognizes the possibility of trade-offs between length of stay and cost per patient-day. This arises because cost per day is highest immediately after admission when care is most intensive and declines as stay is prolonged. Long stays, as we shall see, also raise occupancy and reduce the time during which the bed is vacant between patients at high levels of overhead. If cost is used as the measure of input and the patient-day as the measure of output, it is possible to create a spurious picture of high productivity or efficiency by simply lengthening stay. This cannot be done if cost per case is the measure of productivity or efficiency. In fact, the most efficient solution may be one that raises costs per patient-day through the provision of more intensive care, provided shorter stay more than offsets the increase, and results in lower costs per case. It must be recognized, however, that this analysis in its entirety deals only with the internal operations of the hospital and does not take account of the influence of these on the demand and need for care in the community.

A final aspect of the definition of output pertains to the manner in which stand-by capacity is to be handled. Whenever services provided or cases processed are used as the measure of output, no account is taken of the investment in holding hospital beds or ambulatory care personnel and facilities ready for action when the call for their services arises. As we shall see, this is a question which has attracted considerable attention where hospitals are concerned. This is because of the preponderant magnitude of fixed costs, as compared to variable costs, in hospital operations. The same kinds of considerations should, however, also be applicable to evaluating the productivity of other resources, including that of physicians in office practice. For example, Wolfe et al. have reported that in one group practice each physician put in 42 hours of work plus 28 hours of "active stand-by on call" per week (166, p. 119). This means that 40 percent of the physician's weekly output is in stand-by services. Yet the usual measures of physician output (and most measures of hospital output) ignore the stand-by service component. One important reason may be the difficulty of estimating what amount of stand-by service is necessary and legitimate, and what amount merely represents oversupply. In a subsequent section we shall discuss how this question has been answered for hospitals. To the author's knowledge, no similar answer has been offered for the services of physicians and other health personnel in independent practice.

The fact that the product of health resources may be defined in several ways, including (1) services produced, (2) episodes of illness cared for, and (3) increments (or decrements) in health, leads to a modification in our model as shown in Fig. IV.1. "Productivity," depending on how the product is defined, may be seen as the intervening factor between "supply" and "service capacity" or between "supply" and "need-satisfying equivalents." Furthermore, it should be pointed out that one needs to distinguish potential productivity from productivity as realized in actual practice. "Productivity" accordingly appears at different points in the model as seen in Fig. IV.2, which shows only part of the total model. The factors that influence productivity will, of course, also vary depending on its position in the model.

COMPARABILITY OF OUTPUTS. Comparisons of productivity require measurement of standard product. Unfortunately, whether one selects services or health outcomes as the measure of product, problems of comparability occur. The usual measures of service output are the visit to the physician or the patient-day in the hospital. It is clear, however, that the content of a visit or patient-day has changed considerably over time and differs markedly from case to case and, on the average, among individual providers or categories of providers. Some examples are to be found in a study of hospital care made for the American Medical Association. Among these is the finding that between 1946 and 1961 there were large increases, as shown in Table IV.17, in the use of selected

Fig. IV.2.   A partial model for evaluating supply modified to accommodate several definitions of actual and potential productivity

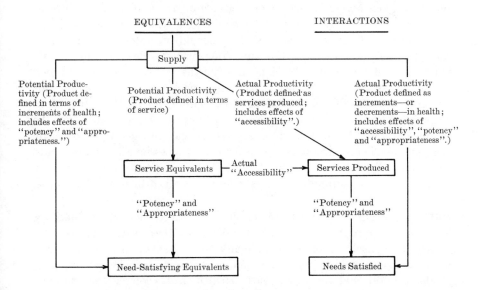

Table IV.17.   Percent increase in the use of specified
hospital services per patient-day. Nonfederal, general,
short-term hospitals, U.S.A., 1946–1961

Services[a]	Percent Increase 1946–1961
Operating room	16
Pathology reports	72
Generic drugs	107
Laboratory procedures	164
X-rays	169
Consultations	231

SOURCE: Reference 131, Tables 21–27, pages 27–29.

[a] The measure of services per patient-day has been adjusted for differences in length of stay using a ratio of
mean length of stay 1961/1946.

hospital services per patient-day in a nationwide sample of nonfederal,
general, short-term hospitals.

Related to secular changes and contemporaneous differences in the
content of care, are expected changes and differences in other dimensions
of "quality." These include the accuracy of diagnostic and therapeutic
decisions. Changes and differences in effectiveness are also involved in
the data of Table IV.17. All of these differences need to be taken into
account if a standard or comparable service product is to be defined. It is
generally believed that the problem of defining a comparable product is
removed when states of health or well-being are used as a measure of
output. Unfortunately, this may not be the case; there are merely different problems. These arise because the morbidity states that are to be
cared for differ from time to time and from place to place. If the product
is health, it is necessary to standardize for the states of ill-health which
are to be converted into health. Strictly speaking, the output in this
instance is not health, but a specific modification in health status. Since
amenability to modification depends on several characteristics of the
original state, this must be standardized if the product is to be made
comparable. There are also differences in professionally defined and
technologically determined expectations of the end-points of care. As new
knowledge and techniques accrue, the acceptable health product changes.

MULTIPLE PRODUCTS. A third problem in the measurement of productivity
is the presence of multiple products. We have already emphasized that
patient care itself is made up of many components that represent the
input of many health personnel and other resources. There are, also,
products additional to patient care. Health professionals, for example,

may be engaged in teaching, research, or administration. The activities of a hospital are also multifarious and its products correspondingly varied. In a very perceptive analysis, Codman, many years ago, examined the product of a great institution, the Massachusetts General Hospital. For the year 1912 he identified the following as the products of the Hospital as shown in Table IV.18.

Table IV.18.   The Product of the Massachusetts General Hospital for the year 1912 as estimated by Codman

A. Administration
  1. 6896 patients treated
  2. $3 per patient per day
  3. 16 days average stay
  4. 320 beds; each bed served 22 patients

B. Education
  1. 61,000 student hours
  2. Graduate and summer teaching
  3. Example to clinic visitors
  4. 34 nurses graduated
  5. 18 assistants graduated
  6. 53 social service assistants

C. Important by-products
  1. 115 medical and surgical papers
  2. The influence on medical standards
  3. Important ideas demonstrated

SOURCE: Reference 113, figure on page 406.

Codman had a full appreciation of the multiple nature of the product, even though the specification of the several outputs was not very precise. Particularly noteworthy is the emphasis he placed on the discovery and dissemination of new knowledge which included more effective ways of treating illness. He considered this to be a product that was multiplied many-fold through use by others who were unrelated to the hospital. In this sense, part of the product of many physicians and hospitals might be attributable to the Massachusetts General Hospital.

DEFINITION OF INPUTS. The definitions of input and output are as two sides of a coin. We have already said that services may be considered either as outputs, or as inputs mediating an ultimate output: health. Furthermore, the presence of multiple outputs predicates the partitioning of inputs so that inputs and outputs correspond. An input that requires special attention is time. Physicians may increase their production either by working longer hours or by organizing their work in a way that permits them to accomplish more during a given period of time. Accordingly, Garbarino has distinguished the "output effect," which is the effect of operating at different percentages of capacity, and the "methods effect," which is the effect of changing methods of production (89, p. 47). It is standard to express the productivity of labor in terms of a fixed unit, usually a man-hour. This excludes the effect of longer or shorter hours of work except as they indirectly influence performance while at work. In analogous studies of the productivity of health manpower, it would be useful to distinguish the two factors of "output" and "method" and to gauge their separate effects on production. This is especially important because hours of work are more subject to variation in independent practice. In all instances it should be made clear whether the measure of health manpower productivity that is used includes or excludes variation in time as an input. In studies of the productivity of hospitals, the time factor is usually not recognized as a separable input. This may be because the hospital is supposed to operate at peak capacity round the clock, every day of the week—an assumption that is known not to be true. Furthermore, the complexity of the hospital operation would make it difficult to isolate time as a separate input. Nevertheless, certain variations in the methods for measuring hospital productivity have a bearing on the "output effect." One could argue, for example, that the inclusion or exclusion of the effect of low occupancy in estimating economies of scale, is analogous to including or excluding that portion of time during which the hospital is not actually engaged in patient care.

Our definition of productivity specified that inputs and outputs be measured in real physical units, for example, man-hours of physician labor. However, because a given health service or output usually requires several inputs, including the labor of many health professions and other workers, as well as buildings, machinery, and equipment, the need often arises from combining these inputs into a single measure. Hence, in many studies of productivity the cost of producing a given output is used as a measure of input. Cost is by definition the variable used in measuring economic efficiency. Irrespective of why cost is used as a measure of input, the essential requirement when it is used is that cost be accurately and appropriately measured and allocated to the various inputs. This is far from being a simple matter, especially in the health industry where cost-accounting practices tend to be primitive and variable (112, 119).

DEFINITION OF THE SERVICE-PRODUCING ORGANIZATIONAL UNIT. So far, we have spoken of the productivity of the physician and of the hospital as if these were fully separable. It is obvious that hospital productivity is determined to a large extent by the contribution of physicians, the bulk of whom are in private practice. Similarly, the productivity of physicians in private practice is greatly influenced by the way in which they use the hospital. Inpatient and outpatient hospital services can almost fully substitute for services in the patient's home or the physician's office. The reverse is also true, though not to the same extent. There is some evidence that, within a certain range, as the supply of physicians diminishes, more hospital days of care are used per unit population (95). There are, obviously, advantages to grouping patients at one site and making use of the resources that the hospital places at the disposal of the physician. Penchansky and Rosenthal have argued that part of the increase in physician income in recent decades is the result of the contribution made by the hospital to the physician's practice; and that this contribution is significantly higher for those physicians (surgeons, for example) who are more than usually dependent on the hospital for their practice (92). In a recent paper, Johnson has analyzed very perceptively the role of the physician in hospital productivity and the actual or potential contributions of the hospital to the productivity of the physician as he serves the interests of the hospital as well as his own (94). Johnson points out that narrow preoccupation with the productivity of the physician alone, or of the hospital alone, will not provide incentives for maximizing the joint productivity of both. He further offers specific suggestions for bringing about increases in joint productivity. The implication of all this to our present concerns is that the unit of analysis in studies of productivity needs to be carefully considered. In some cases (for example, for most dentists) the practitioner's office is the relevant organizational unit or firm. For some purposes it may be appropriate to limit analysis to the office practice of physicians. For other purposes it is necessary to consider the hospital-physician complex as the producing unit. In any event, it is important to choose the unit of study with full understanding of its organizational and functional context. Both the design of the study and the interpretation of the findings are dependent on this more general context.

Measuring Physician Output

In this section we shall consider the measurement of physician output with special emphasis on ambulatory care. The usual measure of physician output is the physician visit. The visit, however, is an extremely heterogeneous unit in both content and quality. Important considerations are whether the visit must involve contact with a physician and whether the contact has to be in person or may include telephone conversation. The definition adopted by the National Health Survey may serve as an example:

A physician visit is defined as consultation with a physician, in person or by telephone, for examination, diagnosis, treatment, or advice. The visit is considered to be a physician visit if the service is provided directly by the physician or by a nurse or other person acting under a physician's supervision . . . Physician visits for services provided on a mass basis are not included in the tabulations . . . Physician visits to hospital inpatients are not included. If a physician is called to the house to see more than one person, the call is considered to be a separate physician visit for each person about whom the physician was consulted. A physician visit is associated with the person about whom the advice was sought, even if that person did not actually see or consult the physician (75, pp. 51–52).

Visits are further classified by location. The National Health Survey distinguishes five varieties as follows: (1) home, (2) office, (3) hospital clinic, (4) company or industry health unit, (5) telephone contact, and (6) other, including school, insurance office, and health department clinic. As already mentioned, the survey does not include a sixth most important location, the hospital. The inputs into a visit vary by the function of the visit. It is therefore customary to distinguish initial visit, follow-up visit, consultation and complete physical examination. Follow-up visits, for example, are considered to require much less input than do consultations or initial visit. More detailed categorizations, presumably related to physician input, have been developed for the purpose of determining prices. For example, the "relative value scale" developed by the Michigan State Medical Society recognizes 7 categories of office or home visits, 4 categories of consultations, and 7 categories of inpatient hospital visits each of which is further subdivided into four classes according to the day of the hospital stay during which it occurs (77). Similarly, the California relative value scale recognizes 9 categories of office visits, 8 of home or nursing home visits, 6 of hospital visits, 4 of consultations and 3 of infant, child, and adolescent care (76). The wide variations in presumed input are indicated by the fact that office visits in the California scale range from 0.8 to 6.0 units in value, and inpatient visits in the Michigan scale from 0.8 to 8.0 units. Table IV.19 gives examples excerpted from these two sources. The relative value scales also include extensive listings of many discrete procedures of a diagnostic or therapeutic nature that are part of the product of outpatient (or inpatient) care additional to the "visit" per se. Kovner, in his scheme for measuring outpatient office visit services, recognizes the distinction between

Table IV.19. Categories of office visits and corresponding relative values, California and Michigan Relative Value Studies, 1964 and 1968

Office Visits, California		Office or Home Visits, Michigan	
Initial office visit, routine, new patient or new illness, history and examination	2.0	Brief. (such as: routine injection or dressing. May or may not require the presence of the physician)	1.0
Initial (or subsequent) office visit, complete diagnostic history and physical examination, established patient or minor chronic illness, including initiation of diagnostic and treatment programs	3.5	Routine limited. (such as: routine initial or follow-up visit with history, physical examination and initiation of diagnostic and treatment programs for a single or minor complaint not requiring complete history or physical examination)	1.5
Initial (or subsequent) office visit, complete diagnostic history and physical examination, new patient or major illness, including initiation of diagnostic and treatment programs	6.0	Routine extended. (such as: routine initial or follow-up visit with history, physical examination and initiation of diagnostic and treatment programs requiring study of more than one system or extended study of one system)	2.0
Follow-up office visit, brief; e.g., routine injection, minimal dressing, etc.	0.8	Intermediate. (such as: periodic health examination or initial or follow-up visit requiring extensive professional care less than the equivalent of Routine Complete)	3.0
Follow-up office visit, routine	1.0	Routine complete. (such as: routine complete history, physical examination, evaluation and initiation of diagnostic and treatment programs)	4.0
Follow-up office visit necessitating professional care over and above routine visit	1.5	Comprehensive intermediate. (such as: comprehensive, intensive resurvey of complete history, physical examination, evaluation and diagnostic and treatment programs in an established patient)	5.0
Follow-up office visit, prolonged, over and above the preceding	2.0	Comprehensive complete. (such as: comprehensive complete intensive history, physical examination, evaluation and initiation of diagnostic and treatment programs characteristic of services rendered by a specialist)	6.0
Follow up office visit necessitating complete re-examination and re-evaluation of patient as a whole (continuing illness)	3.0		
Re-examination, comprehensive diagnostic history and re-evaluation, established patient (annual type)	4.0		

SOURCE: References 76, p. 9, and 77, pages 1–2.

"office visit services" and all other services, but only because different sources are used to derive the weights that permit the construction of a single measure of output (81). Bailey, on the other hand, attaches great theoretical importance to the difference. He distinguishes "physician products" as those where "the dominant input is physician time," and "ancillary products" as those "that are produced by others." He argues that the products of ambulatory care are not one, but many; and that the production function of each must be examined separately. This is because each may vary quite independently of the others and be differently influenced by factors, such as size of operation, that influence productivity (105). The empirical evidence that bears on this will be briefly described in a subsequent section.

It is clear that the measurement of physician product would require that all the relevant variability, as described above, be in some way standardized. Some have felt that physician time per visit may serve as a rough indicator of differences in the content and quality of the visit, or that part of it exclusive of "ancillary services." If physician pricing were perfectly competitive, price would serve as a proxy. Since this is far from being the case, relative value scales may serve as a rough approximation. One must be aware, however, that relative values reflect, in part, established pricing in a highly noncompetitive market and, in part, normative judgments about the relative worth of different services. What precisely underlies current prices and judgments of worth has not, to the author's knowledge, been systematically explored. In spite of these limitations, both dollar income to the provider and relative value units have been used as measures of output.

Recently, Blendon published a list of 53 operations rated for surgical complexity by a panel of 80 surgeons and anesthesiologists who were in active practice in a leading university hospital (79). Since the term "surgical complexity" was not defined for the judges, it was not known precisely what characteristics of surgical procedures were taken into account in arriving at the ratings. Nor is it known whether surgeons in a given subspecialty were likely to regard procedures in their own field as more or less complex than those in another. It may also be that surgeons in a teaching hospital experience an unrepresentative selection of cases and therefore have a view of the complexity of procedures that cannot be generalized. Nevertheless, it would be very instructive if comparisons were made of these ratings with relative value scales and with actual fees charged, in the latter instance after corrections were made for relevant patient and surgeon characteristics, including geographic location.

A method for weighting services devised by Boyd in order to remunerate physicians in fee-for-service practice more equitably has features that lend themselves to the development of a weighted measure of output (80). This is not surprising, since the objective of equitable rewards is presumably to adjust payment to inputs into the product. Among the components of the weighting system (called DIFAM) the following subset would be applicable to the task of product standardization: (1) empirically observed service time per visit or service; (2) "standard service factors" that are meant to reflect "difficulty and responsibility" involved in specified categories of services, and (3) a factor that preferentially weights specialists as compared to generalists in a ratio of 1.5 to 1.

The most ambitious scheme for the standard measurement of the physician's product is that developed by Kovner (81). He uses a model of the clinical decision-making process to define more precisely the contributions of physicians and other health professionals to the patient visit. When these contributions are defined and quantified, it is possible to standardize the visit in terms of its content. Kovner begins by dividing ambulatory care into "office visit services" and other services which include "specific diagnostic services," "therapeutic services," "surgical services," "radiologic services," "laboratory services," and "all other services." According to Kovner, "office visit services" may be seen as a bundle of "identifiable medical procedures (IMP)." Examples of such procedures are evaluation of the patient's previous record, history taking, investigation of a normal organ or a part having a specific function, "mental size-up" and the conveyance of information, advice and reassurance. Each "identifiable medical procedure," or IMP, may involve three phases of decision-making. These phases, somewhat analogous to those conceptualized by Ledley and Lusted (376), are as follows:

(1) an examination phase, comprising examination, investigation, or preparation for treatment of an organ of the human body (or part having a specific function, such as the eyes, heart, legs, hands, or ears) and investigation of any symptoms or of vital signs relevant to the organ; (2) a retrieval phase, consisting in the retrieval of specialized information or medical knowledge related to the elements of information acquired in the examination phase; and (3) an interaction, evaluation, or diagnostic phase, in which the elements of information acquired in the examination and retrieval phases interact to produce a diagnosis or evaluation of the patient's condition (81, p. 113).

It follows that the elements of care may be presented as a matrix with columns composed of "identifiable medical procedures" and rows consisting of the three phases of decision-making. This does not mean that all cells in the matrix are necessarily filled. For example, Kovner has probably alienated the entire nursing profession by deciding that nursing procedures, at least in the context of "office visit services," only have an "examination phase." Quantification is achieved by assigning weights to each cell in the matrix. The weights appear to be derived by a curious mixture of arbitrary assignment and empirical derivation. Each "identifiable medical procedure," complete in all three phases, generates one unit which is also called an IMP. Since this gives each cell a weight of 0.33 IMP, procedures that consist of less than the full complement of phases are correspondingly reduced in weight. Each nursing service, for example, merits only 0.33 IMP. By contrast, the impact of certain procedures is magnified through a process of subdivision. For example, an investigation of outpatient records showed that the average "elements of information" obtained during an office visit was about 3. This meant that the arbitrarily assigned weight of one unit for that procedure (history-taking) had to be divided into three, with 0.33 IMP assigned to each item of information, the assumption being that each item of information is itself subjected to the three phases of decision making. Histories that deviated from the empirical norm of 3 items of information are rated accordingly. For example, a history that elicits 6 items of information is assigned a rating of 2 IMP. Similarly, the process of physical examination is magnified by the number of organs or parts examined as well as by the number of abnormalities found, with one IMP assigned to each organ, or part, and each abnormality. For example, examination of a normal lung rates 1 IMP; but the examination of a lung with a congested area merits 2 IMP: one for the lung and one for the congested area. Adjustments are also made, when services are provided by specialists under circumstances which are presumed to require the higher skill of the specialist—for example, when consultations are requested by the general practitioner. In such situations, the values of the second and third phases of decision-making (retrieval and evaluation), but not the first phase (examination), are increased by a factor equal to the ratio of the years of medical education of the specialist who provided the service to the years of medical education of the average physician who provides outpatient services (5.5 years).

Since, in the Kovner study, the evaluation of service is based on what appears in office records, certain procedures that are not explicitly recorded are likely to be lost to the rating system. This is generally true of two critical elements in care: (1) evaluation of mental state, and (2) imparting information, advice, and reassurance. Kovner somewhat arbitrarily rectifies these omissions by (1) assuming that the evaluation of mental state occurs intuitively in every case, and assigning 1 additional

IMP to each visit to account for this; and (2) by adding to the total of the units assigned to all office services an increment of 35 percent, except when the service is a complete physical examination, where the increment is only 16 percent. These percentages are arrived from judgmental estimates of the proportion of total office-visit time that is devoted to the activity of imparting information, advice, and reassurance. Their application has the effect of establishing an arbitrarily invariant relationship between this critical activity and all other elements of office care.

A final problem in the measurement of outpatient services is the measurement of the non-office visit ambulatory output in units comparable to the IMP so that all inputs can be aggregated. Kovner achieves this by finding the price equivalent of his IMP units using the relative value scale of the California Medical Association. Once this equivalence is established, it is possible to convert prices into IMP units, or the reverse, so that all services can be aggregated either in IMP units or relative value price units. The exchange rate between IMP and relative value price units was established by an empirical study in which both units were used to measure the same volume of "typical office visits." Kovner uses independently derived weights to measure the output of "office visit services" which, according to him, account for approximately 65 percent of the total output of the ambulatory care facilities studied. For other services, it is felt that the California relative value scale of prices provides valid relative weights. The entire system is seen to rest on a model of clinical process and decision-making to which are attached weights derived from a variety of considerations that include: (1) certain arbitrary, quasi-normative, statements concerning the relative importance of different elements in the model of care and of decision-making; (2) empirically derived norms for history taking; (3) empirically derived norms for medical education; (4) quasi-empirical norms for the amount of time spent in imparting information, advice, and reassurance, (5) an arbitrarily fixed quantity assigned to evaluation of mental state; and (6) partly empirical, partly normative, weights derived from prices recommended by the medical profession. This method for measuring output has been described in some detail not because it is fully endorsed by the author. Many questions could be raised about the model and about the derivation of the various weights. It is clear, however, that the approach as a whole is promising. The author believes that careful conceptual and empirical exploration of the process of clinical care and decision-making will lead not only to better ways of measuring output, but also much needed innovation in defining and measuring the quality of care (377).

Measuring Hospital Output

As we have already emphasized, the hospital has many products, only one of which is patient care. Patient care itself is divisible into many components. The argument that various components of office care should be kept separate and treated as products, each of which has a separate production function, should apply with even greater force to the hospital. This is because hospital care has an even larger number of separable patient care components and is formally organized into fairly autonomous units or departments. Accordingly, Rajgrodzki "would define the hospital as a multiproduct (multiservice) health plant. Each of its independent units—for example, laboratory, radiology, dietary, etc.—produces an independent micro-product" (118). There are other axes of classification: for example, medical service, nursing service, housekeeping service, and administration. The patient care units are themselves organized into departments such as medicine, surgery, pediatrics, obstetrics-gynecology, and newborn nursery. It is not only possible, but very likely, that productivities in these various subunits have experienced different secular trends and are currently different from each other, within a given hospital as well as among hospitals. Such differences arise from a variety of factors, which include degrees of administrative rationalization, manpower differentiation, and substitution (as in nursing), and mechanization or automation (as in laboratory services).

It would be not only useful, but essential, to an understanding of hospital productivity as a whole to examine the productivity of its component units and products. There is equal need, however, for a summary measure of hospital output that would reflect the performance of the hospital as a whole. As we have discussed in a previous section, the product may be measured in terms of services, cases, or changes in health status. The usual measure used is the patient-day. This represents actual care provided. Almost always, however, hospitals maintain more beds than are actually used, partly to allow for patient turnover and partly to accommodate peak loads in a rather variable demand. This means that the occupancy of the hospital is usually less than 100 percent, often considerably less. As we shall see later, hospital size and the size of patient care subunits within the hospital, are an important factor in determining the excess in beds that need to be maintained to meet variations in demand. The more important issue here is that a hospital which has assumed responsibility for a roughly definable population must maintain certain stand-by capacity. Since fixed hospital costs are said to be about two-thirds or three-quarters of total costs, the maintenance of stand-by capacity is costly. The issue is whether the provision of such capacity, during the time it is unused, is a hospital "product." The answer to the question has important implications for the measurement of productivity and efficiency (119). If stand-by capacity is a product, a measure of bed-days must either replace or supplement the patient-day measure. However, some adjustment in the bed-day measure must be made to take account of oversupply of hospital beds: beds that exceed reasonable requirements of stand-by capacity for a given population. The considerations that go into a decision of what is reasonable will be discussed in a subsequent section.

Irrespective of what measure is used to measure the patient care product, corrections must be made for its heterogeneity. Heterogeneity stems from a number of interrelated factors that include age, sex, and diagnostic characteristics of patients, the skill and qualifications of the medical staff, the range of equipment and special services available, and the performance of additional functions such as teaching or research which get confounded with patient care. One approach to standardizing for such differences, which applies to the output of the physician as well as that of the hospital, is to use appropriate research design and statistical techniques for analysis. Examples will be given in the section that deals with the relationship between productivity and hospital size. Another approach is to standardize the measure of the product itself. Saathoff and Kurtz have proposed a method for standardizing hospital output by distinguishing a number of hospital services and assigning weights to each, as shown in Table IV.20. Stated as an equation: adjusted units of service = (adult, pediatric, and newborn days) + 2

Table IV.20.   Weights proposed for specified hospital services judged to correspond to time and money inputs for these services

Services	Weights
Medical day	1
Pediatric day	1
Newborn day	1
Obstetrical day	2
Surgical day	2
X-ray diagnostic procedure	0.3
Laboratory test or tissue examination	0.1
Outpatient visit	0.2

SOURCE: Reference 115.

(surgical plus obstetrical days) + 0.3 (X-ray diagnostic procedures) + 0.1 (laboratory tests and tissue examinations) + 0.2 (outpatient department visits). The authors justify the relative weights as follows:

Weights were assigned on the basis of what were considered to be logical time and cost relationships of these services in total hospital operations. Pertinent literature was examined and numerous discussions with informed individuals were also held in arriving at these decisions. Although the formula itself is obviously arbitrary, the authors submit that the underlying concept is sound and realistic (115, p. 14).

The application of this system to 13 Nebraska hospitals within the size range of 50 to 99 beds, showed that the standardized units of service were from 23 to 63 percent higher than the adult plus pediatric patient-days for the corresponding hospitals. This indicates considerable reordering in hospital output as a result of standardization (115, p. 16, table).

Instead of arbitrary weights, price or cost may be used as a proxy measure of the inputs into the product of a hospital in a manner analogous to the use of price to weight the services of physicians. A simple example is the development, by the American Hospital Association, of a measure of "adjusted patient days" that combines two patient-care products of the hospital: outpatient visits and inpatient-days (116). "Dividing the inpatient revenue per patient day by the outpatient revenue per outpatient visit produces a ratio, a correction factor, indicating the number of outpatient visits necessary to equal one day of inpatient care in terms of level of effort" (116, p. 467). This ratio varies by hospital size and by year, appearing to be larger as hospital size increases, and also tending to be larger in more recent years. This means that inputs into inpatient care have increased at a somewhat faster pace than inputs into outpatient care and that the larger hospitals are distinguished from smaller hospitals by devoting relatively more of their resources to inpatient care as compared to outpatient. This method, as well as the interpretation of its results, depends, of course, on the assumption that revenues are proportionate to cost, that cost is accurately allocated to various activities, and that cost represents value of resource inputs. All of these are questionable assumptions in the hospital field.

Cohen has further refined the standardization of hospital output by actually obtaining empirical data on the cost of several hospital services that, collectively, define the hospital's product, at least insofar as patient care is concerned (128, 129). Cost data were obtained from member hospitals of the United Hospital of New York for 1962 and for 1965. As in the weights assigned by Saathoff and Kurtz, the cost for an adult or pediatric day was assigned a value of 1, and all other costs expressed in proportional terms. Table IV.2 gives the weights for the two years and, for comparison, the more arbitrary weights assigned by Saathoff and Kurtz to more or less comparable items. Cohen has proposed an addi-

Table IV.21.   Alternative sets of weights assigned to specified hospital services that are intended to be proportionate to inputs used to produce these services

Services	Cohen		Saathoff and Kurtz
	1962	1965	
Physical therapy treatments	0.15	0.12	
Electrocardiograms	0.20	0.16	
X-ray therapy treatments	0.39	0.41	
Blood transfusions (and plasma)	0.90	0.56	
Electroencephalograms	0.73	0.62	
Radio isotope treatments	—	0.75	
Operations, weighted[a]	4.75	3.90	2.00 (surgical day)
Deliveries	2.36	2.15	2.00 (obstetrical day)
X-ray, diagnostic[b]	0.16	0.12	0.30
Laboratory examinations	0.07	0.04	0.10 (includes tissue)
Newborn days	0.53	0.49	1.00
Outpatient visits	0.28	0.25	0.20
Emergency room treatments	0.16	0.16	
Ambulance trips	—	0.34	
Adult or pediatric patient days[c]	1.00	1.00	1.00

SOURCE: References 129, Table II, page 12, and 115, page 16.
[a] Major operations plus $\frac{1}{3}$ minor operations.
[b] $\frac{1}{20}$ dental films plus other films.
[c] Arbitrarily fixed at unity.

tional adjustment that recognizes the ''quality'' factor in certain hospitals. He proposes that total output in university-affiliated hospitals be increased by a value from 10 to 30 percent to recognize that each unit of service in a teaching hospital represents that much ''more care.'' Presumably, this recognizes dimensions of quality (for example, our category of ''appropriateness'') not already reflected in differences in cost. The rationale for using cost as a basis for weighting output is that cost is presumably a measure of the resources put into the product. Lave points out that in a perfectly competitive market this would be true (112, p. 79n). Because hospitals are far from being perfectly competitive, differences in cost can be accepted only as a first approximation to differences in input. There are, in addition, serious problems in hospital cost

accounting, which Cohen recognizes. The group of hospitals chosen for
the determination of weights use rather uniform, though not identical,
cost allocation procedures. Nevertheless, it is not clear to what extent the
weights continue to reflect rather arbitrary procedures in the allocation
of costs to the several services (119). A final issue is the extent to which
the hospitals selected are representative of all hospitals. There is no
reason to expect that the relative inputs into the several services will be
the same in all hospitals. For example, the cost of laboratory services
might be a smaller fraction of the cost of the adult patient-day in a
poorly equipped hospital that cares for simple cases and performs the
simplest tests. Similarly, the cost of the newborn day will be relatively
increased if there is a unit for the intensive care of premature and
otherwise distressed infants. Cohen notes, for example, that the omission
of certain rare, but costly, services from the calculation of weights, tends
to favor the smaller hospitals that do not provide these services. Geographic differences in relative prices may also be significant. Cohen notes,
for example, that the weights he has derived reflect the unusually high
price of blood and blood transfusions in New York City. Similarly,
"since . . . hospital services are not equally labor-intensive geographical wage variations will affect the ratio of their costs" (128, p. 363).

Factors in Productivity

OTHER INPUTS. We have already presented the notion that many inputs go
into the production of patient care. We have emphasized that when only
one input, such as physician man-hours, is used to obtain the ratio of
output to input, the effect is to attribute to that one input the contributions of all other inputs. Other inputs include additional numbers and
varieties of health personnel and other workers, more equipment and
varieties of such equipment, other technological innovations in treatment
and management, and organization of personnel, space, and work flow.
The increasing importance of cooperating and subsidiary health personnel in the production of the services of physicians, dentists, and nurses is
amply documented. Data from the decennial census shown in Table
IV.22 demonstrate the dramatic shift in the relationship between numbers of physicians and all other workers in the health occupations. The
magnitude of functional differentiation within nursing is attested to by
the data in Table IV.23. Weiss has reclassified jobs within health occupations into three levels, based on income and education. The trends are
shown in Table IV.24. Fein has called attention to the importance of

Table IV.22. Number of physicians and all other health personnel, and physicians as percent of all health personnel, U.S.A., each tenth year, 1900–1960

Year	Number in Thousands		Physicians As Percent of Total
	Physicians	All Other Health Personnel	
1900	123.5	73.6	168
1910	152.4	155.1	98
1920	151.3	257.4	59
1930	162.7	438.1	37
1940	174.5	517.9	34
1950	199.9	671.9	30
1960	242.5	897.0	27

SOURCE: Reference 378, page 30.

Table IV.23. Percent distribution of nurses by type of nurse, U.S.A., 1950, 1960, and 1968

Category	Percent Distribution		
	1950	1960	1968
Registered nurses	51	46	37
Practical nurses	19	19	18
Aides, orderlies, attendants	30	35	45
TOTAL	100	100	100

SOURCE: Reference 6r, Table 8, page 2 and Reference 3, page 135.

Table IV.24. Percent distribution of health personnel by levels based on income and education, U.S.A., 1940, 1950, and 1960

Category	Percent Distribution		
	1940	1950	1960
High level	34	29	24
Middle level	45	42	41
Low level	21	28	34
TOTAL	100	100	100

SOURCE: Reference 15, page 97.

looking at the composition of the increment of manpower in order to appreciate the magnitude of recent ("marginal") change. The data in Table IV.25 for the dental occupations, illustrate the point.

Table IV.25.   Percent distribution of dental personnel in 1950
and 1960 and percent distribution of the increment in dental
personnel between 1950 and 1960, by type of dental personnel,
U.S.A.

| | Percent Distribution | | |
Category	1950	1960	Increment 1950–1960
Dentists	51	46	29
Other (assistants, hygienists, technicians)	49	54	71
TOTAL	100	100	100

SOURCE: Reference 83, Table IV–3, page 115.

Technological change in the health industry has been immense. The
Department of Labor has given a descriptive account of such innovation
(73, 74). These include methods of preventing disease, more effective
therapeutic agents, new surgical techniques, including the use of pros-
theses and transplants, partial or complete automation of laboratory
testing and diagnostic screening, the use of computers in clinical decision-
making, patient monitoring systems, systems for information-handling
using computers, and methods for centralizing and distributing drugs
and other supplies in the hospital, including the use of disposable supplies. There are, however, some problems in assessing and interpreting
the effect of technology on productivity in the health industry. If the
measure of output is services rendered, technology has the obvious potential to increase such output. If the measure of output is increments in
health, technical innovations have a mixed effect, including certain
paradoxical effects to which we have already referred. Briefly, there are
diminishing returns because of the accumulation of residual problems
not susceptible to significant amelioration by current technology. If the
measure of output is cases appropriately treated, the dominant effect is
probably to expedite care so that more cases are cured or brought to a
conclusion within a given time period. The remarkable decrease in the
average length of stay in general hospitals is largely attributable to this
effect. However, as the slowing and possible reversal of this trend suggests, the paradoxical effects of technology need to be recognized. These
occur in two ways. New technology creates new standards of care so that
the appropriate conclusion of care for a given episode of illness may in
fact take longer to bring about. Also, the cases that present themselves
for care are increasingly those that technology has been able to maintain
alive but not to cure. In other words, the morbidity mix has changed and

corrections have to be made for this in measuring output when changes in health or cases cared for are used as the criterion. Some simple but cogent examples of the mixed effects of technology may be seen in dentistry (31, pp. 475–482). It is estimated that the introduction of fluoridation of public water supplies will result in a 50 percent reduction in tooth decay in 1975 as compared to 1950, thus reducing need for care. The introduction of high-speed drilling equipment is estimated to reduce the time needed to fill a cavity from 25 minutes to 21, a saving of about 20 percent. On the other hand, it is feared that greater success in caring for and preserving teeth will increase markedly the occurrence in later life of diseases of the gums and tissues surrounding the teeth, thus placing new burdens on the profession. The occurrence of such new needs does not, of course, mean that productivity has not increased, but merely that the nature of the problem which the dentist must ameliorate should be taken into account in estimates of productivity, if the findings are to be meaningful.

PERSONAL CHARACTERISTICS. In addition to the magnitude and nature of associated inputs, certain personal characteristics of physician and health professionals obviously influence productivity. These include training and skill. The studies that pertain to the accuracy of physician decisions have been described in a work on quality control (270) ; but the author is not aware of studies that measure speed and accuracy combined. Such studies are more likely to be found in the literature of dentistry and nursing, with which the author is not as well acquainted.

Age is, of course, another personal characteristic that is likely to influence productivity. This happens in several ways. Peterson et al. have shown that older general practitioners in North Carolina were less likely to provide high-quality care (139). However, since this study was cross-sectional rather than longitudinal, it is not possible to be certain that the phenomenon noted is one of deterioration with age. The volume of service is also likely to be reduced both by reduction in hours of work and in service produced per hour. In the younger age group, productivity may be artificially reduced because of the time it takes for physicians in private practice to build up a full complement of clients. As reported by Pennell (96), in 1932 Leven reported that the amount of idle time consumed in establishing a practice represented at least two full years for the average physician. An argument often made on behalf of prepaid group practice is that it cuts down drastically the time taken to achieve employment at full capacity for the beginning physician. Needless to say, productivity at either end of the working life span would vary by specialty, location, and level of supply relative to demand. The effects of the last of these three factors would suggest that the amount of time taken to establish employment at full capacity is shorter now than it was in 1932.

An indirect way of measuring the effect of age on productivity would be, as Pennell suggested many years ago, to study professional income at various ages. Several studies have attempted more direct measurement of the work load of physicians at various ages. Among the earliest of these studies were those undertaken by Ciocco and Altman for the Committee on Allocation of Medical Personnel of the Procurement and Assignment Service during World War II. These studies were begun in the District of Columbia and Maryland (159). The findings of a survey in Georgia were later added to those in the first (160). Still later, Ciocco et al. conducted a similar study in the 29 westernmost counties of Pennsylvania for the National Security Resources Board (161). The relationships between age and work load found in all these studies, including both urban and rural subdivisions, were essentially similar. The highest work load was regularly reported by the age group 35–44, with a somewhat lower work load in the single younger age group, and progressively lower work load in three older age groups. The hours of work followed a somewhat similar pattern, which, however, showed smaller variations by age. The net effect was a distinctly lower product per man-hour as age increased. The pattern is clearly shown in Table IV.26, which gives data for office visits for white male general practitioners in Baltimore, 1942. Physicians who were not in active practice were excluded (160, Table 4, p. 1337, and Appendix Table 1, p. 1348).

Table IV.26.   Work load of white male general practitioners, according to age of practitioners, Baltimore, 1942

Age of Physician	Patients per Week	Hours per Day	Weekly Patients per Hour per Day[a]
Under 35	102	5.2	20
35–44	113	5.8	19
45–64	67	4.9	14
65 and over	42	4.7	9
All years	82	5.2	16

SOURCE: Reference 160, Table 4, page 1337, and Appendix Table 1, page 1348.

[a] The figures in this column are meaningful only if it is assumed that the number of days worked per week is comparable among age groups of physicians.

Additional interesting findings relevant to productivity were that home visits were relatively more frequently made by the older practitioners and that the work load of female physicians was a fifth to a sixth that of male physicians. Sex can, therefore, be added to age as an important personal characteristic that influences productivity.

More recently, a study by Clute of general practice in two Canadian provinces revealed a similar relationship between output and age as shown in Table IV.27. Unlike the findings by Ciocco and Altman, there

Table IV.27.   Non-hospital visits per week made by physicians in specified age groups, Ontario and Nova Scotia, Canada, c. 1956–1960

Age	Median Number of Non-Hospital Visits per Week	
	Ontario	Nova Scotia
31–35	90.5	97.5
36–45	100.0	84.0
46–61	66.0	74.0
All Ages	86.0	86.0

SOURCE: Reference 165, Table 56, page 240.

were no significant differences in total time worked by age. Differences in output are therefore solely attributable to the pace of work.

Roughly similar findings were reported by Altman et al. for the office practice of a sample of members of the New York Society of Internal Medicine. Instead of age, a highly related variable, year of graduation, was used to show differences in productivity. The findings were as shown in Table IV.28.

Table IV.28.   Work load of internists according to their year of graduation from medical school, members of the New York State Society of Internal Medicine, June 1963

Year of Graduation	Office Visits per Week	Office Hours per Week	Visits per Man-hour
1954–63	59.3	32.7	1.8
1944–53	57.9	36.4	1.6
1933–43	57.8	37.1	1.6
1924–33	52.4	34.1	1.5
1923 and Before	32.3	24.9	1.3
All	54.6	35.2	1.6

SOURCE: Reference 167, Tables 1 and 2, page 668.

In February 1965, Eimerl and Pearson obtained information concerning the work load of general practitioners for one part of England and Wales which included Liverpool and its hinterland. They confirmed, for another time and in another place, the original findings of Ciocco and Altman, which suggest that there are, perhaps, certain constancies in medical care, after all.

The older the doctor the less time he spent in the consulting-room and the fewer patients he saw there—that is, there was a trend towards older doctors seeing proportionately more patients on home visits, and spending more time on them (181, p. 1551).

On the other hand, Mechanic has reported equal hours of work, but at a slackening pace, with increasing age among general practitioners in England and Wales (180).

In 1944, Elliott Pennell, as a part of a long series of manpower studies for the Public Health Service (which Maryland Pennell continued after his death), used unpublished data from the Maryland and Georgia surveys of Ciocco and Altman to construct a hypothetical curve that related relative output to physician age. The average number of patients seen in office, home, and hospital by active physicians in the age group 35–39 was arbitrarily assigned the value of 1, and all other values expressed as multiples of this. The observed values were approximately as shown in Table IV.29. A curve was fitted to these observations which

Table IV.29.   Relative number[a] of patients seen in office, home and hospital according to age of physicians, Maryland and Georgia, 1942

Age	Relative Number of Patients per Week
30–34	0.84
35–39	1.00
40–44	0.97
45–49	0.73
50–54	0.81
55–59	0.64
60–64	0.50
65 plus	0.37

SOURCE: Measured from Figure 1, Reference 96.

[a] A value of 1 was assigned to the number seen by active physicians in the age group 35–39.

yielded detailed relative productivity ratios by single year of life. The empirical observations and the fitted curve are shown in Fig. IV.3. Table IV.30 gives selected values from the full tabulation cited by Pennell.

There are, of course, a large number of assumptions in these determinations of productivity in relation to age. They exclude the product of young interns and residents in full-time hospital work, a feature of medical practice which is much more prominent now than it was when these studies were made. They also assume that the mix of patients, the content of care, and the impact on health status are roughly similar for physicians in all age groups. This is not likely to be the case since age reflects several factors, including the competing effects of professional maturity or prestige, as well as of gradual technological obsolescence. Evidence of the former is the finding that older internists are more likely to receive patients by referral, especially from general practitioners (167). Similarly, Clute has reported that older general practitioners earn

Fig. IV.3.   Relative weekly number of patients seen in office, home and hospital by active physicians engaged in private practice, by age of physician. Maryland and Georgia, 1942 and in the U.S.A. in 1969

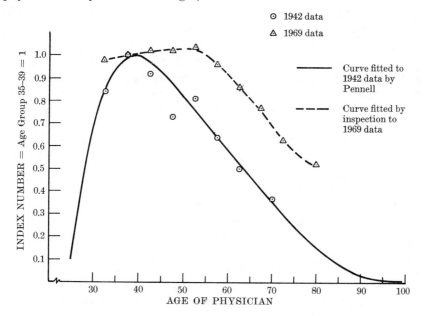

SOURCE: Reference 96, Figure 1, p. 290, and Table 5, p. 298, and reference, 20, Table 22, p. 59.

Table IV.30.   Constructed relative values of
physician workload[a] according to age of physician

Age	Ratio	Age	Ratio
25–26	0.10	65–66	0.47
30–31	0.68	70–71	0.35
35–36	0.95	75–76	0.25
40–41	1.00	80–81	0.15
45–46	0.93	85–86	0.08
50–51	0.81	90–91	0.03
55–56	0.70	95–96	0.01
60–61	0.59		

SOURCE: Reference 96, Table 5, page 298.

[a] Based on empirical observations of numbers of
patients seen in office, home and hospital by samples
of physicians in Maryland and Georgia, 1942. Physicians 35–39 equal 1.00.

more per hour even though they see fewer patients per unit time (165,
Table 30, p. 193). Support for the expectation that age may be correlated
with obsolescence, at least in some situations, comes from the findings of
Peterson et al., who report lower levels of quality in the work of older
general practitioners in rural North Carolina (139). Finally, there may
be differences in the effect of age upon the performance of physicians in
the several specialties. Such differences are obscured when all physicians
are considered together, as if they were homogeneous. Differences between specialties in productivity and in general patient care potential
are also obscured by the process of averaging. Finally, the values developed by Pennell have additional assumptions, which include those
about the age at which physicians enter practice and about the rapidity
with which work load is built up. These assumptions are probably not
applicable today. However, the general approach to the evaluation of
supply and the projection of future needs (to be discussed in a subsequent section) developed by Pennell, represents a degree of methodological sophistication seldom equalled since.

In the light of these observations it is interesting to compare the
productivity data compiled by Pennell with the findings of a recent
survey of the workload of a representative national sample of physicians.
In this sample, physicians in the age group 35–39 did work more weeks
per year and more hours per week than did younger and older physicians. The differences in weeks practiced were very small, whereas those
in hours practiced per week were relatively much larger. The survey

distinguishes hours devoted to direct care from total hours of work. In general, the proportion of total hours devoted to direct care increases with age. In this context, the total product of the physician is best measured by the total number of visits per year, but productivity may be measured either in terms of visits per hour or visits per hour of direct care, depending on whether one is concerned or not concerned with outputs other than visits. Whichever of these measures is used, there is a clear relationship with age, but the peak is found in the age group 50–54 rather than at 35–39 as in the curve hypothesized by Pennell; and the fall to either side of the peak is much less steep. Table IV.31 and Fig. IV.3 compare the findings of the national survey with those cited by Pennell using the age group 35–39 as the standard of reference. In interpreting these comparisons, it should be remembered that the two sets of data differ markedly in the mix of services by location (office, hospital, and home), in the extent and variety of the specialization of physicians, and in their urban-rural distribution. For more accurate comparisons it would be necessary to correct for those differences.

The effect of personal characteristics is relevant not only to manpower projections, but to the assessment of supply in any situation in which age and other characteristics are likely to be atypical. For example, in rural areas the relative preponderance of generalists increases the potential for meeting general medical care needs, but the relative concentration of older practitioners reduces this potential. It was estimated in 1959, that 28 percent of physicians in isolated rural areas were over 65 years of age (6j, p. 28).

FUNCTIONAL DIFFERENTIATION. Several effects stem from the functional differentiation of care-providing resources. Classical economic literature, taking its cue from the celebrated pin factory of Adam Smith, has emphasized the greater *skill and speed,* and hence productivity, of specialized manpower. We have reviewed, in another work (270), the evidence suggesting that specialists are more likely to deliver higher-quality care than do generalists. The information concerning speed is more difficult to interpret. The general expectation is that specialists, after corrections are made for differences in case mix, give longer time per visit and, consequently, see fewer patients per unit time. It is not known to what extent slower processing of patients is due to handling more difficult cases and to what extent it is counteracted by the occurrence of fewer visits per episode of illness and of a higher likelihood of more complete recovery. The empirical evidence bearing on these matters

Table IV.31. Specified measures of workload and productivity in each age group, relative to workload and productivity in the age group 35–39. National sample of physicians, U.S.A., 1969, and physicians in Maryland and Georgia, 1942

Age	UNITED STATES 1969							MARYLAND AND GEORGIA 1942
	Weeks Practiced	Total Hours Per Week	Direct-Care Hours Per Week	Total Visits Per Week	Total Visits Per Year	Total Visits Per Hour	Total Visits Per Hour of Direct Care	Total Visits Per Week
30–34	0.95	0.97	0.97	0.98	0.94	1.00	1.01	0.84
35–39	1.00	1.00	1.00	1.00	1.00	1.00	1.00	1.00
40–44	1.00	1.00	1.03	1.02	1.01	1.02	0.99	0.97
45–49	1.00	0.99	1.01	1.02	1.02	1.03	1.01	0.73
50–54	0.98	0.97	1.01	1.04	1.03	1.08	1.03	0.81
55–59	0.98	0.95	1.00	0.96	0.94	1.01	0.96	0.64
60–64	0.98	0.88	0.95	0.86	0.85	0.97	0.91	0.50
65–69	0.97	0.80	0.85	0.77	0.74	0.95	0.90	—
70–74	0.97	0.68	0.78	0.63	0.61	0.91	0.81	—
75–over	0.98	0.65	0.67	0.52	0.51	0.82	0.77	—
65–over	—	—	—	—	—	—	—	0.37

SOURCE: Reference 20, Table 24, page 59, and Reference 96, Figure 1, page 290.

is rather sketchy. Ciocco and Altman summarize their findings as follows:

The data on the patient load of specialists reveal little regularity of pattern. While specialists of the District of Columbia and Baltimore, with the exception of pediatricians and the ophthalmologists and otolaryngologists, carry a somewhat lower patient load on the average than do the general practitioners, specialists in Georgia consistently have a higher patient load. Neither are comparisons of specialists under 45 years of age with those 45 years of age and older very revealing. The only specialties having the same age difference in all areas—a higher patient load among the younger men—are surgery and eye, ear, nose, and throat work (160, p. 1336).

In 1966, a mail survey of a representative sample of all U.S. physicians in private practice showed the data given in Table IV.32 by specialty.

Table IV.32.   Work load of physicians according to specialty, sample of office-based physicians, U.S.A., 1966

Specialty	Mean Hours Direct Care of Patients per Week	Office Visits per Week
General practice	49.2	130.8
Surgery	45.6	74.0
Internal medicine	45.3	77.2
Obstetrics-Gynecology	47.4	88.1
Pediatrics	46.4	121.5
Psychiatry	38.1	36.6
Radiology	30.3	135.4
Anesthesiology	43.0	27.0
Other	36.6	90.4
All	45.3	—

SOURCE: Reference 162, Tables 8 and 10, pages 521 and 522.

Although differences in hours of direct care are evident, the authors comment that these were "not so great as expected" (162, p. 520). The variations in visits per week are much larger, probably due to differences in case mix. Visits per hour cannot be computed from the data cited because hours of direct care, as given, include time additional to office work. It should also be pointed out that the data were obtained by mail questionnaire and are, therefore, probably based on rather rough subjective estimates whose validity needs to be established. As far as is known, the effect of seasonal differences in work load has not been taken into account. Also not corrected for are differences in scale of operation (for example, solo practice versus group or hospital-based practice) among general practice and the specialties. Most important, however, is the relative meaninglessness of comparing work load and productivity among specialties which produce such a heterogeneous output. What is needed are studies that examine performance (qualitative and quantitative) for generalists and specialists as they care for conditions which both can handle with a reasonable degree of comparability.

While such data are not available, a very rough approximation might be the comparison of physicians who report to be in general practice with those who report that they specialize in internal medicine. Data from the AMA "periodic survey" for 1969, as shown, in part, in Table IV.33, suggest that general practitioners produce more services per week and per hour of direct care than do internists, with the differences being most marked in metropolitan areas. Since general practice includes varying amounts of pediatric care, almost certainly more so in rural than in urban areas, data for pediatricians are also cited in the Table. Unfortunately, even if it were possible to correct for the mix of adult and child services, the products of internists and generalists could turn out to be substantially noncomparable both in terms of inputs into care and ultimate effect on health.

Another consequence of functional differentiation is its effect on *substitutability and interchangeability*. Interchangeability refers to the ability to make short term adjustments through adding or removing units of supply that can serve equivalent functions. Examples are the ability of the professional nurse to do the work of a practical nurse, or the provision of "swing beds" in hospitals in order to accommodate the overflow from whichever service happens to be particularly overloaded. Substitutability refers to the more stable, long term adjustments that are brought about by using one type of service source instead of another. The reason for doing this is that the substituting source of service is more plentiful than the source substituted and/or is easier to produce because it requires much less investment of resources. Examples are using a practical nurse rather than a professional nurse to take temperatures, a nurse rather than a physician to take blood pressure readings, home care instead of inpatient care, or nursing home care instead of hospital care. Nurses are easier to train than physicians and home care is said to be less costly than hospital care.

The effect of functional differentiation (specialization) on interchangeability and substitutability is interestingly complicated. Functional differentiation is necessary for the planned substitution of one

Table IV.33. Specified measures of workload and productivity by selected specialty, sample of physicians, U.S.A., 1969

| Specialty | Weeks Worked Per Year | Hours Worked Per Week | Hours of Direct Care Per Week | Visits Per Week | | | Total Visits Per Hour of Direct Care |
				Total	Office	Hospital	
General practice	48.3	52.0	47.8	167.0	129.5	28.2	3.49
Internal medicine	47.9	52.8	47.7	127.2	86.3	33.5	2.67
Pediatrics	48.1	52.9	46.9	146.5	125.3	19.0	3.12

SOURCE: Reference 20, Tables 16–19, pages 50–54.

source of service for another. However, it may make the system less flexible and less able to cope with variable demand in the short run, or changing conditions over the long pull. For example, functional differentiation in nursing makes possible the substitution of the subprofessional nurse for the professional. Specialization in medicine may make it impossible to substitute the services of a neurosurgeon for those of a dermatologist, to take an extreme example. Pursuing this argument, we have already referred to the reduction in family practice due to specialization in fields other than internal medicine or pediatrics. A characteristic of functional differentiation that appears to be decisive in its impact on interchangeability and substitutability is the presence or absence of what might be called "hierarchical directionality." This refers to the situation in which successively lower levels of personnel can perform only part of the functions of those at the immediately higher level. When such directionality exists, lower-level personnel can assume functions of upper-level personnel, but the latter can always supplement or replace the former in order to cope with variable demand or changing conditions. If differentiation is "horizontal," or on an equal level, components cannot be interchanged, and the system is more rigid. There are certain "mixed" situations in which there appears to be hierarchical differentiation without interchangeability or substitutability. Consider, for example, the position of the physician vis à vis a highly specialized technician in the engineering aspects of electronic monitoring. The reason for this seemingly anomalous situation is that while the technician may be administratively subordinate to the physician, functional hierarchism does not exist.

Functional differentiation, as an inherent property rather than something administratively imposed, is generally thought of as a property of personnel which results from special educational preparation and training. For purposes of schematic symmetry, if nothing else, one could postulate an analogous situation for hospital beds. Imagine a hospital organized to provide progressive patient care. The units set up for self-care cannot readily be used for intensive care should the occasion demand. The intensive care section can, however, be used for self-care patients, although this would be inefficient. It is interesting to note that the rigidity introduced by organizing and equipping the hospital for progressive care is usually counteracted by making provision for a number of "flexible" beds that can be used to provide for overflow from any one of the subunits.

DEPARTMENTALIZATION. Departmentalization imposes administrative barriers to interchangeability and reduces the adaptation of supply to changes in demand. This is true of the hospital in which beds are assigned to departments (medicine, surgery, pediatrics, obstetrics, gynecology, etc.) so that there may be a waiting list for beds in one department while beds go begging in another. As this example suggests, departmentalization and functional differentiation are often related, but they are separable concepts. For example, although the services mentioned above are functionally differentiated, the hospital beds themselves are not differentiated, or minimally so, in most instances. Departmentalization without functional differentiation can occur within a hospital on several grounds, including payment status (ward versus private) and separate provider "firms." An example of the latter occurs in large city hospitals where more than one medical school establishes essentially separate services. One may also consider the several small hospitals, in any one category, that exist in a community, to be an example of "departmentalization." A particularly salient example of the effects of intrahospital departmentalization is the separation of obstetrical from all other beds, which is required both by law and by the conditions for accreditation. Weissman and Sigmond point out that although this separation was necessary when puerperal fever was rampant, there may be no health reason for its maintenance now (134). Currently, the effect of the separation is to perpetuate strikingly low occupancy rates in obstetrical units in the face of rising pressure on beds in other units of the hospital. Weissman and Sigmond cite several demonstrations of the feasibility of admitting selected nonmaternity patients to maternity beds without risk to mothers. In one instance the occupancy rate of the maternity unit was raised by 25 percent. Weissman and Sigmond estimate that if this practice became universal it "would make available for nonmaternity patients at least 20,000 of the 40,000 obstetrical beds vacant on average every day in the U.S., eliminate the need for almost a half *billion* dollars in new hospital construction, and still permit obstetrical units to function at a comfortable 66.6 percent occupancy" (134, p. 91). Unfortunately, we are not told how this estimate was made. Quantitative methods for taking into account the effects of departmentalization have been developed by Blumberg and others. These will be discussed in a subsequent section.

It may be inferred from the above that departmentalization contributes to low levels of hospital occupancy and therefore to lower levels of productivity. However, Goldman et al. have reminded us of certain advantages (281, pp. 119–120):

The principal advantage of bed allocation is the potential efficiency to be derived from grouping patients with similar health problems in the same physical area, convenient to the facilities and services they require. Patient grouping also allows hospital personnel to develop specialized skills in the performance of their patient care functions; and since the practice of medicine is subdivided in the same manner, the physician can decrease his travel time between patients by concentrating his patients in one physical area.

Departmentalization may, however, be excessive, going beyond the legitimate requirements of functional differentiation and efficiency of operations. For example, some authorities have questioned the value of semiprivate rooms that require matching by sex or other patient characteristics. In the opinion of one prestigious group "the semiprivate room may in fact be an expensive anachronism" (221, p. 24). However, a simulation study by Goldman et al. revealed no decisive preference for a policy that allocated all patients to private rooms over one that allocated beds to private rooms, semiprivate rooms, or four-bed wards in accordance with average room-type demand. Under rules specified by the simulation program "average bed utilization" and "average annual total patient days waited" were not significantly different for the two policies. There was, however, less likelihood that the total bed capacity of the hospital would be exceeded when patients were all allocated to private rooms (281). One may also express the hope that through proper design and organization it may be possible to achieve appropriate functional grouping while reducing certain barriers to flexible use of hospital beds.

Analogous situations for personnel have not attracted much attention. One might say that the departmentalization of the hospital may place unequal loads on the resident physicians in the various hospital departments. But in this instance functional differentiation rather than departmentalization is the major obstacle to interchangeability, with the exception of the now less frequently encountered "rotating intern." A more analogous, but largely hypothetical, situation is the imposition of administrative limitations on the use of physicians in one group to help out those in another group in a multigroup group practice plan. A situation much more frequently encountered in real life is the presence of two agencies employing public health nurses (the health department and the visiting nurse agency) in a single community, not only without provision for interchangeability, but with legal and administrative barriers to interchangeability between them. We are not talking here about the issue of coordinated service, but merely about the ability of a larger pool of similarly trained nurses to meet greater fluctuations in service needs than can be met by two smaller pools of nurses with no interchangeability between the pools. On a national scale, state licensure regulations may also produce the departmentalization effect (but on a different time scale) by limiting the ready movement of manpower.

SCALE OF OPERATIONS. Traditionally, economics has accepted the proposition that as the scale of a manufacturing plant becomes larger, costs per unit of product decrease up to a limit after which they rise. The relationship of cost to scale is expressed as a U-shaped or a more flat, saucer-shaped curve. The reduction in unit cost, referred to as "economies of scale," comes about in a number of ways. Division of labor brings about the development of greater skill in the performance of a smaller range of tasks by each employee, as well as more precise matching of skills to task requirements so that highly skilled and scarce personnel (for example, physicians) are not wasted on relatively low-order activities. Large-scale organization also makes possible the greater use of machinery and equipment to help perform tasks at lower cost. Furthermore, since each item of equipment and each professional person is "indivisible," the chances that equipment and personnel do not stand idle, but are utilized to capacity, is expected to be greater as the organization becomes larger in scale. For all the foregoing reasons, economists begin with the strong presumption that larger hospitals will be more productive and efficient than smaller hospitals, larger group practices more productive and efficient than smaller groups, and these, in turn, more productive and efficient than solo practice. This presumption is so strong that Fein, in discussing the economies of scale associated with group practice, concludes that "the 'burden of proof' should be on those who would deny their existence rather than on others to demonstrate that they are present" (83, p. 98n). However, it is also recognized that the economies of scale have a limit beyond which the manufacturing plant experiences "diseconomies of scale." One expects to find, therefore, for each type of plant, a size, or a range of sizes, at which the plant is most productive or efficient, and beyond which there are declines in productivity or efficiency. The reasons advanced for this decline, which is evidenced by the rising limb of the U-shaped or saucer-shaped curve, include increasing difficulties in management and coordination, as well as decreases in personnel morale and productivity.

The foregoing discussion of the economies and diseconomies of scale restricts itself to the internal operations of the plant—be it hospital or practice. There are, of course, additional aspects to determining overall productivity or efficiency which relate to the costs of acquiring inputs and distributing outputs to consumers. As hospitals become larger and physicians become aggregated into groups, often within or adjacent to hospitals, problems arise that relate to the efficient distribution of services. Martin Feldstein describes these as follows:

"Hospital 'distribution costs' per case, including social as well as money costs, increase with the size of the catchment area served. These costs include the operation of the ambulance service, the use of patients' time in transit to hospital, the risk due to distance to be travelled in emergencies, the provision of in-patient care for persons who would have been seen as out-patients if they lived closer to hospital, and the reduction in use of hospital services by persons living at a distance" (2, p. 56).

Millard Long and Paul Feldstein have also called attention to this problem, and have made actual measurements to determine the effect of travel cost on the choice of the most efficient hospital size (353). This factor in the assessment of supply will be discussed more fully in a subsequent section dealing with spatial characteristics of supply in general. Here we will be concerned only with the internal operations of the service-producing resource.

In evaluating the supply of medical care resources, and in planning for the future, the issue is to determine the extent to which the theoretical economies of scale have been actually realized (for example, in group practice or in the larger hospital) or are realizable and, if such economies exist, what might be the most efficient size for each category of resource. It is conceivable, as Bailey has argued (105), that certain characteristics of the organization of health services might minimize the economies of scale and magnify the diseconomies. Among the former is the traditionalism of most physicians and their unwillingness to delegate their functions to others. The labor-intensive nature of health services, the generally low wages in the hospital industry, the difficulties in mechanizing many health service functions, and the noncompetitive nature of the industry might all pose barriers to realizing fully the potential benefits of larger scale. Martin Feldstein has called attention to the rather informal nature of the "production process" in hospitals as compared with industrial production. Since, in his view, "the pace of operations is . . . critically dependent on the attitudes and behaviour of staff members," the diseconomies of scale are likely to set in at smaller sizes and to be more marked (2, p. 59). In support of this view he cites the findings, by Revans, that in larger hospitals there is poor communication between supervisory and staff nursing personnel, more morbidity and absenteeism among nurses, and longer hospital stay per admission for patients.

In the following sections findings will be presented on the relationship between productivity and size, for hospitals and office practice respectively. Various issues of method will also be presented as they become pertinent to the studies and their findings.

The reader should remember that in all instances the studies to be reviewed are concerned only with internal economies or diseconomies. If external costs were to be added, the optimal size of the service-producing unit would be smaller than that indicated by considering internal costs alone. Of equal importance is the fact that in all instances the economic cost of producing services is the measure of productivity. No attention is given to modifications of health status or to client wishes and preferences. One could postulate that clients might have distinct preferences for smaller organizations in which they feel more at ease and which appear to be more responsive to their needs, as they define them. If so, the most desirable size of hospitals and, especially, of ambulatory care units, might be even smaller than that indicated by study of costs, whether internal alone or internal combined with external. This view is supported by the report that the members of the Group Health Cooperative of Puget Sound have consistently resisted the formation of group facilities of excessive size for fear that care in such facilities would become forbiddingly impersonal (390).

Hospital Size and Productivity

We have already discussed the major issues of method that are involved in measuring the relationship between hospital size and productivity, when external costs or the distributional aspects are excluded from consideration. These pertain mainly to the definition and measurement of input, output, and size.

The measure of *input* in all the studies to be reviewed is cost. This immediately raises the question of what elements of cost are included and whether these are comparably measured for hospitals of all sizes. Unfortunately, the published accounts do not always give sufficient information on this point. Obviously, adjustments must be made for differences in cost that are related to size but causally unrelated to productivity, if the discovery of spurious relationships is to be avoided. Differences in the prices paid for labor and material inputs constitute one such variable. Since larger hospitals (excluding psychiatric institutions) tend to be in urban areas, the wages they pay tend to be higher and the prices for material inputs probably lower due to quantity purchasing and lower transportation costs. The smaller, rural hospitals tend to pay lower wages but higher prices for other inputs.

The unit of *output* in all the studies to be reviewed, except one, is the patient-day. The one exception is the use, by Martin Feldstein, of the "case" as the measure of output. The implications of choosing one unit or another have already been discussed. More important still is the problem of making appropriate corrections for the content and quality of the product and excluding products other than patient care. The problems of measurement and interpretation arise from the fact that size is positively related to occupancy rate, to length of stay, and to content and quality of care. These in turn are related to both cost per case and cost per day.

The measure of *size* used in most studies is patient-days per unit of time (for example, a year) or average daily census. Others have used the actual number of beds available for service. These differences introduce certain issues of interpretation that we have not discussed as yet, but which, in part, will prove to be familiar. Whan patient-days or daily census are used as a measure of size, one finds that essentially identical units have been used to measure both output and scale. Martin Feldstein has discussed several computational artifacts that can follow from this practice (2, pp. 60–61). When hospital beds are used as a measure of size, it may not be possible to determine with accuracy what, in fact, is the number of beds actually available for use in any given hospital. As we shall see, reported hospital capacity may be significantly off the mark. Furthermore, there is, in most instances, a positive relationship between hospital size and percent occupancy. Thus, as Carr and Paul Feldstein point out, "using number of beds to measure hospital size overstates the size of small hospitals" (122, p. 52). The effect is to exaggerate whatever relationships are found between cost and scale. For example, the differences in bed capacity between 50 and 500 beds may represent differences in average daily census of 25 to 450.

REVIEW OF STUDIES. The more recent and refined studies of the relationship between productivity and hospital size may be said to have begun with the work of Paul Feldstein, published in 1961 (121). In 1967 W. John Carr and Paul Feldstein published the results of a study of over 3000 short-term, voluntary, general hospitals registered by the American Hospital Association (122). Costs per patient-day, adjusted for differences in wages, were related to average daily census, which was the measure of size. Adjustment for heterogeneity of output was made by using multiple regression to allow for the effect of the number of special facilities and services present in each hospital out of 28 such facilities and services listed in the *Guide Issue of Hospitals*. Adjustments were also made for the presence of a formal educational function by including in the regression analysis the following additional variables: (1) existence of a hospital nursing school, (2) number of student nurses, (3) number and types of internship and residency programs, (4) number of interns and residents, and (5) affiliation with a medical school. The findings fit theoretical expectations concerning the returns to scale. As average daily census increased, average cost per patient-day declined, until it reached a minimum level at about an average daily census of 190, and then began to rise. There was reason to believe, however, that the regression equation underestimated the degree of initial decline and overestimated the amount of rise in cost at large-size levels. Consequently, more detailed analysis was undertaken by dividing the array of hospitals into five groups by the number of special facilities or services each hospital was reported to offer. The original regression analysis was performed separately for each of the service groups. The results showed the following: (1) on the whole, hospitals with more services had higher costs per patient-day than did hospitals with fewer services but comparable size; (2) in all service groups, cost decreased with increasing size, but at a progressively lower rate as size increased; (3) only in the group with most (20–28) services was there a minimum, or most efficient, size (at about a daily census of 350) beyond which cost per patient-day increased. The implications for the assessment of hospital resources, now and in the future, are summarized as follows:

Our findings suggest that small hospitals with high service capability should not generally be built because they are likely to be of uneconomic size. Large hospitals having low service capability are also likely to be uneconomic, since there are few or no additional economies associated with increased size to offset the greater transportation costs incurred (122, p. 64).

Berry has introduced a further refinement in standardizing for differences in the hospital's product (125–126). He grouped over 5000 nonfederal, short-term, general and other special hospitals registered by the American Hospital Association in 1963 into categories according to which of 28 special facilities and services each hospital was reported to have. In any one category of hospitals, all the hospitals had the identical facilities and services. Thus the categories arrived at by Berry differed from those constructed by Carr and Feldstein. Each of the latter had the same *number* of special facilities or services, but not necessarily the same *kinds* of such facilities or services. The method used by Berry identified about 3400 groups, of which 40 were considered to have enough hospitals (between 10 and 92) to warrant analysis. For each group a correlation coefficient was computed between cost per patient-day (the measure of input) and patient days (the measure of size). The correlations were negative in no less than 36 out of 40 groups tested; and in every group that contained 15 or more hospitals. Not all the negative relationships were statistically significant, but the large number of negative correlations, in the author's opinion, "overwhelmingly support the conclusion that hospital services in the short term hospital industry are produced subject to the economies of scale" (125, p. 138). The analysis performed by Berry did not lend itself to the determination of the most efficient size of hospital, or the detection of diseconomies of scale restricted to a limited range of sizes. Furthermore, Berry recognizes that standardization of the product using the availability of special facilities and services as the criterion is only a "second-best approximation for grouping by product homogeneity" (125, p. 135). This is because similarity in the presence of services does not assure similarity in the diagnostic mix of patients or in the actual use of these services.

Quite independently, Martin Feldstein has approached the problem of product standardization by doing what Berry suggests is the preferable procedure: correcting hospital costs for differences in diagnostic mix (127). He does this by using multiple regression analysis to determine how much variability in cost among hospitals is attributable to differences in the number of cases in specified diagnostic categories treated by each hospital. Two sets of computations, using 9 and 28 diagnostic categories respectively, have been published.

Martin Feldstein studied the relationship between cost and hospital size in 177 acute nonteaching hospitals, ranging in size from 72 to 1064 beds, in England and Wales, in 1961. This study is distinctive in several ways. First, the measure of size is the number of available beds. This permits the use of a separate measure of size and of output. However, it also has the potential of introducing the effect of differences in occupancy. This does not happen in this sample because there is no systematic relationship between hospital size and percent occupancy. The absence of such a relationship is unexplained, but it could be due to the predominantly large size of hospitals in the sample, and the lower barriers to intra- and inter-hospital transfers in Britain as compared to the United States. Second, the measure of output is the case rather than the patient-day or the patient-week. The advantages and disadvantages of this measure have already been discussed. Although Feldstein has advocated the use of the case as the measure for output, it is interesting to note that his analysis, by correcting for "case flow," appears to involve a retreat from this position. This is especially true because the major determinant of differences in case flow in his sample was length of stay rather than occupancy.

The measure of input was operating costs, including maintenance and normal replacement of equipment, but excluding depreciation, building costs, and purchase of major long-lived equipment. It was not considered

necessary to adjust for differences in the prices of labor and other supplies because these were considered to be either reasonably uniform or
not to vary systematically with size. The third distinctive feature of the
study is that differences in output among hospitals were handled by
adjusting cost to differences in the proportion of hospital cases in each of
nine diagnostic categories: (1) general medicine, (2) pediatrics, (3)
general surgery, (4) ear, nose, and throat, (5) other surgery, (6) traumatic and orthopedic surgery, (7) gynecology, (8) obstetrics, and (9)
other.

The findings were as follows. As expected, cost not adjusted for case
mix, increased markedly with size. Even when adjustments for case mix
were introduced, there was no conclusive evidence of significant economies of scale; costs appeared unaffected by scale. At best, "if we
disregard the standard errors [the quadratic cost function with case mix
included] indicates a shallow U-shaped curve with minimum average
cost per case at approximately 310 beds" (127, p. 66). The doubtful
nature of the relationship found may result from incomplete correction
for differences in the product, or due to the counterbalancing effect of
diseconomies which Feldstein emphasizes as more than usually applicable
to hospital operations. These include, as we have already said, difficulties
in communication, lowered employee morale, and a slower pace of patient
management with resulting prolongation of stay. The corrections for
diagnostic differences were rather rough and do not represent differences
in input for cases in similar diagnostic categories, but of varying clinical
severity or difficulty. Differences in length of stay may reflect such clinical differences, even after corrections are made for diagnostic mix, rather
than differences in the pace of operations, as Feldstein tends to believe.
The argument can only be settled by direct assessment of the need for
stay, and of the content of care, in hospitals of different size. Failing
this, Feldstein attempted to further minimize between-hospital heterogeneity by dividing hospitals by size, first into two and then into four
groups. The findings were essentially similar, indicating "a slightly U-
shaped curve with a minimum in the range of 250–350 beds" (127, p.
71). A second refinement was to look for a "case flow effect" in all
hospitals, as well as in each of the two and four groups aggregated by
size. In the hospitals studied, the differences in the numbers of cases
processed each year was a function of length of stay and was found to
decrease as the hospital became larger, indicating longer stays in the
larger hospitals. The expectation, therefore, is that cost per patient-day
would decrease more markedly with increasing size than does cost per
case; or, as Feldstein puts it, "if flow rates were uniform, larger hospi-

tals would enjoy lower costs per case'' (127, p. 75). This finding accords
with expectation.

Feldstein summarizes his findings and concludes as follows:

> The average cost function, when adjusted for casemix, is a shallow U-shaped
> curve with a minimum at the current average size (310 beds). Costs rise beyond
> this size but level off after 600 beds at about 10 percent above the minimum cost.
> The failure to achieve economies of scale is primarily due to the lower case-bed
> ratio in larger hospitals, even after adjusting for casemix differences. This prob-
> ably reflects a lower level of 'managerial' or labour efficiency and, in particular,
> a slower hospital pace. When costs are adjusted for case-flow rates, cost per case
> decreases throughout the observed range of hospital size to a value of £49.30 at
> 905 beds, some 12 percent below average cost. Cost curves for individual input
> categories show that the pure labour component—ward staff costs—have the
> greatest diseconomies of scale while direct costs and other indirect costs generally
> enjoy increasing returns to scale when adjustment is made for case-flow rates.
> These results indicate that the medium size hospital of 300 or 500 beds is at
> least as efficient at providing general ward care as are larger hospitals. But al-
> though the medium size hospital must not be rejected as uneconomically small,
> it cannot be defended as substantially less costly than the larger hospital. If the
> case-flow rate of larger hospitals could be improved so that it was not lower than
> the rate in other hospitals—primarily by decreasing average lengths of stay—
> operating cost per case in larger hospitals could be reduced to better than 12
> percent below current average cost. Additional savings in capital costs would also
> be achieved. Further economies could be obtained by larger hospitals if they
> lowered their expenditure on ward staff into line with the rest of the hospitals
> (127, p. 86).

A third study of the relationship between cost and size is that reported
by Cohen (128, 129). We have already described Cohen's adjusted
measure of output based on the relative costs of 13 component services in
a sample of urban hospitals. The returns to scale were tested by relating
total cost, excluding depreciation, to total output as measure in Cohen's
standard units. Thus, the relationship explored is one between actual cost
and an index of expected cost. Such comparisons were made for two
samples: one of hospitals in New York City that were members of the
United Hospital Fund, and another for a sample of 82 accredited hospitals (out of 339 queried) in a six-state, northeastern region of the United
States. For the six-state sample, service output data were available only
for adult and pediatric patient-days, newborn days, and deliveries. The
amounts of the other services, where known to be present, were assumed
to have been provided in the same proportions to "inpatient days" as
they were in hospitals used for the derivation of weighted output. The
effect is probably to inflate the expected costliness of the six-state sample,
especially for the smaller, rural hospitals. As might have been expected,

the correlation between actual cost and the index of cost adjusted for service mix was high in both samples (New York City and the six states). However, there was a "significant increase in the multiple correlation in the quadratic total cost curve." It was concluded that there was a straight line marginal cost curve and a U-shaped average cost curve. The minimum point in the latter was obtained at an adjusted output that corresponded to an average daily census of 230–250 patients or 290–295 beds at about 80 percent occupancy in the New York City sample and to 160–170 beds (presumably at a similar occupancy rate) in the six-state sample.

In a second study of New York City hospitals which were members of the Fund, Cohen used more recent (1965), and revised, estimates of relative weights. He also made a correction for quality (to the extent that this is not already reflected in the service mix differences represented in the weighted output) by arbitrarily increasing the output of university-affiliated hospitals by 10, 20, or 30 percent. The findings were essentially similar to those in the first study. The most reliable estimates (from a subsample of hospitals that provided most complete information) suggest that lowest costs per unit of service occur at a hospital size between 540 and 790 beds at about 90 percent occupancy. The optimal hospital size became progressively larger as the increments of value attributed to quality and attached to university-affiliated hospitals increased. Thus, the optimal sizes were 640, 700, or 790 beds, depending on whether the increment in the value of output attributed to quality was 10, 20, or 30 percent. Unfortunately, Cohen has not compared and synthesized the findings in his two studies, nor does he provide an explanation for the rather wide range of optimal sizes in the several samples even when the quality correction is not made. Most probably, these arise from the many limitations in the samples (especially that from the six states) and in the data, as well as in the assumptions involved in their use.

The final study to be reviewed in this series is that by Ingbar and Taylor (130). It deserves special attention because its findings appear to be not only different from all the others reviewed, but also totally unexpected in the light of economic theory. This is a study of 72 "accredited, short-term, voluntary (nonprofit) general hospital(s) that lacked academic, municipal, and religious affiliations," in the State of Massachusetts (130, p. 15). Information was obtained concerning over 100 variables that measure various hospital operations and activities during 1958 and 1959. These variables were subjected to factor analysis. Fourteen factors were found to account for 85 percent of total variation. Of these, 11 were ''identified'' as follows: (1) size-volume, (2) utilization, (3) length of stay, (4) laboratory activity, (5) radiological activity, (6) surgical activity, (7) maternity activity, (8) pediatric activity, (9) ambulatory activity, (10) private services, and (11) ward services. Obviously, each of these factors included a fairly large number of component measures of hospital activity. The ''size-volume'' factor itself contained 59 disparate (though often related) measures which were grouped into seven categories: capacity, total services, maternity services, radiology treatment services, autopsy rates, medical education, and nursing education (130, Table 3.1, pp. 34–39). Multiple regression analysis was used to determine the effect of each of the factors on total cost, cost per bed-day and cost per patient-day. The variables in the multiple regression equations were items (from among the over 100 available) each of which pertained to one of the 11 factors. The power of each of the different factors, and of the different items that constituted each factor, to explain cost was explored. It was found that a very small number of items (representing a few factors) could explain a very large proportion of the variation in cost per unit of service, either bed-day or patient-day. In this review we are concerned only with the part of the study that deals with the returns to scale (130, pp. 55–60, 98–100).

The measure of input was total cost. The hospitals studied all reported to the Bureau of Hospital Costs and Finances of the Commonwealth of Massachusetts, and used a uniform, audited system for computing and allocating costs. The measure of output for this part of the study was the patient-day. Corrections for output variations were made in part by introducing into the regression equation several items which were known to explain over two-thirds of the variation in cost. The items and the factors to which they pertain were the following: medical and surgical expense rate (factor 1), weighted operation rate (factor 6), outpatient radiology weighted film rate (factor 9), and private patient day rate (factor 10). Two additional items pertained to percent occupancy and to the number of available adult and pediatric beds. The measure of size was available beds. The authors were aware of the problem of defining this unit, but decided to accept the number of beds as defined and audited by the Massachusetts Bureau of Hospital Costs. ''These are allegedly the annual average of those that are fully staffed and otherwise immediately available to receive patients on each day'' (130, p. 32). By this criterion, hospital size varied from 31 to 332 beds. For some unknown reason, there was no relationship between bed size and percent occupancy in this sample—a finding similar to that in the sample in England and Wales used by Martin Feldstein. Computations were made for data from 1958–1959 and again, for a slightly smaller sample, for data from 1962 to 1963. The findings were essentially the same in both cases. There was a relationship between cost and patient-day, holding the other variables constant, which had an inverted U-shape. In other words, as size increased, costs per patient-day first increased and then decreased. Maximum costs per patient-day were obtained at a size of 150 beds for the 1958–1959 data and 190 beds for the data 1962–1963. In both computations, the effects of size were rather modest, as shown for the 1958–1959 data in Table IV.34, in which the cost per patient-day at 150

Table IV.34.   Extent to which cost per patient-day in hospitals of specified size differs from cost per patient-day for hospitals of 150 beds. Short-term, voluntary hospitals without academic affiliations, Massachusetts, 1958–1959

Number of Beds	Differences in Costs per Patient-Day
75	−$0.74
100	− 0.33
125	− 0.08
150	—
175	− 0.08
200	− 0.33
225	− 0.74
250	− 1.31
275	− 2.05
300	− 2.95
325	− 4.01

SOURCE: Reference 130, Table 44, page 59.

beds is taken to be the base. Unfortunately, the authors do not give the dollar value for the cost per patient-day at size 150, so that the relative changes cannot be computed. They conclude, however, that "these savings . . . approach 10 percent only when hospitals reach 300 beds. Since there were few institutions of this size among the community hospitals studied, these results must be viewed with caution" (130, p. 58). Furthermore, the authors emphasize that their findings apply only to the kind of hospital and size range (31–332 beds) represented in their sample. Nevertheless, their quite unusual findings have prompted many attempts at explanation and interpretation. Perhaps the most satisfactory interpretation is that offered by Berry, which Ingbar and Taylor also accept as plausible (125, pp. 129–130, and 130, p. 111). In essence, this assumes that the method used did not adequately adjust for differences in service capability. Consequently, as hospitals increase in size, and add a large number of services that they are able to offer, cost rises faster than the economies possible as a result of expanding size. It is only after a certain size is exceeded and, perhaps, the addition of new types of services is not so large, that economies of scale become evident. This interpretation is partially supported by the findings of Ingbar and Taylor that costs within some departments (for example, radiology and laboratory services) did, in fact, show economies of scale throughout the range of hospital sizes. Accordingly, it is possible to postulate that cost-per-patient-day would continue to fall beyond the 300-bed limit reasonably well represented in this sample; and that there could be a second rise in cost due to the onset of actual diseconomies of scale. What the ascending limb of the Ingbar–Taylor curve shows, in other words, are not diseconomies of scale, but diseconomies of service-capability or product differentiation disproportionate to scale.

These speculations highlight the importance of certain distinctions that we have already made, but which may bear repetition and some expansion. The capability to provide service by the acquisition of special personnel or equipment does not necessarily mean that such services or functions are equally used by the hospitals that have them. There may be two sorts of inequality: in the amount of such services used per patient-day or per stay, as well as in the degree to which the available resource is fully used, employed, or exploited. In a highly developed and urbanized area, such as Massachusetts, there are many forces that might lead to the overequipment of small hospitals. These include the large number of autonomous hospitals, the relatively plentiful supply of highly specialized physicians who vie for hospital affiliation, and the high level of client expectation coupled with the financial ability to seek satisfaction of such expectations. Internal differentiation of the hospital will show itself in low occupancy if it involves the creation of "distinctive patient facilities," as defined by Blumberg (213). Thus, a hospital may grow in size through the addition of units of beds with no improvement, and possibly deterioration, in occupancy, if the units do not allow for patient substitution or transfer among them. Furthermore, over-differentiation in terms of ancillary services and equipment, including teaching and research functions, may not be associated with changes in the scale or the differentiation of the bed complement. If this is so, it will not be evidenced in changes in size or occupancy.

A summary of the major features of the studies reviewed above is given in Table IV.35.

Productivity and the Scale of Ambulatory Care

We have already described briefly reasons for expecting greater productivity, up to a limit, with increase in scale of operation. These arguments should apply to ambulatory care as well as to hospital care. In addition, because the productivity of ambulatory care is often measured as a ratio of output to the man-hour input of the key professional (usually dentist or physician) the contributions of all other inputs are attributed to that one category of professionals. A case in point is a study of the relationship between patients seen by the dentist and the number of auxiliary personnel he employs. Assuming that the mean number of patients seen by the unaided dentist equals 100, the relative effects of enlarging the complement of auxiliary personnel are seen in Table IV.36. It is clear that as a dentist increases the number of auxiliary personnel that he employs, the output per dentist per unit time increases markedly. Strictly speaking, this does not necessarily mean that there are economies of scale because, in this instance, as the firm becomes larger, the manner in which services are produced has also changed. However, in studies of the relationship between productivity and the scale of ambulatory care one does not always find a distinction made between size per se and the changes in the modes of production that are associated with size and are attributed to it (84). This confounding of the effects of two related but separable phenomena will be clearly seen in several studies of group practice that we shall presently review. In all these studies attention is focused on output per physician as the measure of productivity. In an analogous manner, output per dentist is the usual measure of the productivity of the dental firm. However, even if this convention is accepted, several further caveats need to be introduced. These relate to the measure of input, the measure of output, and the attribution of output to the dentist. As to the measure of input, one has to be able to make the assumption that the hours of work per full-time equivalent do not change as the firm becomes larger. With respect to output, when the number of patients per unit time is used as the measure, it is assumed that cases are comparable and are comparably managed irrespective of the size of the dental firm. Income has often been used as an alternative measure of output because it includes not only the volume of work performed but is also assumed, through the intermediacy of price, to reflect differences in the content and quality of services. As

Table IV.35. A summary of studies of hospital productivity as related to hospital size

Study	Input	Output	Size	Findings
Carr & Feldstein Reference 122. 3,147 U.S. short-term, voluntary, general hospitals, registered by A.H.A., 1963. American Hospital Association., 1963.	*Costs* as reported to American Hospital Association, adjusted for differences in wages but not for differences in other prices.	*Patient-day.* Output differences adjusted for number of special services available in the hospital, for outpatient services and for educational functions in the hospital.	*Average daily census.*	(1) For all hospitals: U-shaped curve with minimum average daily census of 190 (about 220 beds at 85% occupancy). (2) For hospitals grouped by number of services, as follows:

Number of Services	Minimum Size
0–9	not determined
10–12	not determined
13–16	not determined
17–19	not determined
20–28	Average daily census of 350 (370–390 beds at 90–95% occupancy).

Table IV.35. (continued)

Study	Input	Output	Size	Findings
Berry References 124–126. 40 groups of U.S. hospitals derived from over 5000 non-federal, short-term, general and other special hospitals registered by American Hospital Association, 1963.	*Costs* as reported to American Hospital Association. No correction for prices.	*Patient-day.* Output made more comparable by grouping hospitals so each group offers identical kinds of special services.	*Patient-days.*	There are economies of scale. Diseconomies of scale were not identified. No minimum size identified.
Martin Feldstein Reference 127. 177 non-teaching hospitals, ranging in size from 72 to 1064, England and Wales 1961.	*Operating Costs,* including maintenance and the normal replacement of equipment, but excluding depreciation, building costs and purchase of major, long-lived equipment. Corrections for prices not thought necessary.	The hospital *Case:* discharges, dead or alive, without corrections for transfers. Differences in output adjusted by correcting cost for diagnostic mix using 9 diagnostic categories. Additional adjustments made by grouping by size and correcting for differences in "case flow" by size.	*"Available beds."*	Probably a shallow U-shaped curve with minimum between 250–350 beds, rising thereafter to about 600 beds, after which no change. When adjustments are made for "case flow," costs fall throughout observed range of sizes with lowest value at about 905 beds.

Table IV.35. (continued)

Study	Input	Output	Size	Findings
Cohen References 128–129. New York City hospitals, members of United Hospital Fund, 1962, 1963–1964 and 1965; also a sample of accredited hospitals in a six-state northeastern region.	*Total Costs* for United Fund hospitals which used standard practices of accounting required by the Fund. Corrections for starting wages made in six-state sample.	*Patient-days or units of output* generated by weighting component services by costs allocated to such services in the New York City sample. Corrections for quality in some samples by increasing output by 10, 20 or 30 percent.	*Patient-days or units of service* as described under "output."	U-shaped average cost curve with different minimum points depending on sample, values used to correct output, etc. First New York City sample: 290–295 beds at about 80% occupancy. Six-state sample: 160–170 beds at about 80% occupancy. Second New York City sample: 540–575 beds at about 90% occupancy. When quality corrections made for this sample results were as follows: 10% increment: 640 beds 20% increment: 700 beds 30% increment: 790 beds
Ingbar & Taylor Reference 130. 77 accredited, short-term, voluntary hospitals, without academic affiliations, ranging in size from 31–332 beds, Massachusetts, 1958–1959 and 1962–1963.	*Total hospital costs.* Standard accounting methods of Bureau of Hospital Costs and Finances of Massachusetts.	*Patient-days* (Bed-days used for other analyses) Output differences adjusted for effect of certain factors that account for a great share of variability in cost.	*Available beds:* those that are staffed and otherwise immediately available to receive patients on each day.	Inverted U-shaped curve with maximum at 150 (1958–59 data) or 190 (1962–63 data). 150 or 190 are the sizes to avoid.

Table IV.36.   Relative number[a] of patients seen per
dentist per year, according to the number of auxiliary
dental personnel employed, U.S.A., 1958

Number of Auxiliary Dental Personnel		Relative Number of Patients Seen by Dentist per Year
Full Time	Part Time	
0	0	100
0	1	113
0	2	161
1	0	148
1	1	169
1	2	182
2	0	185
2	1	214
3	0	239

SOURCE: Reference 31, page 45.
[a] Number per dentist employing no auxiliary personnel
is taken to equal 100.

we have emphasized in our review of hospital productivity, there is the
further assumption that the market for dental care is competitive.
Another question is whether gross or net income is the more appropriate
measure. When gross income per dentist is used as the measure of
productivity, the product of the entire firm is attributed to the dentist.
Net income is a more realistic measure of the dentist's own contribution
to productivity. However, even when net income is used, it may be safely
assumed that the dentist (or the physician in analogous situations) will
retain a larger share than is his due because he has such a large measure
of legal, and more general social, control over the system of production.

Data from the periodic Surveys of Dental Practice conducted by the
American Dental Association throw some light on these speculations.
Table IV.37 shows income data related to the number of auxiliary personnel employed. A dentist who employs four or more full-time auxiliary
personnel makes more than three times as much as one who employs no
auxiliary personnel; and the proportion of net income to gross is reduced, but not by a great deal, as the size of the firm becomes larger.
Table IV.38 shows the joint effects of additional equipment (typified by
the dental chair) and assistance. Equipment and assistants can independently and jointly improve productivity measured by gross or net
income, although the increase in the latter is somewhat, but not much,
smaller. Finally Table IV.39, demonstrates the effects of organizing

Table IV.37   Annual income per dentist in nonsalaried practice, according to the number of full-time auxiliary personnel[a] employed by the dentist, U.S.A., 1967

Number of Auxiliary Dental Personnel	Mean Net Income	Mean Gross Income	Net as Percent of Gross
0	$14,411	$22,697	63.5
1	20,470	35,345	57.9
2	27,906	50,959	54.8
3	32,271	63,712	50.7
4 or more	40,495	77,639	52.2

SOURCE: Reference 110, Table 13, page 804.

[a] For simplicity, data on dentists that employ part-time personnel without or with full-time personnel have been omitted from the table.

practice into progressively more complex forms. Several measures of the product (patients, visits, gross income, and net income) are given. Although there are unexplained differences in detail when the different measures are used, the general trend is clear. Higher levels of organiza-

Table IV.38.   Annual income per dentist in nonsalaried practice, by number of dental chairs used and number of assistants employed, U.S.A., 1967

Number of Chairs	Number of Assistants			
	0[a]	1	2	3
Annual Net Income in Dollars				
1	13,864	18,469		
2	18,368	21,442	27,745	
3	24,135	24,346	29,266	35,227[b]
Annual Gross Income in Dollars				
1	21,838	31,757		
2	30,354	38,023	50,726	
3	45,674	45,164	57,877	71,694[b]
Net Income as Percent of Gross				
1	63.5	58.2		
2	60.5	56.4	54.7	
3	52.8	53.9	50.6	49.1[b]

SOURCE: Reference 110, Table 12, page 804.

[a] "No employees" or "no full-time positions."

[b] One assistant, one hygienist, and one secretary or receptionist.

Table IV.39. Yearly workload and income per dentist in nonsalaried practice, according to form of practice, U.S.A., 1967

Form of Practice	Number of Patients		Number of Visits		Net Income	Gross Income	Net as Percent of Gross
	Mean	Median	Mean	Median			
Nonsalaried practice without partners and with no sharing of costs of offices, assistants, etc.	1,288	1,000	3,572	3,122	$24,400	$44,982	54.2
Nonsalaried practice without partners, but sharing costs of offices or assistants, etc.	1,365	1,100	3,426	3,200	24,097	45,420	53.1
Nonsalaried practice as partner in a complete partnership	1,729	1,100	5,143	3,800	31,647	57,845	54.7

SOURCE: Reference 109, Table 5, page 343, and Reference 111, Table 51, page 379.

tion are associated with greater productivity per dentist. As is true for the studies of group practice by physicians, which we shall review next, it is not known to what extent the increased dental productivity that is noted in Table IV.39 is a function of scale and to what extent it is brought about by the use of more auxiliary personnel and more equipment as the firm becomes more formally organized and larger.

The major question with respect to the productivity of physicians has concerned the advantages of group practice over solo practice, and the economies of scale and the more efficient modes of production associated with the former. These economies may be represented as increases in the quantity or quality of care per unit input in group practice itself, as well as for group practice and the hospital jointly. This is one instance in which it becomes particularly important to decide whether the offices of physicians can be viewed as self-contained firms. For example, studies have shown that a major contribution of group practice has been its reduction, apparently appropriately, of the use of the hospital. Furthermore, when the hospital and the group practice are operated jointly, many efficiencies are expected to result in the operations of both. The other side of the argument, made most cogently by Bailey, is that the physician in solo practice need not be robbed of the benefits of large-scale production of certain ancillary services if these are easily available to him or to his patient from large-scale producers such as the hospital or independent laboratories, radiologists, and the like. Fein has written an excellent review of the relationship between productivity and the organization of physicians' services (83, pp. 901–29). Elsewhere, the author has reviewed the literature concerning several aspects of group practice, including its effects on use of service, expenditures for care, and quality (99, 100). What concerns us here are the studies that deal explicitly with productivity or efficiency, usually with little reference to the quality of the product.

Boan has assembled some evidence (Table IV.40) that suggests greater physician productivity for group practice as compared to solo practice in Canada (101). A survey of Canadian physicians performed by the Royal Commission on Health Services has shown that, on a per physician basis, physicians in group practice employ more nurses, technicians, and clerical personnel than do physicians in solo practice. In spite of this, the net income of physicians in group practice is somewhat larger than that of specialists, and considerably larger than that of generalists, in solo practice. The same survey has shown that the average group practice has more medical and office equipment than the average solo practitioner. However, the value of such equipment per physician is less in group practice than it is in solo practice. The same is true for the cost of "paramedical" personnel per physician. This constellation of findings, summarized in Table IV.40 is interpreted by Boan to support the theo-

Table IV.40. Number and cost per physician of specified personnel, value of capital assets and annual income, by type of practice, Canada 1960

Specified Items	Group Practice	Solo Practice	
		General	Specialist
Number of persons employed per physician[a]			
Nurses	0.5	0.3	0.3
Technical staff	0.4	0.05	0.07
Clerical and other	1.0	0.4	0.5
Average annual cost per physician[a] who reported employment of:			
Nurses	$1,740	$2,470	$2,610
Technical staff	1,520	1,850	2,260
Clerical and other	2,540	1,580	1,970
Average depreciated value of capital assets per physician who reported such assets	$4,460	$8,840	$6,160
Average annual total net income[b]	$19,420	$13,820	$18,730

SOURCE: Reference 101. Based on reports in a questionnaire on the economics of medical practice administered by the Royal Commission on Health Services to all physicians and surgeons in Canada, March 1962.

[a] Part-time and full-time employment are not distinguished. As a consequence, the number employed per physician is probably inflated for solo practitioners who tend to use more part-time help. Also, the cost per physician is not synonymous with employee income.

[b] Average annual total net income from medical practice and salaried appointment of active civilian physicians in Canada during 1960.

retical expectation that the physician in group practice is more productive than his counterpart in solo practice. While these findings are suggestive, they are not conclusive. The time factor in physician input has not been considered. Output is not directly measured, nor is there any information on product comparability. Differences in net income of physicians are only an indirect indicator of differences in total productivity. Because of lack of data or limitations in existing data, it is not possible to say how much of the increment in net income of physicians in group practice is attributable to productivity and how much to other factors such as the greater likelihood of group practice physicians being specialists, relative scarcity related to geographic location, wages paid to employees, and the socioeconomic characteristics of clients. Finally, no distinction is made between economies that are attributable to scale per se and those attributable to different modes of production. In fact, the emphasis is almost exclusively on the latter: namely, the ability of group practice physicians to use more non-physician personnel and more equipment, at lower cost per physician, in order to improve their productivity, as measured by higher net income per physician.

Bailey has pointed out additional problems in using net income as a measure of productivity (105–107). His major argument is that "the medical firm" produces a range of products rather than only one product. The increased revenue to group practice is postulated to be due not to greater physician productivity but to a different product mix that includes relatively more low cost, high price services such as X-rays and other diagnostic tests. This hypothesis is supported, according to Bailey, by his own empirical studies in the San Francisco Bay Area (Table IV.41). These studies, which are based on rather small numbers, show that although physicians in larger partnerships and groups are supplemented to a greater extent by the services of other personnel, their productivity in terms of office visits is not increased. What is increased is income, and the proportion of revenue derived from ancillary services which require little clinician input. Other studies suggest that the lack of difference in office visits by size of firm is not brought about by compensatory differences in hospital visits.

Bailey argues cogently for the need to see ambulatory care in terms of many fairly separate component outputs, some produced almost entirely by physicians engaged in patient care and others almost entirely by non-physicians or by physicians not engaged in patient care. His argument that the physician's office need not provide all services internally, but may purchase such services from other large scale producers is also well taken. Fein has pointed out, however, that in such cases, the benefits of large scale organization accrue, at least in part, to the large scale producer, and that the distributional costs of external production have to be taken into account (83). Furthermore, the findings of Bailey with regard to hours of work and visits by physicians are not in accord with other reports in the literature.

In his study of a representative sample of general practitioners in the Canadian provinces of Ontario and Nova Scotia, Clute reported certain findings that provide interesting comparisons with those of Boan and of Bailey. In addition, Clute has that rarest of all things, reasonably valid

Table IV.41. Measures of input and of production, by size of firm, sample of internists, San Francisco Bay Area, April 1967

Measures of Input and Output	Firm Size				
	Solo (N = 12)	2-man (N = 4)	3-man (N = 6)	4 to 5-man (N = 5)	Clinics (N = 4)
INPUT MEASURES					
Average hours per physician	218	222	197	200	197
Average paramedical hours per physician	187	181	225	271	499
Average technical hours per physician	7	11	9	44	122
Average paramedical hours per physician hour	0.858	0.817	1.142	1.353	2.531
Average technical hours per physician hour	0.032	0.050	0.046	0.220	0.619
OUTPUT (PRODUCTION) MEASURES					
Office visits per physician[a]	286	278	291	243	286
Office visits per physician time with patients[a]	3.4	3.0	3.5	3.1	2.9
Gross monthly income per physician	$4,777	—	$6,107	—	$6,725
Average percent of revenues earned by sale of ancillary products	15%	—	34%	—	48%

SOURCE: Reference 105.

[a] Office visits are weighted by assigning to the major categories of regular office visits, annual examinations, and complete histories and physical examinations, weights based upon the amount of time the physician normally devotes to each service output.

information on the quality of care provided by the general practitioners. His findings are summarized in Table IV.42. It appears that physicians in group practice work longer hours in Ontario, but not in Nova Scotia, and earn more per hour of work, especially in Ontario. According to Clute, the differences in quality of care that appear to favor group practice are not significant. There is no information on the number of total visits or visits per hour in solo practice as compared to group practice. If one were to judge by income alone, subject to the limitations pointed out by Bailey, one would have to conclude that with increasing scale of

Table IV.12. Hours of work, quality of care and hourly median net professional income, by type of practice, samples of general practitioners, Provinces of Ontario and Nova Scotia, Canada, 1956–1960

Inputs and Outputs	Ontario	Nova Scotia
Hours of work per week		
Solo practice	44.6	—[a]
Group of two or more	68.2	—[a]
Quality of care, mean score		
Solo practice (29, 28)[b]	54.6	42.4
Group of two or more	62.8	46.2
Median net professional income per hour of work, in dollars		
Solo practice		
Without nursing or secretarial assistance (9, 11)	$4.19	$3.24
With nursing or secretarial assistance (19, 12)	5.17	4.57
Group of two (8, 4)	6.09	4.99
Group of more than two, with assistance (6, 8)	8.17	4.29

SOURCE: Reference 165, page 103; Table 80, page 318; and Table 421, page 194.

[a] No data given, but findings described as not significantly different for solo and group practice.

[b] In parentheses are numbers of respondents in Ontario and Nova Scotia, respectively.

organization, the physician becomes more productive, holding quality of output constant.

Yett used a sample from the A.M.A. list of self-employed physicians under age 65 to study the relationship between yearly "tax-deductible professional expenses" per physician and patient-visits per year per physician (102). These were the measures of input and output respectively. Patient visits were also the measure of scale. The method of analysis was to postulate certain mathematical models of the relationship between professional expenses and patient visits and, using multivariate analysis, to determine which of the models best fit the data. Corrections were made for field of specialization, group versus solo practice, geographic region and price differences as signified by salary figures for nurses, office aides and technicians. The author concludes that the data are consistent with the hypothesis that there are economies of scale. It also appears that at every level of output (patient visits) tax-deductible professional expenses are lower in group practice than in solo practice, suggesting greater productivity in the former. However, as Yett himself recognized, these findings need further confirmation. The response rate to the questionnaire on which this study is based was only 41 percent and, due to additional depletion from other reasons, the final analysis is based on a mere 15 percent of the original sample. Three strikingly different mathematical models of the hypothesized relationship between expenses and visits fit the data about equally, and all three models leave a considerable amount of variation unexplained (R^2 equals about 0.5).

McCaffree and Newman studied the cost of prescribed drugs in a prepaid group practice plan and found that these were 45 percent lower than the national average (103). This figure is reduced to 28 percent when corrections are made for the estimated purchase of drugs by group plan enrollees from outside pharmacies and for the fact that community pharmacies are subject to taxes, must make a profit and, in addition, often perform certain special services that add to the convenience of the purchaser (see Table IV.43). According to the authors, several factors

Table IV.43.   Cost of prescribed drugs to the purchaser in a prepaid group practice plan as compared to average national figures, including specified elements of cost, 1966

Items	Prepaid Group Practice	United States	Difference as Percent of U.S. Gross Average Annual Cost
Gross per capita annual cost	$8.80	$16.00	45%
Decrement from U.S. cost attributed to profit and taxes	—	1.28	8%
Increment of 15% to prepaid plan cost attributed to purchase of drugs outside the plan	1.32	—	8%
Decrement from U.S. cost attributed to special services (credit, delivery, etc.) provided by community pharmacies	—	0.16	1%
Total adjusted per capita annual cost	$10.12	$14.66	28%

SOURCE: Reference 103.

related to organization and to size are responsible for the savings in drug costs. These include reduction of inventory and purchase of lower-priced generic drugs brought about by the institution of a drug formulary, large-volume purchasing, the manufacture of some pharmaceuticals on the premises, precounting and prepackaging of certain medications, and the use of pharmacy clerks in lieu of additional licensed pharmacists. The study makes a fairly good case for greater efficiency of the prepaid drug program partly due to increased productivity of the pharmacist. The case would have been stronger if the comparability of the service provided has been established, the costs under the prepaid program had been compared with costs for a similar population in the same community using identical sources of information, and if the quantitative effects of the several cost-reducing factors had been assessed.

Recently, data have become available for a national sample of U.S. physicians that permit comparisons with findings in several of the Canadian and U.S. studies described above (20). Data on workload are summarized in Table IV.44. If attention is confined to the two extremes, solo and group practice, it becomes clear that physicians in group practice, contrary to the findings of Bailey in San Francisco, and more in keeping with those of Clute in Ontario, work longer hours per week and make more visits in the office as well as in the hospital. Unfortunately, the number of weeks worked per year is not given, so that the total yearly product cannot be compared. However, for each hour of work, and each hour of direct care, more visits are produced by each physician in group practice than by his counterpart in solo practice. Thus if visits per man-hour are the measure of productivity, physicians in group practice are distinctly more productive than those in solo practice. At this point one can, of course, question whether visits are the appropriate representation of output. Even if visits are used to represent output, one can question their comparability across types of practice. Physicians in group and solo practice are known to differ in the ratio of generalists to specialists, in geographic location, and in type of practice. The data do not permit correction for differences in specialty mix. They do indicate that metropolitan versus nonmetropolitan location is not a decisive factor in the differences observed. More important is the difference in the mix of office versus hospital visits produced. Only a fifth of visits by solo physicians are in the hospital, compared to almost a third of those made by group practitioners. It is not easy to say precisely what this means for the measure of productivity. Hospital visits could be both easier or more difficult to make, depending on a variety of circumstances, including distance from the office to the hospital, the number of patients each physician has in the hospital on a given day, the nature and severity of the illness and the availability of resident medical staff and other personnel to help the attending physician. However, even if only office visits per

Table IV.44.   Measures of work load according to type of practice and location, national sample of physicians,[a] U.S.A., 1969

Hours and Visits per Physician	Type of Practice			
	Solo	Two-Man Partner- ship	Informal Association	Group Practice
Hours per week				
All areas	50.5	54.5	53.7	54.2
Nonmetropolitan	53.5	56.2	55.6	55.3
Metropolitan	49.8	54.1	53.5	53.9
Hours of direct care/week				
All areas	45.6	47.9	46.9	47.5
Hours of direct care as percent of total				
All areas	90.3%	87.9%	87.3%	87.6%
Visits per week				
All areas all visits	121.5	154.4	125.8	145.9
All areas office visits	91.8	109.1	96.4	98.6
All areas hospital visits	25.1	43.6	30.7	46.9
Hospital visits as percent of all visits				
All areas	21%	28%	24%	32%
All visits/hour of work[b]				
All areas	2.4	2.8	2.3	2.7
Office visits/hour of direct care[b]				
All areas	2.0	2.3	2.1	2.1
All visits per hour of direct care				
All areas	2.8	3.8	3.0	3.6
Nonmetropolitan	3.5	5.7	3.7	3.4
Metropolitan	2.6	3.3	3.0	3.6

SOURCE: Reference 20, Table 24, page 61, and Table 25, page 62.

[a] Excludes interns, residents, federally employed physicians and inactive physicians.

[b] Computed from data in source tables.

hour of direct care are considered, one finds that group practice has a slight edge in productivity over solo practice.

Table IV.45 provides data on income, expenses and prices which may be compared with the finding of Boan (101), Bailey (105), Clute (165) and Yett (102). Taking all these into account, one finds that there is general agreement that group practice is financially more advantageous to the physician. The data from the U.S. national sample agree with the

Table IV.45.   Measures of income, expenses and price, according to type of location and type of practice, national sample of physicians,[a] U.S.A., 1969

Income and Expenses per Physician and Price per Procedure	Type of Practice			
	Solo	Two-Man Partner-ship	Informal Association	Group Practice
Net income (dollars)				
All areas	$35,049	$39,858	$39,537	$39,065
Nonmetropolitan	34,652	38,378	31,979	34,978
Metropolitan	35,131	40,245	40,482	39,978
Expenses (dollars)				
All areas	19,711	22,889	21,343	20,910
Nonmetropolitan	21,008	19,062	28,229	20,265
Metropolitan	19,445	23,890	20,482	21,055
Income plus expenses[b] ($)				
All areas	54,760	62,747	60,880	59,970
Nonmetropolitan	55,660	57,440	60,208	55,243
Metropolitan	54,576	64,135	60,964	61,033
Income as percent of Income plus Expenses[b]				
All areas	64%	64%	65%	65%
Nonmetropolitan	62	66	53	63
Metropolitan	64	63	66	66
Net income/hour/week[b]				
All areas	$ 694	$ 731	$ 736	$ 721
Nonmetropolitan	648	682	575	633
Metropolitan	705	744	757	742
Net income/hour of direct care/week[b]				
All areas	769	832	843	822
Expenses/visit/week[b]				
All areas	162	148	170	143
Expenses/office visit/week[b]				
All areas	215	210	221	212
Selected prices, all areas (dollars)				
Initial office visit	11.53	11.37	11.49	12.55
Follow-up office visit	7.30	7.21	7.46	7.26
Follow-up hospital visit	8.55	7.75	8.65	7.81

SOURCES: Reference 20, Table 24, page 61, Table 25, page 62, Table 30, page 73, Table 31, page 74, and Table 79, page 79.

[a] Excludes interns, residents, federally employed physicians and inactive physicians.

[b] Computed from data in source tables.

Canadian data reported by Boan in showing group practice to have lower expenses per physician and to yield higher net income per physician. Thus, gross income per physician would also be higher for group practice in the U.S. national sample, as was true for the practices studied by Bailey. More interesting is the relationship between net income and a measure of input such as hours of work. As was reported by Clute for Ontario and Nova Scotia, and as can be shown to be the case for the data assembled by Bailey, income per hour of work is higher for group practice than for solo practice. Thus, if income could be taken as the representation of the quantity and quality of the physician's product (which it cannot be without serious reservations) group practice would seem to be more productive than solo practice. It is also possible from the national sample to compute expenses per visit per week. The reader will recall that Yett used an analogous measure to study physician productivity. When expenses are related to all visits, group practice exhibits remarkable economies in the production of visits. However, when expenses are related only to office visits, the two types of practice appear to be comparable with a very small, possibly negligible, advantage to group practice. This suggests that the greater use of the hospital is probably responsible for a share of the financial advantage enjoyed by the physician in group practice. It is unfortunate that it has not been possible to separate income and expenses attributable to office practice from those attributable to practice in the hospital.

As a preliminary conclusion, subject to the many cautionary statements that we have made concerning each of the studies reviewed, it appears that in general these studies support the view that group practice renders the physician more productive. This is true whether one measures the product in terms of hours worked, visits made, or income earned. What remains unclear is precisely what brings about the phenomena observed. As Berki has pointed out, none of the studies reviewed has examined the effect of scale divorced from associated changes in methods of production (84). In fact, most of the studies have emphasized the contributions of the latter. Boan has emphasized the use of equipment, nurses, technical staff, and clerical personnel. As shown in Table IV.41, Bailey has documented the large increase in the contribution of "paramedical" and "technical" personnel as the size of the ambulatory firm becomes larger. He has explicitly attributed the larger income of physicians in the larger firms to the sale, as it were, of the services of these personnel. Clute also has demonstrated (see Table IV.42) how net income per hour increases as the physician uses more assistance, as well

as when more doctors undertake to work together McCaffree and Newman have emphasized the economies brought about by methods of prescribing, preparing, and dispensing drugs in a group practice. A recent
study by Yankauer et al. has given particular attention to the use of
auxiliary personnel, and the propensity to delegate activities to such personnel, as factors in the productivity of physicians in different types of
practice (108). From their data it is possible to make some distinctions
concerning the effects of size of firm and the effects of using auxiliary
personnel and delegating tasks to them.

The study by Yankauer and associates reported findings from a mailed
questionnaire survey of 90 percent of board certified pediatricians who
graduated from medical schools after 1930 (108). Productivity was
viewed in terms of median hours spent in the office per week, median
total visits per week, and a ratio of the second measure to the first, which
gives a rough measure of visits per unit time. All these measures of
production tended to show increases with number of physicians and
number of other health workers per practice, and with the propensity to
delegate tasks to persons other than the physician. The presence of at
least one registered nurse among these persons had a significant enhanc-
ing effect on task delegation and production. The effect of differences in
case mix was also evident. The production of visits was negatively related
to percent of cases that were for health supervision (as distinct from the
care of illness), and the percent of health supervision visits that lasted 15
minutes or more. Contrary to expectation, the category of multispecialty
groups (those with 5 or more physicians and 5 or more other health
workers of whom at least one was a registered nurse), was not the most
productive in terms of the indicators used. Table IV.46 shows selected
findings from this study which document the relationships described
above. To a degree these findings support the views and findings of
Bailey as described earlier in this section. According to Yankauer et al.,
task delegation, hours of work and the pace of work were influenced, not
so much by "administrative theory or organizational opportunity," as
by demand. In parts of the United States characterized by a relative
paucity of certified pediatricians, the pattern seemed to be for one or
more private pediatricians to employ several additional workers, with or
without including a registered nurse, to delegate many tasks to these
workers, to work longer hours, and to see more children per unit time,
partly because relatively fewer well children are seen and less time is
spent with them. The other extreme was exemplified by the category of
pediatricians in northeastern cities who worked with one additional
worker who was not a registered nurse, who saw preponderantly well

Table IV.46.   Aspects of the practice of board-certified pediatricians, by type of practice and number of other health workers employed, U.S.A., 1967

| Aspects of Practice | Solo Practice, Employing Additional Workers as Indicated Below | | | | Multispecialty Group Practice[a] |
	One non-RN	One RN	Two includes RN	Three includes RN	
Median hours in office	31.0	33.4	35.0	36.7	37.3
Median total visits	81.5	93.1	108.5	131.1	105.1
Median total visits divided by median hours in office	2.60	2.78	3.10	3.57	2.82
Percent respondents delegating one or more tasks	6.1	10.8	16.5	27.4	7.5
Ratio of health supervision visits to illness visits	1.5	1.2	1.1	0.9	0.7
Percent of health supervision visits of 15 or more minutes	76	68	57	52	63

SOURCE: Reference 108, Tables 1 and 2, pages 39 and 40.

[a] Five or more physicians with 5 or more other health workers at least one of whom is a registered nurse.

children, and spent a great deal of time wth each well child. The authors regard this type of practice to represent, not so much quality, as "luxury" or waste. "Preventive services can be overdone as well as underdone."

The authors recognize the several limitations in their study. The reports by physicians may be of varying degrees of accuracy or validity. The category of "multispecialty groups" does not necessarily represent the larger, and better organized, prepaid groups. Differences in case mix and in quality are not adequately adjusted for by merely distinguishing preventive from curative visits. Nevertheless, the findings raise important questions about the assumptions concerning the greater productivity of group practice, especially since they support the contentions and findings of Bailey.

One may conclude from the above that the important consideration in physician productivity is not so much the size of the firm, as measured by number of physicians, as is the use of larger numbers of auxiliary personnel and the delegation to them of tasks ordinarily performed by the physician. As we have already remarked, this is a viewpoint that is consistent, though not identical, with that held by Bailey. It is also consistent with findings in the national sample of U.S. physicians to which we need now to return. A re-examination of Tables IV.44 and IV.45 shows that in most instances it is not the group practice but the two-man partnership that has the highest values for hours worked per week, visits per week, and net annual income per physician, and the lowest value for expenses per physician per office visit per week. The group practice does, however, generally perform better than the informal association. The explanation for these observations could be that the two-man partnership uses relatively more auxiliary personnel and delegates more functions to them. Anecdotal support of sorts comes from the report of an expert group that evaluated the operation of the Kaiser Foundation Medical Program. The experts concluded that Kaiser-Permanente groups had indeed lowered the costs of providing medical care but that this was almost entirely due to the elimination of unnecessary health care, particularly hospitalization. No significant innovations were observed in the use of auxiliary manpower. The production process was notable for being highly traditional rather than otherwise (104). These observations should not, however, obscure the fact that the average group practice is more likely to use equipment and auxiliary personnel than is the average solo practitioner. What is deplored is that group practices do not appear to have lived up to their potential to make radical departures in the manner in which labor and capital resources are used to provide care. It should also be remembered that pure economies of scale in group practice are presumptively present, though they have not been empirically confirmed. According to Berki, the data reported by Yankauer et al. lend themselves to such an interpretation (84). Table IV.47 constructed from Yankauer's data are certainly consistent with this interpretation. Reading vertically in each column of the table, one notes the augmenting effect of adding auxiliary personnel on the visits produced per hour. However, reading diagonally one notes the effect of increasing the size of the firm while holding constant the ratio of physicians to non-physicians. This also is seen to increase the number of visits per office hour. Further studies of this kind are necessary to establish the occurrence and relative importance of the two factors: changes in the modes of production and changes in size holding the method of production constant.

Table IV.47.   Visits made by each board-certified
pediatrician per hour of work in the office,[a] according
to number of physicians and number of other workers[b]
in each practice, U.S.A., 1967

Number of Other Workers[b]	Number of Physicians	
	1	2
1	2.78	
2	3.10	3.25
4		3.39

SOURCE: Reference 108, Table 1, page 39, and Reference
84.
   [a] Median total visits ÷ median hours in the office.
   [b] At least one of these workers is a registered nurse.

Trends in Productivity

There will be no attempt in this section to discuss the general evidence
that has a bearing on the subject of productivity trends in the health
services industry. Since our interest is mainly in methods of assessment,
we will confine ourselves to a brief description of the major published
studies of trends in the productivity of health personnel and hospitals.

PHYSICIANS AND DENTISTS. Klarman has reviewed and evaluated the
rather meager literature dealing with measurements of trends in the
productivity of physicians (72, pp. 150–157). The earliest studies were
made by Dickinson for the American Medical Association (86, 87).
Because he lacked information on the actual number of services provided
by physicians, Dickinson had to use an *indirect method* to arrive at this
figure. He did this by using national data on expenditures for physicians'
services and deflating these by the prices of physicians' services as obtained from the Consumer Price Index. Very simply, the operations were
as follows:

(1) $\dfrac{\text{Expenditures for physician care}}{\text{Prices of physician care}} = \text{Physician services}$

(2) $\dfrac{\text{Physician services}}{\text{Number of physicians}} = \text{Services per physician}$

More recently, Garbarino has used annual physician income, rather than
expenditures for medical care, in a similar way (88).

(1) $\dfrac{\text{Annual income of physicians}}{\text{Price of physician care}} = \text{Physician services}$

(2) $\dfrac{\text{Physician services}}{\text{Number of physicians}} = \text{Services per physician}$

(If the data are in terms of average income, the denominator in the second fraction is obviously 1.) In the near future, information will have been collected by the National Health Survey for a sufficient length of time to permit the use of a more *direct method* for estimating productivity trends, as follows:

$$\frac{(\text{Physician services per person}) \cdot (\text{Number in population})}{\text{Number of physicians}} = \frac{\text{Services per}}{\text{physician}}$$

Before presenting the findings of the studies by Dickinson, Garbarino, and others, it would be well to review briefly some of the limitations in the methods they use. It is clear that all these estimates purport to measure labor productivity alone. In other words, the production of all other inputs is attributed to physicians or dentists. The rationale for this practice has already been discussed. Furthermore, neither Dickinson nor Garbarino made corrections for the number of hours worked by physicians. There is sufficient explanation for this omission in the absence of valid data on hours worked by physicians. In these studies, the input is physicians rather than man-hours. Garbarino did, however, explicitly consider the distinction between the "output effect" and the "methods effect" in interpreting his findings. We have already pointed out the possible implications of using gross versus net income as representations of the physician's product. Expenditures for physician care, the measure used by Dickinson, corresponds to gross income. Garbarino, on the other hand, made two computations using net income in one and gross income in the other (88, Table 3, p. 11). Even more important than the foregoing, no corrections were made for changes in the content and quality of the output, which is measured in terms of the number of services provided. Once again, one can hardly fault the investigators for not doing something that is hard to do even when the necessary data are available. Finally, the basic data are themselves open to question. The data on expenditures are fairly rough approximations (301). Valid data on the professional income of physicians are hard to obtain. The Consumer Price Index in general and its medical care component in particular are open to a great deal of criticism (302–304). It follows that the data on the labor productivity of physicians and dentists are, at best, extremely rough approximations.

As might have been expected, all trends in the productivity of physicians and dentists have shown striking increases. Dickinson has estimated that between 1940 and 1950 there was an increase of 30 to 50 percent in physician productivity. Garbarino has estimated an increase of 142 percent between 1935 and 1951, using gross income in the computation, and an increase of 128 percent between 1936 and 1951 using net income. This suggests that in the early 1950's compared to the mid-1930's, the physician was able to retain nearly as much of the total earnings of his practice in spite of the increasing complexity of provid-care. There was a very rapid increase in productivity during World War II which Garbarino attributes mainly to longer hours of work ("output effect"). Since the war, the increase has been slower and has been attributed mainly to changes in productivity proper ("methods effect"). Apparently using the Dickinson method, Garbarino has reported a 10 percent increase in productivity during 1949 to 1954.

More recently, Weiss has used the Dickinson method (deflating expenditures by price) to study the productivity of dentists. He has gone one step further by making corrections for hours of work put in by dentists. Weiss estimates that between 1950 and 1963, there has been a 44.2 percent increase in the productivity of dentists active in private practice, an average increase of 2.85 percent per year. Hours worked per dentist have apparently changed very little during this period, so that the changes in productivity are to be attributed to what Garbarino calls the "methods effect." Between 1950 and 1961, the average yearly increase in productivity per dentist was 3.2 percent and per dentist-hour only slightly less—3.1 percent (15, pp. 122–136).

All the above studies have used what we called an indirect method to arrive at the number of services produced by each physician during the year. The direct method would use data on services, if a time series of these were available. The National Health Survey begins to provide such a series based on household interview reports of visits to physicians excluding hospitalization. In Chapter III we have discussed the general limitations of data obtained in the Household Interview Survey. A more specific limitation, germane to our present concern, is that physician visits include visits made in the office, clinic, or home, as well as telephone "visits," but not visits made in the hospital. Even if one were able to standardize for differences in the mix of services that constitutes the output of visits from one time period to another, there would still remain differences in "appropriateness" and "potency," as we have discussed in a previous section. The Periodic Survey of Physicians, conducted by the A.M.A. does include hospital visits, but the surveys, which began in

1966, do not as yet give us a time series of sufficient duration (20). They do, however, indicate the magnitude of loss from not including hospital visits. For all physicians, 26 percent of visits are in the hospital (20, Table 19, p. 54). This is, of course, a percentage that varies by specialty of physicians, by age of patients, and by other factors. An alternative source of information on physician workload are the reports of periodic mail questionnaire surveys conducted by the journal *Medical Economics*. However, the rates of return in these surveys are so low that some have questioned whether the findings are representative.

Jones et al. have used data from the National Health Survey to compute the changes in the productivity of physicians (97). They find that between 1959 and 1964 there was an increase of only 4 percent in patient visits as compared to an increase of 8 percent in the number of physicians. Taking the figures at face value this would mean a decrease in the number of visits per physician and hence a reduction in productivity. During the same period there was a 40 percent increase in personal expenditures for physician services and a 15 percent increase in prices. This would mean a 12 percent increase in productivity using the indirect method of computation. The difference in the conclusions using the two approaches highlights the problems in the basic data and in the assumptions that are used in arriving at estimates of productivity. A review of a number of additional studies of productivity and of their findings may be found in a recent paper by Klarman (98). He notes that the range in reported values is large. "For the 1960's the annual rate of increase is between 2.4 and 4.5 percent. For a decade, these figures translate into increases of 27 to 55 percent" (98, p. 370). But take with a large grain of salt!

HOSPITALS. The literature on measurement of trends in the productivity of hospitals is even more meager than that for physicians and dentists. The one study usually cited is that by Lytton (114). This is an investigation of eight agencies or major components of agencies in the federal government, of which only one, the Veterans' Administration hospitals, had experienced no increase in productivity. On the contrary, productivity during 1947–1958 had declined 11 percent. The measure of input for the hospital study was average employment, "including consultants and attendings" at Veterans' Administration hospitals, "adjusted for common services in 1956–1958." The measure of output was "in-patient daily load at VA hospitals." The major lesson to be drawn from this study is the importance of using the appropriate measures of input and output and of correcting for changes in these. For example, Rajgrodzki has pointed out that during the relevant period, there was a marked shift in the patient load of VA hospitals away from long-term care (tuberculosis and neuropsychiatric care) to more short-term care (general medical and surgical and neurological) with higher service content. This is confirmed by an increase in admissions disproportionate to the smaller increase in the number of beds. Similarly, Lytton makes no corrections for the changes in the mix of hospital employees and for the reduction in the hours of work that is expected to have taken place during that period (118).

SERVICES PRODUCED IN RELATION TO CAPACITY TO PRODUCE

Introduction

The reader will recall that the first step in the assessment of supply, as called for by our model, is classification into categories meaningful to the particular purposes of the assessment, followed by enumeration of those units that one wishes to assess. Enumeration is the first step in quantification. The next step is a determination of the capacity to produce service. Hence, in a previous section we discussed those attributes of supply that influence productivity, the output being defined as services. A third step, which we will discuss in this section, is the comparison of the services actually produced with the services which could potentially be produced. The purpose is to find out whether the currently available resources are overburdened or if, on the contrary, they are underutilized. It is obvious that if present resources are overburdened, the need for expansion is pressing, whereas if present resources are underutilized, it is necessary to take up the "slack" before expansion of resources is considered.

The comparison of services actually produced with services which could potentially be produced requires analysis of the present "service load" and, possibly, of secular trends in "service load." There are, obviously, aspects to the analysis of service load which go beyond comparisons with potential service load. In this section our attention will be focused on that comparison; however, it may be convenient to introduce other considerations as the occasion arises. It is hoped that if the reader is forewarned of these occasional excursions he will not be confused by their having exceeded the confines of our model.

Another reason for confusion could be the absence of terminology that clearly distinguishes the use of service by persons from the use of the resources to produce services. Obviously, these are two sides to a single coin, but the distinction between them is important. The context generally indicates what is being considered at any given time. However, it would be useful if "use of service" and "utilization" were confined to the demand side of the coin and some other term were available to describe the supply side. Perhaps the most descriptive term for the latter would be "exploitation," if the pejorative connotation of the word could be ignored. Failing that, the word "employment" might denote the extent and manner of resource use; but "employment" introduces its own ambiguities, especially where manpower is concerned. The author has been unable to find a fully satisfactory terminology, but will attempt to keep the two phenomena described above as clearly distinct as possible.

Finally, the distinction into steps which involve first the assessment of capacity to produce and then of actual production (or the reverse), while important conceptually, is not necessarily applicable operationally. In real life, the assessment of the two is often inseparable or intertwined. Accordingly, in the following presentation the two steps will not be always kept distinct.

General Framework

The discussion in this section will be organized around a conceptual framework which is shown graphically in Fig. IV.4. According to this model, examination of a resource, such as a hospital, is likely to show that a part of its capacity is occupied or in use whereas another part of it is unoccupied or unused. The portion in use produces a given output which may be referred to as the "service load." Further examination of this portion is likely to show that it is divisible into normatively definable components. One part consists of patients who require the services of the resource in question and may therefore be said to account for a portion of capacity that is being used appropriately. Another part consists of patients that should not be cared for by the resource in question because they require care by another kind of resource or no care at all. They represent, therefore, inappropriate use of the resource. As we shall see later in this section, the general tendency is for patients to be cared for by a resource that provides levels of care higher than that required by the patient. Less often, the appropriate level of care is higher than that which the resource is capable of providing. The important point is that if this portion of the service load could be eliminated, by arranging for appropriate disposition of the patients, capacity that had hitherto been in use would be released to be used more appropriately. We con-

Fig. IV.4.   A model for assessing services produced in relation to the capacity to produce service

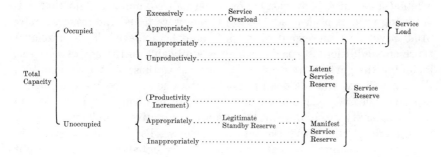

clude, therefore, that there is a reserve of service which is hidden or "latent" but which can be released by appropriate means.

Let us now look at that portion of capacity that is unoccupied or unused. Here again, we may conclude that a portion is appropriately unoccupied. This is because a portion of capacity is being held in reserve to meet urgent and unpredictable demands. Since it could be claimed that all unused capacity is being held back for this purpose, it is necessary to use some normative guides (to be discussed later in this section) to determine how much capacity it is legitimate to keep as standby reserve. The remainder of unused capacity can then be judged to be inappropriately unoccupied. Needless to say, all unoccupied capacity is subject to being put to use. For that reason, it is referred to, in our model, as apparent or "manifest service reserve." One could make a very good case, however, for considering "legitimate standby reserve" as part of the "service load." As we have pointed out before, it is quite proper to say that the product of the hospital is so many days of care plus so many days of readiness to provide care. If this viewpoint is adopted, "manifest service reserve" would include only that portion of capacity that remains inappropriately unoccupied.

A special situation exists when a resource is so intensively used that the service load exceeds some normatively defined limit. We can then postulate that a portion of the service load is excessive and constitutes "service overload." The definition of what constitutes excessive use of a resource raises some difficult questions which we shall consider later in this section. In the meantime, we should point out that the excessive portion of the case load can itself be made up of patients or services that are appropriate to the resource and those that are not. In terms of our model, there can be "latent service reserve" even in situations of excessive resource use. This means that the classes under our category "occupied" are, unfortunately, partially overlapping. Finally, irrespective of whether a resource is overloaded or underutilized, one may find that it is not being used at peak productivity. If one were to use the resource more productively, an increment of output could be achieved. This increment represents additional capacity which is applicable to the entire resource, including the portions that are in use as well as those that are not in use. We can now expand the definition of "latent service reserve" to include capacity released by removing inappropriate use and that increment to service capacity brought about by its more productive exploitation.

Throughout the description of our model we have tended to see it in terms of the hospital, so that capacity is represented as beds and output as patients or patient-days. This is because beds are such an easily identifiable representation of capacity, so that one can see at a glance whether beds are full or empty. Needless to say, the model is offered in the hope that it is more generally applicable, so that it can apply to health personnel as well as facilities, and accommodate alternative definitions of output as patients or services. In subsequent sections we shall see whether this is indeed the case or whether the model needs to be modified, and in what ways.

The model so far described has a static property in that it represents the average relationships between services produced and the capacity to produce, or a cross-sectional view of these relationships at a given moment in time. However, an important characteristic of need, of demand, and of service load is that they vary significantly in time. There are variations by hour of day, by day of the week, and by month or season. It is important therefore to consider fluctuations in case load and relate these to fluctuations in capacity. While it is easy to see how need, demand, and case load can fluctuate, it is sometimes forgotten that capacity may also be inconstant. This occurs, for example, when the hospital is not fully staffed and operational at all hours of the day and every day of the week, or when the physician is unavailable, evenings, nights, and week-ends. The time dimension should therefore be added to the model. In subsequent sections there will be repeated reference to specific instances in which this dimension becomes critical.

Measuring Service Capacity and Service Load

GENERAL FRAMEWORK. In attempting to measure service capacity and service load, and the adjustment of one to the other, it is useful to think of capacity as a container and of service load as a flow of material into the container, where it is processed and then discharged. There are, of course, certain important properties that govern the operations of this model. Certain of these characteristics concern the inflow of material. This is discontinuous, variable in rate, and only partially subject to control or regulation by the providers of care. Discontinuities arise because of the very nature of the "raw material," which is patients. Each patient is discrete and must be handled as such by the system. This means that there are likely to be gaps between the arrival of one unit and the other, as well as between the processing of one unit and another within the "container." The frequency and duration of these gaps is an important determinant of the capacity to provide service and of the degree to which this capacity is exploited. The inflow is not uniform because it is subject to the influence of two sets of factors: (1) the occurrence of illness or other situations that require care, and (2) the decisions of patients and physicians concerning entry into the system that provides care. The occurrence of illness in a population is generally a random and rather infrequent event. There are, however, important nonrandom aspects which, as we have discussed in our chapter on need, bring about a patterned distribution of illness in time, place, and person. These factors include contagion and a variety of ecological factors that influence the susceptibility of the host, the virulence of the agent, and the opportunities for interaction between the agent and the host. The decisions of patients and physicians concerning entry into the system can also be nonrandom to the extent that an element of discretion exists in whether care is or is not received or offered. Where the element of discretion is marked, care may be designated "elective." The need for care may, however, be urgent. Hence it is important to distinguish degrees of urgency in assessing the capacity of the medical care facility to respond to demands for service. Another aspect of patient and physician decisions is their relative importance in determining entry to care. As we have already emphasized, entry into the medical care system is usually, but not invariably, initiated by the client. However, further use is subject to considerable control by the physician and other primary health professionals. It is therefore important to consider who governs the inflow of material and the processing of such material, and what factors influence the decisions and alter the behavior of those who serve as "gate keepers" or "governors."

A second important set of characteristics pertains to the nature of the hypothetical container in our model. It is obvious that the word "container" is a misnomer that is used only as a first approximation in describing the model. The "container" is, in fact, a manufactory or a generator of service. It does, however, have an additional storage function in the sense that it holds the patient while he is being serviced. Part of the time during which the patient is held is necessary for the provision of service and for observing the effects of service. However, there may be, and often are, unnecessary idle periods during which the service function is not being exercised and the patient is merely held or stored before service is initiated or after a service phase is concluded, with or without anticipation of future services. The distinction between service and storage is obviously a matter of degree. The difference is very clear when intensive servicing is in progress or when no significant service is being provided for appreciable periods of time. At other times the distinction is blurred. This ambiguity is heightened by the fact that a certain amount of holding may be necessary in order to marshal a sufficient number of patients for efficient processing. These ambiguities notwithstanding, it is useful to make the following distinctions, at least conceptually. The time during which the patient is subject to care may be considered to constitute "holding time." In the hospital literature this is called "length of stay." It is the time that elapses between "admission" and "discharge." Therefore, it is necessary to define precisely what constitutes "admission" and "discharge" under specified circumstances. "Holding time" is itself divisible, at least in theory, into two portions: "service time" and "waiting time." The time that elapses between the admission of one patient and the admission of another to a discrete service-producing unit, such as a hospital bed, represents the length of the care cycle and may be called "cycle time." Included in "cycle time" is "holding time," and, in addition, the interval between two cases during which capacity remains idle or is being replenished or reordered, so that it is capable of providing service afresh. This interval has been referred to in the hospital literature as "turnover interval" or "turnover time," a term which can be adopted for more general use.

In keeping with the model described above, we shall be concerned in this and subsequent sections with (1) the measurement of inflow and outflow, (2) the measurement of time spent within the "container," which is designated as "holding time," (3) the determination of what proportion of this time is devoted to service functions and what proportion merely represents "storage," (4) the determination of gaps or idle time between patients, and (5) the comparison of service load to service capacity. Because systematic measurement of these aspects of service load has been developed largely in the hospital field, we shall begin with hospitals. We shall then attempt to apply the same model to analysis of the service load of physicians. It is mainly for this purpose that we have attempted to develop a more general model and terminology. It is a major objective of this book to test the utility of models stated in more general terms to generate comparable and sometimes new ways of analyzing a range of medical care phenomena that have been up till now considered in isolation.

HOSPITAL CAPACITY AND SERVICE LOAD. In measuring the service capacity of a medical care resource it is first necessary to recognize the several functions that a resource may perform and to segregate that portion of capacity that is employed for purposes other than patient care. The capacity of the hospital to provide inpatient care is generally measured by the number of beds that it contains. Hospital beds are further differentiated in a number of ways which we have discussed in a previous section. These include the distinction between "beds" for adults, "cribs" for children, and "bassinets" for the newborn. It is also necessary to specify whether the number of beds cited refers to "bed capacity" or to "bed complement." "Maximum bed capacity" is defined as the number of beds that can be placed in the hospital area designed for beds, excluding temporary holding areas such as recovery rooms, labor room, and the like. "Bed complement" refers to the number of beds actually provided. This may be more or less than the number for which the hospital was designed. It is clear that "bed capacity" is relevant for certain aspects and "bed complement" for other aspects of assessment. The distinction between "bed complement" and "maximum bed capacity" is fundamentally a distinction between empirical and normative definitions of capacity. For many purposes—especially the investigation of service overload—a normative definition is necessary. Poland and Lembcke borrowed the notion of normal bed capacity from the 1946 Commission on Hospital Care and related it to the minimum standards for space required by the Public Health Service for hospitals constructed under the Hill-Burton Act. They based normal bed capacity "on a minimum of 100 square feet of open space for 1-bed [rooms] and 80 square feet per bed for multiple-bed rooms—private closets, lockers, toilets and showers excluded; provided that regardless of size the maximum capacity will not exceed that for which (the hospital) was designed" (366, p. 88). Unfortunately, the designation of normative capacity is not so simple. It is becoming increasingly evident that hospital services are limiting factors that are equally, if not more, meaningful than mere living space. Hence, for most purposes it is necessary to introduce the additional notion of the "operational bed" or the "immediately available bed." This is necessary because the limiting factor in the supply of inpatient services may not be space for beds, or actual beds installed, but staff necessary to service the beds, as well as the ancillary services needed to render the bed operational. In keeping with this concept, the American Hospital Association reports hospital capacity in terms of "beds" defined as the "average number of beds, cribs, and pediatric bassinets regularly maintained (set up and staffed for use) for inpatients during 12 month period." Bassinets for newborn infants are not included in the bed count, but are reported separately (42, p. 460). It is obvious that this and similar definitions leave room for considerable ambiguity. There are a variety of interpretations of what is adequate staffing and what scale of ancillary services is necessary to make a certain number of beds operational. By and large, one has to accept the hospital's own view of its own operational capacity as defined within broad limits set by state licensure and other professional standards. Disparities between capacity as defined and actual operations, as revealed through service load analysis, are then attributable to differences in productivity and efficiency. The relevance of this factor to the identification and measurement of economies of scale has already been discussed in some detail. It should be clear, therefore, that certain conclusions about the productivity or efficiency of hospital use, as derived from service load analysis, depend on the definition of capacity to begin with. For example, a large hospital with many empty beds may be running efficiently if staffing and ancillary services have been cut down to the number of beds most frequently in use. Such adjustments, which may not be apparent in service load analysis, should become obvious if cost data are also considered.

A more rigorous approach to the definition of the service capacity of a hospital is proposed by Dowling, who distinguishes three types of capacity: physical, institutional, and experienced (220, pp. 178–203). The "physical capacity" of the hospital and of its several departments is determined by assuming that certain key physical resources are used continuously. For the hospital as a whole the key physical resource is the bed. For other departments it could be the x-ray machine or the operating room. The assumption here is that continuous operation is feasible and that staff and supplies can be made available to service the key resource. The "institutional capacity" of the hospital and of each of its component units is determined by hospital policies concerning staffing and operations. It is obtained by accepting these policies but by assuming that staff and equipment are so used that certain production norms are met. Finally, "experienced capacity" is simply the level of output observed during the busiest month for each of its component units. The assumption here is that the hospital is either actually staffed to meet this peak demand on its services or could be staffed to do so. The former is said to be usually the case. It is obvious that all the three definitions of capacity are normative in nature, although they differ in the demands they make upon the hospital. Physical capacity is the highest attainable while experienced capacity is the lowest, as well as the most realistic. Actual average capacity will fall short of all three. It is necessary to find out to what extent and for what reason. It should be remembered, however, that operation at the highest possible capacity is not necessarily the most efficient, since beyond a certain point costs may rise faster than output.

Assuming that some satisfactory determination of bed capacity has been achieved, the operational service capacity of the hospital may be expressed in bed-days during a given interval of time, usually a year. Bed-days represent potential output at full employment. Actual use of the hospital is determined by two variables: the frequency of admissions and the average length of stay in the hospital. From these three variables (bed-days, admissions, and length of stay) may be derived a number of measures of hospital service load. We shall first give these measures and their manner of derivation, and then discuss how these measures may be used to gain insight into a hospital's operations.

Table IV.48 gives the basic hospital data and the measures derived from these data for two hypothetical hospitals which have similar capacity but operate at different paces, as shown by different lengths of stay. Although, analytically, the three basic items of information needed to derive all the other measures are bed complement, admissions, and length of stay, in actual operations the hospital keeps records of daily census (usually at midnight) and may derive length of stay from census and admission data. Table IV.48 makes allowance for this practice by showing daily census and length of stay twice: once under "basic data" and again under "derived measures." The following is a discussion of the major entries in Table IV.48.

We have already discussed the questions that pertain to the specification of the hospital's bed capacity (item A). The admissions to the hospital are officially reported as the number accepted for inpatient service during a 12-month period, excluding births (42, p. 460). The number of admissions to the hospital equals discharges when equilibrium has been attained; hence equal values are assigned to these in the table (item B). Discrepancies will arise when, during a given period, there is either depletion of hospital occupancy or buildup. It is usually more

Table IV.48. Measures of hospital capacity and of service load in two hypothetical hospitals

Measures	Hospitals I	Hospitals II	Units of Measurement
BASIC DATA			
A. Operational bed complement	200	200	beds
B. Admissions or discharges per year	7,300	3,650	
C. Average daily census	160	160	patients
D. Average length of stay	8	16	days
DERIVED MEASURES			
E. Bed-days per year $(A)(365)$	73,000	73,000	bed-days
F. Patient-days per year	58,400	58,400	patient-days
G. Average daily census $\dfrac{BD}{365}$ or $\dfrac{F}{365}$	160	160	patients
H. Average length of stay $\dfrac{(C)(365)}{B}$	8	16	days
I. Occupancy ratio $\dfrac{C}{A} \times 100$ or $\dfrac{F}{E} \times 100$	80	80	percent
J. Discharge ratio: discharges per 1000 bed-days per year $\dfrac{B}{(A)(365)} \times 1000$	100	50	discharges
K. Discharge ratio: discharges per bed per year ("case flow") $\dfrac{B}{A}$	36	18	discharges
L. Turnover interval (vacant bed-days per discharge) $\dfrac{E\text{-}F}{B} = \dfrac{(365\ A) - (365\ C)}{B}$	2	4	days
M. Unused bed-days per bed $\dfrac{E\text{-}F}{A} = \dfrac{(365\ A) - (365\ C)}{A}$	73	73	bed-days
N. Average hospital cycle $\dfrac{(A)(365)}{B} = D + L$	10	20	days
O. Occupancy ratio adjusted for minimum turnover interval of 1 day $\dfrac{(B)(H + 1)}{E} \times 100$	90	85	percent
P. Occupancy ratio adjusted for standby reserve (1) using Poisson probability tables (p = 0.01)	96	96	percent
(2) using $\dfrac{C + 3\sqrt{C}}{A} \times 100$	99	99	

convenient to work with discharges because these are associated with an already completed, and therefore more precisely definable, length of stay. The average daily census (item C) is a valid measure of the service load during a given day, provided differences in content and quality are ignored or standardized, as already described in a previous section. However, it is only when one measures the occupancy ratio (item I) or the number of unused bed-days per bed (item M) that one obtains a measure of the relationship between service load and capacity. The occupancy ratio, therefore, is often used as a rough measure of the efficiency with which a hospital is used. The rationale for this, as we have already discussed, is the relatively large fixed cost of maintaining empty, but operational, hospital beds. Such use of the occupancy ratio may, however, be very misleading unless several factors are taken into account. We have already referred to the need to have an accurate, or comparable, definition of bed complement so as not to include beds which are essentially nonoperational and that, consequently, do not represent truly idle capacity. A further requirement is concurrent examination of average length of stay (item D). As we have already said, it is possible to raise occupancy simply by keeping persons in hospital for longer periods of time. Longer stays add to the patient-days of hospital care generated by a given number of admissions and, furthermore, reduce the number of times during a year when gaps must necessarily occur between the discharge of one patient and the admission of another to occupy the same bed. In the hypothetical example cited, such interruptions occur twice as frequently for Hospital I as for Hospital II. It is necessary, therefore, in comparing occupancy ratios, to adjust for the influence of different lengths of stay. The average length of stay has, itself, been used as a rough indicator of hospital productivity or efficiency. This is because length of stay is a measure of one time input and a proxy for other inputs in time and resources. If the output is taken to be the case treated, then time per case (which is average length of stay) is the reciprocal of the productivity ratio. Here again, the pitfalls are many. Corrections need to be made not only for differences in case mix, but also for differences in services offered by the hospital and used for patient care. An additional consideration is that length of stay, as a proxy for service input, is not a uniform quantity. The intensity of service is at its highest soon after admission to the hospital, and tends, on the average, to decline progressively thereafter unless there are exacerbations in the patient's clinical condition.

Length of stay is one measure of the pace of hospital operations. Another is the length of time between cases during which a bed remains vacant. This is the "turnover interval" (item L). Together with the length of stay, it determines the total length of the average hospital cycle (item N). The hospitalization cycle is a measure seldom used in the hospital literature. More frequently, the phenomenon to which it relates is measured as a discharge ratio, either per 1000 beds per year, or per bed per year (items J and K). Obviously, the discharge ratio is inversely related to the length of the hospital cycle. For that reason it may be a more satisfactory measure of "case flow" since it increases as the pace of flow of cases through the hospital becomes more rapid. The discharge ratio contains all the pitfalls associated with interpretation of length of stay and of defining operational bed capacity. The turnover interval would seem to be a simpler measure because it merely concerns itself with idle time in relation to service load. However, as we have already emphasized, idle beds do not necessarily mean that other hospital resources are also idle.

One use of the turnover interval is to introduce an adjustment in the occupancy ratio. If it is assumed that a gap of one day is an acceptable turnover interval between cases, this figure may be used to adjust the occupancy ratio. For the hypothetical hospitals in Table IV.48, the occupancy ratio is equal, but the hospital cycle is twice as long in Hospital II. In this hospital both the length of stay and the turnover interval are twice as long as they are in Hospital I. It is clear that, provided case mix and outcome are comparable, Hospital I is more productive and perhaps more efficient, assuming the cost of the more rapid pace is not disproportionate to the gains in output. In spite of this, the occupancy ratios for the two hospitals are identical for the reasons that we have already described. If, however, one day of minimum idle time is added to the patient-days in each of the two hospitals, an adjusted occupancy ratio can be computed (item O) which reveals, though only in part, the differences between the two hospitals.

A final adjustment to the occupancy ratio may be made to account for desirable standby reserve (item P). The adjustment is based on the assumption that the occurrence of disease is random and rare and, hence, that admissions to the hospital are approximated by a Poisson distribution. That this can be only an approximation may be deduced from our own discussion of the random and nonrandom elements in the occurrence of illness and in admissions to service. As far as we can determine, the Poisson distribution was explicitly offered as a mathematical approximation of the demand for hospital beds by D. J. Newell, who used the Poisson assumptions to estimate requirements for emergency care (210). The demand for emergency beds is, of course, most likely to conform to the Poisson assumptions that the events be rare, unrelated, and random. Nevertheless, even in this instance, the observed data did not conform to expectations until the demand on Sundays, which was lower than average, was separated from demand on weekdays. Each of these two components of demand, over a period of three years, did, however, conform reasonably well, though not completely, to the Poisson distribution. More recently, Young has reported that the daily admissions to each of several inpatient units of the Johns Hopkins Hospital and, in some cases admissions to an entire service, could be described "quite well" by the Poisson distribution (279). Long and Feldstein tested admissions to maternity units in the Chicago region. They conclude: "While the Poisson arrival assumption is not rejected, a better model seems to be a Poisson process with a shifting parameter; there is a monthly seasonal, and there appears to be daily variation as well" (353, p. 122n). Young has also demonstrated theoretically that if it is accepted that admissions are Poisson-distributed and that average length of stay can be described, as Bailey has suggested, by a negative exponential distribution, the daily average census must also be Poisson-distributed (279). The soundness of these assumptions, and of the conclusions that flow from them, is supported by the work of Blumberg, who has reported several empirical studies which show that the average daily census over a period of time is Poisson-distributed. Blumberg does point out, however, that the distribution will depart from this pattern (1) for elective procedures, (2) for diseases that are epidemic or markedly seasonal in their incidence, (3) when facilities are frequently overcrowded, with long waiting lists, and (4) when there is rapid growth in average daily census (213). In spite of these limitations, the Poisson distribution appears to be reasonably descriptive of the frequency of average daily censuses in a given institution or of subparts of these censuses. A characteristic of this distribution is that its variance equals its mean. Accordingly, the entire distribution of daily censuses can be reconstructed given only the average daily census. From this frequency distribution it is possible to tell what is the probability that a hospital's capacity will be exceeded during a given period of time.

This information can obviously be put to use in planning for hospitals, as we shall see. Here we wish to use it to correct the occupancy ratio so as to allow for desirable standby capacity. To do this, it is first necessary to decide how often (every how many days, on the average) one can tolerate demands on the hospital that exceed its capacity. Blumberg suggests that a frequency (p) of $1:100$ or $1:1000$ is acceptable. Given this value (p) and the value for the average daily census, it is possible, using the formula for the Poisson distribution or, more simply, an appropriate table, to determine the number of beds which would be needed. Using a table provided by Blumerg (213, p. 79) it is seen that for an average daily census of 160 patients, and a *p*-value of 1:100, the size of the hospital would be 191. The difference between 191 beds and 160 beds represents justifiable standby reserve. This means that the product of the 31 additional beds must be added to that of the 160 beds that are occupied, on the average. It follows that the adjusted occupancy ratio for each of the two hypothetical hospitals is $191/200 = 0.955$, or 95.5 percent.

A somewhat different method, using the same rationale, is the application by Long and Feldstein of the "Erlang loss formula" to determine how frequently hospital capacity is fully occupied (353, p. 122). An alternative rule-of-thumb computation, suggested by the Commission on Hospital Care many years ago is to add to the average daily census a number of beds equal to 3 or 4 times the square root of the daily census.

$$\text{Desirable capacity} = \text{average daily census} + 3, \text{ or } 4\sqrt{\text{average daily census.}}$$

The factor of 3 results in a hospital operating at a "high level of occupancy," whereas the factor of 4 results in a hospital that operates at a "low level of occupancy" (209, pp. 277–278). The formula used is equivalent to adding to the mean of the Poisson distribution 3 or 4 times the standard error of that distribution. Unfortunately, because of the characteristics of the distribution, there is no fixed value, expressed as units of standard deviation, which corresponds to any given probability of capacity being exceeded. This varies for different distribution means (average daily censuses). Hence, as Blumberg has pointed out, the foregoing formula will yield values that may differ considerably from those derived from the Poisson distribution itself (213, p. 79, footnote to Table 2).

It is clear from the above that the occupancy ratio, adjusted for standby capacity, depends very much on the normative decision concerning what is an acceptable price to pay, in terms of unused capacity, in order to gain a specified level of protection against the risk of having demand exceed hospital capacity. If, for example, the decision had been to provide enough beds to ensure that capacity were not exceeded more than once every 1000 days ($p = 0.001$), the number of beds to be maintained would have been 201. The conclusion, under this assumption, would be that the hypothetical hospitals in our example had an adjusted occupancy ratio a little over 100 percent. There are also a number of technical considerations that influence the results obtained. We have already pointed out the fact that the Poisson distribution may not represent the distribution of daily censuses, and that its use is predicated on certain assumptions, as well as on the convenience of reconstructing the total distribution given only one readily available value: the average daily census. If data were available on the actual frequency distribution of daily censuses, these empirical data could themselves be used to obtain a direct estimate of how frequently the capacity of the hospital is likely to be exceeded. Obviously, this would remove the need for making any assumptions about the shape of the distribution of daily censuses.

The importance of this added degree of precision has been pointed out by Drosness et al., who examined the frequency distribution of daily censuses, during a representative period, in departments of all twelve hospitals in Santa Clara County, California, ranging in size from 24 to 2188 beds (214). They found that the normal distribution fitted the observed distributions better than did the Poisson distribution in all instances except for the large medical-surgical units in four hospitals. Although these latter were better approximated by the Poisson distribution, they were, in fact, "truncated" through the absence of the long right tail of the Poisson. Allemand and Turney have also reported a normal distribution for the daily census in a maternity unit (215). Similarly, Phillip has reported that the frequency distribution of admissions to the ambulatory emergency service of one hospital were better described by a normal than by a Poisson distribution (216). He suggests that while the occurrence of morbid events may be Poisson-distributed, intervening events that influence admissions might distort the original pattern. For emergency units he postulates the following three factors that might be responsible for the departure from the Poisson pattern: "(1) If the emergency unit serves primarily a specific segment of a larger geographic unit characterized by high accident and violence rates. (2) If emergency cases are funneled into a unit by an administrative fiat. (3) If the cases handled by an emergency unit are an admixture of true and pseudo-emergency cases" (216, p. 46). Whenever the actual frequency distribution of daily censuses is normal in shape, the application of the Poisson estimate will yield a larger requirement for standby reserve. Unfortunately, the mere knowledge that the distribution of daily censuses is normal in shape does not help in arriving at an estimate of standby capacity. One needs also to know the standard deviation of the daily census in order to estimate, using the appropriate table, how frequently a given census is likely to be exceeded. In other words, the normal distribution does not have the conveniently fixed relationship between mean and standard deviation that characterizes the Poisson distribution.

Another aspect of the correction for standby capacity is the need to take into account the division of the hospital into "distinctive patient facilities" (213). When variability in total daily census is used as the basis for the estimate, irrespective of whether one uses the Poisson distribution or another empirically derived distribution, the assumption is made that there is interchangeability among beds in the hospital. Since this is known not to be true in most cases, the estimate thus obtained is an underestimate of standby capacity required.

A final refinement in the estimate of standby capacity is the adjustment for the proportion and timing of elective admissions. Theoretically, standby capacity is necessary only for the rather small, though variable, proportion of urgent conditions. For all others, it is possible to postpone admission, thus creating a reasonable waiting list. One aspect of this process is the scheduling of elective admissions in such a manner as to reduce to minimum fluctuations in the daily census. It is possible, in this way, to improve the efficiency of hospital operations and reduce the bed capacity held open for emergencies. Querido has reported a mathematical method developed by Professor P. de Wolff to allow for the development of waiting periods that are normatively defined for each diagnosis (218, pp. 122–127). Apparently the effect of this refinement on estimates of hospital capacity is rather small as compared to the adjustment necessary to account for daily fluctuations in census. Accounts of techniques, generally using computer simulation, to develop various scheduling strategies include those by Young (279, 280), Parker (282), and Robinson et al. (283). For further information, the mathematically inclined reader is referred to these papers and the further references that they cite.

PHYSICIAN CAPACITY AND SERVICE LOAD. In previous sections we have discussed some aspects of the measurement of the physician's capacity to produce service and of the measurement of the physician's output. The capacity to produce service has been defined in terms of man-hours of physician input. A variety of factors that influence the productivity of this input have been discussed. Output has been defined in terms of services and in terms of cases who have received service. The services themselves have been categorized in a manner that relates to their content. We have accordingly distinguished first visits from follow-up visits, complete examinations from partial examination, and client-initiated visits from referrals or consultations. Because the place of the visit may also be related to its content, we have distinguished office visits, hospital visits, home visits, telephone consultations, and the like. Other categories that are germane to the evaluation of the physician's work load deal with (1) urgency, (2) necessity, (3) whether scheduled or unscheduled, and (4) correspondence with regular working hours. Hence, one distinguishes urgent from non-urgent calls; necessary from unnecessary; visits by appointment from drop-ins (when the patient presents himself at the doctor's office), or call-ins (when the patient calls to say he is coming but without prior appointment); and regular visits from evening, night, or weekend calls. One scheme for classification is described by Spenser (149, Table I, p. 42).

In all the foregoing categories, the visit is the usual unit of enumeration. For many purposes this suffices. For other purposes, especially when the object is to determine the extent to which time is appropriately used, it is necessary to divide the work load into another set of categories that corresponds to functions or activities. Such functions and activities include face-to-face patient contact, indirect contact by telephone, administration, research, teaching, learning, travel to and from patients, and time-out for personal activities including meals, socializing, and the like. Functions and activities can, of course, be cut much finer. Van Deen has made a study of his own practice, using, in addition to the usual classification by type of visit, a division into "work cycles" such as "taking a case history, estimating hemoglobin in a blood sample, stitching a wound, writing a letter, making out a bill, etc. Work cycles can be executed in the consulting room, in the laboratory, or in the patient's home. The number of different work cycles was smaller than expected. It was found that 63 different groups of work cycles sufficed. The most frequent and important were included in only 32 groups of work cycles" (140, p. 278). In addition to enumeration, time is an essential dimension of all the measurements cited above. However, valid time data are difficult to obtain.

We have so far emphasized those aspects of the physician's practice that appear to pertain to evaluations of volume and capacity. Another important set of concerns leads to analyses of the demographic and morbidity characteristics of the physician's load. Still others focus on location of patient and travel to the physician. In all these studies the unit of observation may be the visit, the patient, or both.

There is a considerable literature that pertains to physician work load, with special emphasis on office practice. For some reason, a great deal of it emanates from England where the College of General practitioners has acted as catalyst and sponsor. Wolfe et al. provide a useful bibliography (166, pp. 123–129). Lees and Cooper have reviewed 37 studies and reported in a detailed table what items of information concerning general practice can be found in each (176). In a subsequent paper they summarize the findings (177). A review of this literature reveals a considerable diversity of methods and findings. A striking characteristic is the marked variability in practice among countries as well as among seemingly similar physicians within a locality. The reasons for such differences are very poorly understood. Logan and Eimerl comment on this phenomenon as follows:

> The case load of any sector is mainly influenced by the distribution of all facilities for care in the country, and so it is the outcome of many interacting forces. Even in developed countries without economic or geographical barriers to medical care, the clinical need of the patient in its translation into demand can be deflated or inflated by personal and family attitudes, on the one hand, and those of the medical profession, on the other. Such attitudes will reflect the medical culture of the nation as this is seen in its medical institutions. Thus, the case load of a hospital or clinic or general practice does not measure the underlying clinical need for care, nor the epidemiology of disease or disability; nor does it indicate the size of the need for further facilities, or the obsolescence of those that are outdated (174, p. 302).

The literature on physician case load is very difficult to summarize and interpret. There are many reasons for this. Perhaps most important, the studies reported tend to be merely descriptive. They are usually not developed in relation to some organizing theoretical or conceptual framework and hence do not often address themselves to answering fundamental questions relevant to medical care administration. What one gets are repetitions of descriptions which tax the mind without enlightening it. This is not to say that the studies do not contain valuable information; but only that the information has to be laboriously mined, sorted out, and related to some conceptual framework before it becomes generally meaningful. Another shortcoming that is often encountered is the nature of the sample and hence of the general applicability of the information. Many studies deal with the practices of a single physician, almost always that of the author, or of small groups of nonrandomly selected and unrepresentative physicians. Among the studies of single practices by their principals have been those of Crombie (182), Eimerl (145, 146), and Fry (183, 184). The issues involved in the sampling of general practice have been reviewed by Bevan and Draper with special reference to the British scene (137). An earlier study by A. Bradford Hill provides a model (136). One important feature that is generally true is the need to make allowance for the large fluctuations in case load by day of the week and by season. Jacob has described a method for selecting a portion of his practice for more intensive analysis of morbidity and work load, with special emphasis on the characteristics of high and low utilizers (151–153). He recognizes, as becomes clear in the analysis, that what he calls the "artificial practice" is not representative because it is drawn from patients rather than from persons in the population. A principle of general import is that a random sample of patients is more likely to include those who make more frequent visits. Even when a reasonably good sampling design has been employed, the low response rate that is generally characteristic of studies of ambulatory practice weakens confidence in the general applicability of the findings. Finally, the methods used for obtaining information may be faulty.

The methods used to obtain information include routine records, the use of special recording procedures by a sample of physicians for sample periods, questionnaires and interviews, and observation and recording by others who are often physicians or medical students. Peterson et al. and Clute combined direct observation of the general practitioner at work with the administration of a lengthy questionnaire (139, 165). Backett et al. developed a simple form which permitted the physician to record a minimum of information on all his cases. "In addition, every six weeks, for one week, members of the research team 'sat in' on all consultations and recorded in greater detail what went on" (138, p. 109). Thus, it was possible to relate the sample of more detailed information to the more general background provided by information on all cases. Observation and analysis of one's own work appears to be a not infrequent enterprise among curious and self-critical physicians. Van Deen used a watch to time the cycles of activity which were the units for his analysis (140). Jeans reports on the use of a tape record of office sessions from which it was possible to arrive at time estimates for various activities. Jeans also used simple scale diagrams of the examining room floor plan to plot the patient's and the physician's movements during the day, and to arrive at modifications that reduce physician walking (141, pp. 271, 272, and 274). The author has not encountered descriptions of the use of videotape recording, a method that appears to have many possibilities. Needless to say, the veracity of findings depends on the method used to obtain them. Time estimates of work load and of its components are especially open to doubt when obtained by questionnaire or interview. One must also consider the possible effect on practice of the presence of an outside observer. The need to resort to special methods of study is partly a consequence of the rudimentary nature of recording in most ambulatory practice. Special methods of recording more adapted to office practice need to be developed. For example, the standard unmodified International Classification of diseases used in hospital practice has been found to be of limited usefulness in office practice. The College of General Practitioners has provided considerable support to the development of simple methods for recording clinical and administrative data in general practice. Methods which they have encouraged or helped develop have included the picturesquely named E-Book, W-Book, F-Book and L-Book (143–150). The reader is referred to the literature for further information concerning these.

There will be no attempt in this section to summarize the unwieldy volume of information that may be gleaned from the literature on physician work load. Rather, the purpose is to develop an approach to analysis, using as a guide the general framework already described and, in particular, to test the applicability or lack of applicability of measures that have been developed in the hospital field. It is believed that the attempt to use analogous measures in the analysis of inpatient and outpatient work load will improve understanding of both by revealing significant similarities and differences.

One peculiarity of the physician's work load is that it takes place in many localities: for example, in the office, the hospital or, decreasingly, in the patient's home. The model that we shall develop is geared to the analysis of office care. However, one needs to consider what allowances should be made for the fact that a considerable proportion of the physician's work load is not included in the count of admissions to his office. This could be done by excluding from both capacity and work load of those segments devoted to non-office work. This is legitimate for some purposes. However, where the intent centers, as it often does, on the effective use of total physician capacity, it is necessary to include all elements of case load no matter where encountered. One consequence of this is that it highlights the fact that a significant part of the physician's case load is also part of the hospital's case load.

We have already seen that an examination of the hospital's capacity to provide service reveals unsuspected ambiguities. But these are as nothing compared to the lack of clarity in defining the comparable parameter for physicians and other health professionals in independent practice. The obvious analogue to the hospital bed is physician time or, more precisely, slots of physician time into which patients might fit as they do into hospital beds. But there are serious difficulties in utilizing this analogy. First, as is true of the hospital, the physician may be employed in activities other than patient care. These include teaching, research, administration, and even business activities unrelated to medicine. Second, and much more difficult, is normative formulation of what constitutes an appropriate work day for the health professional in independent practice. Part of this formulation, as Clute has pointed out, involves decisions concerning what is adequate time for leisure, for a satisfactory home life and for continuing education (165, pp. 465–470). Studies of general practice regularly show that physicians work unusually long hours, feel pressed for time, and are unable to keep up with advances in medicine.

Accordingly, Le Riche and Stiver have proposed that the normative service capacity of the physician should be set at 1800 hours per annum and that an additional 200 hours be provided as worktime but devoted to continuing education. This adds up to 40 hours per week for 50 weeks (154). By comparison, Theodore and Sutter report that a national sample of "office-oriented" physicians in the winter and spring of 1966 worked an average of 55.8 hours during the most recent week, of which 45.3 hours was for "direct care of patients." "The largest portion of physicians reported practicing between 40 and 69 hours per week, i.e., more than a full-time 40-hour week" (162, p. 520). One must conclude either that physicians, on the average, are considerably overemployed or that the normative capacity estimate is widely off the mark. This is the case even though no account has been taken of standby reserve, namely, the number of hours during which a physician is readily available when called upon to provide care. In one medical group, Wolfe et al. have estimated that each physician worked on an average of 69.5 hours per week, of which 27.8 hours, or 40 percent, was for "active standby" (166). In solo practice, the hours of active standby would almost be certainly much longer and, in some circumstances, almost unremitting.

It is clear that a normative definition of service capacity is a critical requirement at every step in the model for evaluating the relationship between services provided and the capacity to produce services. Failing some external standard for arriving at such a definition, Ciocco and Altman derived it from subjective estimates by asking general practitioners to "state the number of patients they could see in 1 week and still furnish satisfactory care" (160, p. 1338). They found that 60 percent of urban, and 40 percent of rural general practitioners said they could increase their current patient load. A self-defined standard of capacity has obvious limitations, not the least of which is the relationship between case load, price, and income. However, this approach deserves further exploration. In a survey of general practice in England and Wales, Mechanic found that, second only to remuneration, was concern over the large case loads of doctors and the correspondingly limited time available to provide satisfactory care (180). Ciocco and Altman found that some of the physicians they questioned did express a desire to reduce their patient load. In one of their physician categories, urban physicians under age 35, the desired patient load was, in fact, a little lower than the actual load.

To reiterate, any normative definition of physician capacity should include an estimate of work hours to be devoted to patient care, of hours for active standby, and of hours for continuing education. The sum of the first two of these, work hours allocated to patient care and active standby, correspond to the hospital's operational capacity, but only roughly. To achieve more complete correspondence, it would be necessary to specify the normative length for each visit by type of visit. This is necessary, in part, to maintain the analogy between physician capacity and hospital capacity. The physician's day would be divided into time slots within which patients would be fitted as they are into hospital beds. There is, however, a more fundamental reason. It stems from the ability of the physician to lengthen or shorten the length of the visit to fill whatever time is available. This means that empty stretches of physician time would not show unless the number of patients per day was extremely low. We shall return to this phenomenon in the sections on service overload and service reserve. The methods for arriving at time norms for specific types of services will also be discussed in a subsequent section.

A normative definition of physician capacity is necessary if one wishes to make normative judgments concerning the appropriateness of the relationship between service load and capacity. If, however, the intent is merely to describe service capacity and its relation to service load, an operational definition is all that is necessary. This is merely a statement of how much time is devoted to each physician activity. We have already emphasized that in specifying operational capacity for patient care one needs to exclude those activities of the physician that are not directly related to this function. Such activities are readily identifiable if they occupy appreciable chunks of time, especially if the physician is separately remunerated for them. However, in many cases, activities that do not directly contribute to patient care are unremunerated and so dispersed during the working day that they require special attention to identify and isolate. There are, in addition, a number of ''personal'' activities that do not contribute to patient care and which are therefore not part of net working time devoted to that purpose. These include meals, social activities, personal business, and the like. Not infrequently there may be a question as to what share of what activities is considered an integral part of patient care and what part an extraneous interruption. Such questions should be resolved by careful definition. For example, medical recording, correspondence, and travel to hospital and the patient's home could very well be considered to be part of time available for patient care even though they consume time that is not occupied with direct care.

The literature on physician work load contains many examples of attempts to categorize the physician's work day or work week according to the class of activities which it contains. Unfortunately, there is an almost bewildering variability in the categories and their definitions. This makes comparisons almost impossible and interpretation very hazardous. There are, in addition, serious questions about the validity of some of the data, arising in part from deficiencies in sampling and in part from the methods used to obtain information. The following are some selected findings of selected studies. As already mentioned, Theodore and Sutter found that the average work week of the physician in the United States was 55.8 hours, of which 45.3 hours was for direct patient care (162). Clark et al. have reported on the professional activities, additional to private patient care, undertaken by a sample of internists in New York State. The authors give the distribution of these activities by time devoted to each (169, Table 2, p. 179). Unfortunately, one cannot compute, from the data given, what percent of total physician time these activities collectively consume. Eimerl and Pearson have reported that a roughly representative sample of physicians in a section of England and Wales spent 10 percent of their time on "administration" and another 40 to 60 percent on home visits, apparently including travel time (181). Crombie has reported that in his own practice, in a suburb of a large English city, he spent 16 percent of his time on "administration" and an additional 17 percent for travel. "Administration" was defined to include "consolidating visits and commitments, assembling dressings and other equipment, making entries on N.H.S. record cards, telephoning and dealing with correspondence, discussing mutual professional problems with partner, and referring to patient records or literature" (182, p. 142). Wood has reported that he spends 14 percent of his time on office visits, 41 percent on home visits, 8 percent dispensing drugs, 18 percent writing, and 19 percent driving—an average of 40.8 miles a day. "The annual mileage covered by a doctor is variously put at 15,000, 14,000, 8,784 and 8,000 miles . . ." (cited by Lees and Cooper [177, pp. 426, 427]). Wolfe et al. have reported that in a group practice in Saskatchewan about 10 percent of physician time (excluding active standby) was spent on clinical meetings and an additional 5 percent on "interval between patients, and chart completion" (166, Table 5, p. 115). Parrish et al. have described the activities of 25 general practitioners who served as preceptors in a Department of Community Health. These physicians spent about 9 percent of their time on "personal" and another 16 percent on "administrative" activities (163, Table 4, p. 897). "The personal activities included the following: personal business or telephone calls; snacks and coffee breaks; restroom breaks; visiting with friends, personnel, or visitors; reading personal mail or newspapers; and personal conversations with patients about subjects other than the patient's medical condition." Administrative activities included "preparation of bank deposits; dictating or writing letters; making notations on records and charts; opening and reading office mail; completing and signing insurance forms; making out laboratory reports; telephoning or writing prescriptions; preparing medication to be dispensed to patients; admitting patients to hospitals; calling consultants about patients; personnel management; talking to salesmen of drug companies; ordering supplies; completing birth and death certificates; completing tax forms; and reading medical journals'' (163, p. 894). Bergman et al. studied the activities of four pediatricians with teaching appointments in the Seattle area. These physicians spent 9 percent of their time on paper work, 8 percent on personal activities (mainly meals), and 6 percent on travel between patients (171, Table II, p. 255). All these findings are of interest primarily to the extent to which they may indicate misuse of physician time, a subject to be discussed in a subsequent section.

The reader will recall that specification of operational capacity was the first element in our analysis of service load. The next requirement was specification of two basic characteristics of service load: admissions and length of stay. Here again, the application of the hospital model to outpatient physician care reveals interesting problems. Functionally, the analogue to an episode of hospital care is an episode of ambulatory care. Admissions would correspond to the first contact between the patient and the physician (or his substitute) and discharge the last such contact during a given episode. Length of stay would correspond to the time elapsed between admission and discharge. Obviously, this period would be made up partly of service time and partly of waiting time, as previously defined. It would be interesting to develop a system of case load analysis in these terms. The work of Solon et al., to which we have already referred, could serve as a beginning in this direction (382, 383). It is customary, however, to use a different time scale altogether in analyzing the case load of the physician in the ambulatory care facility. This is because the ambulatory care facility (which could be the office of the solo practitioner as well as the premises of a group practice) is seen as a container which is filled and emptied each day, or each 24 hours, with no carryover from one period to the next. The adoption of this model, and of the vastly accelerated time scale which is inherent in it, has a profound effect on the definition of the unit of service and of the relative importance of the different durations associated with the provision of care.

The unit of service is taken to be the patient visit to the physician or ambulatory care facility. Length of stay, when used for hospital care, denotes the interval between admission and discharge, with the day of admission and the day of discharge counted as one day. Needless to say, admission does not correspond with arrival at the hospital, and discharge need not correspond with departure. Admission to, and discharge from, the hospital are defined in terms of the completion of certain administrative procedures which define the legal and other relationships between hospital and patient. In ambulatory care, admission and discharge procedures differ widely in level of formality, depending on the level of formal organization in the ambulatory resource. Hence, arrival time and departure time are often clearer signals of the initiation and termination of the relationship, and therefore of the length of stay. Even when reasonably formal admission and discharge procedures are present, the total duration of stay is so short that the interval between arrival and admission and between discharge and departure becomes a matter of concern for certain types of case load analysis, notably for the design of appointment systems. Accordingly, one might wish to preserve, at least theoretically, the distinctions between arrival time, admission time, discharge time, and departure time. The strict analogue to length of stay would be the interval between admission and discharge. There is no term that indicates the duration between arrival time and departure time in current medical care usage. The phrase "transit time" has been proposed (384). Transit time is itself composed of waiting time and service time. Service time may be subdivided by type of service, procedure or health professional involved. The time consumed in contact with the physician is usually designated "consultation time." Similarly, waiting time may be dissected to reveal time elapsed (1) between arrival and first service, (2) between arrival and first physician service, and (3) between services. The relevance of some of these intervals to the design of appointment systems will be described in a subsequent volume. In the meantime, it is important not to confuse patient waiting time with idle time of the physician or other service-producing units in the ambulatory care resource. Patient waiting time and physician idle time could be directly related as a result of inefficient operations. More often, they are inversely related, waiting time being an indicator of service overload.

Finally, one ought to appreciate the difficulties involved in obtaining a measure of transit time and of its components in ambulatory care. Hospitals that maintain a computerized statistical system such as that offered by the Commission on Professional and Hospital Activities, are able to implement direct measurement of length of stay. Other hospitals derive this datum, as indicated in a foregoing section, from information on discharges and average daily census. In ambulatory care operations the organizational apparatus that permits the routine measurement of basic case load data is usually lacking. Even when ambulatory care is organized, the routine, direct measurement of transit time is not easy since it requires the introduction of arrival and departure time into the record. Nor can transit time be derived from average daily census and admission, since average census fluctuates widely during the day and is therefore extremely difficult to measure. More detailed measurement of the components of transit time is almost always a matter for special sample study.

The census in ambulatory care may be defined as the number of cases waiting to be served plus those being served at any moment in time. The average census for the day would be the mean of all such observations. It excludes, as does the average daily census for hospitals, those who have not been admitted to the facility but are on the waiting list. If, however, one were to consider the episode of care as the unit of service, the average daily census of the ambulatory facility would include all patients, no matter where located, who were under current active care by the physician. This would include patients seen in the hospital, in the emergency clinic, and in the home. It is customary, however, to restrict the analysis to the patients in the physician's office. This is because the average daily census is not used as a measure of work load. Its major, perhaps only, use is in relation to studies of patient waiting and the design of an appointment system. The value for the average daily census can be derived in a manner analogous to that used for hospitals, as follows:

$$\frac{(\text{patients per physician working day}) \ (\text{transit time in minutes per patient})}{\text{physician working time in minutes per day}}$$

As we have already pointed out, this measure cannot be obtained routinely because of the difficulty in measuring transit time. Consequently, one views with more than usual interest the description by Rossiter and Reynolds of a device that permits automatic monitoring of the patient census in an ambulatory care facility (155). The device is actuated by two parallel beams of light, in a horizontal relationship to one another, projected across the entrance of the physician's waiting room. Depending on the order in which the two beams are interrupted, one unit is added or subtracted from the count of persons that cross the entrance. A continuous graphic recording is maintained. A correction needs to be made to allow for the proportion of persons who enter and leave the room who are not themselves patients but who accompany patients to the physician's office.

Perhaps the most critical aspect of case load analysis is the relationship between case load and capacity. For hospitals, the measures of this relationship include (1) the occupancy ratio, (2) the number of unoccupied bed-days per bed, and (3) the number of unoccupied bed-days per admission or the turnover interval. The development of similar measures for physicians and ambulatory care facilities leads to certain interesting observations. The most important of these pertain, as we have pointed out, to the definition of physician capacity and the different meanings and uses of descriptive and normative measures of capacity. Another distinction, which we have also mentioned, is that which needs to be made between the work of the physician in his office and that in the hospital and elsewhere. Finally, one needs to distinguish measures of the exploitation of the physician's capacity as distinct from those of the exploitation of the ambulatory resource as a whole. An "occupancy ratio" (or "exploitation or employment ratio") can be developed for physicians as follows:

$$\frac{\text{Used consultation time}}{\text{Available consultation time}} \quad \text{or} \quad \frac{\text{Patients seen}}{\text{Patients that could have been seen}}$$

Although seemingly different, this derivation is fully analogous to the hospital occupancy ratio, which is the ratio of beds actually occupied to beds available to be occupied. In the formula cited above, the numerators correspond to the hospital measure of patient-days and the denominator to the hospital measure of bed-days. As already emphasized, the denominators may be descriptively or normatively defined. The magnitude and the meaning of the occupancy ratio would differ accordingly.

The usual measure of case flow in ambulatory care is visits or patients per unit time, for example per hour. This is generally a descriptive measure, but a normative analogue could be devised by using visits actually produced during a specified number of normatively defined consultation periods. A value of 1 would be the standard value. Values above 1 would indicate an undesirably high case flow, possibly associated with poor quality, and values below 1 a wasteful use of physician resources. The turnover interval could also be measured in a manner analogous for hospitals, as follows:

$$\frac{\begin{array}{c}\text{Available}\\\text{consultation time}\end{array} - \begin{array}{c}\text{Consultation time}\\\text{actually used}\end{array}}{\text{Number of admissions or discharges (visits)}}$$

We have already given reasons for believing that the turnover interval in ambulatory practice will be small and will not adequately reflect differences in case load as related to capacity. It is also important to remember that the interval between seeing patients is not necessarily idle time for physicians, a point fully analogous to that made about the interval between filling beds in a hospital.

Important considerations in the evaluation of hospital capacity were adjustment of the occupancy ratio for minimum turnover interval and for stand-by capacity. These considerations have not received attention in the analysis of physician case load for a number of reasons. The minimum turnover interval is handled by defining the visit to include the necessary activities of preparing for the reception of the case and of attending to business created by the case after the patient has left the physician's presence. Corrections for active standby are handled by deducting the period of active standby from both output and input. In other words, case load during regular working hours is analyzed separately from the case load during other times when the physician is on call. However, as ambulatory care becomes more organized, it will be useful to analyze occupancy in terms of the capacity of the facility and all its personnel to provide total coverage, including active standby. This would render the situation for the ambulatory care facility fully analogous to that which now holds for the hospital.

As a summary of the preceding discussion, Table IV.49 gives

Table IV.49.   Possible measures of the capacity and service load of an ambulatory care facility and corresponding measures used for hospitals

A. Operational bed complement	A. Descriptively defined as hours allocated to patient care or number of consultation periods actually available, given a defined case mix.
	A_1. Normatively defined as desired hours allocated to patient care or as a specified number of consultation periods to correspond to a given case mix.
	(Descriptive or normative estimates of stand-by capacity and time for continuing education may or may not be included depending on purpose of the analysis.)
B. Admissions or discharges per year	B. Patients or visits per day.
	(This is the usual measure of case load and may, therefore, include cases seen elsewhere than in the office. In any event, item B and item A must relate to the same segments of case load.)
C. Average daily census (observed)	C. Average number of patients waiting to be seen and being seen in the ambulatory care resource. Generally excludes patients under care elsewhere. Direct data generally not available.

Table IV.49.   (continued)

D. Average length of stay (observed)	D. Could be defined as average "transit time" which is the time between arrival and departure, or as average "holding time," which is the time between "admission" and "discharge." In many situations the distinction cannot be made. Usually requires special study to determine.
E. Bed-days per year	E. Visits that could be provided during a working day using either empirical or normative standards.
	E_1. Time available for consultation during a working day using either empirical or normative standards.
F. Patient-days per year	F. Visits actually provided during a working day.
	F_1. Time actually used for consultation during a working day.
G. Average daily census (derived)	G. Derived as follows if a direct measure of transit time or holding time were available. $$\frac{BD}{\text{Physician working time in minutes per day}}$$
H. Average length of stay (derived)	H. Derived as follows if a direct measure of average daily census were available: $$\frac{(C)\ (\text{Physician working time in minutes per day})}{B}$$
I. Occupancy ratio	I. Might be designated as "occupancy ratio" "exploitation ratio" or "employment ratio" $$\frac{F}{E} \times 100 \text{ or } \frac{F_1}{E_1} \times 100$$
K. Discharge ratio	K. Visits per unit time
L. Turnover interval	L. Problems in interpretation discussed in text. Derived as follows: $(E_1 - F_1)/B$
M. Unused bed-days per bed	M. $(E_1 - F_1)/A$

measures used to analyze hospital case load and their analogues for physician case load. The items cited are keyed to the items in Table IV.48.

Service Overload

There are certain ambiguities in the concept of "service overload." If one conceives of capacity as the volume of a rigid container, then capacity can be fully loaded, after which there will be an overflow. There are analogues in this model for the concept of a completely loaded capacity and the concept of demand exceeding capacity. "Service overload," however, is a concept somewhat different from either. It postulates, as it were, some elasticity in the container, so that it can adjust to a limited degree to work load that exceeds its "usual" or "normal" capacity, but not without the development of "strain." Operationally, therefore, the evidence of such strain is the pathognomonic sign of service overload as distinct from "service overflow." On the other hand, certain phenomena, while not conceptually identical with "service overload," are so closely related as to be presumptive evidence that such overload exists.

Presumptive evidence of service overload exists when there are very high occupancy measures in a hospital or ambulatory practice. These measures of occupancy, and the considerations that need to be taken into account in their derivation and interpretation, especially where physician capacity is concerned, have been fully discussed in the foregoing section. Evidence of high occupancy includes high average values as well as the frequent occurrence of 100 percent, or near 100 percent, occupancy. Evidence for demand exceeding supply is the rejection of admissions and the presence of waiting lists. Average time between application for admission and admission would constitute one measure. Isaacs has examined the demand for geriatric beds, with special attention to the discrepancy between the number of patients accepted for admission and those actually admitted during a given period of time, as well as the proportion of admitted persons who have waited longer than 28 days after acceptance (217). He proposes the following measure of overload:

$$\frac{(\text{accepted patients}) - (\text{admitted patients})}{\text{number of beds}} \times 100$$

However, as we have said, the excess of demand over capacity is only presumptive evidence that "service overload" exists. This is so because it is conceivable, though not likely, that a hospital can limit admissions to such an extent that it can continue to operate within its capacity without evidence of strain, even though there may be a long waiting list. This may be also true for a physician who may practice comfortably through limiting his appointments. Whether this rather fine distinction between "service overload" and "excess of demand over capacity" is worth making will depend in part on empirical studies of how service producers respond to excessive demand. Another caution, of a more operational nature, concerns the interpretation of the waiting list itself. It is necessary to examine carefully the manner in which the waiting list is generated and maintained. After some time, the need for care may have disappeared or satisfied in some other way, or at some other facility, even though a person's name may remain on the waiting list. Patients may also have moved away or died. Airth and Newell discuss the uses and limitations of waiting lists in estimating demand for hospital beds. They cite a study in Cardiff in which, of the total number of persons on the waiting list, 3 percent were there because of duplication of names, 15 percent had already been treated or died, and 15 percent said they did not intend to seek admission (357, pp. 78–80).

Certain phenomena are considered to constitute direct evidence of service overload. These include the following: (1) decline in efficiency, (2) expansion of capacity beyond normatively set limits, (3) reduction in capacity allocated to non-service functions, (4) changes in case mix, (5) changes in internal service and waiting times, (6) deterioration in quality, and (7) dissatisfaction among personnel and patients. Measurements of efficiency and quality tend to be rather difficult. Expansion of capacity beyond normatively set limits is easier to detect. The physician will work longer hours. The hospital will put beds where they are not supposed to be. The bed in the hall is a dead give-away. Under these circumstances, the occupancy ratio, using normatively defined capacity, will exceed 100 percent at least part of the time. Accordingly, the frequency distribution of occupancy ratios becomes an important tool in the detection of service overload. Closely allied to the expansion of service capacity is reduction in capacity devoted to non-service functions such as continuing education or research. This is certainly true for physicians in private practice. One might also look for analogous phenomena in the hospital: for example, curtailment of rounds and other educational activities, reduced attendance at clinical conferences, and the like. A fourth phenomenon to look for would be changes in case mix. The ratio of urgent to non-urgent cases should change in favor of the first. One would also expect changes in length of stay. Two factors are at work here. First, service time is likely to be reduced and, second, waiting time is likely to be lengthened. The effect on length of stay,

holding time, or transit time will vary depending on the relative preponderance of the two effects on their two components: service time and
waiting time. In the physician's office the prominent effect will be considerable curtailment of consultation time, with or without a lengthening
in transit time. Incidentally, there may be certain paradoxical secondary
effects on case load characteristics that result from inadequacy of
management during the initial visit or from unwillingness of patients to
use an overcrowded facility. For example, there may be more return
visits as well as greater demand for home visits or for visits out of
regular scheduled hours. The hospital length of stay could be shortened
or lengthened depending, in part, on the relative capacities of the bed
complement and their ancillary services. If the ancillary services become
overburdened first, or to a greater extent, it is conceivable that patients
will wait longer for service and hence that the length of stay will, paradoxically, be prolonged in the face of high demand. Finally, overload will
manifest itself in dissatisfaction among personnel and patients. This is
an especially critical sign in office practice, where the greater flexibility
of capacity may conceal the fact that it has exceeded desirable limits.

It would be interesting to compare the theoretical expectations detailed
above with the findings of empirical studies concerning the response of
hospitals and physicians to high levels of demand. Published accounts of
such studies are rather rare. Martin Feldstein has given particular attention to the relationship between supply and demand concluding, in
general, that supply plays an important role in determining demand. As
one aspect of his exploration of this area, he has measured the extent to
which the availability of hospital beds in a region influences admissions
and length of stay (222–224). A ''responsiveness index'' analogous to
the economic measure of ''elasticity'' was developed for this purpose. It
is derived as follows:

$$\text{Responsiveness} = \frac{\text{Percent change in ''bed use''}}{\substack{\text{Percent change in beds available} \\ \text{per 1000 population}}} \times 100$$

Bed use may be measured in terms of the number of beds used per 1000
population, the number of cases treated per 1000 population, and the
mean stay per case (222, p. 562). This measure of responsiveness has
several advantages. ''First, since it is a ratio of two percentage changes,
it is independent of both unit of measure (bed day, cases treated, etc.)
and of the scale (per 1000 population, per 10,000 population, etc.) . . .
Secondly, it permits us to divide the responsiveness of 'beds used' (R_b)
into a 'mean stay' responsiveness (R_m) and a 'cases treated' responsive-

ness (R_c) so that $R_b = R_m + R_c$" (223, p. 67). In short, it is possible to measure how responsive is hospital use to relative scarcity of hospital beds and how much of the response can be attributed to adaptation in admissions and how much to adaptation in length of stay. The data pertained to the supply and use of non-hospital beds in 11 hospital regions outside London. The findings were at variance with the expectation that the length of stay would exhibit the greater responsiveness. There was "50% greater effect on the number of cases treated than on the average stay per case" (222, p. 562). Of several possible explanations he considers, Feldstein favors the hypothesis that physicians are more concerned with giving what they consider to be appropriate care to patients who are already in the hospital than with modifying their practice to accommodate the greatest number of patients. This tendency may be reinforced by the organization of medical care under the National Health Service in a manner that brings about a considerable degree of administrative and financial insulation of hospital practice from the large mass of general ambulatory care. In the United States where the admission of a physician's private patient to the hospital may depend on his making room by discharging another of his patients, the pattern of response could be different. In view of these speculations, it is interesting to note that Feldstein has reported similar responses to variations in the supply of general hospital beds in the United States (225). Apparently one has to look further for an explanation.

Feldstein found that total responsiveness, as well as the relative contributions of admissions and length of stay, varied by diagnosis in a manner only partly predictable from the urgency or the seriousness of the condition. As might have been expected, appendectomies were largely unresponsive to bed scarcity, and whatever responsiveness was present was due to variation in length of stay. Less urgent medical and surgical conditions, such as respiratory infections, hemorrhoids, and varicose veins, were highly responsive, with a greater part of the response due to variations in admissions. On the other hand, medical conditions subsumed under the heading of arteriosclerotic heart disease were very responsive to bed scarcity, whereas tonsillectomy and adenoidectomy were not. For maternity cases, responsiveness was intermediate in magnitude with strong preponderance of variability due to admissions. These aberrant findings are difficult to interpret. Feldstein is aware of the noncomparability of cases, especially within a broad category such as arteriosclerotic heart disease. He points out that, where beds are plentiful, less serious cases might be admitted, producing a shorter average stay and thus helping to conceal the lengthening of stay expected where there is no scarcity. The relative nonresponsiveness of tonsillectomies and adenoidectomies may have resulted from a lack of correlation between overall bed scarcity and the scarcity of beds allocated to the ear, nose, and throat service. In other words, the definition of supply must take into account the interchangeability of beds within a hospital. In our own discussion of the possible effects of overload we have suggested that scarcity might have a mixed and contradictory effect on length of stay by shortening service time but lengthening waiting time. All these factors are subject to investigation in future studies. Finally, it is clear from Feldstein's findings that the different levels of responsiveness exhibited by different diagnoses would result in differences in case mix as a response to scarcity. Vaananen et al. have reported data from Finland that support this conclusion. Among the communes in one hospital region there were great variations in hospital ownership and a partially related variation in hospital use. Where hospital use was very low, the proportion of urgent use was much higher than in communes where hospital use was high. Interestingly enough, the length of stay decreased as the number of hospital beds per unit population increased. Unfortunately, the data cited do not permit a direct relationship to be drawn between supply and variations in case mix. The evidence for the relationship as interpreted above remains indirect (226).

Systematic study of the response of physicians to increases in work load is even more lacking than comparable studies for hospitals. It is generally believed that the initial, and perhaps most important, response of physicians to service overload is to work longer hours with neglect of continuing education, leisure, and family life. That this may not be fully true, at least beyond a certain level of overwork, is suggested by a study by Eimerl and Pearson of the work load of two groups of physicians, one during one week in August when the load was low and one during February when the work load was high. The major response noted was a reduction in time per consultation and a smaller increase in total work time. The findings also suggest a possible curtailment in the relative frequency of home visits, but this cannot be proved because the case mix during the two periods is not comparable. The data were as shown in Table IV.50. The conclusions concerning the response to increases in work load are, unfortunately, somewhat weakened by the fact that the data do not pertain to the same physicians observed at two time periods, but to two samples of physicians neither of which was fully representative. Furthermore, differences in type of case encountered during the two time periods might explain, at least to some extent, the observed differences in consultation time. Nevertheless, the findings are interesting.

Table IV.50.   Seasonal change in specified measures of the work load of general practitioners. Merseyside and North Wales, England, August 1964 and February 1965

Measure of Work Load	Percent Change Compared to August
Average number of patients seen	
In consulting-room	+34
On home visits	+17
Average time spent per week	
In consulting-room	+9.5
On home visits	+1.5
Average time per consultation	
In consulting-room	−18
On home visits	−13

SOURCE: Reference 181, Table VII, page 1552.

They also demonstrate that neither visits nor hours worked are, by themselves, a complete measure of work load. Crombie and Cross have documented differences in hours worked by month in one suburban practice. The range, excluding the very unusual month of August, was 20.4 hours per week in July to 31.8 hours in March. Unfortunately, the number of cases per week is not given by month, so that time spent per visit cannot be computed. Crombie and Cross do note, however, that "when the demand for patient care was heavy during a particular week, the time spent on administrative duties was reduced for that week, but was increased in the subsequent week" (182, p. 142). The work load analyst should be alert to the possibilities of such displacements in time. Mechanic related work load, in hours, to practice size as determined by the number of persons for whom the general practitioner has accepted responsibility. He concludes as follows:

What is particularly interesting, however, is how little of the total variance in work load can be explained by practice size—probably no more than 5 percent . . . One factor affecting time spent concerns the way in which the doctor distributes his time between surgery and domiciliary visits, but a more important explanation of the weakness of size of practice in predicting work time lies in the manner in which doctors with large numbers of patients adjust to their work loads. Size of practice is more important in how it affects the pace and style of the doctor's work pattern than it is in affecting the number of hours he devotes to his practice. Doctors respond to large practices not by continually increasing the length of the work day, but by practicing at a different pace and style, in which they pack more work into any period of time and take various shortcuts (180, pp. 250–251).

It is possible that response of physician to the excess of demand over capacity depends on several factors, including type of case, organizational characteristics, and personal attributes of the physicians themselves. As we have suggested, it is possible that in some instances the physician will maintain his normal operations and either refuse to accept additional work or decide to place patients on a long waiting list. The possible influence of clinical characteristics is suggested by White and Pike. In the process of constructing appointment systems based upon service data from a variety of hospital clinics in Great Britain, it was noted that in certain services—a fracture clinic, for example, the physician appeared to adjust time per case so that he would see all patients during the clinic session. By contrast, data from general medical and general surgical clinics showed that time per case was not usually affected by the number of patients in the clinic (157). One assumes that in these circumstances it is possible to make alternative arrangements for patients who cannot be seen or that they are simply turned away.

An interesting approach to the analysis of response to different workloads is offered by Haussmann in a study of hospital nursing services (158). If it is assumed that nursing services are ordered in a scale of priorities from most urgent and important to least, and that nurses arrange their activities so that highest priority tasks are performed first and others wait, and if it is further assumed that demand for the services in the several priority rankings is either random or reasonably so, one can then construct a mathematical model that can predict what happens to the time that patients must wait for services of specified levels of priority. It turns out that as workload is made to increase, either by assigning more patients to each nurse or by assigning patients who generate more demands for service, waiting time for service responds in a manner characteristic of each priority class. Time elapsed between demand and delivery of services in the highest priority class is very short and changes hardly at all as workload increases. By contrast, services in the lowest priority class, which may be summarized as the giving of emotional and physical support, experience a very rapid increase in waiting time, which soon becomes infinite. In other words, such services cannot be given, with consequent deterioration in the quality of nursing care. As workload increases, services that are intermediate between most urgent and least urgent are postponed for moderate lengths of time. It can be said, of course, that these findings are implicit in the assumptions that underlie the mathematical model. These assumptions are, however, reasonably true to life. The priority rankings of nursing services were provided by the nurses themselves. The approximately random occurrence of demand not only for unscheduled but also for scheduled services was empirically confirmed, as were the general rules of behavior when nurses had to make choices among demands for services of differing priority. The utility of the model is that it identifies and displays in precise quantitative terms the consequences that flow from the underlying characteristics of the situation.

Service Reserve

The reader will recall that our model for the analysis of the capacity to provide service postulated the possibility that some "service reserve" would remain under most circumstances, including situations characterized by considerable service overload. Service reserve was itself divisible into several components as follows:

Service reserve
Manifest
Underemployment
Standby capacity

Latent
Misuse
Productivity potential

In this section we shall pursue the discussion of service reserve with special attention to the several components identified above.

MANIFEST SERVICE RESERVE. Manifest service reserve refers to identifiably vacant or unoccupied capacity. Its magnitude is most conveniently measured by the complement of the occupancy ratio after correction for minimum turnover interval, as follows:

$$100 - \frac{\text{Corrected occupancy}}{\text{ratio in percent}} = \frac{\text{Nonoccupancy ratio}}{\text{in percent}}$$

Part of the capacity that appears unoccupied may be held vacant intentionally in order to meet the unforeseen or unscheduled demands for service generated by fluctuations in demand and other factors. We have already pointed out that it may be erroneous to consider capacity held vacant for this purpose as unoccupied or unproductive. A reasonable level of standby reserve is a service that needs to be taken into account in measurements of occupancy and productivity. Accordingly, corrections of the occupancy ratio have been proposed to take account of the standby reserve of hospitals. The rationale for this correction and the method of computation have been described in a previous section. It should be emphasized, however, that this correction might involve an overestimate. Since the likelihood of future censuses is based on the average of past censuses, there is an implicit assumption that past censuses represent necessary hospital use. As we shall see below, this is an unjustified assumption. What is being suggested is that the hospital can probably get by with a smaller standby capacity than the usual computation would indicate if only urgent cases were admitted. This would be true, however, only if the underestimate due to the assumption of bed interchangeability had been first removed. Whatever nonoccupancy remains after corrections are made for minimum turnover interval and for legitimate standby reserve is considered to represent unused capacity.

The analysis described above applies most immediately to hospitals. We have already discussed the reasons why it cannot be applied, without modification, to the services of physicians. These reasons include: (1) the absence of a normative definition of physician hours except in salaried practice, (2) the ability of the physician to lengthen or shorten service time in response to fluctuations in demand, and (3) the ability of the physician to exchange service time for time devoted to other functions such as administration or continuing education when service load increases. The effect of these characteristics is that whatever service reserve physicians may have is most likely to be latent rather than manifest. However, if one were able to define the length of the regular work day for the physician and the minimum turnover interval between patients, one could compute the nonoccupancy ratio as described above. Another possible approach to the discovery of unused capacity or "manifest service reserve" is to ask physicians themselves to indicate the limits of their capacity to provide care. Ciocco and Altman used this approach to determine service reserve among general practitioners in Georgia during the week of December 13–19, 1942. Table IV.51 gives the findings for the average physician. It is clear that service reserve, based on the physician's own estimate of his capacity, varies by age and place of residence of the physician. In one category (physicians under 35 in urban counties), there was an overload. The overall service reserve was 13 percent of capacity in urban counties and 10 percent of capacity in rural counties. These estimates are, of course, not expected to be applicable to the current situation. The study is cited merely as an illustration of method. From this viewpoint one might question whether the week chosen is representative of the entire year and whether Georgia is representative of the nation. More fundamentally, one might question whether self-

Table IV.51.   Comparisons of actual and desired work-loads of general practitioners, according to location and age of physicians, Georgia, 1942

A Residence and Age Group of Physician	B Patients Seen	C Patients That Could be Seen	D Difference: B − C	E D As Percent of C
Urban counties				
Under 35	120	116	+ 4[a]	+ 3[a]
35–44	168	181	−13	− 7
45–64	108	132	−24	−18
65 and over	55	65	−10	−15
All ages	112	129	−17	−13
Rural counties				
Under 35	145	153	− 8	− 5
35–44	155	159	− 4	− 3
45–64	113	128	−15	−12
65 and over	62	70	− 8	−11
All ages	111	123	−12	−10

SOURCE: Reference 160, Table 5, page 1339.
[a] Actual workload is more than that desired.

estimates of capacity can be accepted as substitutes for socially defined normative standards. Finally, these estimates do not deal with the question of corrections for standby reserve.

Physician standby capacity could be of two forms. One form could be time left uncommitted during regular working hours in order to accommodate clients who come without an appointment. It should be possible to estimate how many such calls for service are likely to be made and what proportion of these are likely to need immediate care. Accordingly, the suitability or unsuitability of time left vacant for this purpose could be determined. While this is an interesting theoretical question, the need for such a refinement in analysis is not likely to arise with any frequency. The provision of standby capacity outside regular working hours is more of an issue. With respect to this, it might be argued the only reasonable time allocation for the solo practitioner is complete availability at all times. This would lead to the conclusion that all physicians are fully occupied at all times providing either service or standby potential— a conclusion that does not appear to be analytically useful. A more productive approach might be taken to a number of physicians in a group practice or to all physicians in a community or locality, taking into account factors such as specialization (the analogue to bed inerchangeability) and the availability of ambulatory care (but not home visits) in hospital emergency rooms. The fundamental question to be answered is what amount of physician standby time is adequate to meet the needs of the group or the community. If this answer were available, one could then determine whether the current allocation in the group or community were excessive or insufficient. This is a problem that needs and deserves further work.

In conclusion, it might be pointed out that the application of a community-wide model, such as proposed for physicians, to the analysis of hospital capacity would also bring about significant changes in the estimates of legitimate standby reserve and therefore of service reserve. It should be clear from our description of how the magnitude of standby capacity is determined, that if all the hospitals in a community were considered to constitute a single pool in which beds were interchangeable, each hospital would need to maintain a much smaller number of vacant beds to meet fluctuations in demand.

One important aspect of manifest reserve is the temporal variability in its occurrence. We have already referred to increases in hospital efficiency that can be brought about by smoothing out variations in demand through appropriate scheduling. Studies of hospitals have shown interesting variations in occupancy by day of the week which suggest that appreciable hospital capacity is underutilized during weekends. London and Sigmond studied occupancy in 14 hospitals in Western Pennsylvania (227). Highest occupancy occurred on Monday and Tuesday and lowest occupancy on Saturday and Sunday. For all hospitals, the range was from 2.5 percent above average occupancy on Mondays to 4.3 percent below average occupancy on Saturdays. However, the range between highest and lowest values varied by hospital from 3.0 percent to 10.7 percent. Fluctuations were smaller for hospitals with higher average occupancy. Variability was largest in the pediatrics service and least in obstetrics. There were much larger reductions in occupancy during holidays: 15 percent below average for Thanksgiving day, 40 percent below average for Christmas day, and 18 percent below average for New Year's day. For some reason, possibly elective discharges, even occupancy on the maternity service was significantly depressed during these holidays: by 17, 33, and 7 percent respectively. The effect of holidays, for all cases was apparent some days before and after each holiday, lasting 6 days for Thanksgiving and 22 days for the Christmas–New Year season. Drosness et al. have reported similar fluctuations in average daily census, by day of the week, in 12 hospitals in Santa Clara County, California (214, Fig. 1, p. 66). Here, however, the peak in occupancy came later in the week, on Thursday, in all major services except pediatrics, which appeared to maintain a high census Monday through Thursday, but sank to the lowest level of all—about 18 percent below average—on Saturday. For all services combined, the range was from about 5 percent above average on Thursdays to 8 percent below average on Saturdays.

The precise meaning and consequences of fluctuations in hospital occupancy by day of week and during holidays have not been fully explored. If hospital staff are proportionately reduced during weekends and holidays, the hospital may be operating at comparable levels of productivity during these periods of time. If the hospital remains fully staffed and operative at all times, periods of low occupancy denote low productivity and inefficiency. In either case it is felt that periods of low occupancy represent a reserve that could be utilized and, in so doing, relieve some pressure for the building of new hospitals. Some studies have revealed an additional component of service reserve during the weekend occupancy slump: a reduction in service capacity even larger than that in bed occupancy. The evidence comes from studies of length of stay by day of admission. Lew has made a study of admissions, by day of the week, to hospitals in Western Pennsylvania (228). The results confirm the presence of a weekly rhythm for the flow of elective cases: admissions tending to be most frequent on Sundays and discharges on Saturdays. Emergency cases, as might be expected, arrive randomly throughout the week, but fall into rhythm by observing the Saturday discharge ritual. More significant, however, was the relationship between day of admission and length of stay. When cases were classified by diagnosis, whether medical or surgical, and whether emergency or elective in nature, it became clear that the length of stay was significantly longer for cases admitted during the second half of the week. The effect was not demonstrable in all cells of the classification, the frequency diminishing in the following order: medical elective, medical emergency, surgical elective, and surgical emergency. In the last category, the effect was more often absent than present. Crystal and Brewster made a similar study of 308 hospitals that participate in the statistical program of the Commission on Professional and Hospital Activities, using data for July to December 1964 (229). The findings for each of 5 diagnoses (without distinction as to degree of urgency) showed longer stays for admissions on Fridays and, especially, those on Saturdays. The effect was present irrespective of the mechanism used for paying hospital expenses. These findings confirm suspicions that during weekends the service capacity of the hospital is reduced to levels even below those of its bed capacity. The low occupancy ratio is therefore not evidence of service reserve in the true sense, but it does show the presence of unused or inoperative beds. Any increase in bed occupancy alone would merely decrease the efficiency of the hospital operation unless the ability of the hospital to service the additional patients were also increased. This is an excellent instance of the discrepancy between the measure of bed capacity and the actual service capacity of the hospital. The discrepancy apparently results from reductions in the pace of operations in the ancillary services such as laboratories, x-rays, operating rooms, etc. To sum up, there are during weekends and holidays more vacant hospital beds than is usual. In addition, the filled beds are not fully operative, in the sense that they are being serviced at a lower level than usual. Needless to say, this phenomenon is a concession to the cultural and social organizational characteristics of a society. Whether hospitals should be isolated from the prevailing rhythms of social life, and what might be the benefits and costs of such isolation, is a matter for debate. No doubt, factors other than the efficiency of the hospital itself would have to be considered.

Analogous phenomena of fluctuations in occupancy or nonoccupancy would be expected for ambulatory resources. The dimension of timing is especially significant in the analysis of the hospital emergency service. The literature includes some information on this matter. See, for example, Barry et al. (202), Skudder et al. (199), King and Sox (208), and Vaughan and Gamester (200). These studies, unfortunately, do not relate case load to service capacity. Hence no conclusion can be drawn about service overload or service reserve. The information is important, however, in planning for appropriate staffing and organization to meet demand. A similar situation prevails with respect to studies of the office practice of physicians, except that it may be easier to make some rough estimate of capacity. However, as we have already discussed, manifest reserve may be difficult to detect. Fluctuations of demand by day of the week have been reported for office practice. Eimerl and Pearson have reported, for a group of English and Welsh practitioners, that patient consultations on Mondays were almost double those for the next busiest day of the week. They conclude that "such pressure on Monday cannot bring advantages to either patient or doctor; further study is indicated" (181, p. 1151). Forbes et al. have reported that one-third of all "urgent" attendances, as requested by clients, occurred on Mondays and that there was a progressive decline each day thereafter (190). Hardman did not find such a systematic relation between day of the week and "late calls," but Monday was a day on which relatively many such calls were received (189). Baker has reported little fluctuation by day of week in his practice, except for the weekend and when the physician was off-duty (186)

Clute reported similar findings for general practitioners in Ontario and Nova Scotia (165, Table 19, p. 102). Monday was a busy day, but not strikingly so in comparison to some other days in the week. There was, however, a suggestion of bimodality, with a peak during the early part of the week, a trough on Wednesdays, another peak on Thursdays, and a decline to the lowest point on Sundays.

The significance of all this is somewhat ambiguous. One might make the same remarks concerning the need to adjust load to capacity for physicians as have been made for hospitals. One can be clear, in other words, about the need for capacity and load to vary in concert. Furthermore, one can suspect from fluctuations in the ratio of cases to normative capacity, the presence of either overload or latent, or manifest, reserve. Unfortunately, the data are seldom presented explicitly in this form. Even if they were, one would be hard put, in the absence of normative standards, to say what represents overload and what underemployment. With respect to fluctuations in capacity itself much less can be said. Some have argued that the hospital must oparate at an even, high capacity throughout the week and be fully staffed and operative to achieve this goal. The author has not heard the same argument applied to ambulatory care resources. This is because the model does not apply to the solo practitioner, although it might apply to the group practice. We have pointed out, furthermore, that it may not be possible or desirable to disengage fully the operations of medical care resources from the rhythms inherent in the social and cultural life of the community. This is a concept that requires further exploration and justification. In the meantime, at least one economist, Burton Weisbrod, has suggested that hospitals might smooth out fluctuations in demand by appropriate pricing policy (230). Possibly, the weekend and holiday bargain sale may yet become a feature of hospital prices. But what of the effect on clients, hospital staff, and their families?

LATENT SERVICE RESERVE. The notion of latent service reserve is a recognition of the fact that although a service-producing resource may appear occupied, a certain proportion of its effort may consist of activities that are either unnecessary or could be more efficiently or appropriately produced elsewhere. Latent service reserve is therefore detectable through a lack of fit between the needs of the client and the functions of the service-producing resource, both normatively defined. It manifests itself as a "misclassification" of patients under care by a resource. As already implied, at least two components go into the normative definition of fit: one is economic efficiency and the other medically or socially defined aspects of appropriateness. Generally, these two criteria are not in conflict, but they could be; hence the need to consider them separately.

Some degree of misclassification in the patient load is a characteristic of all service-producing resources. In the following discussion we shall not attempt anything near complete coverage. We shall be concerned almost entirely with hospital and physician care, partly because these will serve as examples of a more general phenomenon. Furthermore, the emphasis will be on hospitals. The greatest amount of work has been done in the hospital field. This is because the organized nature of hospital activities lends itself to critical study and because the increasing costs of hospital care have stimulated the search for less costly, but at least equally effective, alternatives. Studies of patient misclassification have taken one of several forms. These include (1) the need for admission, (2) the justification of repeated admissions, (3) the justification of length of stay, and (4) the justification of the patient's being under care at any given point in time. It is obvious that all these variants are concerned with two fundamental questions: Should the patient have been admitted at all, and at what point should he have been discharged? In some studies a further attempt has been made to determine what alternative resources would be more appropriate as a source of care. Naturally, this requires the development of a scheme for classifying patient needs and another, congruent, scheme for classifying resource functions. When such classification of patients and resources is carried out, a consequence is the generation of need estimates for resources other than the one under study. Accordingly, a reclassification of patients and resources is often a necessary first step in planning a more rational reordering of the medical care in a community (255). In this section we shall discuss the subject of misclassification by (1) presenting the findings of the major hospital studies known to the author, (2) discussing those aspects of method that are most critical in evaluating the findings of past studies and the design of future studies, and (3) summarizing the findings and methods of studies of misclassification of physician care.

Studies of the necessity for hospital admission recognize the presence of a discretionary element in the decision to admit. There are two elements of discretion: (1) whether the hospital, or some other resource, is the most appropriate site for care, and (2) whether admission must be immediate or may be scheduled to fit better into the hospital's capacity. These decisions, in the case of the hospitals, are largely under the control of the admitting physician. The physician's behavior is influenced, however, by a large number of factors that include the wishes of the client, the manner in which clients and physicians are related, including the method of remuneration, and the nature of the organizational linkage between the physician and the hospital, including methods for administrative control of physician behavior. For example, patients are admitted to the hospital more readily and kept there longer .when the supply of hospital beds is plentiful, there is no immediate financial penalty to the client, and there is a financial incentive to the physician. Certain aspects of these factors will be discussed in chapters on methods of remuneration and administrative controls in a subsequent volume.

Several studies have dealt with the necessity for admission to the hospital. Anderson and Sheatsley studied a representative sample of 50 general and special hospitals in Massachusetts during 1960–1961 (231). In the opinion of the admitting physicians, 70 percent of admissions were absolutely necessary and in 70 percent of cases admission was considered to be needed immediately. For the rest, there were various degrees of discretion. However, in only about 4 percent of cases did the physicians consider a site other than the hospital to be equally appropriate. For those for whom care in the hospital was not considered absolutely necessary, the patient had been admitted, nevertheless, for medical reasons in about 80 percent of cases, personal characteristics of the patient in about 20 percent of cases, and other factors in the patient's situation in about 15 percent. Since more than one factor was present in some cases, these percentages (80, 20, and 15 percent) exceed the total of those for whom admission was not absolutely necessary. Only 9 percent of physicians reported that patients exerted pressure ''fairly often'' or ''very often'' to be hospitalized. In interpreting these findings it ought to be realized that this is a study of the manner in which physicians perceive and report on their own decisions to admit patients. Evaluation by outsiders, possibly using a different set of criteria, could yield different results. One such study was conducted in Michigan general hospitals in 1958 (233). An important feature of this study was the formulation of standards for admission and for length of stay for about 20 diagnoses that accounted for the major share of hospital care. Hospital records were then used to determine justification for admission and length of stay. When admission or length of stay were judged to have been questionable, the patient's physician was interviewed and given an opportunity to explain his reasons for admitting the patient or for keeping him in the hospital for a period shorter or longer than provided for by the standards. The proportion of cases admitted unnecessarily was rather small: 4.3 percent, omitting 5 diagnoses in which admission was considered always mandatory. Comparable findings were later reported from a study of 5 general hospitals in Nassau County, New York, in which a similar method was used (247). In this instance, physicians from the surveyed hospitals judged that 3.4 percent of cases had been admitted unnecessarily. An outside consultant who had been instrumental in developing the standards (Dr. B. Payne) reviewed the same hospital records and judged that 4.6 percent of admissions had been unnecessary. However, because of the nature of the sample, the figures cited cannot be considered representative of all cases in all the general hospitals in Nassau County.

A distinctly greater degree of unnecessary use was found by Morehead et al. in a sample of hospital care received by families of the Teamsters Union in New York City. For all diagnoses, 15 percent of admissions were judged to have been unnecessary. This percentage varied markedly by department, with a range from 12 percent for medicine to 40 percent for pediatrics. Of even greater interest are the differences noted by type of hospital and type of physician (234, Tables 8–10, pp. 52–54). We have described these differences in a monograph on administrative control of quality (270). Here we need to note a major difference in the method used between the study of Michigan hospitals and the study by Morehead et al. In the second of these two studies, no specific standards were formulated. Two physicians of high reputation independently reviewed the complete hospital record for each patient. Differences between them were later resolved, in almost all cases, through joint discussion. How much of the difference in findings noted between the Michigan and the Teamster studies can be attributed to these differences in method cannot be said.

Reports of unnecessary hospital use have also come from other countries which differ markedly from the United States in the manner in which medical care is organized; where there is, in particular, a sharp separation of the physicians who are responsible for specialist care in the hospital from the general practitioners who are responsible for ambulatory care outside the hospital. Querido has reported the findings of a study of 290 requests for hospital admission which were made in 1954 by general practitioners in Amsterdam, Holland (235, pp. 52–58). Since the general practitioners who participated in the study were not a representative sample of all general practitioners in Amsterdam, the following findings should be viewed with some caution. The findings were that of all the requests for admission, 14 percent were rejected by the "screening physician" of the Municipal Medical Service, whose function it is to approve admissions after examining all cases either in the patient's home or in the offices of the Medical Service. The general practitioner who made the evaluation, in consultation with the screening physician, judged that, in an additional 51 percent, the pre-admission work-up by the general practitioner had been inadequate, taking into account the investigative resources available to the average practitioner. These judgments, which did not rest on explicitly formulated criteria, were subsequently challenged by the general practitioners on the grounds that they involved a misconception of the appropriate role of the general practitioner when, in his opinion, hospitalization was indicated.

Several studies of patient misclassification have emanated from Great Britain. Notable among these are the studies of the needs of patients in mental and chronic hospitals which began with the work of Lowe and McKeown in 1949 (264) were later pursued by McKeown and his associates at the University of Birmingham (266, 267) and, eventually, led to the formulation of the concept of the "balanced hospital community" (268). More specifically concerned with the need for admission is a study by Mackintosh, McKeown, and Garratt of patients in all general, special, and chronic hospitals in Birmingham during parts of 1958 and 1959 (236). "The appropriate hospital physician was asked to consider whether, on medical grounds alone, each patient required admission to hospital" (236, p. 815). Only 4.7 percent of the sample of patients evaluated were judged not to have required admission. The percentage of unnecessary admissions was 1.6 for general and special hospitals and 11.8 for chronic hospitals. These findings were at variance with those of other studies by Crombie and Cross and by Forsyth and Logan (269) (cited by Mackintosh et al.) which showed much higher prevalence of unnecessary use: about a quarter in each case. Dr. Crombie was therefore asked to review independently the records of 158 cases in one Birmingham hospital. The hospital physicians had judged 3.8 percent of these to have been admitted unnecessarily; Crombie judged 22.2 percent to have been so admitted. Further discussion of these cases with the hospital physicians revealed that an important reason for the discrepancy was the inclusion, in the hospital physicians' judgment, of social factors that justified hospital admission. This happened even though the original instructions had asked the physicians to exclude such factors from consideration. When such factors were excluded, the hospital physicians arrived at an estimate of unnecessary admission in 13.3 percent of patients in this hospital—a figure midway between the original estimate of 3.8 percent and the figure of 22.2 percent found by Crombie. The significance of these differences in judgment will be discussed in some detail below.

Another approach to the study of misclassification is to focus on multiple admissions to the hospital and, as we shall see, on unusually high utilizers of physician services. The National Health Survey regularly reports data on the frequency of admissions to the hospital in representative samples of the population (237). Woosley has reported a study of repeated hospital admissions among Michigan Blue Cross members (241). Acheson and Barr have demonstrated one aspect of the usefulness of an existing system of record linkage by publishing their findings on multiple spells of inpatient treatment during one year in Oxford County Borough, England (242). Their study includes, but also distinguishes, transfers among hospitals and readmissions from a non-hospital site. Earlier, Roemer and Myers reported on the occurrence of multiple hospital use in Saskatchewan with special emphasis on the characteristics of multiple utilizers (238). Querido has reported a study by van Wermeskerken of the psychodynamics of families whose children are repeatedly admitted to the hospital (248 pp. 208–214). Most studies of unusually high utilizers have focused on demonstrating the presence of a group of consumers who are persistently high utilizers and on elucidating the factors that account for this phenomenon. Our own interest, within the present context of measuring latent reserve, derives from the suspicion that repeated use may signify some defect in the organization of service or in the content or quality of care. Furthermore, the relatively few cases who are unusually high utilizers account for a disproportionately large share of services produced. For example, the National Health Survey reports the yearly data for 1960–1962 (Table IV.52). It

Table IV.52.   Percent distributions of persons, admissions and patient-days by number of yearly hospital admissions per person, U.S.A., 1960–1962

Frequency of Admissions	Percent of Persons in Population	Percent of Hospital Admissions	Percent of Hospital Days
None	91	—	—
Once	8	86	68
Twice	1	11	22
Three or more	0.3	3	11
TOTALS	100	100	100

SOURCE: Reference 237, Tables 1–3, pages 15–16.

is clear from these figures that only a little over 1 percent of persons in the population are admitted to the hospital more than once during any one year. These persons account for only 14 percent of hospital admissions, but for 32 percent of hospital days. Naturally, the frequency with

which multiple admissions are recorded depends, in part, on the length of
time during which observations are cumulated. This is an important fact
to keep in mind in comparing the findings of the various studies mentioned above: the longer the period of observation, the greater becomes
the relative weight accorded to the effect of multiple use. Table IV.53

Table IV.53.   Percent distribution of hospital admissions by frequency
of admissions per person, during specified periods of time in specified
locations

Period and Population	All Admissions	Once	More than Once
1 year U.S.A., 1960–1962 (Reference 237)	100	68	32
2 years, Michigan Blue Cross, 1956–1958 (Reference 241)	100	27	73
5 years, Saskatchewan, 1950–1954 (Reference 238)	100	24	76

SOURCE: As specified in the table.

gives the percent of hospital days accounted for by persons who have
experienced one or more than one admission during the periods specified.
    Having described roughly the dimensions of the phenomenon of mul-
tiple hospital use, the question that interests us in particular is the
magnitude of unnecessary use associated with this phenomenon. Unfortunately, information on this is very fragmentary. Acheson and Barr
reported that readmissions and transfers were strikingly more frequent
among the aged and somewhat more frequent for females than males at
all ages. Readmissions were not influenced by marital status or social
class, but transfers were more frequent for patients without spouses and
for persons in less favorable social circumstances. The most important
factors, however, arose from the natural history and treatment of the
disease process itself. Transfers are believed to have a larger social and
administrative component in their causation than do readmissions. The
study reported by Querido shows a distinct relationship between family
characteristics and the frequency of hospital admissions for children,
suggesting, by implication, that the reason for admission may be not
strictly medical. It is possible, however, that psychopathology in the
family might have been the result rather than the cause of multiple
admissions. Roemer and Myers paid more attention to social and medical

factors in the causation of multiple admissions in Saskatchewan. They summarize their findings as follows:

From this study, some of the characteristics of the hospital-repeaters can be defined. In the prairie setting in Saskatchewan, at least, they seem to be predominantly residents of the smaller towns and villages, rather than the large cities . . . The hospital repeaters are, indeed, more frequently old persons in any place of residence, who not only are more subject to chronic disease but whose home and family situation may be less satisfactory. They are, moreover, more often lonely persons—that is bachelors, widowers or divorcées—as distinguished from married individuals living with a spouse. They are persons predominantly with serious chronic disorders—heart disease, cancer, bronchial asthma and bronchitis, arthritis, cerebrovascular disease, non-infectious disease of the gastrointestinal and the genital organs, etc. Small part is played by the hypochondriac with changing ailments about whom we hear much complaint. They are persons whose repeated admissions are associated with progressively longer periods of hospital stay and eventually, after three admissions, with the likelihood of a surgical operation.

The epidemiological significance of these findings is easy enough to state, but extremely difficult to apply. It means that if we wish to make inroads on the causes of high hospital utilization, and large hospital expenditures, efforts should be concentrated on these hospital repeaters. It means more and more attention required on the effective management in the home and office of the chronic degenerative diseases. It means more and more attention to the aged. It means more and more attention to the housing and living conditions of people. It suggests the need for more prepayment of medical services, more home-care programs, more health education, and more research on methods of primary prevention of the chronic diseases (238, p. 480).

One may conclude that persons who experience multiple admissions are generally in need of some form of care, but that this form of care may not be necessarily, hospital care. This conclusion is supported by the findings of a study of extremely high hospital utilizers conducted for the medical program of the United Mineworkers Union by Koplin et al. (243). A salient characteristic of these patients was repeated surgical intervention and frequent change of physicians. Some patients had been under the care of 17 different physicians during the previous four years. A group of such patients were referred to three internists who undertook to review the cases, provide personal care, and to integrate all additional medical care received from other sources. Before-and-after comparisons showed 44 percent reduction in yearly hospital admissions and 48 percent reduction in yearly hospital days, representing substantial financial savings. Unfortunately, the study design did not provide for contemporaneous controls. Furthermore, it is not possible, from the experience of this highly selected group, to generalize about the magnitude of unnecessary use among all hospital repeaters. Nevertheless, it is reasonable to conclude that repeated hospital use corresponds to a segment of hospital capacity where latent hospital reserve is very likely to be revealed.

Another approach to the identification of misclassification is the justification of length of stay. Both unusually short and unusually long stays are believed by many to be particularly likely to involve unnecessary hospital use and, therefore, to reveal the presence of latent service reserve. The interest in unusually long stays in reinforced by the observation that a relatively small proportion of these account for a disproportionately large number of hospital days. For example, in 1963–1964, stays of 31 days or longer in short-term hospitals in the United States constituted 3 percent of discharges but accounted for 22 percent of hospital days. The relative saliency of long stays is even more marked among the aged. For the age group 65 and over, stays of 31 days or longer occurred in 6 percent of discharges and accounted for 26 percent of days (245). There are others, however, who believe that short periods of overstay associated with the much larger number of patients who fall between the extremes of length of stay, account, in the aggregate, for a much larger share of latent service reserve. Hence, attention has been directed to the justification of length of stay in all cases that depart from normatively defined limits set for each type of case. Concerning this, the reader may wish to consult another publication by the author that is exclusively devoted to this subject (270). Here it will be sufficient to mention briefly some of the major studies and their findings so that the reader may have some impression of their methods and of the scale of latent reserve due to inappropriate length of stay.

The study of admissions and length of stay in Michigan hospitals, to which we have already referred, revealed the findings shown in Table IV.-54 concerning the appropriateness of stay. On balance, unnecessary days

Table IV.54.   Percent of hospital discharges and hospital days judged inappropriately short or long, Michigan, 1958

Length of Stay	Percent of Discharges	Percent of Hospital Days
Inappropriately short	6.8	2.3
Inappropriately long	9.6	6.8

SOURCE: Reference 233, page 474, and Table 219, page 488.

exceeded inappropriately short days by 4.5 percent, indicating the magnitude of latent reserve generated by this phenomenon. The Nassau County study, which used similar methods, revealed roughly similar findings.

However, the precise percentages reported cannot be generalized because of the manner in which the sample was drawn. Of greater interest in this study was the degree of disagreement on appropriateness of stay between the hospital physicians who made the initial evaluation and the outside consultant (Dr. B. Payne) who reviewed each hospital record for a second time. Physicians from the several hospitals surveyed judged 13.4 percent of cases to have had inappropriate stay whereas the outside consultant, using the same explicit criteria, judged stay to have been inappropriate in 30.6 percent of cases. As already emphasized, this very large estimate of misclassification applies only to selected diagnoses in selected hospitals and cannot be generalized (247).

Other estimates of the extent of latent service reserve associated with unnecessary hospital use may be derived from the reported effects of administrative controls based on reviews of length of stay (249, 250, 270). One such estimate was the release of the equivalent of 900 hospital beds in the State of New Jersey. This corresponds to a little over 4 percent of the capacity of voluntary short-stay hospitals in that state. It should be clear, however, that this figure is an underestimate of latent service reserve actually present, since it represents only partial success in the less than universal application of administrative controls on length of stay.

A fourth approach to the study of misclassification in hospital use is to examine whether at any given time, usually during a single day, those who are in hospital need to be there. Such studies often involve analysis and classification of the service needs of the patient and their comparison with descriptively or normatively defined service functions of the institution in which they are. Sometimes there is the further attempt to determine what alternative institutional placement or kind of care would have been most appropriate. This means that descriptive or normative service functions have to be specified for the alternative sources of care. In some studies there is the further attempt to find out why patients who are in the hospital without current need for hospital services have not been more appropriately placed. All these evaluations may apply to all patients present in the hospital or only to a segment of these. A segment that has attracted special attention comprises all patients who have remained in hospital about 30 days or longer. The major reason for selecting this group of patients is, as we have said, the large number of days consumed by such patients and the presumption that long stay in a general hospital is often unnecessary. An additional reason is that, after prolonged stay, the needs of the patient are likely to be well documented and sufficiently stabilized to permit a valid judgment concerning the need for hospital stay and the assignment to an alternative facility. No matter what patient population is examined, a sample of patients in the hospital will not be representative of hospital discharges, since it will contain a larger proportion of patients with longer stays than is found among discharges. This is because patients in hospital are to some extent a residue of those who pass through the hospital. The "cross-sectional" view of the hospital service load obtained by studies of patients who are in hospital on a given day needs to be adjusted before it can be considered to represent the service load as a whole. Keeping these aspects of method in mind, it might be useful to review briefly the findings of some studies that have used this approach to the assessment of hospital use.

Rosenfeld et al. studied a sample of patients in four hospitals in Boston, Massachusetts, who, on a given day, were found to have been in hospital 30 days or longer (252). A physician evaluated each patient using predetermined guidelines pertaining to patient needs and facility functions. He judged that 42 percent of these patients did not require active hospital care. The 42 percent who did not need active hospital care comprised 14 percent who needed no medical facility, 12 percent who needed an "intermediate care facility," and 16 percent who needed an "extended chronic care facility." Of those who were in hospital without current need for active hospital care, 38 percent were there because the home was considered unsuitable, 28 percent because the family was reluctant to accept the patient, 25 percent because there were no suitable alternative facilities, and 9 percent for medical research. Needless to say, these findings, deriving as they do from a study of four selected hospitals, are not representative of the total community. However, a more recent study by Van Dyke et al. has shown an essentially similar picture for the ward services of the larger hospitals in New York City (254). Nine municipal and voluntary hospitals were studied. On a given day, 26 percent of patients in municipal hospitals and 21 percent of those in voluntary hospitals were found to have been in hospital for 30 days or longer. Of such patients, 41 percent were judged by the surveying physicians not to require the services of the general hospital on medical grounds. The proportion of those in hospital unnecessarily was 50 percent of long-stay patients in municipal hospitals. The proportion varied between 15 and 59 percent of long-stay cases in voluntary hospitals, with an average of 29 percent. The 41 percent of long-stay patients who were judged not to require active hospital care comprised the following segments as judged by physicians who assessed their needs: 19 percent who could have been discharged to their own homes or a substitute, 11 percent who needed a nursing home, and 10 percent who required care in some other institution. Patients were still in hospital unnecessarily because over one-third were waiting for hospital discharge arrangements to be made. In another third there were problems of finding a suitable place for the patient to go. A variety of factors, which included the need to increase the hospital's census, accounted for the final third of those who remained in the hospital without medical justification. To reiterate, this study pertains to ward patients only and does not represent the entire population of hospital patients in New York City. It does, however, concern a very large population for whom a considerable degree of public responsibility has been assumed.

Several studies of patient misclassification have emanated from Rochester, New York, under the stimulus of active community planning toward a more rational allocation of resources. Wenkert and Terris report the findings of one study in which a team composed of an internist, a public health nurse and a social worker reviewed the needs of patients in hospitals and other facilities. The study was confined to patients who had received at least 30 days of care in a general hospital or more than three months of continuous care in another institution or at home. In the opinion of the survey team, 70 percent of patients in general hospitals required short-term hospital care (less than 30 days), 15 percent required long-term hospital care (more than 30 days), and 3 percent were allocated to each of skilled nursing homes, unskilled nursing homes, and organized home care programs. The proper disposition of the patient was undetermined in 3 percent of long-stay cases. Varying degrees of misclassification were present in other facilities, as well: 11 percent of patients in nursing homes, 56 percent of patients in long-term hospitals, and 50 to 60 percent of patients under the care of public health agencies in the home, for periods of three months or over (255, Table 2, p. 1291). A second study of Rochester hospitals, conducted by Browning and Crump, concerned itself with all patients on the medical and surgical services of general hospitals rather than only those who had remained 30 days or longer (256, 257). In addition to this important difference, the study is notable for a number of interesting refinements in method. These include (1) the use of two teams of physicians, one recruited from the hospitals surveyed and one from outside the community, to survey the same hospitals; (2) the allocation of judges to hospitals in a manner that assures a random sample while it corrects for the effects of variability in judgment among the surveyors; and (3) the development of a scheme for specifying patient need as well as the characteristics of the resources to which patients were to be assigned. The teams of physicians and surgeons recruited from the local hospitals arrived at the

Table IV.55.   Percent of general hospital beds that, on a representative day, were occupied, occupied unnecessarily or occupied by an elective admission, according to hospital service, Rochester, New York, 1961

Characteristics of Occupancy	Medical Service	Surgical Service	Both Services
Percent of surveyed beds that were occupied	89.6	90.1	86.6
Percent of occupied beds that were occupied unnecessarily	20.1	9.6	14.3
Percent of occupied beds that contained an elective admission	18.5	46.0	33.4

SOURCE: Reference 256, Table 4.

judgments shown in Table IV.55 concerning the appropriateness of general hospital use, on the medical and surgical services respectively, having regard to the range of alternative resources available in the Rochester community. Assuming that surgeon surveyors are no different in their judgments from physician surveyors, there are interesting differences by type of service. Surgical patients are less likely to be in the hospital unnecessarily but more likely to be there for non-urgent conditions. For both medical and surgical services combined, on a given day in Rochester, the general hospitals contain 13 percent manifest reserve uncorrected for minimum turnover interval and standby capacity (unoccupied beds), 11 percent latent reserve (beds unnecessarily occupied), and 29 percent of beds which represent a margin of flexible use since they are occupied by patients whose admission is elective. The patients who did not need to be in hospital had service needs as follows: home (no service) 17.5 percent, ambulatory service 36.8 percent, home care (private physician and visiting nurse) 14.0 percent, organized home care 7.0 percent, nursing home care 12.3 percent, long-term hospital care 10.5 percent, and other, 1.7 percent.

The Rochester surveys are an excellent illustration of the use of patient classification studies to generate estimates of need for various services in a community. It should be emphasized, however, that what is achieved is a more appropriate rearrangement of the total current service load without reference to that portion of need that remains undiscovered within the population. Preston et al. have modified this general approach to generate an estimate of bed needs for a university hospital, classified by type of bed (261). Concurrent daily census studies were made of nursing and medical needs of inpatient, outpatient, and emergency room patients. Classification, with certain guidelines provided, was entrusted to those professional persons who were operationally responsible for the decisions concerning the care of patients. The authors consider this approach to have a certain operational validity since it is such decisions that determine the manner in which the hospital is to be used. There were no estimates of reliability. It is concluded that "7 percent of the mean daily census was composed of patients who in the opinion of the responsible physician could have been cared for most appropriately outside the traditional hospital" (261, p. 769). About 30 percent of the remaining patients were assigned to the "self-care" category. The mean daily demand for hospital care was 241, with 215 already in hospital, an additional 21 generated by the outpatient department, and another 4 generated by the emergency service. The total of 215 cases was distributed with respect to type of care as follows: intensive care 10.4 percent, intermediate care 49.3 percent, self-care 28.7 percent, long-term care 7.5 percent, observation and care 0.8 percent, and overnight care 3.3 percent. From these data the authors project bed needs for each type of service. The method for doing this is described in a report of an earlier study that used a similar procedure to determine the need for overnight facilities for ambulatory patients (262). Essentially, this consists of adding to the estimate of need an appropriate number of beds to allow for fluctuations in demand (standby reserve) under the assumption that the average daily census in each category of service (and combination of these categories) is Poisson-distributed.

Similar studies of misclassification, based on evaluation of single-day censuses, have been reported from Britain. We have already referred to the studies by Lowe, McKeown, and their colleagues at the University of Birmingham. These studies focused, however, on the classification of the need for service of patients in mental and chronic disease hospitals. By comparison, misclassification in general hospitals was considered to be negligible, as illustrated in the estimates of Table IV.56 which form the basis for regrouping patients in Birmingham hospitals according to type of facility needed for their care.

As we have shown in the foregoing discussion of the justification of admissions to hospital, other studies from Great Britain, including one by the Birmingham group itself, have demonstrated that misclassification in general hospitals is far from negligible, contrary to the assumption incorporated in the table cited above. Forsyth and Logan, working at the University of Manchester, have reported the findings of a survey of a sample of patients in Barrow and Furness Group of hospitals in the Manchester Hospital Region. The nine "hospitals" in this group range in size from 10 to 189 beds and include institutions that in the United States might be classified as general hospitals, chronic disease hospitals,

Table IV.56.   Percent distribution of patients in specified facilities by type of care needed, Birmingham, England, 1957

Reassessment of Type of Care Needed	Present Location			
	Mental Hospital[a]	Chronic Disease Hospital	General and All Other Hospitals	Total
Full hospital care	13	20	100	54
Limited hospital care without mental supervision	2	53	—	9
Limited hospital care with mental supervision	73	20	—	31
Hostel only	12	7	—	6
TOTALS	100%	100%	100%	100%

SOURCE: Reference 268, page 701.
[a] Patients in mental deficiency institutions are excluded.

nursing homes, and homes for the mentally defective. The classification of patient service needs was made by a physician attached to the research team who made quarterly rounds of the hospitals and discussed each case with the physician in charge of the patient or his deputy. On this basis the surveying physician determined the "clinical necessity for admission," assuming a certain level of general practitioner care available outside the hospital. The findings for four quarters combined, by type of service and by sex are shown in Table IV.57.

Table IV.57.   Percent distribution of male and female patients in specified hospital services by type of care needed, Barrow and Furness Group of Hospitals, England, c. 1967

Classification of Patient Needs	General Medicine		General Surgery		Pediatrics
	Male	Female	Male	Female	Both Sexes
In need, on clinical grounds, of care that could only be given as an in-patient	54	43	81	84	67
Not on clinical grounds alone, in need of in-patient care	25	42	9	9	23
Doubtful of classification	21	15	9	6	10
TOTAL	100%	100%	100%	100%	100%

SOURCE: Reference 269, page 83.

These findings fully confirm the expectation of significant misclassification in general hospitals and other institutions. The relatively small extent of misclassification in the pediatric service is at variance with the findings by Morehead et al., who reported that pediatric admissions were the least likely to be necessary when compared with other hospital services (234). The relatively lower levels of misclassification in the surgical services is, however, similar to the finding by Browning and Crump in Rochester, as shown above (256).

As we have already pointed out, studies of misclassification that focus on persons who are already under care fail to reveal that portion of need that remains undiscovered within the population. A more recent survey in the Rochester area has met this objection by sampling persons 65 years of age or over irrespective of where they may have been (258–260). A standard method was developed for assessing health care needs which involved placing each person in the appropriate position along two scales. One scale described physical need in a progression of "no care," "congregate living," "at home, with public health nursing," "coordinated home care," "nursing home care," "intensive nursing care," "chronic-illness hospital care," and "general hospital care." A second scale described mental status as "no mental impairment," "intermittent supervision needed," "continuous supervision needed," "marked depression," or "menace to themselves or others." Depending on where a given person was at the time of the survey, he was evaluated by one or more of a public health nurse, an internist and/or a psychiatrist. It was then concluded whether each person needed care and, if so, at what level. Perhaps the single most striking finding of the survey is the level of autonomy and good health enjoyed by the elderly. As many as 83 percent lived at home without receiving care from any health service organization, and an additional 7 percent lived at home but received services from a nursing agency. Furthermore, fully 75 percent of the elderly had neither "mental impairment" nor needs for "physical care." The second important finding, and the one germane to our current concern, was the remarkable degree of misclassification (or "misplacement," to use the terminology of the investigators) that was evident wherever the elderly were found to be. This was true for the entire sample. It was also true in a sample of new admissions to chronic disease institutions which was studied to determine whether "misplacement" occurred *ab initio* or was mainly the result of changes in the condition of the patient without corresponding changes in the placement. Table IV.58 shows the findings for the two samples. It is remarkable how many admissions to long-stay facilities start out by being in the wrong place. Another finding is the markedly different proportions of misplacement among the several institutions: ranging from 7 percent of the aged in general hospitals to 94 percent of the aged in the state mental hospital. The survey also found that the risk of becoming misplaced was not equally incurred by all the aged. Misplacement occurred more frequently among the aged who were relatively younger, were male (except in nursing homes), and who belonged to the lower socioeconomic groups. "In the state mental hospital, all patients in social classes 4 and 5 were misplaced" (259, p. 50).

The data in Table IV.58 indicate the magnitude of latent service

Table IV.58. Percent of persons in specified locations judged to require care at a level different from that considered appropriate to each location, Monroe County, N.Y., 1964 or 1966

Location	All Aged[a]	New Admissions[b]
All locations	41	47
At home	42	—
Boarding homes	59	—
Homes for the aged	14	—
County home	25	—
County Infirmary	37	41
Nursing homes	19	47
State hospital	94	88
General hospitals	7	—

SOURCE: Reference 258, Tables 1 and 2, pages 330 and 331.
[a] Sample of all persons 65 or over.
[b] Sample of persons 65 or over who were newly admitted to chronic-care institutions during 5 months in 1966.

reserve in each type of facility considered independently. It is necessary, however, to consider the net effect of the reapportionment of patients among facilities, since some patients will require higher levels of care, whereas others will require lower levels, or no care at all. In this survey, the dominant fault was for patients to be placed in settings that provided higher levels of care than they required. Of all aged patients in chronic disease institutions, 37 percent required lower levels of care and 2 percent required higher levels. Of all admissions to such institutions, 37 percent required lower levels and 11 percent higher levels of care. There are, in addition, persons who do not receive care but who require care of specified levels. When theoretical reallocations were made, one could compare current use of facilities and optimal usage, indicating where the net surplus and net deficit were to be found at the community level of accounting. Table IV.59 shows the findings. It is clear that, as far as this population is concerned, there was no surplus of resources except in psychiatric inpatient care, and the major deficits were in resources for congregate living and public health nursing services in the home.

Table IV.59. Percent distribution of persons aged 65 or over by the level of care they receive and the level of care they are judged to require, Monroe County, New York, 1964

Level of Care	Those Who Receive Care	Those Who Require Care[a]
All levels	100.0	100.0
Acute medical care	0.8	0.8
Subacute medical care	0.1	0.1
Psychiatric inpatient care	1.4	0.1
Intensive nursing care	0.4	0.3
Institutional nursing care	2.6	2.7
Congregate living	1.6	5.9
Public health nursing service at home	2.4	6.7
No physical care from health service organization	90.7	83.4

SOURCE: Reference 259, Table 6, page 49.

[a] Includes those who receive care appropriately at each level plus those who do not receive care but require it at the indicated level.

Our next task is to consider how much credence can be placed in studies which generate estimates of latent service reserve, how errors in such estimates may arise, and how they may be minimized. It is clear that the discovery and measurement of latent service reserve involves judgments about the appropriateness of admission and of length of stay, having regard to the descriptive or normative functions assigned to the resource that provides care. The author has considered the appropriateness of admissions and length of stay to be one component of estimates of the quality of care and has, accordingly, discussed the problems of method in detail within that context (270). Here we shall deal with only selected aspects of method that pertain directly to the assessment of latent service reserve. The first question to consider is who makes the estimates. This is important because the professional identification of the surveyor determines the whole approach to evaluation, including the internalized values and criteria that are used to make the judgments. In the studies that we have reviewed there has been a wide variety of surveyors, including physicians, nurses, and social workers, acting separately or as a team. It is not likely that the representatives of the several professions will evaluate patient needs or facility functions similarly, nor that their knowledge of the potential of alternative resources will be similar. Needless to say, within each profession there are further distinctions by specialty. For example, most physicians are not sharply aware of the rehabilitative needs of many patients. The source of information is another variable in method that is likely to influence the resulting assessment. Information may be obtained from the medical record with or without supplementation by nursing and social service records, interview with the attending physician, interview with other professionals such as nurses, social workers, physical therapists, and the like, and from actual examination of the patient by one or more of the foregoing professionals. While all these aspects of method can be expected to influence the findings, actual evidence concerning their effects is fragmentary, to say the least. In the study of stay in Michigan hospitals it was estimated that additional information obtained by interviews with the attending physician brought about reclassification in 12.6 percent of the total number of cases studied (233). Zimmer has reported no difference in judgments concerning need for hospital stay between physicians who only had access to the patient's record and physicians who were also permitted actually to examine the patient. However, since it is not known how often patients were, in fact, examined, this finding cannot be accepted at face value (277). In a study by Zimmer and Groomes of the appropriateness of stay in nursing and boarding homes, the agreement between two nurses, on the one hand, and two physicians, on the other, was of a very low order. However, the two nurses agreed between themselves to a greater extent than did the two physicians. Nurses were more critical of the use of nursing homes and boarding homes than were the physicians: 40 percent questioned by one or both observers versus 16 percent (278).

In the most recent of the Rochester surveys, Berg et al. report high levels of agreement among nurses, internists, and psychiatrists in assigning aged persons to specified levels of care. For example, there was a correlation coefficient of 0.95 percent between the judgments of two teams, each consisting of one nurse and one internist, who evaluated the same patients in chronic care facilities. In the study of patients in a state mental hospital, the correlation coefficient was even higher between judgments of psychiatrists on the one hand and of a nurse-internist team on the other. In the study of admissions to chronic disease facilities, independent judgments by a nurse and a physician agreed in 90 percent of judgments made. Since for the remaining 10 percent, in which there was disagreement, the final adjudication was as likely to be in favor of the nurse as of the physician, it was concluded that "nurses make such judgments about as reliably as physicians" (259, pp. 46–47). Unfortunately, levels of agreement among members of a single profession or between members of different professions are not often reported to be so high. For example, in a study reported by White et al. (263), nurses agreed with the physician in 67 percent of cases involving the allocation of patients in a general hospital to one of three levels: intensive care, intermediate care, and self-care. The frequency with which the nurse agreed with the physician differed according to certain patient characteristics, but did so most markedly according to level of care as determined by the physician. The nurse was in agreement in 58 percent of cases assigned by the physician to intensive care, in 88 percent assigned to intermediate care, and in 35 percent assigned to self-care. Nurses were as likely to assign patients to intensive care as were physicians, except that very often they bestowed this distinction on different patients. Out of 194 patients assigned to intensive care either by the nurse or by the physician, there was agreement in only 40 percent of cases. Physicians were significantly more likely to estimate that patients were ready for self-care. Here the disagreement levels were very high. Concerning persons thought to be ready for self-care, either by the nurse or by the physician, both agreed in only 27 percent of cases. Such disparities among studies in reported levels of reliability require an explanation. The critical factor appears to be the extent to which procedures are standardized, so that all assessors use the same criteria to classify patients. Berg et al. took pains to assure comparability in this respect. White et al. did not, because their intent was to determine to what extent judgments by physicians, which were assumed to be valid, could be replicated by carefully structured nursing evaluations. The findings were disappointing, to say the least. It would not be proper to conclude, however, that the nurses were necessarily wrong or the physicians necessarily correct in their evaluations. An external criterion of validity is notably lacking in this instance.

As we have suggested, part of the difference between the judgments of different observers is likely to be explained by differences in internalized values and criteria. The nature and content of the criteria used to arrive at judgments of misclassification are of central importance. Almost all the studies of misclassification that we have reviewed specify that judgments be made on the basis of the presence or absence of "medical" or "clinical" need, often with the additional specification that psychological, social, and other situational factors be excluded. We have also seen that such factors are precisely those that account, at least in part, for admission and for continued stay. In the study reported by Mackintosh et al. (236), social factors were also the major reason for the discrepancy in judgment between the attending physicians and the external reviewer. Accordingly, one must consider, first, whether the distinction between "medical" factors and "psychological or social factors" is sufficiently clear to permit disentanglement in the assessment of individual needs. Second, one must consider whether psychological and social needs are not perfectly legitimate reasons for the use of the facility in question. The manner in which these questions are answered, conceptually as well as operationally, is expected to influence profoundly the assessment of latent reserve. Another significant characteristic of the criteria used is the extent to which they are formalized and explicitly stated. Such specification applies not only to the elucidation of service needs, but also to the specification of the legitimate service functions of the several medical care resources to which the patient could be allocated. Furthermore, specification includes at least two components: one concerns the manner in which the evaluation is to be made, what aspects of need are to be considered and the like, and another concerns the specification of the decision rules that determine congruence between patient needs and resource functions. Examples of specification that merely structure the process of evaluation without specifying the decision rules are to be found in the reports by Rosenfeld et al. (252, p. 143), and by Browning and Crump (256, pp. 9–15). Van Dyke et al. provide guides to the classification of service resources as well as decision rules for referral to a public health nursing agency (254, pp. 107–112). The method used in the Michigan study, especially as further developed by Payne, tends to emphasize the decision rules concerning admission and length of stay (233, 271). A serious difficulty in the formulation of such decision rules is the rather fluid and imprecise nature of medical opinion concerning length of hospital stay for specified diagnostic categories. Regional differences in length of stay for the same diagnoses have been reported in this country (272, Table 2, p. 69). Logan and Eimerl have assembled information on the remarkable, and largely unexplained, differences in diagnosis-specific length of stay in different countries. These are accompanied by equally unexplained differences in the incidence of hospitalization by diagnosis (174, Tables 3 and 4, pp. 305, 307). Acheson and Feldstein have examined some of the factors that seem to influence decisions concerning length of stay of maternity cases in British hospitals (273). Innes et al. have assembled data that demonstrate variability in seemingly acceptable length of stays for specified diagnoses, and have shown that, under defined conditions, length of stay can be considerably shortened without injury to the patient (274). Similarly, Berg et al. have reported that it is possible to halve the hospital stay of healthy newborn infants with low birth weight without apparent injury and with possible benefit to the infant and mother (275). This suggests that widely accepted criteria that govern length of stay may not rest on valid grounds but may themselves need to be revised. Needless to say, well-controlled studies are required for this purpose.

Certain difficulties arise in the specification of the service functions of the resources to which patient needs most clearly correspond. In the opening sections of this chapter we referred to the remarkable difficulty of classifying the large number of facilities that go under the rubric of "nursing home." Indeed, some studies of misclassification have had to devise or adopt special, hypothetical classifications of the kind of facilities to which patients might be assigned. Rosenfeld et al. have devised and described the following hypothetical types: "facility for active medical care," "facility for extended chronic care," "facility for intermediate care," and "non-medical facility" (252, p. 143). Van Dyke et al. adopted for one phase of their study the "Columbia Village" classification, developed by the District of Columbia Department of Public Welfare, which comprises: "essentially outpatient care," "total organized program at home," "institutional–protective environment," "institutional–mainly personal care," "institutional–skilled nursing care in addition," and "institutional–special nursing care in addition" (254, p. 81). An important consideration, then, is precisely what alternative the assessor has in mind when he decides that a resource other than the hospital is most appropriate for a given patient. Does the assessor decide on the basis of what exists in the community or on the basis of what should exist? If he decides on the former grounds, is he aware, on the one hand, of the problems of effecting a successful transfer and, on the other, of the limitations and capabilities for care of the alternative resource? Studies that have explored the effects of these distinctions include those by Van Dyke et al. and by Browning and Crump. Van Dyke et al. compared the judgments of the physician assessors, who base their recommendations on service needs "without regard to socioeconomic problems" with those of social workers who were asked to consider "whether or not the study physician's plan was feasible in view of the social problems they uncovered . . . The social worker's discharge plan of choice reflected what seemed to her to be practical and available, in view of her added investigation of the case. Her decision was not qualified by known shortages or waiting periods of certain types of care"

(254, pp. 69–70). Table IV.60 gives the percent of 248 patients allocated to specified sources of care by the survey physicians and by the social workers respectively. It also gives, for comparison, whatever plans for discharge the hospital staff had developed at the time of the survey (254, Table 5–1, p. 102). Social workers appear to be less certain of the ultimate disposition of several of the cases and of the ability of the patients' family to cope. Insufficient discharge planning appears to be an important failing of the hospital staff. In evaluating this piece of information the reader should remember that all patients had been in the hospital at least 30 days!

Table IV.60.   Percent distribution of patients in hospital 30 days or longer, according to plan for care recommended by physicians, social workers, and hospital staff. Selected hospitals, New York City, 1961

Plan for Care	Physician	Social Worker	Hospital Staff
Home or substitute	47	38	32
Nursing home	28	31	20
Other institution	25	19	17
Unascertained	0.4	12	1
No plan	—	—	30
TOTAL	100%	100%	100%

SOURCE: Reference 254, Table 5–1, page 102.

Browning and Crump asked their physician and surgeon surveyors to make two estimates of unnecessary care for all patients in the medical and surgical services of general hospital on any one day, one estimate based on what alternative resources were currently available in the community and another on the basis of the presence of "optimum facilities" as defined in the study. It is likely that the estimates based on current resources took into account simply the types of facilities available and disregarded the quantitative capacity of such facilities to absorb an additional load. The findings of locally recruited physicians and surgeons were as shown in Table IV.61. It is clear from the table, that the degree of misclassification depends on the nature of the assumptions concerning alternative resources. Forsyth and Logan specify their assumptions as follows (269, pp. 82–83) :

Certain assumptions were made as well; for example it was assumed that general practitioners were fulfilling their role inherent in the structure of the National Health Service and were willing, aided by the domiciliary services of the local authority, to undertake home care. It was assumed also that out-patient departments could be organized as polyclinics and had all the diagnostic facilities readily available. In fact, of course, none of these assumptions applied. Never-

Table IV.61.   Percentage of persons unnecessarily hospitalized, Rochester, New York, 1961

	Percent of Beds Occupied Unnecessarily	
Service	Present Facilities	"Optimum Facilities"
Surgical	9.6	11.0
Medical	20.1	30.2
Both services	14.3	19.6

SOURCE: Reference 256, Table 4.

theless, the assessment of clinical need does indicate some of the possibilities inherent in the present structure of the Health Service, for we must assume that future policy can only aim at bringing the promise to reality.

Another problem in evaluating the appropriateness of hospital admissions and length of stay is raised by the large extent of disagreement among judges. Because the majority of cases are judged to be appropriately placed, the amount of agreement appears to be reasonably high. It is when one considers the extent of agreement on cases concerning which doubt has been raised by at least one assessor that the magnitude of disagreement becomes evident. Table IV.62 summarizes the findings of

Table IV.62.   Reliability of judgments on appropriateness of hospital use

Source and Nature of Study	Percent of Cases Questioned by One or More Judges	All Full Agreement as Percent of All Cases	Full Agreement on Inappropriate Use as Percent of Questionable Cases
Morehead (234): two judges	26	88	53
Browning (276): two judges	18	86	20
Zimmer (277): charts only. Two judges	19	85	23
Zimmer (277): pooled data, four judges	27	73	6
Zimmer and Groomes (278): two outside physicians	8	84	0
Zimmer and Groomes (278): two nurses examining same cases as above	20	76	40

several studies that have measured the reliability of judgments concerning the appropriateness of admissions, of length of stay, or both. It is claimed by some that explicit formulation of criteria governing judgment will improve reliability. While this appears to be a reasonable expectation, it has not been proved by actual observation. Browning and Crump believe that they were able to minimize the effect of observer variability, as well as other factors associated with sampling, through rotating all observers through all hospitals in a manner determined by a Greco-Latin square (256).

An interesting aspect of disagreement between observers that has attracted some attention is the possibility of bias resulting from the nature of the association between the assessor and the patient or institution under study. It is reasonable to believe that physicians will be less critical of their own practice, or of the practice of their immediate colleagues, than they will be of the practice of others. This may reflect differences in criteria or standards as well as undue leniency or severity. Table IV.63 compares the findings of several studies which have looked into the difference between "internal" and "external" assessments or audits. One may conclude from these data that persons more or less closely associated with the care under appraisal are less likely to be critical of it. However this is not invariably the case. A very interesting exception is the opposite finding when interns and residents judge the necessity for continued care for long-term patients in general hospitals. This may represent a major disparity in criteria used, since interns and residents may be overly sensitive to their own need to learn as they provide care. In examining the data cited above, the reader should be careful not to use the value of the percentages as an indication of the level of misclassification. The nature of the sample used may not justify such generalization. Furthermore, in some of the studies cited (for example, that by Wenkert and Terris) the difference observed is not one merely between internal and external assessment but includes other differences, such as that between a physician and a team including a nurse and a social worker.

Finally, it is important to consider carefully the problem of representative sampling in studies of latent service reserve. Misclassification is likely to vary widely by type of hospital, hospital department, and case mix. As we have already emphasized, the evaluation of patients in hospital on any given day does not yield a representative picture of misclassification among hospital discharges. Furthermore, because only the presence or absence of misclassification on a single day is determined, there are no estimates of the bed-days of hospital capacity lost due to

Table IV.63.   Percent of cases judged to represent unnecessary hospital use, according to method of assessment

Source of Data and Nature of Study	Percent of Cases Considered to Represent Unnecessary or Inappropriate Use	
	Internal Assessment	External Assessment
Mackintosh et al. (236). Need for admission judged by physicians for their own patients compared with judgment of external assessor who reviewed medical records		
a. Initial comparisons	3.8	22.2
b. After reconsideration of social factors by the patients' physicians	13.3	22.2
Nassau County Study (247, Tables 1a and 1b). Local hospital physicians compared with outside consultant using same criteria		
a. Admissions	3.4	4.6
b. Length of stay	13.4	30.6
Browning and Crump (256, Table 4). Physicians recruited from hospitals surveyed compared with physicians recruited from outside the community. Appropriateness of being in hospital on a given day		
a. Assuming present community facilities	14.3	18.8
b. Assuming optimal community facilities	19.6	23.8
Wenkert and Terris (255, Table 2).		
a. Residents and interns compared with survey team of physician, nurse and social worker. Patients in general hospital 30 days or longer	57	15
b. Agency staff compared with survey team of physician, nurse and social worker. Patients receiving nursing service at home for 3 months or longer.	19[a]	55
Zimmer and Groomes (278, p. 17). Physicians in charge of the patient compared with outside physicians. Patients in nursing and boarding homes.	14.7	14.9

[a] Visiting nurse service considered adequate substitute for organized home care.

misclassification. Such estimates would require information on how many days in each completed stay are unnecessary.

It is now time to return to our classification of service reserve and consider the second component under latent service reserve: that portion of capacity that could be released through the introduction of more productive and efficient ways of running the hospital. We have indicated in a previous section some of the ways in which this may be done. In a subsequent section we shall have more to say about the more productive use of personnel. However, the author has limited knowledge of studies which have measured the amount of capacity released through the introduction of more productive ways of using the hospital. One exception is a study, reported by Querido, of unproductive use of time during hospitalization (248, pp. 127–134). This was a study of 10 hospital departments in Amsterdam, including surgical, medical, and other services in private, municipal, and university hospitals. All patients were observed by one physician throughout their stay. The medical regimen prescribed was not questioned; hence the quality of care is not at issue. The object was to measure delay in effectuating the medical regimen. Delays that did not contribute to lengthening stay were not included. If two or more delays were concurrent, only the longest was counted. "As ineffective days were counted 24-hour units in which—without medical grounds— no progress was made towards the purpose of the hospital admission" (248, p. 130). Using these guidelines, it was found that of 389 patients studied, 260 (67 percent) had some delay that added up to 1339 "ineffective" days, or 17 percent of the total length of stay for all patients. The causes for delay are cited in some detail. Table IV.64 presents a summary. The single most important reason was "lack in decision" which accounted for 37 percent of ineffective days. The second most important reason was "needless or useless admission" which accounted for 10 percent of ineffective days. If this last cause is excluded, ineffective days constitute 15 percent of total stay for this group of patients. The factors that contribute to "lack in decision" are poorly understood. Querido comments as follows: "It may be that physicians, working under fairly heavy stress have a tendency to postpone decisions in which circumstances allow this, as a reaction to the frequent situation in which a decision must be instantly forthcoming" (248, p. 132). Accordingly, there were personal variations in such behavior. The distribution of reasons for delay also varied by department. There were, however, no clear differences between teaching and nonteaching hospitals or between municipal and private hospitals. These findings are extremely interesting because they provide elegant confirmation of certain features in our

Table IV.64.   Percent of hospital days judged ineffective, by factors that caused delay in effective care, Amsterdam, Holland, c. 1955

Cause for Delay	Percent of Ineffective Days
Bottlenecks in Treatment and Diagnostic Facilities: clinical laboratory, anatomical laboratory, x-ray department, operating room, etc.	26
Delay in Consultation	4
Lack of Communication and Decision: lack of contact between staff members, lack in decision	46
Factors Outside the Hospital: waiting for information, needless or useless admission, patient not in condition, delay in transfer, delay in discharge	24

SOURCE: Reference 248, Table 53, page 131.

model. First, they sustain the distinction between "waiting time" and "service time" as two components of length of stay or "holding time." They also suggest that bed capacity may be out of balance with the capacity of service facilities, thus creating the "bottlenecks" which generate about 26 percent of ineffective days. This lack of congruence may, of course, be a matter of scheduling rather than of disparity in total capacities. Deficiencies in communication and decision-making may also explain part of the diseconomies associated with hospital size. Since control over physician decisions and schedules is even more tenuous in most U.S. hospitals, it would be interesting to pursue such studies here in hospitals of different size and with differing modes of organization.

So far we have confined our attention to the ferreting out of latent service reserve in hospitals. We shall now turn our attention to seeking out such misuse of the service capacity of health personnel, with special emphasis on physicians providing ambulatory care. We shall, however, mention other health professionals as well and refer to the misuse of personnel potential in a variety of settings. Before we reach the substantive part of our subject, it would be well to point out some peculiarities that distinguish the analysis of latent service reserve for physicians from that for hospitals. First, the initiative for beginning care generally belongs to the patient or a person acting on his behalf. These usually determine not only whether care is to be initiated, but also, to a varying extent, the time and place of care, as well as the physician's first impression of the urgency of need. Professional control over the exploitation of the ambulatory care resource is therefore somewhat attenuated, and a great deal of attention focuses not on the efficient operation of the resource, but on the psychological and social factors that influence the behavior of clients. This is not to say that the efficient operation of the ambulatory care resource is any the less important, but that additional considerations of a complex nature, not so amenable to administrative control, enter the picture. Where hospitals are concerned, it is easier to think that administrative control over the behavior of physicians and other staff will bring about the desired level of efficient operations. Other distinctions need to be made, where health personnel are concerned, irrespective of the place of their employment. One is the provision of unnecessary care, often referred to as "abuse." The second is the performance of tasks by the health professional which are either beyond or beneath his level of training and competence. There are therefore two variants of misuse which together correspond to the notion of "misclassification" in the use of the hospital. Incidentally, the fact that one component of misclassification is known as "abuse" highlights our first contention, that the client is seen to be a more active and exigent participant in the system under evaluation. One seldom hears speak of hospital "abuse," even though it takes place. Needless to say, the notion of "abuse" of the services of the physician or of the hospital should be widened to cover unnecessary care for which the physician himself is responsible. Or, preferably, one should speak of unnecessary or inappropriate care. Finally, certain modifications to the evaluation of latent service reserve derive from differences in ways in which capacity and service load are viewed for the hospital as compared to the physician providing ambulatory care. These differences have already been discussed in a previous section. In Table IV.65 is a listing of analogous, though not necessarily identical, variables for hospital and ambulatory care, which can be the object of study in seeking latent service reserve.

With respect to initiation of care, two questions arise: (1) whether care is necessary or appropriate in terms of the physician's role as normatively defined, and (2) how large an element of discretion exists in the timing and site of care as related to need? There is a dearth of rigorous, or even not so rigorous, studies of both these aspects of the demand for ambulatory care. Nevertheless, the protest that many patients seek care for inappropriate reasons or with trivial complaints is

Table IV.65.   Aspects of the utilization of hospital and ambulatory care facilities that can be studied to reveal latent service reserve

For Hospitals	For Ambulatory Care
Admissions	Initiations (or episodes)
Multiple admissions	Multiple initiations (or multiple episodes)
Long stays	Multiple visits per episode
	Lengthy transit time or holding time
Patients in hospital on given day	Case load, usually for longer period than a day

frequently voiced by physicians, especially in prepaid group practice (99). Mechanic reports that 48 percent of general practitioners in England consider that there is a very serious or fairly serious problem of "having too many patients who present trivial or inappropriate problems" (180). This is indeed the second most frequently cited reason for dissatisfaction with general practice. Turning to more systematic studies of inappropriate use, Van Deen, after careful analysis of his own practice in Holland, concluded that only 2.1 percent of all his work could be considered "unnecessary." This proportion was somewhat higher, 5 percent, for "health insurance patients" (140, p. 281). Krass, in a paper provocatively titled "Is There Abuse in General Practice?", made a study of 1000 consecutive attendances in his practice in North London, England, during mid-August to mid-September (188). He was able to classify the reasons for attendance into 9 groups and an additional 5 subgroups (188, pp. 126–127). Attendances in following groups and subgroups were considered "unnecessary work":

Group 2B—Presenting with small symptoms causing no distress with no apparent or negligible physical findings. Short duration—This group contained minor bruises and abrasions, the early negligible cold and mild catarrh. It gave benefit of the doubt to some possible psychological cause, or organic basis for complaint.
Group 5—Minimal or negligible presenting symptoms with nonexistent or negligible physical signs.
Group 8—Presenting certificates (other than group 4), letters and signature. Coal certificates, housing and sanitary inspection letters, ambulance ordering, maternity forms, passports, etc.
Group 9—Direct request group. No complaint, but a direct request for some appliance or medicine, e.g. stockings, holiday travel tablets, reducing weight remedies, etc.

The attendances in these groups comprised 19.2 percent of all work in the physician's office. To these could be added all attendances in Group 4B and half of the attendances in Group 6B described below:

Group 4B—Prolonged recovery due to gain from extended certification or other reason.
Group 6B—Repeat prescriptions, not necessary on account of definite physical or psychiatric diagnosis.

Krass concludes that at least 25 percent of work in the physician's office is "unnecessary." Several aspects of this study are to be noted. First, the 25 percent estimate for attendances does not necessarily correspond to 25 percent of physician time. This distinction must always be kept in mind in case-load analysis of ambulatory care. Second, a great deal of work perceived as "unnecessary" by the physician is related to the provision of documents or certificates of one kind or another. We shall have more to say about the "certification function" of the physician in a subsequent volume. Third, there is some ambiguity in the definition of the concept "unnecessary," since Krass himself concedes that about half of the work could be done by "well-paid staff in the form of trained nurse-secretaries" (188, p. 131). Seemingly, then, about half of "unnecessary" work is within the normatively defined ambit of the general practitioner's function. What is at issue is whether it can better be done by less trained persons working under his supervision. In other words, about 10–15 percent of the practitioner's work is unnecessary, and an additional 15–20 percent was considered necessary but not to require the attention of the physician himself. This raises the final and most fundamental issue of all, the need for a normative definition of what is the general practitioner's or any physician's, function. We noted in our discussion of hospitals and related institutions the problems of arriving at such a definition for these facilities. These problems are, if anything, more vexing where the physician of first recourse is concerned.

Information on the urgency of demand for ambulatory care is also rather meager except for investigations of the use of hospital emergency services where the degree of urgency is an important social justification for the maintenance of the service. Several studies, from here and abroad, have shown that one-half to one-third of the case load of hospital emergency services is, in fact, not urgent, and that one-half or more consists of nontraumatic conditions. In fact, the emergency service has increasingly tended to approximate, in case load and in function, the office practice of the general physician. This is particularly true for the urban hospitals that serve underprivileged populations with limited access, or tenuous attachment, to a private physician. Skudder et al. reported for a sample of U.S. hospitals in 1958 that 42 percent of admissions to the emergency services were for "non-emergency" conditions and only 30 percent for trauma (199). A survey of emergency care in Michigan hospitals during one week in 1965 showed that 57 percent of attendance was for traumatic conditions and 43 percent for nontraumatic conditions (200). Turning to urban hospitals, Lee et al. reported that during 1957 attendance at the emergency service of the Beth Israel Hospital was for emergency conditions that required immediate attention in 6 percent of cases, and for urgent conditions that required early attention in 44 percent of cases. The rest, excluding 4 percent of doubtful classification, were for non-urgent conditions or scheduled procedures (201). A report from the Grace-New Haven Hospital indicates that only 26 percent of cases admitted to the emergency service required immediate care (205). However, when a system of "triage" was instituted which consisted in screening by a resident physician with arrangements being made for alternative care where indicated, the results roughly were as shown in Table IV.66.

Table IV.66.   Percent of total cases admitted to emergency service by disposition of cases,   Grace–New Haven Hospital,[a] 1963

Disposition		Percent of Case Load
All patients		100
Treated		85
Immediately	42	
After two hours	42	
"Triaged out" to :		15
Home	8	
Clinic	3	
Private care	2	
Elsewhere	1	

SOURCE: References 203 and 204.
[a] Now known as Yale–New Haven Hospital.

The studies cited above, and especially the one described last, correspond to the single-day census studies of misclassification in the hospital. They involve a classification of the need for care of the patient and an implied or explicit statement about the function of the emergency service and of alternative sources of care. All these studies raise the question of what is the socially defined function of the hospital emergency service. If the purpose is to care only for cases that require immediate care (which itself needs to be defined) considerable latent service reserve will be revealed, possibly even after corrections are made for standby capacity. However, there is reason to believe that the emergency service functions to a considerable extent as a substitute for physician care and as standby capacity for physicians in private practice who have effectively renounced their standby function.

Information concerning the urgency of care in home and office practice is harder to come by. Hardman has studied the occurrence of late calls in his own practice on the "suburban fringe of Liverpool" between March 1963 and February 1964 (189). "A late call is defined as a home visit following a request made after 12 noon for a visit on the same day" (189, p. 54). Of these calls, 15 percent were classified as "emergencies," 20 percent as "urgencies," and 64 percent as "non-urgent." Non-urgent conditions were defined as "any disease where the immediate prognosis is not altered for the worse without rapid treatment" (189, p. 55). Needless to say, this is a criterion that the client cannot be expected to apply to his own demand. Late calls were most frequent among children below 10 and old persons 70 or older. However the degree of urgency, as judged by the physician, was lowest among children below 10 (17 percent emergent or urgent) and increased fairly systematically with age, reaching a level of about 70 percent emergent or urgent in age groups 50–59 and 60–69. Among the oldest, those 70 or above, the urgency ratio declined once again to 38 percent emergent or urgent. Hardman compares his findings with three other studies from Great Britain. Apparently there is general agreement that about two-thirds of late calls are not urgent. However, there are large, but unexplained, differences in the incidence of late calls in the several studies compared (189, and 177, Table XI, p. 427). Wolfe et al. have reported on the demand for home calls in a prepaid group practice in Saskatchewan (166). During 1964, about 9 percent of visits were in the home. "In the opinion of the physicians making the calls, 12.3 percent of calls could have waited or were not justified; 26.7 percent were elective; 10.8 percent represented emergencies; 17.4 percent represented urgent conditions and 32.8 percent were categorized by the doctor as 'fair enough'" (166, p. 111). The comparability of these various studies depends, of course, on the definitions of urgency and on the frequency with which home calls are made. It is interesting that in Saskatchewan, where the frequency of home calls is possibly about a third of that in Great Britain, a roughly similar proportion of home calls (about a third) were considered emergencies or urgent. It would be interesting to see if this ratio also holds for the United States, where the frequency of visits is nearer 5 percent of total visits.

Forbes et al. have published the findings of a study of office attendances, excluding prenatal and well-baby visits, in one practice in a small market town in England (190). About 27 percent of all attendances were ostensibly "urgent," defined to mean "when a patient made contact with the practice and stated that his condition was such that he required medical advice on the same day" (190, p. 856). In such cases, the physician's estimate of urgency was as shown in Table IV.67. It would appear,

Table IV.67. Percent distribution of attendance at office of general practitioner, by degree of urgency[a]

Reason for attendance	Percent
Merited treatment urgently	34
Need for immediate reassurance	41
Patient inconsiderate or frivolous	21
Other reasons	4

SOURCE: Reference 190, page 856.
[a] Probably around 1965.

therefore, that about 20 percent of all demands for office care (with certain exclusions) need to be attended to during the same day through treatment (9 percent) or reassurance (11 percent). However, it was judged that with some experience and judgment a trained nurse could "treat, or at least temporarily reassure, a large proportion of patients in this group." Needless to say, these data cannot be generalized.

Certain characteristics of urgent demand are of interest for the planner and administrator of ambulatory services. In the study by Forbes, urgent attendances varied by age and sex, being lowest among the elderly and highest among children of preschool age. Sex differences varied by age group, with a small net excess in females in all age groups. Urgent attendances also varied systematically by day of the week, being highest on Mondays and lowest on Saturdays, an observation that is pertinent to the design of appointment systems. There appeared to be no systematic relationship to distance of place of residence. A few patients and families accounted for most urgent demands. Only 146 families, consisting of 500 persons (7 percent of all persons), were responsible for 47 percent of all urgent demands. The "urgent demanders" must apparently join the high utilizers as populations that require special attention in the administration of health services. Whether urgent demanders are also high utilizers is a question concerning which the author has no information.

As in the evaluation of hospital use, the study of high utilizers, and of their true need for care, offers one approach to the search for misclassification in ambulatory care services. Unlike studies of hospital care, usually no distinction has been made, in studies of ambulatory care, between high utilizers due to repeated admissions (episodes) and high utilizers due to many attendances during any one episode. This is unfortunate, because the factors that determine initiation may be different from those that determine the volume of care during a given episode. Jacob has developed a classification for the study of high and low utilizers which explicitly recognizes these and other factors in determining overall attendance (151–153). Although this classification appears, in part, to be unnecessarily complex, it deserves further testing. The actual findings concerning the utilization of ambulatory services leave no doubt that during any given year, a relatively small number of patients use a disproportionately large number of services. There is some doubt, however, whether there are, in fact, separable categories of persons or of families who remain high or low utilizers over an extended period of time. Densen et al. have studied patterns of utilization among members of a prepaid group practice plan (Health Insurance Plan of Greater New York, HIP for short) over a three-year period (191). During a single year, 4 percent of members used one-fourth of the visits, and 12 percent of members used half the total visits. "HIP members followed for the 3-year period 1954–1956, were more likely to remain at the same utilization level from year to year than would be expected if one year's experience were independent of the previous year's. This was true for all utilization levels—low, medium, and high" (191, p. 227). Of those who were high utilizers in Year One, 36.5 percent were high utilizers in Year Two, and 20.9 percent high utilizers in both years Two and Three. The nonutilizers also tended to maintain their pattern over the three-year period. Of those who were nonutilizers in Year One, 46 percent were nonutilizers in Year Two and 31 percent were nonutilizers in both years Two and Three. Certain characteristics were correlated with stability in utilization patterns. The tendency to continue as high utilizers was greater among the aged, males, and those who had been in the plan for a longer period of time. The tendency to remain as a nonutilizer was greatest among females and the aged. While these findings suggest that there is a real distinction between low and high utilizers, they say nothing about the appropriateness of use, which is our immediate concern. Kessel and

Shepherd examined the characteristics of low utilizers in the practice of Dr. John Fry in a "middle class dormitory suburb" of London (193). They found that 3 percent of persons had not visited the general practice for ten years. They concluded that low-utilizers tended to be healthy and self-sufficient, and found no evidence of significant unmet need among them. Wamoscher examined the other end of the utilization spectrum in his practice in Israel: namely those patients who returned repeatedly for care (192). In this practice, the average level of utilization was 4.8 visits per person per year. The study focused on high utilizers, who were defined as those who made 10 or more visits per year. These persons constituted 14 percent of the population served, but accounted for 50 percent of all visits. They averaged 16.2 visits per year as compared to 2.9 visits per person per year for all the remaining persons at risk. Among the high utilizers, 43 percent attended for "organic" complaints, 12 percent for "functional" complaints, and 46 percent for both "organic" and "functional" complaints. There is no suggestion in the study that high utilizers attended unnecessarily; but this was not the precise focus of the study. Unfortunately, there was no comparison with low utilizers. From all of this, no clear conclusion may be drawn about the relationship between level of utilization and unnecessary or inappropriate use of ambulatory services. The matter is open for further investigation.

One component of misclassification in the services of health personnel, whether in an ambulatory care or an inpatient facility, is the employment of personnel for tasks which are either beyond or beneath their level of knowledge, training, experience, and competence. The use of health personnel for tasks which they are not well equipped to perform is, generally, in the domain of quality control. However, it is conceivable that productivity and efficiency will also be impaired. More clearly related to our current concern with latent service reserve is the use of highly trained personnel for tasks that could be performed as well, or even better, by personnel with less training and therefore at lower cost. We have already discussed several considerations relevant to this matter in our sections on "productivity" and "substitutibility." Here we shall refer briefly to some studies that give a rough impression of the scale of misclassification and, consequently, the magnitude of the gains in capacity of a given health profession, should misclassification be rectified. Among such studies are those that classify work load according to time spent on various activities. We have already reviewed some of these and shown that physicians in office practice spend considerable time in activities other than direct patient care. These include travel, administration, and personal matters. The question can be raised about the extent to which these activities can be reduced and whether some, such as those involved with administration, cannot be delegated to someone else. More fully on target are studies which examine patient care activities themselves in the light of levels of skills needed to carry them out. Fry has estimated that 20 to 30 percent of the work in his own general practice could be performed by a "trained auxiliary" working under his supervision. He refers to similar proportions cited by Crombie and Cross and by Cartwright and Scott (183, p. 633). We have already referred to the estimate by Krass that 15 to 20 percent of attendances in his practice could be handled by "trained nurse-secretaries" (188, p. 131). Unfortunately, the validity of these estimates cannot be determined. However, similar results have been reported for other health personnel in other settings. A study by the Division of Nursing Resources, Public Health Service, showed the following, based on findings in 34 hospitals, as of August 1956 (see Table IV.68). In this study, the time not accounted for by

Table IV.68. Percent of time spent by specified personnel in activities considered appropriate to each category[a]

Personnel Level	Percentage of Time Spent in Appropriate Activities
Head Nurse	61
Professional Staff Nurse	78
Practical Nurse	69
Nursing Aide or Orderly	79
Clerk	78
Housekeeping Maid	94
Dietary Maid	100

SOURCE: Reference 196, Table 1, page 42.
[a] Consolidated findings of several studies conducted in 34 hospitals during the decade prior to 1956.

appropriate activities was predominantly occupied by activities at a lower level than appropriate. The head nurse, for example, spent 16 percent of the time doing professional staff nurse work and 16 percent doing clerical work; whereas the staff nurse spent 8 percent of the time doing clerical work.

A more recent study of nursing personnel in New York City schools showed considerable misclassification, with only 36 percent of all time of staff (including physicians, nurses, and public health assistants) spent on direct services to children (198). An attempt was therefore made to reorganize the delivery of service and a comparison made between a group of schools operating as before and another in which the new scheme was introduced. The findings for the year 1966, as cited in Table IV.69, are extremely interesting.

Table IV.69.   Percent distribution of time of public health nurses and staff nurses by specified level of activity, New York City Schools, 1966

	Percent Distribution of Nurses' Time			
	Public Health Nurses		Staff Nurses	
Level of Activity	Control	Experimental	Control	Experimental
Professional	58.3	72.1	54.8	66.2
Subprofessional	30.4	14.4	33.5	23.3
Incidental	11.2	13.5	11.7	10.5
Other	0.1	0	0	0.1
Total	100	100	100	100

SOURCE: Reference 198, Table 2, page 732.

It is clear that only about two-thirds of the time of professional nurses is spent on professional activities. It is also clear that the gains brought about by reorganization of the system of delivery to utilize a "team . . . designed to enable each member to devote the largest possible percentage of time on duties appropriate to his training and experience," brought about only small amelioration in misclassification. The medical care administrator is cautioned, therefore, not to consider demonstrable misclassification as equivalent with realizable service reserve. There may be something even more fundamental than organizational structure underlying misclassification in the use of personnel time: the incapacity of professional people to perform at their highest levels for prolonged periods of time. It is quite likely that, to perform effectively, professional people need the relief brought about by the admixture of less demanding work. In addition, there are issues of scheduling and effectiveness in bringing about change in the client that should be considered in the allocation of duties to professional personnel. Hence, it is important not to be misled by simple studies of misclassification. One must supplement these by studies of the productivity, efficiency, and effectiveness of a care delivery system in actual operation. However, studies of misclassification are an essential first step in designing and setting in motion alternative systems.

According to our model for the study of capacity and service reserve, there is a component of latent reserve that can be generated through increases in the productivity of health personnel. Our review of misclassification suggests that a reordering of tasks and responsibilities of health personnel should be one approach to increasing productivity. This takes us back to our earlier discussion of trends in productivity as well as of the relationship between productivity and scale of organization, with special reference to group practice. We may conclude this section with some comments on the more efficient use of physician time through exercising greater control over the time and place of visits. We have already reviewed some of the information on the urgency and necessity of late calls and home calls. The ratio of home calls to all visits varies to a remarkable extent among countries and among physicians within a given locality. Logan and Eimerl have assembled data from several countries that indicate a range from 9 to 10 percent in the United States, Sweden, Czechoslovakia, and the Federal German Republic to as high as 50 percent in Scotland (174, Table 6, p. 309). The fact that neighboring England, under the same National Health Service as Scotland, averages about 25 percent, raises fascinating questions which are not easy to answer (175). In the British studies reviewed by Lees and Cooper, the reported range was from 12.0 to 68.2 percent (177, p. 416). More recent data from the United States indicate that home visits are now nearer 5 percent of all visits, including telephone consultations. These figures raise sharply the question of the gains of productivity that would occur if home visits were reduced to the indispensable minimum. Eimerl and Pearson, in a study of general practitioners in Merseyside and North Wales, found that "between 40 and 60 percent of working-time is taken up with serving only one-sixth to one-third of patients," and wondered whether the community can "afford the luxury of having the doctor acting merely as a chauffeur for so much of his time" (181, p. 1552). Wolfe et al. have estimated, for their group in Saskatchewan, that a home visit, including travel time, averages 34 minutes in duration as compared to 15.5 minutes for the average clinic visit (166, p. 111). Needless to say, these time relationships would vary by the geographic characteristics of the practice and should be corrected for differences in case mix. One should also consider the financial and other costs to the patient and his family of making the trip to the physician's office. Finally, the economic calculus is not the only, nor necessarily the major, consideration. There are questions of where the patient may be best served as well as of what patients desire and expect. As we shall see in a subsequent volume, clients continue to expect home care to be available and are distressed by the increasing difficulty in obtaining it.

CAPACITY TO PRODUCE SERVICE IN RELATION TO NEED AND DEMAND

As we have shown, the evaluation of service-producing resources involves first, the proper specification of the particular resources under review and, second, the determination of the capacity of each resource to produce services. A third aspect of assessment, which is the subject matter of this section, is the degree to which the resources in question, and the services they actually produce or are capable of producing, correspond to the volume and distribution of need and demand. Several dimensions of assessment, included in this brief statement, require emphasis. First, it is necessary to distinguish the actual services produced from the potential to produce services under certain specifiable conditions. We have, in our previous section, dealt at length with the identification and measurement of unused or misused potential for service. Second, it is important to distinguish need for service from demand for service. The several definitions, levels, and measures of need have been discussed in a previous chapter. We have also discussed the degree to which need and demand are congruent, with emphasis on the extent and sources of lack of congruence between need and demand. Third, there is a distinction between the aggregate volume of need or demand and certain distributional characteristics of these. Distributional characteristics are, in turn, relevant to the dimensions of space and of time. In other words, there is concern not only with whether total supply is in balance with total need or demand, but with whether services are available where they are needed (or demanded) and at the proper time.

Relationship to Aggregate Need and Demand

A central question in the assessment of supply is whether there is an "excess" or a "shortage." Of these two, the possible presence of a shortage has attracted by far the greater attention, especially with respect to the supply of physician manpower. This preoccupation with the "shortage" of physicians and other health personnel, including nursing, suggests that this may indeed be the area of greatest weakness in the medical care system as presently organized. It may also reflect the interesting conceptual and methodological issues raised by the attempt to define a "shortage" of manpower in the medical care field. The literature concerning this has been reviewed briefly by Klarman (1, pp. 88–101) and by Fein (289, pp. 13–21 and 54–60), and by Butter (285).

The determination of "excess" or "shortage" presupposes a comparison between at least two things: a measure of supply and a measure of calls made upon that supply. It follows that we must determine, first, what is the appropriate measure of supply. In general, studies have used a count of the service-producing resources themselves: the number of physicians or nurses, or of hospital beds, for example. When this is done, all the factors that mediate the actual production of services and their effectiveness are assumed to be constant, an unwarranted assumption. Furthermore, the possible presence of service overload or of service reserve is not always taken into account. Turning to the measure of the calls made upon supply, two approaches are possible: one is a measure of need and the other a measure of demand. Because, in practice, need and demand are interrelated, it may not be possible to say of any given measure that it represents one to the exclusion of the other. There are, nevertheless, fundamental differences, conceptually and methodologically, between a determination of shortage based on need and one based on demand.

UNSATISFIED NEED. Persons with a primary commitment to one of the health professions, or to the public health movement that may be considered their extension, tend to define a "shortage" in terms of unsatisfied need for health care. More specifically, a shortage is said to exist if the service equivalents of need exceed the current or potential capacity of resources to provide service. In other words, "shortage" differs from "unmet need" by postulating that need exceeds the *capacity* of the system to satisfy that need. This definition, while eminently congenial to the traditional health orientation, leads to a number of difficulties. First, whose definition of need is the one relevant to definitions of shortage: that of the health professional, that of the client, or perhaps that of some social instrumentality that includes them both, but with some adjustments to both? Second, there are the problems of measuring need, irrespective of what definition is used, and of translating measures of need into their equivalents in services adequate to satisfy need. There are technical difficulties in accomplishing these requirements, some of which we have discussed and some which we shall take up in a subsequent chapter. Furthermore, some have asserted that need, viewed in this manner, is virtually infinite and, therefore provides no fixed benchmark against which to compare the capacity to provide service. Third, assuming that service equivalents are definable and that services can, in fact, be made available, what assurance is there that the services would be used? The arguments that need is at once infinite and not fully convertible into effective demand appear to be contradictory. Both may, however, hold if planning for the supply of service is divorced from provision to make that supply accessible to use. Finally, assuming the capacity to make services available and usable, the question arises whether this is the best possible allocation of national resources, or whether the "general welfare" might not be better served if less of the national wealth were devoted to health services and more to some other employment. One might even argue that health itself might be better served if resources were allocated to things like education, job training, nutrition, recreation, and environmental control, rather than to personal health services as traditionally conceived.

So much for a general statement of difficulties encountered in the evaluation of resources based on a notion of need. In a subsequent chapter we shall present in detail methods which, given certain assumptions, make it possible to translate need into service equivalents and these, in turn, into service capacity.

UNSATISFIED DEMAND. The second method for the determination of whether there is "excess" or "shortage" is to compare the capacity to provide service, actual or potential, to the demand for services. Simply stated, the question asked is whether there are more or less of a particular health service (for example, the services of physicians) than people are willing and able to pay for at current prices. As Boulding has pointed out, this is an approach more congenial to the libertarian orientation, whereas the criterion of need appeals more to the egalitarian (284, p. 217). Consequently, the use of demand as the touchstone for adequacy is favored by traditional economics. Often implicit in its use is the assumption that, by and large, medical care is similar to other goods or services which consumers desire and that its optimal distribution may best be left to market forces. However, such assumptions are not a necessary concomitant of the use of demand as the criterion in the assessment of the adequacy of supply, since demand itself is subject to social control by instrumentalities other than, or additional to, the free market. Nevertheless, those who emphasize the primacy of demand as opposed to need, tend to believe that the sum of individual preferences is the best criterion for the allocation of resources and that, given free reign, the market will achieve the best possible equilibrium between all demands and resources.

The paradigm in Table IV.70 shows, in a simplified manner, first, two

Table IV.70.   Hypothetical situations of imbalance between supply and demand
for television sets and ways in which imbalance could be restored

States of Imbalance and Ways of Restoring Equilibrium	Market Variables		
	Television Sets for Sale	Price per Set	Persons Willing to Buy
A. Situations of imbalance			
1. Excess	1000	$800	500
2. Shortage	1000	200	2000
B. Equilibrium established by:			
1. Change in price			
a. Direct, monetary	1000	400ᵃ	1000
b. Indirect monetary, or			
non-monetary	1000	300 plus waiting	1000
2. Change in production			
a. Downward	500	800	500
b. Upward	2000	200	2000
3. Change in consumer preference			
a. Upward	1000	800	1000
b. Downward	1000	200	1000

ᵃ The italicized values indicate the changes by which equilibrium is established.

hypothetical situations of disequilibrium in the market for television
sets, one definable as an "excess" and the other as a "shortage." It then
shows several ways in which equilibrium may be established so that
either "excess" or "shortage" are wiped out.

The hypothetical model demonstrates clearly the essential characteristics of definitions of "excess" and "shortage," respectively, as shortage of buyers or an excess of buyers in relation to the quantities offered
for sale, at the prices specified. It also shows that equilibrium can be
established by a variety of mechanisms. The first of these, and the one
most readily altered, is price. It is clear that by simply raising price it is
possible to disuade a sufficient number of buyers and thus to eliminate a
"shortage," even though the quantity of goods offered for sale remains
unaltered. In certain situations which may be particularly relevant to
medical care buyers are dissuaded not by increases in price but by
hardships associated with the receipt of service—for example, long
waiting periods—which may also involve monetary loss to the client.
Such factors can be considered tantamount to a change in price. Somewhat slower to respond to states of imbalance are changes in the production of goods offered for sale either downward or upward, depend-

ing on whether there is an excess or shortage. Over an even longer period of time it may be possible to alter the preferences of the potential customers themselves, so that they may come to value certain things more or less than others and in this way to redress previous imbalance of long standing or to create new states of imbalance.

While the model presented above embodies a perfectly reasonable construct, certain of its features are unpalatable to the health professional. The notion that a shortage can be erased by an increase in prices appears to be a contradiction in terms, since such an increase would make care even less available to persons in the low income groups, who need it most. But the conflict is more fundamental than a disagreement over terminology. It arises from the concept of need for medical care as a professionally definable reality, and from the commitment to need as the primary criterion for the equitable distribution of health services.

Having presented the concepts of "excess" and "shortage" as states of imbalance between the quantities offered for sale and the quantities that persons are willing to buy at specified prices, it is necessary to turn to the kinds of empirical evidence that may be sought as indicators of balance or imbalance. In the course of doing so we shall also summarize the findings about manpower shortage in the recent past. Such studies follow one of two lines of inquiry. The first attempts to show, as Fein has put it, that "the supply of services offered is less than potential producers would be willing to make available" (289, p. 16). The second is that, at current prices, potential consumers would be willing to buy more medical care services than are now made available to them.

On the supply side, evidence has been assembled to suggest that, at current yearly incomes, more persons would be entering the profession of medicine in preference to some alternative line of work than are now doing. Such findings are based on an analysis of the investment that individuals make in their education as compared to the returns to them on that investment. The outlays for education consist of two categories: (1) direct expenditures for tuition, supplies, and so on, and (2) opportunity costs, or income foregone while engaged in study rather than gainful employment. The returns are income earned over a lifetime from the particular employment to which the education is relevant. Since both expenditures and incomes, especially the latter, occur over variably prolonged periods of time it is necessary to make certain adjustments to account for this. Such adjustments may be made in one of three ways. First, it is possible by applying over the relevant period of time a discount rate that is considered appropriate, to determine the value of returns of outlays and of the difference between the discounted values, at a given moment in time, usually the time when professional career choices are likely to be made. This, in brief, is the expected value of the investment in each alternative career at that time. Clearly, other things being equal, the investment with the highest present value is to be preferred. Second, it is possible, given data on outlays and earnings, to determine the rate of discount (internal rate of return) which will render the expected outlays and earnings equivalent at the time career choices are made. The internal rates of return are therefore the discount rates that make the current value of outlays plus returns equal to zero. It follows that the investment (in this case, career choice) which must be discounted most heavily to be reduced to a value of zero is the one that is most profitable. A third approach is to determine the "rate of discount over cost," which is the single discount rate that equalizes the present values of any two alternative investments. Above this rate, one investment has a higher present value than the other, whereas below this rate the relative positions of the two alternative investments are reversed. Using this method, the criterion of choice of investment is not fixed, since it depends in part on how the investor evaluates the rapidity with which returns are realized in relation to the total sum eventually realized, and in part on the prevailing interest rate. There are examples of the application of these three methods to study of the incentives for entry into the health professions. Friedman and Kuznets have studied the present value of the investment in medicine and dentistry (286). Hansen has reported on the internal rates of return for physicians, dentists, and male college graduates (288). Yett has compared various levels of nursing preparation and college education for women using both the internal rate of return and the rate of discount over cost (296). The findings of these studies will be described and discussed below.

Friedman and Kuznets, in a classic work, compared the incomes of physicians and dentists (286). After the necessary adjustments were made, the income of physicians was 17 percent higher than that of dentists. This indicated that persons contemplating entry into one of the two professions should be choosing medicine in preference to dentistry. Friedman has elaborated on this analysis in a more recent publication (287). Also more recently, Hansen has compared physicians, dentists, and male college graduates in 1939, 1949, and 1956. Rather than comparing adjusted incomes, as did Friedman and Kuznets, he determined the discount rates that would render the three groups comparable by making the sum of the current values of outlays and returns equal to zero. The higher this rate, the more favorable is the financial balance sheet of the group. Hansen's findings are summarized in Table IV.71. In this table,

Table IV.71.   Absolute and relative[a] internal rates of return on investment in education for specified occupational categories, U.S.A., 1939, 1949, and 1956

Personnel	1939		1949		1956	
	Rate	Ratio	Rate	Ratio	Rate	Ratio
Male college graduates	13.7	1.00	11.5	1.00	11.6	1.00
Physicians	13.5	0.98	13.4	1.16	12.8	1.10
Dentists	12.3	0.90	13.4	1.16	12.0	1.04

SOURCE: Reference 288, page 86.

[a] Relative to the rate of return for male college graduates.

the ratios are constructed by equating the rate of return for male college graduates to 1.00 in each year, so that other rates in that year can be compared to it. From these data it is seen that in 1939 the rate of return was lower for physicians and dentists than for male college graduates. In other words, during that year the economic returns did not justify choosing medicine or, even more so, dentistry, over occupations open to male college graduates, assuming that the then current situation would continue into the future. In 1949 the situation had altered in favor of medicine and dentistry, the prospects for each having become equally better than that for college students. By 1956 medicine enjoyed the most favorable financial returns, with dentistry second and college graduates third. However, the superiority of medicine and dentistry over male college graduates was greater in 1949 than it was in 1956.

Under certain assumptions such comparisons may be construed to mean relative excess or shortage in the production of service. If it is assumed that persons at the point of choosing a career know the ultimate financial balance sheet of the alternative careers and that their choices are determined by this knowledge, it might be inferred that more people stand ready to enter the relatively more remunerative profession in preference to one that is less remunerative. This excess in potential production over actual production is, as we have indicated, one definition of "shortage." By the same token there is a relative "excess" in the alternative profession for which the financial balance sheet is less favorable.

There are serious limitations in this approach. First, one might question the two fundamental assumptions: that potential entrants into a profession know the balance sheet and that this is the determining factor in choice. The assumption of thorough rationality is in itself merely an assumption. Furthermore, one may question whether the balance sheet is correctly drawn. Clearly, the losses and gains under consideration so far have been primarily monetary. The inputs into professional training and its rewards or consequences include physical and intellectual effort, psychological stress, social dislocation, moral hazard, responsibility, autonomy, social status or prestige and, perhaps, even life span. These inputs introduce into the calculation of outlays and returns factors difficult, if not impossible, to assess. This is especially true because different candidates for training may, by virtue of differences in temperament or ability or values, view the losses and gains as differently balanced. Friedman and Kuznets, in comparing medicine and dentistry, concluded that the nonmonetary balance sheet also favored medicine and that the relative shortage in medicine is therefore even greater than indicated by the 17 percent excess in adjusted average lifetime income. However, this conclusion can be only accepted as an opinion, limited by the availability of information and deeply colored by the subjective biases of the investigators themselves.

Another limitation is the relative nature of the conclusions. The information obtained is in the form of relative excess or shortage rather than excess or shortage in comparison with some standard of what is good or appropriate. The conclusion that there is overinvestment in medicine relative to dentistry could equally well be stated as underinvestment in dentistry relative to medicine. Furthermore, the accounting is purely personal and does not include the social investment in education nor its social returns. Finally, there are a number of more technical considerations that influence the findings. These have been well summarized by Klarman (1, pp. 90–93) and include (1) whether hourly wages rather than total income is the more appropriate measure of professional returns; (2) doubts concerning completeness and bias in reporting income; (3) the effect of the personal income tax as it is modified not only by average income but also by the frequency distribution of incomes within each profession; and (4) the appropriate discount rate to be applied in arriving at the present value of past and future expenditures and incomes. For example, a high discount rate will reduce the present value of long-deferred income and therefore present medicine in a less favorable light. If the income of physicians is underreported as compared to that of college graduates, for example, the relative pecuniary advantages of medicine are thereby understated. It is also conceivable that part of the secular changes in relative positions of several professions may be due to changes in reporting income. If hourly earnings are used in lieu of average income, the profession with the longer hours of work (probably medicine) will lose in relative rank. Klarman cites Friedman to the effect that ''a progressive income tax collects more revenue from the occupation with the more variable and more widely fluctuating income. It also enhances the nonpecuniary (hence untaxed) advantages of an occupation. In the case of physicians the two factors operate in opposite directions" (1, p. 92). In the opening portion of this section we also raised the important issue of whether supply should be measured in terms of manpower or in terms of some measure of the output of manpower. Friedman and Kuznets used the individual practitioner (physician or dentist) as the unit of supply because "the quantity of service any practitioner stands ready to offer depends but little on the 'price' he can get, although, of course, the quantity he actually renders doubtless does depend on the 'price' the consumer must pay . . . Economic factors affect the supply of service through their effect on the number who try to enter the profession" (286, p. 155). In other words, the relevant phenomenon is not the services produced but the capacity to produce service. Friedman and Kuznets also use the individual practitioners as the unit of demand since, in their opinion, the demand is for a physician or dentist rather than for any specific bundle of services.

So far we have described some rather indirect ways of determining whether there are more or less persons willing to provide service than are currently providing such service. A more direct measure of this may be the number of applicants to medical school. Since applicants to medical school exceed those accepted by a ratio of two to one, it may be concluded that there are more persons willing to enter medicine than are permitted to do so. Klarman cites Friedman and Samuelson among the economists who believe that "the persistence of a large number of rejected, but qualified, applicants constitutes clear proof of a shortage" (1, p. 94). The issue, then, is not simply willingness but also ability to provide service. This second question—of ability as distinct from willingness—leads to a succession of thorny questions, which include (1) the accuracy with which admission procedures can predict the capacity of prospective students to complete successfully the medical curriculum; (2) the relevance of the medical curriculum itself to the good practice of medicine, as defined by the profession; and (3) the relevance of professional standards of medical practice to the acceptability of the medical product to the public. There are serious doubts about the first of these questions and some doubts concerning the second, even within the medical profession itself. Even the third question cannot be dismissed out of hand, as shown by the significant success enjoyed by chiropractic, which is anathema to physicians. Needless to say, one cannot raise, in the calculus of supply and demand in a free market, the most fundamental question of all, that is, the social responsibility for maintaining certain levels of medical competence. This would take us back to the concept of need and of the capacity to satisfy that need, as socially defined.

The reader will recall that the other side of the coin to the definition of shortage is the presence, at current prices, of unsatisfied consumer demand. In other words, what is sought is evidence that people are willing and able to buy more services than are being offered at current prices. The most direct evidence of unsatisfied demand is the appearance, on a more than localized basis, of the phenomena associated with service overload, as described in a previous section. Fein comments as follows concerning some of these (289, p. 54) :

Most of the evidence is impressionistic. Everyone is aware that many persons complain that it is difficult to reach a physician, that often they are discouraged from coming to the office and treatment is prescribed over the phone, even though the patient would prefer to visit the physician and pay accordingly, that physicians are not available for home calls and night calls, that care in hospitals is often provided by interns and residents, and so on. Furthermore, many physicians say they are "overworked," that is, that they would prefer to work fewer hours even if that meant less income.

There are, in addition, certain responses in the system for the provision of care that, collectively, indicate the pressures of demand in excess of supply. These include (1) increases in the price of service, (2) increasing use of substitutes, (3) importation of professional manpower, and (4) the presence of budgeted vacancies. Rayack has assembled information concerning these phenomena as they pertain to medicine (290), and Yett has made similar studies of nursing (294–298). To these might be added the phenomena that we have already discussed as indicators of the readiness of more potential suppliers to enter the market. Thus, the fundamental circularity of our model becomes—perhaps embarassingly— evident!

In our hypothetical market for television sets, a rise in prices was one way in which demand was reduced so as to correspond to supply. In the interest of simplicity, supply was considered fixed. In real life a rise in prices is likely to diminish demand, while at the same time it stimulates supply. Thus a rise in prices is evidence of a shortage in the process of being corrected by a dual effect on demand and on supply. If the rate of increase in price is sufficiently rapid, it will attain a new point of equilibrium between demand and supply, provided it does not overshoot the mark. In recent decades the consumer price index for medical care and all of its components, with the possible exception of drugs, has increased at a rate significantly more rapid than that for goods and services in general (299). Immediately before and after the institution of Medicare there were unprecedented increases in price (300). Although the medical care price index has many limitations, including its inability to correct adequately for changes in the quality of the product, its continued, and recently accelerated, increase suggests a continuing shortage in all medical care services, with the possible exception of pharmaceutical services.

The income of health professionals in independent practice is to a considerable extent, though not completely, determined by the price of their services. It follows that a study of relative incomes in the several professions, as well as of trends in income and in the relative positions of incomes, will give some indication of the relative shortage or excess in the supply of these professions. Accordingly, Rayack has assembled information on the incomes in several professions and occupations, as given in Table IV.72. The data cited above show (1) the rise in incomes over time and (2) the increasing gap between medicine and other professions and occupations, in favor of medicine. However, the reader should be aware of the many doubts concerning the veracity of the income data, especially for professional persons in independent practice. Furthermore, income data are determined not only by the price of services, but also by the other factors that influence productivity and effectiveness, which we have discussed in a previous section. Finally, the use of price (and hence of income) as an indicator of shortage or excess presupposes a market in which prices are free to respond to imbalance between demand and supply. The importance of this assumption will be illustrated when we discuss the special situation in nursing, where the assumption is most transparently inappropriate. The comparative use of income data also suffers from the limitation we have already mentioned in discussing the returns to investment in professional education: namely, that while the relative position of a profession can be determined, it cannot be said with assurance which of the professions being compared is nearest to a state of balance between demand and supply. Secular trends suffer from the same disadvantage, since it is not easy to tell whether rising prices or income mean a developing shortage or the correction of a previous state of excess. Rayack contends, however, that the stability of professional incomes between 1929 and 1939 suggests strongly a state of equilibrium and therefore sets the reference point for all subsequent changes, which have been steadily upward (290).

A second set of phenomena that has been offered by many, including Rayack, as evidence that consumer demand exceeds supply, may be assembled under the heading of "substitution." These include the use of

Table IV.72.   Relative incomes of specified occupational groups, U.S.A.,
for specified periods

| | Index Numbers: 1939 = 100 | | | |
| | 1939–1951 | | 1939–1959 | |
Occupational Groups	Mean Income	Median Income	Mean Income	Median Income
Nonsalaried physicians	318 (341)		(534)	
General practitioners			(546)	
Full specialists			(433)	
Nonsalaried dentists	253			
Nonsalaried lawyers	202			
Professional, technical, and kindred workers		225		348
Managers, officials, and proprietors (nonfarm)		194		312
Full-time employees, all industries	256		361	

SOURCE: Reference 290, Tables 1 and 4, pages 224 and 227.

Figures in parentheses are from surveys conducted by *Medical Economics*. Other data are from publications of the Department of Commerce or the Bureau of the Census. See original reference for details.

nurses to perform the functions of physicians, and of subprofessionals, in general, to perform the functions of professionals including nurses, physicians and dentists. Some—Rayack, for example—also include the increasing use of interns and residents to perform tasks that would otherwise fall upon the practitioner in private practice, as one form of substitution. Klarman reinforces this argument by citing evidence, assembled by Adams, that salaries have risen faster for interns and residents than for persons in other forms of employment. In a previous section we have commented upon the changing structure of the health professions and discussed the effects of substitution on productivity. Other forms of substitution involve the use of one service for another that is in shorter supply. Fein mentions the virtual disappearance of home visits and the substitution of telephone consultations for personal visits. The use of hospital emergency services in lieu of visits to the private practitioner may be considered another example in this category. One effect of substitution is to dampen the increase in the prices of the services affected.

A third piece of evidence, related to substitution but involving additional considerations, is the importation of foreign physicians to serve, first, as hospital house staff, and then to continue as physicians in permanent residence in the United States. In recent decades this has been a slowly but steadily increasing practice. In 1950 graduates of foreign schools, excluding those in Canada, held about 10 percent of internships and residencies and constituted about 5 percent of those who received initial licenses to practice medicine. In 1969 the corresponding figures were approximately 31 and 23 percent respectively (21, 24).

Of the market responses to shortage mentioned so far, increases in price have the effect of dampening demand, whereas the use of substitutes and the importation of manpower tend to augment supply. However, these three responses to shortage do not necessarily indicate the presence of a shortage at any given moment in time. This is because it is not clear to what extent the response lags behind the generation of the shortage. It might be argued, for example, that at any moment a near balance has been achieved between demand and supply. Since the trends in most of the phenomena described continue to be upward, it is difficult to deny that the potential for shortage is continually being generated. But it is difficult to show how far behind is supply in relation to demand. Hence particular interest attaches to the last phenomenon on our list of indicators: the presence of unfilled vacancies in hospitals, other facilities, and medical care programs. Budgeted vacancies represent demand by organized producers of service that is derived from consumer demand. The number of such vacancies and the lag in filling them represent one measure of the discrepancy between demand and supply. However, the reader must be warned that neither this phenomenon, nor any of the others mentioned, can be taken at face value as an indicator of shortage without a thorough understanding of the characteristics of the medical care market as a whole. There are many factors, some of which will be described below, that interfere with the free play of market forces in the provision of medical care services. Furthermore, the phenomena, as measured above, indicate response to actual services produced and usually do not include corrections for the presence of service reserve, either latent or manifest. Ginzberg has discussed briefly this and other limitations in estimates of shortage based on demand or need (293).

With the exception of some dissenters, such as Ginzberg, the conclusion that has been drawn generally from studies of supply in relation to demand, as well as to need, is that there is a shortage of physicians. There are, however, different estimates of the magnitude of the shortage and differences of opinion on whether it is getting worse or better. Hansen has concluded that the relative shortage of physicians was not as large in 1956 as it was in 1949. Rayack, on the other hand, using different indicators, has concluded that the situation has grown steadily worse during this time period. If the general conclusion that there is a shortage of physicians is provisionally accepted, the question arises of why such a shortage persists. Two general explanations are offered. One is that prices do not rise sufficiently to smother the excess of demand over supply; the other that there are restrictions on the entry of physicians into the market. It is not clear what are the restraints on prices. Greenfield and Anderson have reported that, historically, "physicians' fees fluctuate less violently than do prices of other cost-of-living items. In other words, physicians' fees are relatively less sensitive to general economic changes. It is also interesting that, except for the inflationary period during the War of 1812, physicians' fees responded (with some lag) to upward movements in other prices (e.g. Civil War and World War I) but not readily to downward movements (e.g. 1812–1850; 1856–1859; 1929–1932). Of course, these are stated fees, and during downswings, collection of fees by physicians would decrease" (302, p. 11). An explanation commonly advanced for the apparent reluctance of physicians to increase prices to a degree sufficient to control excess demand is the tradition of service and the ethical code that governs the behavior of physicians in response to expressed need for their services. Fein has suggested that, in addition to the foregoing factors, the private practice of medicine fragments the market into little compartments. This inhibits the exchange of information among suppliers of service and, consequently, the generation of generalized price movements. The prevalent use of fee schedules by health insurance, including Blue Shield, may also have put a brake on prices. The rapid rise in prices that coincided with the advent of Medicare, which uses "reasonable charges" as a basis for paying physicians, suggests two things: that the method of payment may be important, and that the private practice of medicine is not so fragmented that it cannot respond rapidly and decisively to an increase in purchasing power (300). However, in spite of such increases in price, the net effect of Medicare has so far been a modest but significant increase in the use of service (385). This illustrates a second, and more important, effect of health insurance. The separation of payments from use interferes with the mutual adjustments between price and use. This separation occurs because an agency other than the consumer often pays all or part of the premium and/or part of the bill. Even when the consumer pays the entire premium, the level of premium is seldom perceived as a deterrent to use in individual cases.

The second factor charged with handicapping the market in its response to increased demand is restrictions on the entry of new recruits into the medical profession. Here again there is considerable lack of clarity, as well as a goodly amount of controversy, concerning the presence of restraints and the manner in which they are exerted. There is a widespread belief in the field of medical care administration that organized medicine, through its influence and control over medical schools and state medical licensure, has acted to discourage sufficient expansion in medical manpower. Most recently, Rayack has assembled historical evidence to support this argument (291).

One set of studies of the relationship between supply and demand has been put aside for separate consideration because the studies illustrate certain limitations of the methods described so far, in particular the need to understand well the specific market in question. These are the studies of nursing supply developed by Yett (294–298). These studies illustrate very well the problems of obtaining valid data over a sufficient length of time so as to permit a study of the trends in the relationship between supply and demand. The large number of assumptions and approximations necessitated by the paucity of data necessarily weaken the confidence to be placed in the findings. Certain peculiarities of nursing increase the difficulty of the task and influence the interpretation of the findings. First, nursing is extremely heterogeneous, being made up of persons with widely differing types of education received at different sites, including hospitals, junior colleges, and colleges or universities. It is necessary, therefore, to consider a large number of nursing variants. This being the case, it is also necessary to provide a range of comparably educated non-nurses for purposes of comparing outlays and returns. Second, nursing students, especially in diploma schools, have provided varying amounts of service. Furthermore, both students and hospital nurses receive remuneration partly in kind, in the form of maintenance. Third, at any given time, large proportions of nurses are inactive, with the proportion varying by age group and also over time. This makes it difficult to estimate the number of active nurses at any given time. Furthermore, it complicates the interpretation of changes in services offered in response to changes in price. This response is due, in the short run, to trained nurses becoming active in the profession and, in the long run, to young women being recruited into nursing. Any particular response that is observed is therefore a mixture of the two effects, without the components being easily distinguishable. Finally, the fact that nurses are relatively infrequently committed to a full life of nursing practice makes it difficult to estimate the returns on the investment in training. The phenomenon of less than lifetime commitment to employment is, of course, prevalent among women in all types of work. Hence, it becomes difficult, a priori, to tell what economic considerations motivate women to choose one line of work in preference to another. In particular, should one postulate that any particular profession is evaluated in terms of full lifetime employment or on the basis of some less than complete employment which the potential recruit has in mind? If the latter is the case, what is the pattern of employment that is relevant to choice?

Yett has made a valiant attempt to handle all these complications with reasonable success. His work is interesting because he used several methods for exploring shortage. These include comparisons of nursing with other types of employment for women, contemporaneously and over time, with respect to (1) real income, (2) internal rates of return, and (3) the rates of return over cost. The findings are too complex to be summarized by any brief statement. The reader is referred to the original references for details. There are, however, some findings of general relevance to the methods advocated to study economic shortages. These will be mentioned briefly. First, when nursing and other forms of employment for women are compared, the profitableness of nursing is less when comparison is in terms of potential lifetime earnings than when the comparison is in terms of earnings predicted on the basis of the pattern of employment characteristic of each of the types of employment being compared. In other words, part of the attractiveness of nursing rests on the ability, or the greater propensity, of the nurse to remain employed. This finding notwithstanding, Yett concludes that potential earnings from full-time employment is probably the more important factor in deciding among alternative career choices (296, p. 51). A second finding of perhaps greater methodological significance is that the different indicators of shortage (incomes, internal rates of return, and rates of return over cost) yield roughly similar findings. A third conclusion of considerable significance is that the methods chosen to demonstrate shortage yield findings that are in accord with the impressions of experts: that there has been a serious shortage of nurses during most of the period since and including World War II. The one important exception is the period between 1949 and 1959, during which the economic indicators of profitableness show an excess of nurses relative to other roughly comparable forms of female employment. During this period there were smaller increases in the real income of nurses and nursing was clearly a less profitable investment. The explanation offered for this discrepancy is an imperfection in the market, so that nursing salaries did not reflect the shortage of nurses which is demonstrable through other indicators, such as the existence of budgeted vacancies and the growth of substitution.

The particular mechanism responsible for this is the control of wages by hospitals, which is made possible because they ordinarily operate as monopsonists or oligopsonists. Yett reports that 40 percent of all general hospitals are in Hill-Burton service areas that contain three or fewer hospitals. In the larger metropolitan areas, where there are more hospitals, the hospital associations apparently control nursing salaries through "wage stabilization" programs. Of 31 such societies surveyed by Yett, 15 responded. Of these 15, all but one had a well-developed "stabilization" program. "The one that did not already have such a program asked for information on how it could set one up" (294, p. 100n). It is believed that, since 1959, the ability of the hospitals to maintain nursing salaries at artificially low levels has been weakened partly by the large new demands created by Medicare and partly by the growth of collective bargaining or the threat of such bargaining by nurses. Consequently, the economic indicators of profitability once again are in accord with other economic and non-economic indicators of shortage. In other words, profitability is rising, although it has not risen sufficiently high to indicate a clear preference for nursing over alternative female employments. Yett's findings for this period include those shown in Table IV.73.

Table IV.73.   Specified rates of return for nurses with specified levels of training, according to assumption concerning propensity of nurses to be employed, U.S.A., 1959 and 1966

Type of Training and Measure of Profitability	100% Labor Force Participation		Occupation-Specific Participation	
	1959	1966	1959	1966
Internal rates of return				
4 years of college	7.1	6.7	11.3	10.0
4 years nurse training	4.2	7.3	9.7	9.8
Rate of return over cost 4 years of nursing compared to 4 years of college	Returns for nursing inferior up to discount rate of 80%	Returns for nursing inferior up to discount rate of 39.7%	Returns for nursing inferior up to discount rate of 80%	Returns for nursing inferior up to discount rate of 80%

SOURCE: Reference 296, Tables 1 and 2, pages 44–47.

These findings illustrate several points which have already been made. First, occupation-specific rates of participation in labor force show nursing in more favorable light than does 100 percent labor force participation. In spite of this, almost all entries in the table, except one, show nursing to be less profitable than the alternative choice. This means, according to one interpretation, that nursing is in relative excess. However, the changes in the relative positions of nursing between 1959 and 1966 show that nursing is less in excess in 1966 than it was in 1959. In this sense, the shortage of nurses is being revealed. As already mentioned, the degree of hospital control over nurses' salaries is believed to be responsible for the fact that nursing appears to be in excess, even though a shortage is believed to exist.

Accessibility

GENERAL CONSIDERATIONS. It is necessary once again to return to the model for evaluating supply as discussed in the opening section of this chapter and as shown graphically in Fig. IV.1. It may be recalled that our model postulated the presence of intervening factors that influenced the capacity of resources to produce services and of services to neutralize need. These factors have already been discussed. There remains a third set of factors—those that intervene between the capacity to produce service and the actual production or consumption of services. These factors are subsumed under the rubric of "accessibility." They are themselves a subset of a larger set of factors that influence the use of service. They are singled out for discussion here because they are conceived as characteristics of the resources themselves that make these resources more or less readily usable. There is a certain degree of arbitrariness in conceiving of accessibility in this manner. The reader will have to judge for himself whether this aspect of the model, as well as all others, are reasonable and useful.

"Accessibility" is viewed as something additional to the mere presence or "availability" of the resource in any given place at any given time. It comprises those characteristics of the resource that facilitate or obstruct use by potential clients. Two kinds of accessibility are distinguished: socio-organizational and geographic. Needless to say, these two components of accessibility are highly interactive. In subsequent sections we shall first consider briefly some aspects of socio-organizational accessibility. Next there will be a more lengthy discussion of geographic accessibility and related aspects of the spatial organization of health resources. In both sections there will be frequent occasion to refer to the interrelationships between social and spatial organization.

SOCIO-ORGANIZATIONAL ACCESSIBILITY. Under this heading might be grouped all characteristics of resources, other than spatial attributes, that either facilitate or hinder efforts of the client to reach care. For example, where physicians are concerned, factors influencing socio-organizational accessibility include such diverse attributes as sex, color, specialization, and level of fees. The reluctance of some men to see a woman physician and the refusal of some white dentists to treat black patients are examples of inaccessibility dependent on socio-organizational rather than geographic factors. Similar factors are operative with respect to organized ambulatory care, hospitals, and other facilities. Of special importance in this context are formal or informal admission policies that exclude patients by color, economic ability, or diagnosis. Among the last are restrictions on admitting persons with mental illness, alcoholism, drug addiction, tuberculosis, and contagious diseases in general.

There is rich anecdotal knowledge of the existence of such barriers and of their consequences. Unfortunately, reports of systematic study are much more difficult to find. For this reason one notes with great interest a study by Gorwitz and Warthen that has looked into the consequences of desegregating state mental hospitals in Maryland (307). Prior to January 1963 white patients were admitted to three such hospitals and black patients were admitted exclusively to a fourth. In 1963 the decision was made to open all four hospitals to all patients irrespective of color, thus reducing social barriers as well as distance to the nearest accessible hospital. As shown in Table IV.74, unduplicated admission rates during 18 months prior and subsequent to the adoption of this policy show that total admission rates for all diagnostic categories to all hospitals increased for both Whites and Blacks, with both relative and absolute increases larger for Blacks. There were also changes in the diagnostic mix of admitted patients. There was almost no change in the rate at which white persons were admitted for schizophrenia and other psychotic disorders, suggesting that for these serious conditions no appreciable change had taken place in the accessibility of services for white patients. There was, however, a 10 percent increase in the rate of admission for schizophrenia and other psychotic disorders in Blacks. Furthermore, admission rates were increased by 21 percent among Whites and 45 percent among Blacks for nonpsychotic disorders, which include mental diseases of old age, alcoholic intoxication, psychoneurotic reactions, and transient personality disturbance. These relative percentage increases are even larger in absolute terms for the black population, which experiences larger rates of admission in almost all of these categories, whether psychotic or nonpsychotic. It is not clear to what extent the changes described above can be attributed to changes in distance to the nearest accessible facility before and after desegregation. Investigation of this

Table IV.74. Unduplicated admission rates[a] of Whites and Nonwhites to four regional state hospitals 18 months before and after desegregation of state facilities, Maryland, July 1, 1961, to June 30, 1964

Diagnosis	Whites				Nonwhites			
	Before	After	Change in Rate	Percent Change in Rate	Before	After	Change in Rate	Percent Change in Rate
All diagnoses	286	324	+38	+13	478	594	+116	+24
Schizophrenic reactions and other psychotic reactions	107	106	− 1	− 1	211	233	+ 22	+10
Selected non-psychotic conditions[b]	154	187	+33	+21	197	286	+ 89	+45

SOURCE: Reference 307, Table 4, page 42.
[a] Rate per 100,000 estimated population 5 years and over.
[b] Diseases of the senium, alcoholic intoxication, psychoneurotic reactions, and transient situational personality disturbance.

feature, with the limited data available, was inconclusive, although the changes were in the expected direction. Subject to limitations in the study, which the authors point out and which include the likelihood that a number of changes occurred concurrently with desegregation, the suspicion remains that the change in accessibility may have been more than a matter of distance alone. The authors conclude as follows:

> It is our opinion that hospitalization is optional for some persons with certain types and levels of conditions—it occurs if the facility is accessible and does not occur if it is not. Since desegregation increased the accessibility of hospital facilities for many more Negroes than whites, state hospital admissions of Negroes rose more than those of whites, with a resultant shift from community to inpatient care (307, p. 44).

The distinction between the barrier effects of distance and of social factors has been examined by Bashshur, Shannon, and Metzner in a study in which specific hospitals, physicians, dentists, and pharmacies are selected as the source of care by a sample of persons who reside in metropolitan Cleveland (308). The critical measure is the percent of people who do not seek care at the nearest resource but travel to the second nearest or beyond. The propensity or necessity to bypass nearer hospitals was higher for black persons than Whites, and higher for Jews than for non-Jews. There were also clear gradients by education and income, with those in the higher groups showing least propensity or necessity to go beyond the second nearest hospital. These findings have been interpreted to indicate that Jews are more selective in the choice of a hospital than are non-Jews, and that Blacks and persons with lesser income and education encounter barriers in access to some hospitals that may be nearest to them. While these interpretations are eminently persuasive, it is important to understand that other interpretations are possible. Without calling on external evidence, it is not possible to say whether barriers to access or selectivity by the client brings about the behavior observed. Population density, the resource-population ratio, and the aggregation or the dispersal of the resource are additional factors that influence the frequency with which the bypassing of the nearest resources occurs. Interactions amongst these several factors can explain further observations concerning the choice of physicians, dentists, and pharmacies. The racial, ethnic, religious, and other socioeconomic gradients in the bypassing of the nearer resources were less for physicians than for hospitals, less for dentists than for physicians, and virtually absent for pharmacies. There were no clear gradients by income either for choice of physicians or dentists. This could have arisen through the interactive effects of two opposing forces: barriers to access in the lower economic groups and greater selectivity in the higher. The factor of client selectivity is probably responsible for the observation that in a sample of 57 person-trips made by Jews, every one involved travel beyond the first two dentists in seeking the preferred dentist. By contrast to all other sources of care studied, pharmacies are relatively evenly distributed, do not discriminate to a significant degree among customers, nor are they subject to as critical choice by clients. Hence, average travel distance to pharmacies was short, and relatively few clients bypassed nearer pharmacies to seek those that were at greater distance.

The attractions created by religious preference and the barriers posed by low income and black color are clearly evident in an earlier study of travel patterns in the Chicago Metropolitan area reported by Morrill et al. (309). Graphic representations of travel by patients from predominantly Jewish communities reveal unusually long and seemingly "irrational" trips to distant hospitals. Negro patients have to travel, on the average, twice as long in order to receive hospital care as they would have to travel if they had equal access to care. The actual figures are 6 miles as compared to 3. Finally, close to 50 percent of poor patients in Cook County "must travel long distances, often by bus, beyond closer intervening hospitals to have the dubious privilege" of receiving care at Cook County Hospital and nearby Veteran's Administration hospitals.

Important among the socio-organizational factors that influence accessibility to resources are those that arise from peculiar configurations in the medical care system itself. For example, the ability of physicians to obtain affiliation at one or more hospitals and their location relative to the hospitals of major affiliation, as well as to potential clients, must play a significant role in influencing the distances which patients travel in order to receive hospital care. Morrill et al. found that in the Chicago Metropolitan area 55 percent of physicians direct patients to only one hospital, and most other physicians direct patients to only two. Although 48 percent of physicians practice at the hospital nearest their offices, as many as 35 percent practice at hospitals beyond the two that are nearest to their offices. Only 33 percent of trips to physicians are made to the physician closest to clients' homes; and only 41 percent of patients seek care at the hospital closest to their homes. Compared to what occurs in the City proper, suburban physicians are more likely to locate nearest to the hospital in which they practice (62 percent versus 34 percent), and clients are more likely to receive care by the nearest physician (46 percent versus 18 percent) and at the nearest hospital (53 percent versus 23 percent). Needless to say, these conditions are only in part caused by patterns in the relationship between physicians and hospitals and the further influence of the physician on the choice of hospital by the patient. The point that Morrill and his associates wish to make, and which will become abundantly clear as we proceed in this chapter, is that features of the medical care system further interact with client preferences, with barriers to free choice, and with the geography of physicians, hospitals, and categories of the population. Such interactions are, of course, most involved in urban areas, which are characterized by concentrations and diversities of people and of health resources, and by other complexities of structure.

A more recent study by Weiss, Greenlick, and Jones illustrates the possible importance of additional characteristics of the organization of care in the choice among alternative resources (330). The study documents the frequency with which members of a prepaid group practice, in an urban setting, receive care at the nearest of three alternative clinics. The observation that as many as 36 percent of visits are to the clinic that is not the nearest to home indicates the importance of factors other than distance alone. The most obvious is that certain specialized services are available only at the clinic that serves as a center for its two satellites. However, when one considers only those services (internal medicine and pediatrics) that are available at all three clinics, as many as 31 percent of visits are still made to the clinic that is not nearest to the clients' homes. The nature of the clinic itself, whether a center or a satellite, appears to be the most important of the several factors that are shown to be related to the bypassing of a nearer clinic to receive care at one that is more distant. For services available at all three clinics, 49 percent of visits to the central clinic are made by persons who live nearer to another clinic; the figures for the two satellite clinics are 18 and 2 percent respectively. This suggests that possibly the prestige of the central clinic or the network of referrals among physicians is a potent influence, at least in an urban area where distance differentials are not so great and transportation facilities are reasonably good.

These examples serve to illustrate the distinction made in our model between attributes of resources and the social, cultural, economic or psychological characteristics of clients that influence the recognition of need and the seeking of care. We are concerned here not with the propensity to seek care but with a "lack of fit," even when the source of care and the client are brought together. The examples also distinguish socio-organizational from geographical barriers. One could, however, draw a certain analogy between these two by saying that either social distance, or miles, poses the obstacle. Morrill and Earickson have expressed the lack of fit, between client and resources, brought about by religious preference, in terms of equivalent barriers that might have been created by distance. In an ecological study of the use of Chicago hospitals they conclude as follows:

Analyses of actual flows and experimental operation of the model suggest that on the average Jews evaluate distance to non-Jewish hospitals as about three times farther; Catholics evaluate distance to non-Catholic hospitals as about twice as far; Protestants evaluate Catholic and Jewish hospitals as about twice as far but evaluate nonreligiously oriented hospitals as about the same as Protestant hospitals (352, p. 134).

There is also a temporal aspect to accessibility that could be discussed either here, as one feature of social organization, or in conjunction with the spatial attributes to be discussed under the heading of geographic accessibility. Time and space are closely, perhaps inextricably, entwined. Together they form major aspects of ecological organization (305, pp. 288–316). Very simply, the hours during which the physician holds office sessions, or the ambulatory care facility remains open, influences the ability of clients, especially working people, to obtain care. A more elegant model would seek to compare the periodicity of the health resource with the social, and perhaps biological, rhythms that govern human populations. For example, we have alluded in a previous section to the daily, weekly, and seasonal variations in hospital occupancy and speculated on the appropriateness of smoothing out such fluctuations. In the following section we shall refer to fluctuations in travel time over the same distance, depending, among other things, on volume of traffic which itself is geared to the spatial and social organization of work, leisure and domicile.

GEOGRAPHIC ACCESSIBILITY: MEASURES OF THE FRICTION OF SPACE. In his classic text on *Human Ecology*, Amos Hawley gives a lucid account of the spatial aspects of ecological organization (305, pp. 234–287). The application of this general framework to an analysis of the organization of health services would be beyond the more limited scope of this section. For a brief review the reader is referred to the paper by Shannon et al. (306). Here the emphasis will be on only one aspect: access to the source of care. In this context the central notion is the simple observation that space creates resistance to motion. Ecologists, following the lead of Robert Haig, have referred to this phenomenon as the "friction of space" (305, p. 237). The resistance so created can be measured in a number of ways, each suited to some particular purpose. These measures include (1) linear distance, (2) travel distance, (3) travel time, (4) total elapsed time, and (5) travel cost. Shannon et al. emphasize that what is sought is, ideally, some measure of total effort associated with overcoming the friction of space, and that the measures enumerated above are only approximations, some better than others (306, p. 145). The concept of "effort," however, is more subjective than the measures of distance, time, and cost. It includes factors such as familiarity with the route traveled and perceptions of distance or travel time. It also includes the suffering and inconvenience occasioned by moving patients stricken with painful or disabling illnesses. As such, "effort" includes the psychological, and perhaps social, valuation placed on spatial attributes.

A number of considerations pertain to the more conventional measures of the fricton of space enumerated above. In most instances of surface travel, linear distance can be taken as only a crude approximation of distances traveled. However, linear distance can be readily measured on a map, and such measurements, crude as they are, have been shown to be related to important differences in the use of health services (325). Given a map showing major highways, it is also possible to measure travel distance. Generally, this is not distance actually traveled but a hypothetical distance, under the assumption that persons tend to choose the shortest distance between two points, or the route that takes the shortest time to travel. The earlier studies of Jehlik and McNamara (320) and of Altman (323), and the more recent studies of Lubin et al. (312), have used this resistance-minimizing assumption. Other studies have accepted a similar assumption by selecting, on a map, the route that is most commonly traveled (326–328) or the route that is thought to be the one most likely to be selected on grounds of "accessibility rather than miles" (329–330).

Another simplifying procedure is not to measure from the actual point of origin or termination but from or to central points of population concentration and concentrations of health resources. Altman measured the distances between large cities "from the center of the town" (323, p. 25). Lubin et al. examined spatial relationships between clients, physicians, and hospitals by locating in each census tract, or parts of larger census tracts, centers of population density, clusters of physicians' offices, and individual hospitals (312). In one study, the location of each physician was assumed to be at the population "centroid" of his census tract (343). Schneider used the "approximate geographic center of the residential use of each of 97 postal zones" to represent all patients who lived in that postal zone (351). Sohler and his associates measured distances to mental hospitals from the population center of each of 169 townships in the state of Connecticut (326). Using centers instead of actual locations results in the loss of detail which may or may not be important depending on the level of aggregation at which a given problem is being considered. For example, clustering may be appropriate in a study of travel patterns within large regions but not within smaller metropolitan areas. Similarly, assumptions concerning the route traveled remove from study factors other than distance or average travel time that could be part of a more realistic measure of the friction of space, whether objective or subjective. As we have seen, even larger errors may result from an assumption that individuals always use the health resource that is nearest to the place where they live or work.

Travel time is generally considered as a more accurate measure of the friction of space than either travel or linear distance (312). Kane has reported that in a rural setting respondents seem to think more in terms of time than distance when asked what factors would most determine the accessibility and convenience of a new facility (331). Unlike distance, travel time shows decided secular trends and random as well as highly systematic variations by which the more static aspects of spatial organization are linked to the development of technology and the rhythms of social life. For example, travel time will vary with time of day, being slower during morning and evening rush hours when most cars are on the road (312). Travel time will also reflect the influence of seasonal, climatic, and other geographic factors not evident from consideration of distance alone. Information on travel time, as on distance, can be obtained directly from surveys of those who use services. It is more customary to measure distances off a map, under the assumptions of minimum effort and central location, and to convert distances into time equivalents. However, such conversion requires additional information and additional assumptions. These include information about modes of transportation, average speeds during different parts of the day on each segment of highway, and legal speed limits. For any given locality such information may be available from studies of transportation relevant to highway construction or safety, or to the more general needs of urban planning. For limited studies it is possible to obtain the necessary information more directly, by actually traveling over the relevant routes, at the relevant times, armed with stopwatch, pencil and a simple form for recording observations (310). The measurement of travel time, however achieved, is only one component of the time used for the receipt of care. The total time elapsed between interrupting one's activities to seek care and returning to those activities includes, in addition, time waiting for transportation at the point of origin as well as at the point of receipt of care. When traveling by private conveyance, the availability of convenient parking may become critical. When public transportation is used, the location of the scheduled stops and the frequency of runs influence both travel time and time lost in waiting. Needless to say, an accounting of elapsed time could, for certain purposes, also include some or all components of time spent within the facility, either waiting or receiving care. The analysis of time lapse within the health facility has been described in a previous section of this chapter.

Money cost may well be the most comprehensive and versatile representation of the friction of space short of some measure of total "effort." The distance-related considerations of cost include direct and indirect as well as internal and external elements. Direct costs include actual costs of transportation as well as "terminal costs" such as those incurred for parking (350). Indirect costs include those of arrangements necessary to release the client from his ordinary duties—baby sitting, for example. More important, however, may be the opportunity costs or the value of time lost. This may be clearly evident if there is actual loss of income attendant upon absence from work. Usually the loss is less noticeable because it is in the form of lost working potential. The value of lost product raises the issue of the differential social valuation placed on the time of the several participants in the medical care transaction. The decision of whether, given an option, physician travel or patient travel is to be minimized depends, in part, on differences in the value placed on time loss for clients and physicians. Schneider (350) provides a brief discussion of this issue and refers to the work of Moses and Williamson for a more complete presentation (311). The relationship between distance, internal costs, and external costs will be discussed in a subsequent section on "locational efficiency." There are also certain relative considerations in evaluating the impact of travel cost. Subjectively, the cost of travel relative to the cost of care itself may be significant. This may represent perceptions of a more fundamental issue: the cost of travel relative to the benefits, actual or expected, to be derived from the receipt of care.

Another consideration in the measurement and evaluation of cost is the partitioning of costs among several uses of a single journey. There are obvious savings in time, money, and effort when a trip to town can include, for example, a visit to the dentist, the hairdresser, and the supermarket. Similarly, travel costs are reduced if several medical care transactions can be completed at one place during one visit. This is a potent argument for the centralization of certain medical care functions. In a more general sense, it points out the importance of assuring congruence between travel for medical care and travel for other, everyday purposes. Such congruence may be more important because it reduces psychological and social barriers than because it also reduces monetary cost. Mountin and Greve were aware of these several factors, and of the additional need to reduce barriers within the health establishment itself, when they recommended "a plan for coordination" of health departments and hospitals.

In other words, local health units should be patterned so that people move in the same direction to secure preventive medical services as they do to obtain curative medical services, hospitalization, and, indeed, the everyday necessities of life (359, p. 5).

A discussion of the financial cost of overcoming the friction of space is not complete unless one re-emphasizes what it leaves out as well as what it includes. The psychic and social "costs," which are excluded, should be major considerations, even though it may not be possible to assign a precise money value to them.

Our discussion of the measurement of the friction of space has, of necessity, included mention of the factors that influence the magnitude of the resistance to motion. A more systematic discussion of such factors might classify them under the following headings: (1) properties of space, (2) properties of technology, (3) properties of persons, and (4) properties of social organization. The properties of space include topographic features such as mountains and rivers which act as natural obstacles. Gravitational gradients, uphill or downhill, can be important, especially when powered vehicles are not available. Climatic conditions could be included as properties of space; as can man-made barriers, such as superhighways, that may interfere with local access while facilitating travel to more distant places. De Visé has described, for the Chicago area, the facilitating and obstructing effects on travel for medical care and other purposes, of such man-made as well as natural features of the environment.

Comparison of these (origin-destination) maps with transportation maps would show that elevated and suburban rail lines appear to serve as axes of location, while industrial rail lines and waterways act as barriers obstructing crosstown traffic. At least five sectors are thereby defined: northwestern, western, southwestern and southern. Among the barriers to movement, the Chicago Sanitary Canal and Lake Calumet effectively arrest development to the southwest and south of these bodies of water (368, p. 18. See also text and Fig. 16, p. 28).

Among the properties of technology are the development of roads and means of transportation. The latter include travel by foot, animals, non-powered vehicles, powered vehicles, etc. In the past, modes of transportation, and the relative performance of land versus water transportation, have been decisive factors in ecological organization (305, pp. 200–201, and elsewhere). The advent of air transportation has obvious implications for the organization of health services, in general, and emergency services in particular. Jolly and King have pointed out that in many primitive locales, the effective range of health services is limited by the distance which persons are willing or able to walk (332, chap. 2, sec. 7). Hogarth has reported fascinating examples of the manner in which properties of terrain and transportation become reflected in formal fee schedules (386). For example, the Swedish fee schedule provides for fee increments according to distance, if travel is by car, and according to time elapsed, if travel is not by car. The Norwegian fee schedule differentiates travel allowances by distance and type of travel combined. The four categories recognized cast an interesting light on the conditions of practice. They are (1) travel by car, motorcycle, or train, (2) travel by motor boat, regular boat service, reindeer, or bicycle, (3) travel by ordinary boat or on horseback, and (4) travel by foot. In the 1959 fee schedule the proportionate weights per unit distance for these four categories of travel were 0.5, 1.5, 2.0 and 5.0 respectively. In France, a distinction is made by type of terrain; travel in level country, mountainous country and high mountains are weighted in the proportions of 5, 6 and 7 respectively. In all three countries, travel allowances are modified by a variety of stipulations that illustrate several of the factors that we have considered in measuring the friction of space or which we shall discuss under the heading of "locational efficiency." For example, the Swedish schedule allows for time necessarily spent in waiting for public transportation. The Norwegian schedule specifies that payment is made only for the least expensive of alternative methods of transportation. In both Sweden and Norway it is specified that when several visits are made in the course of one journey, the travel allowance is to be shared among the visits. In both Sweden and France, allowances are not paid for distances that exceed (or exceed by a specified amount) the distance to the nearest physician. In this way spatial patterns of use are, presumably, adjusted to the spatial configuration of resources (386, pp. 176, 579, 587–588, and 597).

We have already alluded to the properties of persons and of social organization, including economic factors, that influence the resistance of space. Under personal characteristics might be included illness and disability as well as demographic and psychological attributes that influence mobility or the propensity to venture out. The complex of factors that influence the cost of movement have already been discussed in fair detail. The social organizational substrate that determines the flow and ebb of traffic has also been mentioned. Once again, one needs to emphasize the congruence or incongruence of the location of the source of health care with the centers around which the daily or more occasional activities of a community are organized. Perhaps one might also include, as aspects of social organization, the observation that places are not neutral, but have social and psychological meaning. Some places are unfamiliar, threatening or, even, holy. This is in addition to the more concrete dangers that might be encountered, for example, in certain sections of our cities. An interesting example of the more subtle connotations associated with place is the report by Hodges and Dörken of reluctance to use an ambulatory mental health facility because it was placed in the local mental hospital (324). Even more directly relevant are notions, current since ancient times, that some locations are harmful to health and others salubrious—being, therefore, locations where healing may be sought (387, 388). The present location of some older hospitals and sanatoria may owe not a little to these beliefs.

GEOGRAPHIC ACCESSIBILITY: GRAPHIC PRESENTATION. For analysis and planning it is often useful to have a visual picture of the location of resources and of access to them. If linear distance were the measure of the resistance to motion each medical care resource would be shown surrounded by a set of concentric circles, each with a specified radius. The many factors that influence the resistance to motion do, in fact, cause considerable distortion in this simple picture. For example, lines of equal travel time surrounding a resource are likely to be pulled outward along major routes of transportation. Figure IV.5 shows two such lines, called "isochrones," surrounding a hospital. Considerable departure from circularity has occurred. Similarly, it should be possible, under certain assumptions, to draw lines of equal cost ("isodapans") surrounding a resource, although the author has not seen such maps in the medical care literature. In the following section we shall describe relationships between geographic accessibility and the use of services. Based on these relationships, Jolly and King have shown lines of equal care ("isocare" lines) surrounding resources in a geographic area (332, chap. 2, sec. 8). Needless to say, when there are several resources in a locality, lines of equal distance, travel time, cost or care will tend to intersect, identifying zones of equal access to more than one resource.

Bashshur et al. have given a brief description of graphic methods used in describing and analyzing ecological distributions of health-related phenomena (313). These may be classified into "locational descriptive" and "locational analytic" methods. The descriptive methods may show

Fig. IV.5.   Isochrones showing 5 and 10 minutes of travel time from a hospital in Santa Clara County, California

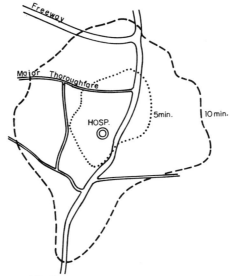

SOURCE: Reference 312, Figure 2, p. 774.

the actual locations of ungrouped phenomena—for example, in the form of a "dot map." They may also show the geographic distribution of grouped data, with each class distinguished by some visual code such as color, shading, stippling, cross-hatching or the like. The analytic methods combine "elements of both geographic representation and statistical areal measurement." They include "the standard deviation ellipse," and "standard distance circle," the "sectorgram" and "three-dimensional analogue models."

For any distribution, including distribution of locations, there are two principal measures: one of central tendency and another of dispersion. The methods used for locating, measuring, and depicting these for places on a map are analogous to the methods used in nonspatial statistics, except that each place requires measurement along two dimensions (for example along an X- and a Y-axis) in order to be located on a surface. The mean center of a distribution of places can be computed by measuring distances along Cartesian coordinates centered on any arbitrary location on the surface over which the places are distributed. The algebraic sum of distances along the abscissa, divided by the total number of places, locates one coordinate of the mean center. The Y-coordinate is obtained in the same way. The Cartesian coordinates can now be redrawn to run through this mean center, which is the center of gravity of the distribution. The standard deviation of the distribution of places relative to this center can be computed along either axis. The axes could also be rotated, so that the standard deviation can be measured from the mean center in any desired direction. According to Lefever, "the locus of the standard deviation value as the axis rotates around the mean center is an ellipse. In order to plot the ellipse on the map it is necessary to locate the major and minor axes (of the ellipse) and to calculate the corresponding standard deviation values" (315, p. 90). Thus, "the standard deviation ellipse" shows on a flat surface the degree of dispersal or concentration of resources around a geographic mean point. The directions of the major and minor axes and their relative lengths indicate differences of dispersal in different directions. The amount of dispersal may be indicated by the magnitude of the standard deviation and by the unit locations within the ellipse expressed as a proportion of all unit locations in the distribution (315). An alternative and simpler measure of dispersal is the "standard distance," which is the standard deviation of all places in a distribution from the mean or median center without reference to any axis. As a visual representation of dispersal, a "standard circle," with radius equal to the standard distance, may be drawn around the center of the distribution. The "standard circle" gives a less realistic representation than does the "standard deviation ellipse" because it assumes that dispersal is equal in all directions around the center. This defect can be remedied to some extent by dividing the circle into equiangular sections, computing the standard distance for all the unit locations within each sector and drawing an arc with a radius equal to the standard distance within each sector. The figure that results from joining these arcs is a "sectorgram." An illustration, with additional details of the method, is provided by Schneider (351, pp. 38–39). A more complete exposition is given by Cherniak and Schneider (369).

Summary representations, such as the standard deviation ellipse or the standard distance circle, because of their very nature may not adequately represent important differences that would be discerned if the entire distributions were plotted. It is, of course, possible to show concurrently, on a single map, both the location of each phenomenon (or a frequency distribution of a phenomenon) and the summary representation of that distribution. Bashshur et al., in their paper on graphic methods, show the distribution of hospitals, physicians, dentists, and pharmacies in Cleveland, using for each distribution both standard deviation ellipse and a three-dimensional model. The three-dimensional models give a picture of the concentration of resources, clients, or other populations over a surface shown as a grid in which each cell represents a standard unit of area. The number of resources or persons in each unit area is represented by a peak-like elevation over that area. Thus one obtains a picture, not unlike a three-dimensional representation of mountainous terrain (313, 338). It is possible to plot rectangular prisms, instead of peaks, over each unit area, which results in a picture similar to that of a city with buildings of varying height (see, for example, 316, Map 12, p. 40). For further details about the more complex analytic graphic methods the reader should consult the papers cited and the sources to which they refer.

Increasingly, the labor involved in the construction of maps and other visual representations of spatial factors is being reduced through the use of computers. In a previous chapter we referred briefly to computer methods for locating or showing the distribution of births, deaths, and similar events that denote need (316, 317). These same methods can show distributions of population characteristics, including use of service. In this section we have referred to computer methods, described by Lubin et al., for plotting isochrones under certain assumptions concerning travel routes and travel conditions (312). Programs have also been developed that enable the computer to draw standard deviation ellipses and three-dimensional representations (313, 338, 316). The reader can readily appreciate that by using such graphic methods, with or without computer assistance, it is possible to obtain a picture of the spatial correspondence —or lack of correspondence—of need, use of service, and supply.

GEOGRAPHIC ACCESSIBILITY AND USE OF SERVICES AND RESOURCES. In this section we shall describe some studies that have examined the relationship between geographic accessibility and the use of services and resources. Before actually doing so, it might be useful to begin with a discussion of considerations that influence our evaluation of such studies and the interpretation of their findings.

There are two perspectives on the relationship between access to service and the friction of space. One is to study the use of services by clients in relation to their spatial separation from the sources of care. The other is to study the employment of the resource according to the spatial separation of its clients from it. The first is a survey of utilization, the second an example of case load analysis. One or the other may be the more appropriate approach, depending on the focus of concern and responsibility. Sometimes it is possible to construct one from the other. For example, if a large number of resources serving a given area are surveyed, it may be possible from the analysis of their combined case load to obtain a picture of how people travel to receive care—if it can be assumed that all, or substantially all, of the care received is confined to the resources surveyed. In precisely this way, Altman constructed data on use of service by clients from reports by physicians concerning their case loads during a given day (323). However, irrespective of whether one focuses on the use of service by a given population or the manner in which a resource is used, a major limitation remains: there is no information about services not received or produced. It is not possible, using either approach, to obtain a picture of services not used because of geographic barriers, unless one assumes that need remains constant irrespective of distance, and that decrements in use, related to distance, represent unmet need. This assumption cannot be safely made because distance from central places in which resources tend to congregate is also correlated with differences in ecology, including social and economic characteristics of the residents, that may influence the occurrence of need, the type of need, and the propensity to seek care. Such characteristics include education, income, occupation, and other attributes associated with rurality as contrasted with urban styles of life. All these correlates of distance influence the interpretation of utilization studies as well as analyses of case load. In addition, data on proportion of case load by distance from a resource cannot be interpreted without knowledge of the gradients of population density surrounding the resource. One aspect of population density is the "nuclearity" of the population, or the extent to which it is aggregated in localities, so that there are relatively few inhabitants in between (332, chap. 2, sec. 8). In any case, it is important to remember that proportions of case load by distance from a resource do not correspond to proportions of inhabitants, by distance from a resource, who use that resource. To derive the latter from case load data it would be necessary to know the number of persons who live in each distance zone surrounding the resource. Adjustments would also have to be made for multiple use by individuals during any given period of time. Case load analyses in terms of visits or other units of service have different connotations from case load analyses in terms of persons who use service one or more times.

Data on proportion of case load by distance from a resource give disproportionate weight to regions further away from the resource. This is because the further one moves away from the center, the larger is the area in each concentric distance zone. Given radii of the set of concentric circles, it is possible to compute the area of each concentric zone and to present case load data in terms of cases per unit area in each zone. Implicit in this procedure is the assumption that the population is evenly distributed *within* each concentric zone. If it were possible to make the further assumption that the population were evenly distributed over the entire set of concentric zones surrounding a resource, the set of data on number of cases per unit area in each distance zone would represent the propensities of persons in each of these zones to use the resource. However, it is not often that one can make such an assumption of homogeneity in population density as distance from a resource increases.

An additional factor that influences observed relationships between distance and use of service is the spatial distribution of resources. It is quite likely that the established distribution of such resources in any given area has been brought about, in part, by the willingness of consumers to travel to these resources. There are, however, other causative factors, such as the dependence of certain specialists on medical centers (343) and the attraction of urban locations for health professionals and health facilities, in general (344). The point to be made is that the existing spatial configuration of resources, no matter how it has been brought about, places limits on the range of observable health behaviors in respect to the friction of space. For example, if general practitioners are closely and evenly distributed in a given population, it may be impossible to say what proportion of persons would travel how far to see a general practitioner if he were the only one in the area in question, and what the effect on use of really long distances would be. However, as we have described, when a choice among alternative resources is possible, the propensity to bypass intervening resources in order to receive care at a resource that is further away, is a useful measure of selective attractions or barriers to care (308, 309, 330). But it should be remembered that this measure does not distinguish whether the patterns observed are due to the preferences of clients, obstacles created by the providers of care or both.

The foregoing aspects of perspective and of method are presented by way of introduction to a description and interpretation of the findings of selected studies that have dealt with the relationship between use and spatial characteristics. By way of additional background it may also be useful to postulate certain expectations and to examine the extent to which these are met by the findings. These expectations, or hypotheses, may be derived from a simple model of "attractions and blocks," such as that postulated by Metzner (318). In this instance the "blocks" are erected by the resistance of space and the factors that contribute to it, as already described. The "attractions" are the quality and reputation of the resource, its specialized nature, its uniqueness or scarcity, and other desirable attributes of the resource or of its location. There are also a number of "propelling" factors related to the perceived threat of illness in terms of urgency and severity. It may be further postulated that the blocks, attractions, and propulsions enumerated above influence not only client behavior, but the behavior of the provider as well (see model of the Medical Care Process as presented in Chapter III). Thus one would expect that use of service and resource employment decrease with distance from the resource and that unmet need increases in parallel fashion. The diminution with distance would be more marked for preventive services as compared to curative services, for generalist care as compared to specialist care, for physician services as compared to hospital services, and for mild illness as compared with severe illness. The effect of urgency might be mixed and therefore difficult to predict. Extremely urgent conditions might be referred initially to the nearest source of care even though it might not be the most appropriate. However, the seriousness of certain urgent conditions might lead to bypassing nearer resources in favor of a more distant resource with the required critical facilities. The outcome of these several factors would be that any given resource would be used differently by persons who live near it as compared to those who are more distant. Furthermore, different resources would differ in outreach, depending on their attractiveness to particular population groups and on the degree to which they perform scarce, highly technical, and specialized functions. It is likely that physician behavior, through referral or failure to refer, would play a significant role in bringing about the patterns of expected use, as described above. Finally, one might find reflected in measures of health and welfare the consequences of the manner in which clients and providers use or fail to use service, as influenced by the friction of space.

Shannon et al. have given a brief account of the development of concepts and methods for studying the effects of distance and have reviewed the findings of several studies in the health field (306). Sohler and his coworkers have recently reviewed the considerable body of literature concerning the relationships between distance and the use of mental hospitals, in this country as well as abroad, and have added important findings of their own (326–328). In general, the findings support the expectations that distance reduces use of service and that the magnitude of the effect differs by type of service and type of resource. These tendencies have been remarkably well documented in the field of mental health, where the inverse relationship between distance and admission to mental hospitals has been recognized as "Jarvis' Law" because it was first reported by Dr. E. Jarvis of the Worcester State Hospital in Massachusetts as long ago as before the Civil War (326). However, there are several studies, some cited by Shannon et al., that have not shown the expected diminution of use by distance (306, 321, pp. 25–26; 322, pp. 67–68; 343, p. 17). In some instances this may have been due to relatively small differentials in the resistance to motion. For example, Altman suggests that the large number of general practitioners relative to population, and their even distribution, may have accounted for the lack of significant correlation between distance and the use of general practitioner services in Western Pennsylvania (323, p. 30). Morrill and Earickson have postulated a two-mile "region of indifference" within which distance has no appreciable effect on physician use in Chicago (352, p. 131). In at least one study, however, there is reason to believe that the apparent lack of relationship between use and distance obscured a more fundamental relationship between unmet need and distance. Hoffer et al. found no difference in the number of office calls and home calls per person in areas classified as open country, village, metropolitan and urban (321, pp. 25–26). However, "unmet need," as judged by the reporting of one or more untreated symptoms, decreased in frequency with increasing urbanization (321, Table 2, p. 15). Unmet need was also related to distance from the nearest town having a physician, as shown in Table IV.75.

Table IV.75.   Percent of persons with one or more untreated symptoms, according to distance from nearest town having doctor, Michigan, 1948

Distance from Nearest Town Having Doctor	Percent of Persons with One or More Untreated Symptoms
0–5 miles	24.1
6–10 miles	28.8
11 miles or more	37.4

SOURCE: Reference 321, Table 2, page 15.

A number of studies may be cited to illustrate the extent to which relationships postulated by our model are, in fact, observed to occur. In a study of medical care in rural Missouri, Jehlik and McNamara show that as distance from the physician increases there is a relative decrease in visits to the physician per unit population in spite of a concurrent increase in the amount of "bed illness" experienced (320). Table IV.76

Table IV.76.   Percent of difference in use of specified services associated with residence of more than 5 linear miles from a physician, rural Missouri, 1949

Measure of Use or Morbidity	Percent Difference Associated with Distance
Physician visits per 1000 persons	−13
Bed-days of illness per 1000 persons	+28
Physician visits per 100 bed-days of illness	−32

SOURCE: Reference 320.

gives the percent difference associated with residence more than 5 linear miles from the nearest physician. Further analysis would be needed to determine whether the differences observed are due to distance alone or are at least partly due to socioeconomic differences associated with distance. No data are given about hospital use in relation to distance. However, there was no relationship between distance to hospital and the frequency of bed illness. Jehlik and McNamara report that "a partial explanation lies in the fact that there is not as much choice between whether a patient shall or shall not be taken to a hospital, as is the case in whether or not the services of a physician shall be used."

Altman used a one-day census of the case load of physicians in Western Pennsylvania to study the relationships between location and use of service (323). He noted a statistically significant correlation between the use of specialist services and distance from specialists, but no significant correlation between the use of general practitioner services and distance to the general practitioner. The difference is attributed by the author to the large number of general practitioners per unit population and their more even distribution throughout the study area. As one might expect, specialists were relatively fewer in number and more likely to be aggregated in urban centers. This may be largely responsible for the observation that specialists had a longer outreach: a larger proportion of their patients came from further away. The differential prevalence and spatial distribution of specialists and generalists may also account for the observation that there were large differences in distances traveled to the specialist by place of residence of patients, while the differences for general practitioners were relatively small, as shown in Table IV.77.

There is no information to indicate the extent to which the longer distances traveled to specialists may also be due to (1) the greater perceived uniqueness and, therefore, lower interchangeability of the services of individual specialists; (2) the greater seriousness of the conditions for

Table IV.77.   Distances traveled to general practitioners and specialists by persons residing in counties of specified characteristics, Western Pennsylvania, 1950–51

County Group of Residence of Patients	Average Miles Traveled to	
	General Practitioners	Specialists
Greater metropolitan	3.0	3.1
Lesser metropolitan	3.6	6.0
Adjacent to greater metropolitan	4.3	10.4
Adjacent to lesser metropolitan	5.3	14.1
Other	5.0	14.4

SOURCE: Reference 323, Table 3, page 28.

which specialists are consulted; or (3) the higher socioeconomic status of those who consult specialists. An elucidation of the role of these factors would require further information about the characteristics of those who seek service, as well as information on the extent to which persons bypass a generalist to see a specialist a further distance away, or seek a more distant specialist in preference to a similar one nearer home.

Sohler et al. have reported on the manner in which distance influences first admissions and readmissions to, and length of stay in, mental hospitals in Connecticut during the period of July 1, 1959, through June 30, 1963 (326–328). An odometer was used to measure distances on a map, along most commonly traveled routes, between the center of each of 169 townships and one of three mental hospitals that serve the state. Although Connecticut is a small state, so that few towns were more than 50 miles distant from a mental hospital, a marked inverse relationship was observed between distance and first admission rates, thus confirming the original observation by Jarvis as reported in 1852. First admission rates in townships that were 0–9 miles distant from the mental hospital in their district were, on the average, triple the rates in townships that were 50 or more miles distant. This relationship was altered in magnitude, but not eliminated, when a number of factors were taken into account singly or in selected pairings. Jarvis' Law held for males as well as females. It was operative in each of six age groups, including the group 65 and over. In fact, for females aged 65 and over, the admission rate for towns 0 to 9 miles distant from the mental hospital was almost ten times the rate for towns that were 50 or more miles away. The effect of distance was also observed for Whites as well as Nonwhites, though it was not as marked for the latter. Age adjusted admission rates for Whites who were younger than 65 continued to show the effect of distance when townships were grouped into two categories of size and two of income. However, "the slope tended to be steeper among the large towns, owing chiefly to differences in proximal rate. This is similar to findings in Norway, where Jarvis' Law is more pronounced when the inner zone contains a large town" (326, p. 508). The effects of diagnostic categories were examined, but not in sufficient detail. Differences in the first admission rate by distance were marked for functional psychoses as well as for all other diagnoses combined, although somewhat less so for the former as compared to the latter. The effect of the presence or absence in the community of sources of psychiatric care alternative to the state mental hospital was also examined. The conclusion was that this variable does not account for the manifestations of Jarvis' Law in Connecticut (327). However, this is a factor that requires further study in order to disentangle two possible effects that may act in opposite directions. The presence of alternative sources of psychiatric care, such as psychiatrists in private practice and psychiatric clinics, could both reduce the need for state hospital care and generate demand for such care. The conclusion to be drawn from the work of Sohler and her associates is that proximity is a very important factor in first admissions to mental hospitals, independently of a variety of associated factors. If the rate for first admissions experienced in the innermost metropolitan zone were to prevail in all zones, first admissions would have been eight times higher for the state as a whole than were currently experienced. The increment would be even higher if readmissions were included in the computation, since the readmission rate has a slightly higher slope when related to distance than does the first admission rate. It should be remembered, however, that findings concerning admissions need to be coupled with information about length of stay in order to measure the full impact of the effect of distance. Sohler et al. used several indirect approaches to their investigation of the relationship between length of stay and distance (328). They conclude that length of stay tends to be longer as distance from the mental hospital increases. This means that patient-days of care would not increase as rapidly as would admissions should hospitals become more accessible. The increment would, however, still be considerable, though its precise magnitude is not yet known. The implications to the planning of health services is obvious. The provision of geographically more accessible resources will generate significant increments of effective demand, though the magnitude of the increment will probably vary by type of service and by type of community.

That different types of resources have different capacities to overcome the friction of space is supported by several studies. Jolly and King have

assembled data from several sources to show that the average number of
outpatient attendances decreases more rapidly with increasing distance
for smaller units, such as an "aid post," than for large units, such as a
hospital (332, chap. 2, sec. 7, fig. 6). As we have already mentioned,
Weiss et al. have shown the greater attractiveness of a central clinic as
compared to its satellites, even for services that are available in all clinics
(329). More often, evidence comes from case load analysis of different
resources. For example, Morrill and Earickson (334) used factor analysis to classify Chicago hospitals into several categories. The data on case
load by distance from each hospital, and category of hospitals, were
converted to admissions per unit area for a consistent set of distances: 1,
3, 5, and 10 miles respectively. Figure IV.6 shows the findings for a
subset of hospital categories plotted so that the frequency per unit area
at a distance of one mile is set at 100 and frequencies at all other
distances are expressed as percentages of this. In all instances there is a
rapid decay with distance, but there are significant differences by hospital type. For example, four research hospitals definitely draw from
further away than do the three hospitals in satellite cities. Schneider has

Fig. IV.6.   Relative frequency of admissions per unit area, by type of
hospital and by distance from the hospital, Chicago Metropolitan area,
1965

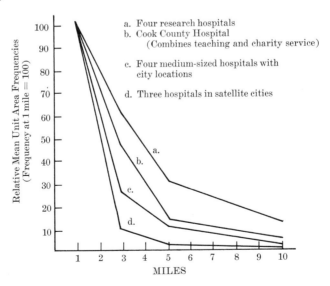

shown differences in distance between patient residences and hospital location by type of hospital service (351). It is sometimes possible to show differences in drawing power among facilities that appear to be reasonably similar in scale and intended function. For example, Hodges and Dörken have reported the frequency distributions of patients treated at three mental health centers by distance of the patient from the center (324). Figure IV.7 shows the findings. Of special interest is the observation that one center, located in the state mental hospital, was more likely to draw patients from farther away than from its immediate vicinity. In further interpreting these data, the reader should remember the considerations presented in the opening paragraphs of this section. For example, the cumulative percentage distribution given by Hodges and

Fig. IV.7.   Percent of patients terminating outpatient treatment at each of three mental health centers who live at specified distances from the respective centers (Minnesota, 1957–58)

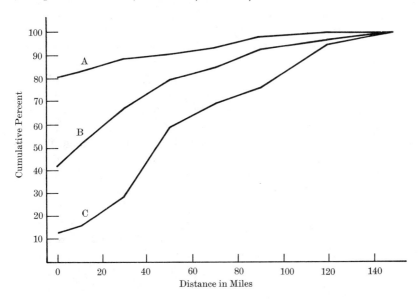

A. Duluth Center. Duluth has a population of 105,000 and is located in St. Louis County which has 230,000 residents.

B. Albert Lea Center, located in a town of 13,000 and a county of 36,000 in rural Minnesota.

C. Fergus Falls Center, located in a town of 13,300 and a county of 50,000. Location of the center in the State Hospital created local resistance to its use.

SOURCE: Reference 298.

Dörken do not correct for differences in population density related to distance from the center, nor do they correct for the fact that the farther one moves away from the center, the larger is the area in each concentric distance-zone. Morrill and Earickson correct for the latter phenomenon by computing frequencies per unit area, in each distance zone, but do not appear to correct for differences in population density, if any.

Drosness and Lubin were able to compare concurrently two aspects of hospital use in relation to the friction of space. They studied 10 general hospitals in Santa Clara County, California, varying in size from 24 to 445 beds. Around each hospital, zones were drawn at three-minute intervals of minimum travel path time. For each hospital two curves were constructed: (1) a cumulative percent of admission by time zone, and (2) for each time zone, admissions to this hospital as percent of admissions to all hospitals. Inspection of the graphs (364, Fig. 2) shows that the curves of cumulative percent of case load are generally similar and indicate rapid "decay" with travel time. In almost all cases, 75 percent or more of the total case load comes from within 15 minutes away. On the other hand, admissions to a given hospital as a percent of all admissions, though inversely related to travel time, show very marked variation by hospital, indicating large differences in dominance of hospitals over their surroundings. As expected, hospital size is clearly a factor directly related to dominance. However, one small 50-bed hospital appears to exert greater dominance over a longer travel span than any other hospital among those studied. There are obviously factors other than hospital size for which the presence of competing adjacent hospitals is likely to be critical. In a subsequent section on the delineation of service areas we shall have more to say about the two ways in which the relationship of a resource to its surrounding may be depicted: in terms of case load and in terms of hospital use.

The counterparts to differences in outreach of different resources are differences in willingness to travel according to perceived need for service. A survey of households in rural Kentucky, reported by Kane, has shown a clear differentiation between perceived priorities and preferences (331). Figure IV.8 shows marked differences in the percent of respondents willing to travel specified distances to obtain different services, apparently based on the perceived seriousness of the situation or condition. Low income (below $3000) did reduce willingness to travel. Sex and education had no influence; nor were the very few households who did not own a car or truck different in expressed willingness to travel for medical care. The study of attitudes as reported by Kane is supported by observations on the manner in which a state mental hospital

Fig. IV.8.   Percent of respondents expressing willingness to travel specified distances or more, by type of service. A rural county in Kentucky, June and July, 1968

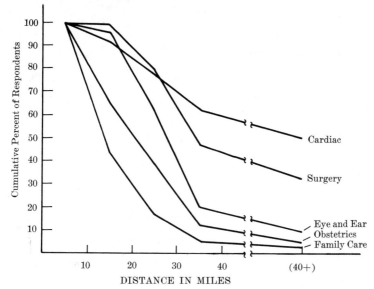

Based on a probability sample of 171 households which constituted about 15 percent of the county's families, with a response rate of 92 percent. The gradient for obstetric care is very similar to those of x-ray services and dental care. The latter have been omitted to simplify the figure.
    SOURCE: Reference 331.

is used by populations living at varying linear distances from the hospital as reported by Person (325). As shown in Fig. IV.9, distance between place of residence and the hospital does not influence the rates of first admissions for a severely disruptive condition such as schizophrenia. On the other hand, milder, though intractable, conditions such as mental deterioration associated with age, decrease in rate of first admissions as place of residence becomes more remote. The rate for all first admissions combined also shows a marked decline. More recent studies of mental hospital use provide at least partial support to the earlier observations made by Person. In our earlier description of the findings of Sohler et al. in Connecticut we emphasized the regularity with which the effects of distance were observed irrespective of other variables, including crude diagnostic categorization and age. It should be noted, however, that the effect of distance was less marked for the functional psychoses, as a

Fig. IV.9.   Relative first admission rates to a mental hospital, by diagnostic category and distance of the hospital from the patient's place of residence (Warren, Pennsylvania, 1948–1952)

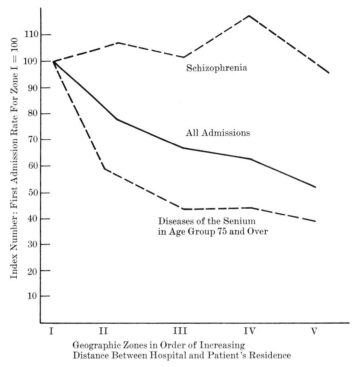

SOURCE: Reference 325.

group, than for all other diagnoses combined. The ratio of first admission rate in the most proximate zone to the rate in the most distant zone was 2:1 for functional psychoses and 3:1 for all other diagnoses (326). "Only 17 percent of persons admitted from the innermost 10-mile zone are schizophrenic. Of those admitted from a distance of 40 miles or more, 30 percent are schizophrenic" (328, p. 76). In a previous section we reported that the desegregation of mental hospitals in Maryland had a much greater augmenting effect on admission rates for nonpsychotic conditions than for the category of schizophrenic and other psychotic reactions. Admission rates for schizophrenic and other psychotic reactions in the white population showed no increase whatever (307). Thus, one may conclude that barriers, whether spatial, socio-organizational, or mixed, are most operative when need is least intense and are least operative when need is very salient and severe.

Weiss et al. have reported on the manner in which several factors influence the barrier effect of distance on the receipt of the more ordinary kinds of ambulatory care. Their major findings concern the frequency with which members of a prepaid group practice will bypass a clinic that is nearer home in order to receive care at one that is more distant. Visits for acute conditions appear to be more often made at the nearest clinic than are visits for chronic conditions (70 percent versus 60 percent). However, when the condition is serious, as shown by the necessity for hospitalization, the likelihood of receiving care at the nearest clinic is reduced. Pediatric services were more likely to be received at the nearest clinic than were the services of internists (78 percent of visits versus 67 percent). There were no differences by social class or sex. Younger patients were more likely than older patients to receive care at the nearest clinic, but this effect was confounded with the difference between the services of pediatricians and internists, as noted above. One may conclude from all this that the barrier posed by distance is not uniform for all kinds of need, and that severity, acuteness, and perhaps other characteristics, such as age, influence the extent to which a given distance does pose a barrier to care.

In an earlier paper, Weiss and Greenlick proposed that not only the volume of care but the mode of entry into the medical care system is influenced jointly by distance and socioeconomic status (329). They note, for example, that at a distance of 15–20 miles from the nearest clinic the use of the telephone by middle-class clients increases markedly, whereas regularly scheduled visits to the clinic are appreciably reduced. By contrast, at this same distance from the nearest clinic, working-class clients show a marked increase in the use of the emergency room. Unfortunately, these sharper differences are selected out of a larger matrix of more ambiguous relationships, without there being a prior base in theory from which the observed relationships could have been predicted. Nevertheless, the general notion that the way in which care is initiated varies jointly with distance and with socioeconomic status, or other socioorganizational factors, is attractive and deserves further study.

Weiss and Greenlick were able to examine four modes for initiating care: the regularly scheduled visit, the "walk-in," the visit to the emergency room, and the telephone call. Interestingly enough, the home visit did not, apparently, constitute a significant portal to care. Another aspect of differential use is whether persons who live farther away from their physicians are more likely to demand home visits as a substitute to their coming to the physician's office. One study from England, where home calls still constitute an appreciable segment of general practice, suggests that several factors may enter the picture (346). In this study, there were no regular gradients related to linear distance. However, there was a significantly higher tendency for persons living three-quarters of a mile to a mile from the physician's office to ask for home visits in preference to attendance at the physician's office. Persons living over two miles away were less likely to make office visits or to ask for home calls. The authors attribute this to a process of selection whereby only "considerate" patients were retained on the doctor's lists if they lived more than two miles away.

The findings concerning the willingness to travel in response to needs that have varying degrees of propulsive force have obvious implications for the planning and organization of health services. What services can be centralized and what others placed in more peripheral locations should depend, at least in part, on the differential propensity of potential clients to travel. For example, the study by Kane suggests that "family care" services, if they are to be used, would need to be placed very close to the consumer, especially in low-income areas. The influence of location on the choice of alternative resources or of alternative health plans is another example. Geographic accessibility and convenience have been postulated as a significant factor in the choice of prepaid group practice in situations of "dual choice," as well as of the use of care outside the group practice plan by those who have chosen to enroll in it. In one study, when subscribers were questioned about the reasons for using outside services, 57 percent of the reasons cited concerned the nature of the relationship with the physician in the plan or outside the plan. By contrast, 29 percent of the reasons related directly or indirectly to distance or time: 9 percent that the group practice center was too far away, 5 percent that clients could not get an appointment, 5 percent that too much time was wasted waiting, and 9 percent that the condition was an emergency (335, Chart 32, p. 28). In another study, 49 percent of the reasons given for the use of outside medical services (excluding surgery and obstetrics) involved dissatisfaction with the group practice plan. However, 37 percent of reasons referred to the accessibility of service. About half of these reasons stressed some element of convenience, including physical proximity and fewer administrative impediments to reaching the physician or to receiving service. The other half of the reasons involving convenience stressed ease in obtaining "emergency" care (336, p. 135). More recently, studies by Bashshur and Metzner, have suggested that distance from the central facility is a significant factor in the initial choice to enroll in a prepaid group practice plan in preference to an alternative plan that offers access to all physicians and hospitals in a community. In postal zones adjacent to the group practice facility, the ratio of eligible persons who had chosen the group practice plan in preference to the alternatives offered was twice as high as the same ratio for the rest of the city. The localization of clientele was further enhanced by an administrative decision to limit home calls to a geographic zone surrounding the central facility. Only 9 percent of the total membership lived outside the "home call area" (337, p. 32). Further analysis of the data by Shannon has shown that the localization of membership around this facility corresponds closely to predictions based upon information concerning distances which persons travel in pursuit of usual activities such as going to work or to school, attendance at church, clubs or union meetings, informal contacts with friends, relatives, or coworkers, shopping trips, and the like (338).

So far, the effects of geographic accessibility have been discussed as they act upon the potential client. There is some evidence that the provider of service is also susceptible. There is reason to expect that physicians who provide family care services (general practitioners, pediatricians, and some internists, for example) would follow closely in their location the residential distribution of the families who are likely to use their services because of need, recognition of need, and ability to pay. By contrast, physicians who depend on services provided in hospitals, and/or obtained from other health professionals, would seek to locate closer to "medical centers." It has been postulated that the differential strength of these two influences, clients versus medical centers, may explain the observed spatial distribution of physicians in different specialties (343, 344). Schneider proposes that a more complete model would include location of the physician's residence as a third independent variable, since not all locations in an urban area would be regarded as acceptable by the physician or his family (350). There is, as of now, only partial empirical confirmation of these postulates. The presence of hospitals has been shown to have an effect on the location of physicians when no distinction is made by specialty status. Mountin et al. have reported that between 1923 and 1938 the physician : population ratios for the poorest counties in the United States declined by 7 percent in counties that had 250 or more general hospital beds, by 26 percent in counties with less than 250 beds, and by 33 percent in counties with no general hospital beds (339). Terris and Monk, in the course of documenting secular change in the location of physicians within three cities in upstate New York, found that the presence of hospital beds in an area was associated with a tendency to retain physicians in that area (340). More recently, Dorsey has documented, for the Boston area, the striking tendency of physicians to locate in hospitals (341). Morrill et al. have reported concerning this phenomenon and its consequences, in terms of client travel, in the Chicago Metropolitan Area. The gist of their findings is that physicians locate near the hospitals at which they practice and that, as a result, patients may have to travel longer distances to the physician or the hospital. In the metropolitan area as a whole, 48 percent of physicians practice in the hospital closest to their offices, and 44 percent of patient-physician-hospital trips are such that physician and hospital are closer together than either is to the patient (309). There is also some evidence that hospitals tend to attract specialists more than they do generalists, and that some specialists are more dependent on hospitals than others. Marden has reported the relationship of the number of full-time, nonfederal generalists and specialists engaged in private practice to the size and characteristics of 369 metropolitan areas. The number of beds in short-term, nonfederal hospitals was an important determinant of the number of specialists, but was either unrelated or negatively related (in the smallest metropolitan areas) to the supply of general practitioners (342). Lubin et al. used the amount of time different specialists spend in the hospital to classify physicians into two groups of more or less hospital-dependent specialists. They showed that in the San Francisco Bay Area specialists who spend 25 percent or more of their time in a hospital locate closer to the hospital than do other specialists (312). Weiss attempted to show whether or not counties, classified in one of five groups in a hierarchy of "medical centers," had different powers to attract physicians in different specialties.

The general conclusion that emerges from this study is that the traditional concept of metropolitan dominance best explains the distribution of medical specialists and psychiatrists, whereas the distribution of the surgical specialists shows some support for the notion of dependence on the medical center. The distribution of the diagnostic and supportive specialties indicates that, relative to other specialties, they are affected more by the location of other physicians and general hospitals than by metropolitan or medical center influences. Thus very little support for the notion of dependency was found in the study. This may be due to the fact that dependency was not measured with a sufficient degree of accuracy (344, pp. 196–197).

In addition to its influence on location, geographic accessibility should have an effect on the manner in which physicians conduct their practice. Lubin et al. have shown that physicians who use more than one hospital admit more patients to the nearer hospital (312). Earlier, Peterson et al. had shown that distance from the hospital was related to the propensity of general practitioners in rural North Carolina to actively use hospital facilities. Table IV.78 gives the findings. Also in rural North Carolina,

Table IV.78. Percent of general practitioners who actively use the hospital according to distance from nearest hospital, rural North Carolina, 1953–54

Distance from Nearest Hospital	Percent of General Practitioners Who Actively Use the Hospital
Under 6 miles	90
6–10 miles	78
11–15 miles	82
Over 15 miles	42

SOURCE: Reference 139, Table 27, page 95.

Williams et al. have shown that distance is a factor in patient referral to a university-affiliated consultant and diagnostic center for ambulatory patients. Patients who lived nearer the center were more likely to have asked for a referral and more likely to have been referred for "non-specific reasons." As distance increased, referral was more likely to be physician-initiated and for "specific reasons." When the distance from the referring physician to the medical center was less than 70 miles, 65 percent of referrals were initiated primarily by patients. When the distance was more than 70 miles, only 35 percent of referrals were so initiated. The mean distance from the center was 59.3 miles for referrals initiated primarily by patients, 67.2 miles for referrals primarily initiated by physicians for "non-specific reasons," and 85.0 miles for referrals primarily initiated by physicians for "specific reasons" (345, pp. 1502–1503). Hobbs and Acheson have shown analogous effects of travel time on the use of specialized obstetrical services in Oxford, England (347). In addition, they examined what is the most important single consideration relevant to access: the impact on health and well-being.

The reader will recall that Jehlick and McNamara reported a larger number of bed-days of illness for persons who lived more than 5 linear miles from the nearest physician, in rural Missouri (320) Acheson and Hobbs (347) studied the frequency with which maternity cases were referred to a maternity unit that provided specialist care as influenced by two factors: (1) whether the referring general practitioner was closer to a general practice maternity unit or a specialized maternity unit, and (2) by travel time from the office of the general practitioner to the nearest specialized unit. Travel times were obtained from the official time table of the local bus company. They do not include waiting for the bus to

Table IV.79. Percent of persons referred for specialist maternity care and perinatal mortality by traveling time to the nearest general practice maternity unit and the nearest specialist maternity unit, Oxford Area, England, 1962

Traveling Time to Nearest Unit Offering Specialist Maternity Care	Travel Time to Nearest General-Practice Maternity Unit Shorter than or Equal to Travel Time to Nearest Specialized Unit		Travel Time to Nearest General-Practice Maternity Unit Greater Than Travel Time to Nearest Specialized Unit	
	Percent of Cases Referred for Specialist Care	Perinatal Mortality per 1000 Cases in the Practice of the Referring Physicians	Percent of Cases Referred for Specialist Care	Perinatal Mortality per 1000 Cases in the Practice of Referring Physicians
0–20 minutes	42%	20	60%	18
21–40 minutes	27	28	49	22
Over 40 minutes	9	44	52	21
All travel times	28	28	53	19

SOURCE: Reference 347, Table 4, page 502.

arrive or leave. In addition, data were obtained on maternal risk factors and on perinatal mortality. The effects of travel time are summarized in Table IV.79. When the office of the general practitioner was no farther away from a general practice maternity unit than a maternity unit offering specialist care, there was a significantly smaller proportion of women referred for specialist care. Within this group of general practitioners, referral for specialist care was significantly greater as travel time to the specialized unit was less. There was no significant relationship, according to travel time, within the group of general practitioners whose offices were located nearer to a specialized maternity unit than to a general-practice maternity unit. More important is the impact of these differential referral patterns on perinatal mortality. Perinatal mortality in the total practice of the general practitioners, including cases referred and not referred, varied inversely with the likelihood of referral for specialist care. When mothers were grouped into three categories according to risk, the referral patterns described above could be discerned in each of the three groups. However, significant differences in perinatal mortality were present only in the group at highest risk. It may be concluded that the location of the offices of general practitioners in relation to the relative locations of maternity units offering either general practice or specialist care is of critical importance to the outcome of pregnancy in a group of mothers who are at high risk. Thus, one identifies a link between the spatial configuration of resources and survival itself.

We have reviewed briefly some findings concerning use of services or resources and geographic accessibility. In addition to the interest in whether there are or are not relationships between use and accessibility, there is interest in defining more precisely the nature of the mathematical function that describes the relationship. Shannon et al. briefly describe the manner in which mathematical functions have been derived and provide references to the literature on locational analysis (306, pp. 147–148). One approach has been to derive models that assume an analogy to gravitational fields. One such formulation, the "gravity" or "interaction model," assumes that movement between two centers is proportional to the product of their populations and inversely proportional to the power of the distance separating them. Empirical data on the relationship between distance and travel have been expressed in a number of ways—as normal, long-normal, quadratic, and Pareto functions. The work of Altman is the earliest example known to the author of an attempt to define as a mathematical function the relationship between distance and the use of physician services.

Examination of the frequencies with which people traveled various distances to obtain physician services shows that they are relatively high in the interval under 5 miles, fall off sharply at first with increasing distance, and then tend to level off. This finding would suggest a function expressing the idea that the frequency with which different distances are traveled varies inversely as some power of the distance traveled. The simplest function meeting this description that a priori would appear suitable to the nature of the data is the hyperbolic. Its form is

$$y = \frac{a}{x^b}$$

where y would in this instance stand for frequency and x for distance. It is the value of b which is of principal interest, for it is the index, as it were, of the size of the problem of distance. The smaller the value of b, the more often will longer distances be observed relative to the number of shorter distances observed; the larger this exponent, the fewer the number of people who travel an appreciable distance. The letter 'a' is a constant which fits the curve to the actual observations; examination of the equation shows it to be the value of y when x is 1 . . . For general practitioners, b is to all intents and purposes the same for each county group, about 2.3; that is, the number of visits observed varied inversely as some exponent lying between the square and cube of the distance . . . The same situation holds with respect to travel to the specialist by residence of the greater metropolitan county, Allegheny; the exponent b turns out to be not only of approximately the same value for the different specialties but also of the same magnitude as that for general practitioners. For the remaining types of counties the value of the exponent decreases as the counties become less urban in character, to 0.4–0.7 in the most rural group of counties . . . The curves for all specialists combined have been plotted . . . the curves described the observed data fairly accurately . . . Some utility for this index might be pointed out. If a determination can be made of the desired goal in distribution of physicians, the function can measure progress being made toward that goal (323, pp. 28–29).

Jolly and King cite several examples to show that the relationship between distance and the use of several types of ambulatory care facilities is probably exponential. This "means that attendance drops by a constant percentage with each additional mile that separates the patient's home from the hospital. If a graph is drawn showing distance and outpatient attendances on a logarithmic scale, the relationship between attendance and distance becomes a linear one, and the slope of the line measures the 'outpatient care gradient' for this hospital'' (332, chap. 2, sec. 7). Morrill and Earickson have studied the relationship between distance and use of Chicago hospitals categorized according to several characteristics. Two mathematical functions were tested as to how they fitted the observed data. One was a gravity or power function, similar to the one postulated by Altman, of the form

$$F_{ij} = \frac{A}{D^b_{ij}}.$$

The other was an exponential function of the form

$$F_{ij} = \frac{A}{e^b \, D_{ij}}.$$

In these formulae,

F = number of patients from area i to hospital j
D_{ij} = the distance from area i to hospital j
b = the slope or steepness of decline
A = a constant
e = the base of natural logarithms = 2.7183

The relationship between distance and the number of hospital admissions per unit area (apparently uncorrected for population density) was generally, but not invariably, best described by the exponential function.

In general, the exponential functions . . . provided the closer fit, although the power function did not do badly. The exponential was significantly better for the special-purpose hospitals and Cook County; the power function was somewhat better for small city and satellite hospitals. Neither function alone was able to fit adequately the satellite data (334, pp. 32–33).

In the studies reported by Sohler et al. the relationship between distance and the first admission rate to the mental hospital was linear; no critical distance was identified within or beyond which distance ceased to have an observed effect (326). The investigators comment that the absence of a critical distance in their studies is in keeping with the findings of a similar study by Blumberg in California where, however, much longer distances were observed. Contrary to these observations is the postulation by Morrill and Earickson that there is, in Chicago, a two-mile "region of indifference" within which distance has no appreciable effect on physician use (352). Whether there are distances that are, collectively, so short or so long that differences within each of the two categories become matters of relative indifference to clients is a question of general significance concerning which little is known, at least in the health field. A recent study by Weiss, Greenlick, and Jones throws some light on this question by showing that as the average distance from the nearest clinic becomes longer, the incremental distance to the next nearest clinic becomes relatively less important as a deterrent to bypassing the nearest clinic in order to seek care at one that is more distant (330). Weiss et al. report on the visits made by members of a prepaid group practice plan to one of three alternative clinics in the Portland metropolitan area. When the nearest clinic is an average of 2.4 miles distant from the homes of clients, 23 percent of visits are made to a clinic that is further away than the one that is nearest, even though this entails an additional 7.1 miles of travel, on the average. This means that 23 percent of visits entail traveling 296 percent longer than is absolutely necessary. When the nearest clinic is an average of 14.0 miles distant from the homes of clients, as many as 43 percent of visits are made to a clinic that is further away than the one that is nearest. Presumably, the larger proportion of such visits is explained by the observation that only a small additional effort in travel is needed to bypass the nearest clinic in order to receive care at one that is more distant. This increment was 0.6 miles on the average, or an additional 4 percent of the average distance to the nearest clinic.

LOCATIONAL EFFICIENCY: GENERAL CONSIDERATIONS. According to Schneider, "the term locational efficiency is meant to refer to the costs of operating a hospital which may be attributed directly to its location. . . . The ideal or optimum location for an industrial operation is that point where the competing pulling forces generated by raw material sources, the market, the labor supply, the power supply, and a host of other factors are balanced or in equilibrium" (350, pp. 154, 155). Obviously, the concept of locational efficiency goes beyond consideration of the effects of distance on use of service, though it includes these. It deals with the question of which among alternative locations for a given resource is better or best in terms of cost. Using an even broader context, it deals with how the several resources in a given community can be located so that some measure of social welfare is improved or maximized. Under either formulation there would have to be consideration not only of costs alone or of benefits alone, but of the relationship between costs and benefits. Thus, a more complete definition of locational efficiency would be that it deals with the manner in which the location of health resources influences the costs and benefits of receiving and failing to receive health care. However, as we shall see below, locational efficiency is almost always described and measured in terms that fall far short of this definition. The conceptual complexities of a complete model, the paucity of information, and the difficulties of measurement have required that the investigator be content with partial measures under highly simplifying assumptions.

One criterion of locational efficiency might be the extent to which costs associated with the friction of space are minimized. The application of this criterion alone would lead to the location of a physician at each street corner and a hospital in each neighborhood, an obvious absurdity. It is clear that this criterion can only be applied in conjunction with others, or within a set of constraints. These additional criteria, or constraints, include, first, the condition that aggregate demand, or need, be met but not exceeded. Need, as we have shown earlier, is both difficult to measure and subject to variable definition by clients as compared to providers, and by each of these according to a variety of circumstances which include aggregate supply and location of resources. Demand is subject to similar influences. It is, therefore, difficult to fix precisely aggregate need or demand. It is easier to offer a range. Second, there are technological criteria that relate the size, and associated complexity, of the resource to the quality of care it can offer, or habitually offers. A given magnitude is necessary to provide the equipment and personnel required. Furthermore, a minimum number of patients of any given type is necessary in order to maintain technical skills at the requisite pitch. Even larger aggregates of ''clinical material'' may be necessary or desirable if the object is to conduct research, particularly in the rarer forms of illness. Third, there are economic criteria that include not only the external costs attributable to overcoming the friction of space, but also the internal costs attributable to economies or diseconomies of scale.

In a previous section we have discussed the external costs attributable to the friction of space and shown that these are divisible into direct outlays and indirect losses due to missed opportunity to engage in productive activity. We have pointed out the need to partition both types of cost among several uses of any given journey that includes the receipt of medical care among other transactions. We have also emphasized differences in the value of lost time for the different participants in the medical care transaction. This raises sharply the question of whether the criterion of locational efficiency is to be the loss of patient time, physician time, or the total cost of both, combined with or without weighting. Whether costs are direct or indirect, but especially as concerns direct costs, there may arise the question of who bears the immediate consequences. It is true that, ultimately, all costs are charged to consumers in one form or another; but the manner in which the burden is distributed can be a matter of critical importance. For example, if the cost of travel is absorbed by the providers of care, it is likely to be reflected in higher prices which, in turn, may be met by health insurance or social welfare. This is generally not true if clients have to pay the cost out-of-pocket. Accordingly, another question that can be raised is whether the criterion of locational efficiency is minimum cost to the community or society, or minimum out-of-pocket outlays by the client. The question of who bears the cost also raises the question of differential ability to pay the cost of travel and differential motivation to travel for care. Travel cost relative to income would certainly be higher for persons in lower economic groups, who also tend to have lower motivation to seek care. This raises the social policy question of whether resources should be located in a manner that favors those with less ability and motivation to seek care. In a subsequent section we shall see that, in fact, the location of resources may be such as to further penalize the populations that are most vulnerable.

Considerations of locational efficiency cannot be concerned merely with the external costs of overcoming the friction of space, whether direct or indirect, and with who bears these costs. Internal costs of operating the facility have to be included. The interrelatedness of internal and external costs becomes evident when one considers the choice between providing fewer large facilities and a larger number of smaller facilities. As already discussed in a previous section of this chapter, the first alternative exploits the economies thought to be associated with size, thus reducing internal costs. It does, however, increase the external cost of travel for clients as well as physicians and other health personnel. It may also increase the cost of transporting necessary supplies, unless the economies of hauling larger quantities offset those of shorter distance.

A lower limit is placed on the size of a given facility not only to reduce cost, but also to assure standards of technical performance. Thus the planner may face a dilemma in reconciling the several requirements, especially in sparsely populated areas. Mountin et al. recognized this problem in their work on regional planning:

Good administration dictates that, except in unusual situations, State plans preclude approval of any project for a hospital of less than 50 beds. On the other hand, in the interest of good medical care, it is highly desirable that patients not be required to travel more than 50 miles except for uncommon conditions. There will be areas so sparsely settled as to make these conditions unattainable (360, p. 10).

Mountin and Greve met the same problem once again with respect to health departments. Although they believed that a local health unit should not serve less than 35,000 people, they also believed that "the local health jurisdiction should be limited to a maximum area of 10,000 square miles and that the diameter of the unit should be no more than 100 miles." (359, p. 4). More recently, Hodges et al. have pointed out the "dilemma" in planning mental health centers in sparsely populated areas. Regulations under the Community Mental Health Centers Act of 1963 state that "every community mental health facility shall serve a population of not less than 75,000 and not more than 200,000 persons, except that the Surgeon General may, in particular cases, permit modification of this population range if he finds that such modifications will not impair the effectiveness of the services to be provided (349). A study of population density in rural areas by state shows that such a unit of population would cover widely disparate areas of land. "In keeping with regulations of the act, a comprehensive community mental health center to serve a rural area in Colorado would have to serve an area with a radius between 49 and 80 miles. In Wyoming a rural mental health center would have to serve an area with a radius between 92 and 166 miles" (348, p. 388). Such considerations raise questions about the applicability of the mental health center concept to highly rural areas.

Hodges et al. offer no solution to the dilemma which they pose—except, perhaps, an adjudication by the Surgeon General, as provided in the Regulations! Mountin and Greve considered the spatial criterion to supersede the minimum population criterion in planning public health areas (359). Mountin et al. were more rigid in requiring that no hospital below 50 beds be approved. Certain needs for inpatient care in remote areas were to be met by the inclusion of limited bed accommodation in outlying health centers, supplemented by arrangements for prompt transportation to the nearest hospital (360). Jolly and King see mobile outpatient services as the solution to bringing services to people in sparsely populated, poverty stricken areas of the world (332, chap. 2, secs. 7–10c inclusive). Contrary to the authors cited above, Long and Feldstein have developed a reasonably rigorous model that permits systematic, quantitative analysis of the problem of optimal hospital size taking account of both internal and external costs (353). Their solution to the problem of choice, as posed above, is to select that hospital size that minimizes internal and external costs combined. While this is socially optimal, the reader should, once again, also consider the incidence of social cost: namely, who bears what element of cost.

The criterion of economic cost is, of course, not unrelated to the two criteria of (1) technological requirements and (2) demand or need. To the extent that resources are not adequately used, because they exceed need or demand, there is a rise in internal costs due to inefficient operation of the resource. Losses from poor quality due to technological inadequacy or insufficient professional experience are much more difficult to measure. However, it should be possible theoretically, to assign some cost factor to poor quality based on correlates such as unnecessarily prolonged treatment, the performance of unnecessary procedures, delayed convalescence, prolonged disability, or even death. A more complete cost model would also have to include the effects on cost of the interaction between supply and use of service. Supply should be seen in terms of both the aggregate scale of the resource and the spatial distribution of the resource. The more there is of any resource and the nearer the resource is to its potential clients the more likely it is that there will be increases in appropriate as well as inappropriate use. Both of these could, theoretically, be represented in terms of corresponding costs. The major components are the costs of care, the indirect costs resulting from lost productivity during the receipt of care, and the money equivalent of the benefits that accrue or fail to accrue due to care. In this way it might be possible to conduct a study of locational analysis not only in terms of current levels and patterns of use, but also in terms of those levels and patterns as they might be altered because of relocating sources of care. Finally, to make matters even more complex, there is the likelihood that there are trade-offs between the quantity of care and its quality. For example, a larger number of smaller facilities, each providing somewhat lower levels of care, could conceivably reach so many more people that the net result is better care on the average. Translating such trade-offs into corresponding costs and benefits, while possible in theory, would be almost impossible in practice due to insufficient information.

It is clear that a full analysis of costs and benefits for purposes of measuring locational efficiency, or of proposing more efficient alternative spatial configurations, is a matter of considerable difficulty. The problem is made even more difficult by the fact that willingness to travel varies with the perceived severity of the medical condition, its urgency and, perhaps its rarity. Corresponding to this is the economic feasibility of placing in smaller, decentralized units the simpler and more frequently used services. These considerations dictate that technological and economic criteria be applied to components of resources distinguished by specialty, type of service, and the like. Generally one would expect a positive correspondence between severity of the condition, complexity of the resource, and willingness to travel. This allows for the advantages of centralization without erecting undue barriers to use. However, there may be situations in which this favorable correspondence does not occur. For example, efficient multiple screening may require large-scale, centralized operation, while the motivation to seek such services may be rather low. In this instance the optimal solution may involve making the resource mobile, providing transportation for clients or providing the service at low price, or even offering financial or other inducements to seek care. Urgency of the condition requiring care is another factor in arriving at an efficient solution to the problem of spatial configuration. Care for relatively frequent and relatively minor, though urgent conditions, such as minor trauma, can be readily decentralized. Urgent severe illness or trauma, however, needs centralization of resources and large scale, in order to assure economy as well as quality. Fortunately, the willingness to travel is no obstacle, provided transportation is available. However, the clinical needs of the situation may require peripheral facilities for first aid with subsequent transfer to a central facility, as occurs in military practice. Well-equipped and staffed ambulance services would seem to combine several functions, including first aid, sorting, and transportation. In addition to all this, the planner needs to consider the factors that influence socio-organizational accessibility. Altering the location of resources may not lead to more efficient operation if there remain important social or organizational barriers to access.

As already mentioned, the cost of overcoming the resistance of space is an important component in measuring locational efficiency. We have already discussed several alternative ways of measuring resistance to motion and the considerations relevant to each. What remains is consideration of the several points in the process of seeking and providing care where such measurements need to be taken. A simple model of medical practice would seem to be helpful in identifying these. According to this model, the key person in determining patient movement is the physician. However, the physician himself is dependent, for a share of his activities, on the hospital. The degree of dependence, as we have already discussed, varies considerably by specialty (343) and, possibly, by other characteristics of physicians and clients. There are physicians, notably in central cities or remote rural areas, who have no affiliations, or only tenuous ties, with a hospital and are therefore virtually independent of hospitals for their practice. Any given physician may have affiliations at more than one hospital, perhaps using each to a different extent and in different ways. The physician is also dependent, on the one hand, on his clients and, on the other hand, on his colleagues from whom he receives patients and to whom he refers. Freidson has proposed a distinction between two types of physicians or practitioners: "independent" physicians to whom patients have direct access, and "dependent" physicians to whom patients go mainly by referral (336, pp. 204–205). The services and colleagues whom the physician needs may be located at the hospital or elsewhere in private offices, establishments, or laboratories. The hospital itself is generally dependent on physicians located in private offices for the flow of patients, but only in part. Patients are admitted to hospital directly in case of emergency. Furthermore, many hospitals operate "emergency" and other ambulatory care facilities that often serve as sources of primary care for many persons. There is also a hierarchy of hospitals and related inpatient facilities with flow of services and patients from one to the other. All these interrelationships produce a complex weave of movements of physicians, other health professionals, and clients, as well as of services and supplies, all relevant, though in varying degree to locational analysis.

The relevant locations include (1) the residences of consumers and their places of work; (2) the residences of physicians, their offices, and the hospitals with which they have affiliations; (3) the residences and offices of dentists and other independent health practitioners; (4) the locations of hospitals in general and of other facilities such as nursing homes; (5) the locations of drug stores, private radiology, and laboratory services and the like; and (6) the locations of warehouses and establishments that provide supplies and services to hospital or private practitioners. The movements include those of consumers, physicians, and other health professionals, and of goods and supplies. The movements of consumers include those of patients and others who accompany them or visit them at the locations where care is received. The movements may originate or terminate at home or at place of work for employed persons, or at an inpatient facility. Movements may be direct or through intermediate steps, for example from primary physician, to specialist, to laboratory or hospital, and to drug store. The movements of physicians include journeys from residence to office or one or more hospitals; from office to one or more hospitals; and, with decreasing frequency in the United States, from the physician's residence, his office or the hospital, to the patient's home. The movements of other health professionals or workers, generally from their homes to their places of employment, also contribute to the cost of care. So does the transportation of supplies and of service personnel to doctors' offices, hospitals, and other facilities.

It is obvious that locational analysis that involves measurement of all the variables discussed in the model described above would be impossible in most situations. It is necessary to conduct partial analyses under simplifying assumptions. Unfortunately, there is little information concerning the relative weights of the various factors under usual circumstances. Even if these were available, they would be influenced greatly by local conditions. For example, Jolly et al. report experience at one hospital in rural Uganda where travel cost to outpatients and inpatients combined equaled more than half the total hospital budget. Each outpatient spent $0.35 on transportation in order to receive services worth $0.11 (332, chap. 12, sec. 7, and chap. 2, sec. 9). Long and Feldstein used data reported by Coughlin et al. showing that ''in Philadelphia inpatients accounted for only 5.9 percent of the total trip miles involved with hospitalization. Visitors to inpatients accounted for over half the travel distance; employees, outpatients, and physicians made the remaining trips. Assuming Coughlin's figures hold generally, a reduction in units that adds one mile to the average distance increases total travel roughly thirty-four miles per case'' (353, p. 126). Furthermore, they used the following rough mathematical relationship between change in existing number of facilities and change in average distance traveled:

$$\frac{D_1}{D_2} = \sqrt{\frac{F_2}{F_1}},$$

where D_1 = average distance traveled now;

D_2 = average distance that would be traveled when the number of facilities is changed;

F_1 = number of facilities now;

F_2 = new number of facilities.

This mathematical relation would approximate the true state of affairs only if facilities and clients were evenly distributed and distance were the only factor in client preference (353, p. 126, text and footnote). Schneider has presented, and argued for, a number of assumptions concerning the locations of physicians, employees, trainees, inpatients, clinic outpatients, visitors and suppliers that led him to consider a much more simplified model. He concludes that ''the locational efficiency of any particular hospital or cluster of hospitals can be approximately, but usefully, measured by analyzing the pulling force of only one group of hospital users—the inpatients'' (350, p. 161). Further empirical work is needed to support this conclusion.

LOCATIONAL EFFICIENCY: SOME EMPIRICAL STUDIES AND MEASUREMENTS. In this section we shall briefly review selected studies bearing on locational efficiency. These will illustrate the more concrete application of several considerations previously discussed in the abstract. Furthermore, they will offer certain techniques which the administrator may find useful in his own work. Finally, the findings of the studies will help document the extent to which locational inefficiency brought about by spatial or socio-organizational factors is a current problem. One class of decisions faced by the planner is the placement of a facility where none existed before. This involves, in part, the determination of central places or preferred locations through studies of pattern and range of usual client activities and interactions. The implicit criterion is that the most efficient location of the medical care facility is likely to be one that corresponds with these patterns. Hawley has described some of the earlier studies that have delineated rural and urban community areas. The criteria used have included local newspaper distribution, milk collection, church and high school attendance, public library use, traffic flow gradients, telephone services, electric power service, wholesale and retail distribution, radio listening audience, and so on. While each of these indicators yields somewhat different boundaries, they do, collectively, show how a given area is spatially oriented and organized (305, pp. 245–258). Kane has approached in an essentially similar way the question of locating a health facility in a segment of rural Kentucky (331). Analysis of data from marketing research and the highway department, and of advertisements in the newspaper of the county seat, showed the trade area to be oriented in a direction totally different from the location of the new facility as proposed by the regional health plan for the area. A household survey that included questions on physician use indicated congruence with the trade area and lack of congruence with the proposed location of the health facility. Further information about consumer priorities for medical care and willingness to travel much greater distances for some services than for others could be used in conjunction with information about the market area to determine not only the location but also the size of the facility and the services to be offered there.

Another type of question that the health administrator may wish answered is whether a given facility, perhaps his own, is most efficiently located to serve its clients. Schneider has approached this question with respect to each of several hospitals in Cincinnati (350). Theoretically, what is required is to locate, for each hospital, that geographic point which minimizes travel, or the cost of travel, for all persons who currently use each hospital, including clients and health workers, as well as to minimize the transportation of supplies from current sources. This location is called the "point of minimum aggregate travel," abbreviated as PMAT. A method is available for solving the mathematical problem posed (314). Once this point is identified, its location can be compared to that of the actual location of the corresponding hospital. A line may be drawn that joins the actual location to the optimal location (PMAT). The length and direction of this line indicates the degree and direction of imbalance between optimal and actual location. Hence this line, which has both magnitude and direction, is called the "locational imbalance vector," or LIVOR. This LIVOR, then, is inversely related to locational efficiency as measured by this approach. Owing to the lack of data, Schneider had to make a number of assumptions which permitted him to use the location of patients that constitute the case load of each hospital as the sole criterion for computing the point of minimum travel. The data used were simply addresses of inpatients obtained from hospital records and linear distances from each patient's residence to the hospital which he used, measured on a map. The findings showed differences in the degree of imbalance among hospitals and demonstrated that several hospitals were considerably removed from locations that would be optimal in terms of reducing travel for their inpatients. The fact that the LIVORs of several centrally located hospitals differ in length and direction demonstrates the particularized attraction that certain hospitals have for certain classes of clients independently of purely spatial considerations.

A more general type of question is not whether each hospital or resource is optimally located with respect to its own constituency, but whether the hospitals, and other resources in a community, are most efficiently deployed in relation to the spatial deployment of those who could use them. Schneider applied criteria and methods of spatial analysis to the solution of this problem in Cincinnati (351). First, it was possible to obtain the number of persons admitted to each hospital by type of service and by postal zone of residence. Places of residence represent the spatial location of demand, whereas hospitals where care was received represent the spatial location of supply. The precise location of each hospital was known, but for patient residences the "approximate geographic center of the residential land use of each of 97 postal zones" was used to represent all patients in that postal zone. Linear distances were measured among hospital locations and among residential locations, determined as above. Thus for each hospital service there were two distributions of distances: one of admissions by location of hospital (representing the distribution of supply) and another of admissions by location of residence (representing the distribution of demand). For each distribution it is possible to compute two attributes: (1) the spatial center of the distribution, which is the point of minimum aggregate travel, and (2) the standard distance, which is a measure of the spatial dispersion of the distribution, analogous to the standard deviation. Given these data, it is possible to locate the central point of each distribution on a map and draw around each central point a circle with radius equal to the standard distance of the distribution. Now it is possible to compare the visual representations of the distribution of places of admission (supply) and places of residence (demand) with respect to two properties: the extent to which the centers coincide and the extent to which the standard circles correspond. A criterion of ideal spatial correspondence (and, presumably, of locational efficiency) was assumed to be that the centers be identical or very close together, and that the hospital standard distance be two-thirds as large as the patient residence standard distance (351, p. 32). A single measure of locational efficiency which combines both criteria of locational correspondence may be computed. This is the "locational efficiency index" (LINEX) which is, for each type of service, the distance between the supply center and demand center plus the difference between the two standard distance measures. This, however, is a crude measure and should be interpreted in conjunction with the actual spatial plots as described above. The reader should also note that the LINEX differs from the LIVOR as discussed in the preceding section, in dealing with the correspondence between all hospitals and all patients, whereas the LIVOR deals with correspondence between each hospital and its patients considered separately. Similar methods of analysis can be used to compare for each specialty the locations of physicians' offices, hospital admissions, patient residences, and physicians' residences.

The application of this method of analysis to Cincinnati showed that, on the average, patients traveled 2.07 miles to the hospital for inpatient care and that patient residences were 4.5 times more dispersed than hospital admissions. Furthermore, there were differences by type of service in dispersion of supply, in distance between center of demand and center of supply, and in relative dispersions of supply and demand. While such differences are to be expected, the actual findings are difficult to interpret. For example, patients traveled more than twice as long for tonsillectomies as they did for neurosurgery. There were also interesting disjunctures between actual and expected locations of physicians' offices. Offices of obstetricians and general practitioners were located farther away from the hospital than would be expected from the considerable proportion of time they spend in the hospital. By contrast, internists and psychiatrists were closer to the hospital than appeared necessary from the amount of time they spend in the hospital. The center of the offices of all physicians combined had not moved much during 14 years in spite of the outward spread of the city. Unlike the locations of physicians' offices, the locations of physicians' residences was similar to that of patients, except for being less dispersed. Residences of general practitioners were most dispersed, while those of orthopedic surgeons least dispersed. There were also large differences in distances between the centers of physicians' residences and the centers of office location by specialty: from 2.4 miles for general practitioners to 5.8 miles for urologists. Schneider points out certain changes in location of physicians' offices and hospitals that would reduce the disjunctures noted. He also discusses the limitations of this method of analysis. The most fundamental limitation of the method is that it adopts a rather simplistic and invariant criterion of locational efficiency which does not permit systematic, quantitative consideration of costs and benefits associated with centralization and decentralization, as suggested by the general model offered in our preceding section. For example, there is no systematic analysis of the trade-offs between internal costs and external costs, or of trade-offs between patient travel and physician travel. No account is taken of the possibility that these trade-offs might differ by type of service and that, therefore, the single criterion of locational efficiency (that the standard distance of the distribution of supply be two-thirds as large as the standard distance of the distribution of demand) may not apply uniformly. Schneider is aware of these limitations and adds several considerations to the calculus of costs and benefits. For example, the costs of extending and renovating old hospitals need to be compared with the costs of building and operating new facilities. Dispersion might lead to ''better'' utilization of service by the communities served. It would be expected, however, to reduce the ability of the physician to hold appointments at more than one hospital. Schneider considers this a weakness, in that it might reduce the scope of colleague interaction and reduce flexible use of hospitals, presumably by hampering a more efficient use of standby capacity. On the contrary, some would consider the centralization of all activities of a group of physicians in one hospital an advantage, because it could create the opportunity for more meaningful collegial interaction and control—in addition to reducing travel for the physician.

Morrill and Earickson have developed a simulation method to determine the extent and nature of locational inefficiencies in any given medical care system and how these may be reduced (352). The data required are (1) information on location of persons, physicians, and hospitals; (2) information on constraints in the system—for example, on willingness to accept charity patients or Blacks; and (3) information or assumptions on preferences that influence choice of physician by the patient and choice of hospital jointly by the patient and the physician. The preferences which the system must satisfy to the largest possible extent are, in effect, the criteria of ''efficiency.'' In the choice of physicians the major criterion is the reduction of patient travel, on the assumption that, beyond a two-mile zone of indifference, attractiveness of the physician falls off rapidly. Black patients are assumed to have an additional moderate preference for black physicians. The preference for hospitals is a more complex matter. Equal weight is given to the distance from the patient and from the physician. In addition, white patients are assumed to have specified preferences by religious orientation of the hospital. Constraints that limit the realization of patient preferences include inaccessibility of private physicians to charity patients, the number of hospital beds, and restrictions on admitting charity patients and Blacks. The simulation may be conducted either to indicate what changes need to be made in the location and scale of inpatient and ambulatory care resources, holding population use patterns constant, or what changes need to be made in population use patterns, holding location and scale of resources constant. Either way, one gets a measure of present imbalance as judged by the criteria adopted. The method also can measure the effect of making "external" changes, such as adding hospitals or physicians in given locations, as well as the effect of removing constraints, such as those that limit access of charity patients and black patients.

The findings in Chicago provide striking examples of locational imbalance and of the impact of constraints by color and payment status. Assuming cost and income barriers were maintained, about 1500 physicians (15 percent) would be shifted, mainly from the central business district and other large clusters to smaller clusters closer to the population. Similarly, about 12,000 hospital beds (16 percent) would be shifted, partly to ghetto area hospitals and partly to the suburbs. The current location of physicians puts a burden of excess travel mostly on paying patients in poor communities and patients in rapidly growing communities. The burden of most excess travel to hospitals falls on black and poor patients generally. If barriers of color and pay status were removed, there would be need for an even greater shift of physicians from the business district and from wealthy areas to where the poor live. "This physician shift is a measure of the great latent demand for physicians in low income areas—in other words, of unmet need" (352, p. 137). However, removal of such barriers for hospitals would reduce the need for costly shifts in the present hospital establishment.

The model described by Morrill and Earickson has capabilities beyond those of the model described by Schneider. It allows the simultaneous introduction of a number of preferences and constraints and makes possible measurement of what happens when these preferences and constraints are modified. It is recognized, however, that the quantitative expressions of these preferences need further verification. The two models are alike in the strong emphasis they place on minimizing distance and the small emphasis they place on the trade-offs between travel costs on the one hand, and the economic and technical benefits of scale on the other. It is possible, however, in the simulation program used by Morrill and Earickson, to conduct the analysis separately by type and level of service and to introduce requirements that hospitals or physician aggregates be not below a given size for each type of care.

An example of locational planning under constraints that include size of facility is reported by Godlund (354). The problem was the location of specialized regional hospitals in Sweden subject to constraints that included (1) a desirable population base of 1 million persons, and (2) use of already existing teaching hospitals which represent a large past investment in human and material resources. Under these constraints, there was need for 8 centers of which 5 centers, including 6 hospitals, were already in existence. The problem, therefore, was the location of two additional hospitals in two out of five suitable towns. Several combinations were tested using as a criterion the minimizing of travel distance (and therefore cost) per unit of population. The efficiency of alternative locations was tested by drawing lines of equal travel time (isochrones) by alternative methods of travel, including train, bus, and private car. Isochrones were drawn at 1-hour intervals up to 10 hours. Where isochrones intersected a boundary was drawn between respective spheres of influence. The author believes that the isochrones also roughly represent cost and therefore correspond to equal cost lines (isodapans). The cost consequences of each alternative combination of locations was obtained by estimating the population in each time-cost zone, assuming an arbitrary utilization rate per unit population, and computing total cost as weighted by population size in each zone. Selected findings of some of the alternatives are given in Table IV.80. The conclusion, based on the

Table IV.80.   Values of specified indices of locational efficiency for four alternative locations of a regional hospital, Sweden, 1955

Index of Locational Efficiency	Locational Alternatives Tested			
	I	II	III	IV
Proportion of population within 4-hour traveling time by train or bus	76.1	81.9	76.9	82.7
Travel cost by train and/or bus in millions of Swedish crowns	21.41	19.47	20.37	18.43

SOURCE: Reference 354, Tables 4–6, pages 21, 23, 27 and 30.

findings cited above and on other considerations, was to recommend a stepwise approach to implementing alternative IV.

Trade-offs between internal and external costs are more explicitly considered in a quasi-empirical study by Long and Feldstein to which we have already referred (353). The assumptions in their model are (1) that as hospital size increases, hospital cost per unit of service decreases, at least up to a point; (2) that as hospital size increases, fluctuations in census are reduced, and it is less likely that additional costs (penalty costs) are incurred because a patient who requires care cannot be accommodated at the preferred hospital; and (3) that travel costs are increased. The sum of these three functions is a U-shaped curve with a minimum point that corresponds to the most efficient hospital size. Long and Feldstein applied their model to obstetrical births in the Chicago region under a number of assumptions, including uniform size and optimal location of hospital units, specified quantitative relationships between size and the three variables, including two estimates of penalty costs. "Assuming there are no scale economies, that penalty costs are between $250 and $500 per case requiring special handling and that the value of travel time is between $1.55 and $2.80 per hour, then the optimal system for the Chicago region would have been between 80 and 125 units and 2,534 and 2,963 beds" (353, p. 126).

The model advanced by Long and Feldstein has the distinct advantage of adding consideration of the internal economies of scale to the costs of travel. While the advantages of scale are seen in purely economic terms, there is reason to believe that these may run parallel to differences in quality. There are also many limitations. There are, as yet, no firmly valid data for use in applying the model. While direct travel costs are counted, indirect costs, which may be different for physician and patient travel, are not included. Finally, optimal geographic location, instead of being assumed, must become part of the problem for empirical solution.

A final example in our review of empirical and quasi-empirical studies of locational efficiency is one by Abernathy and Hershey which is notable because it offers several alternative objectives as criteria for locational efficiency and examines their implications when community and resource characteristics are also specified and varied (355). A region is described in which there are three cities that differ by size, morbidity experience, socioeconomic characteristics, and propensity to seek care relative to the distance barrier. The problem is to determine the location of a progressively larger number of sources of primary care given each of several objectives or criteria of locational efficiency. The objectives offered are (1) to maximize utilization, (2) to minimize distance per capita, (3) to minimize distance per visit, and (4) to minimize the percent degradation of utilization due to distance. As expected, the different criteria lead to different decisions concerning the location of primary care resources. For example, when the objective is to maximize use of service, the source of primary care is drawn to the largest aggregation of persons for whom distance is a powerful barrier (possibly because of low income or education), but who would use large volumes of care if the distance barrier were removed. By contrast, the objective of simply minimizing distance to the primary care center places the center in areas of large population density without regard to differential morbidity and utilization patterns. The third objective, the minimization of distance per visit, is most congenial to the status quo because it places the source of care nearest to aggregations of persons who currently are high utilizers of service. At the same time, this may further reduce use of service by persons for whom distance is a significant barrier to care. The differences in location brought about by applying different criteria are most marked when only one center is to be built and become less marked as the number of centers increases. Similarly, the degree of attainment of the objective increases significantly as the number of centers is increased above one, but there is a marked decrease in the rate of improvement as more centers are added. In the hypothetical region examined there was little additional improvement in any of the measures when more than four centers were allocated. It is also shown, as one would expect, that when one objective (utilization of service) is pursued, there is a loss in the attainment of another objective (distance per capita or per visit). Gains in one can therefore be traded against gains in another. Here again, as the number of centers increases, gains in one objective and losses in another both diminish. In other words, the larger the number of centers that the community is able to provide, the less critical is the differential effect of alternative objectives.

It is clear from an examination of the several studies cited above that considerable sophistication is possible in the analysis of locational efficiency. Nevertheless, none of the models used includes all the considerations that need to go into a definitive analysis. Some combination of the economic model advanced by Long and Feldstein with the distance-centered models of Schneider and Morrill and Earickson would go a great way in meeting the major requirements of measuring locational efficiency. In the meantime, more intuitive methods for arriving at planning decisions are likely to be greatly improved if one has in mind the kinds of issues and considerations that we have raised in our discussion of accessibility.

In situations of great complexity such as this the temptation is great to substitute for analysis the use of rather simple, rule-of-thumb guidelines. For example, Mountin and Greve recommend that the jursidiction of a local health unit "should be limited to a maximum area of 10,000 square miles and that the diameter of the unit should be no more than 100 miles,'' even when this contravenes their other requirement—that the population served be at least 35,000 (359, p. 4). Hodges and Dörken assert that for ambulatory mental health services, a range of 40–60 miles, the rough equivalent of an hour's drive, seems to be the practical limit in rural areas (324, p. 2141). According to Mountin et al., ''it is highly desirable'' that patients not be required to travel more than 50 miles for hospital care, ''except for uncommon conditions'' (360, p. 10). Lubin et al. report that hospital planning guidelines in California recommend a limit of one hour of travel time for areas of low population density and a limit of 30 minutes of travel time for more densely populated areas. Guidelines used in Cincinnati specify 25 minutes of travel time in locating new hospitals (312, p. 771). Altman has suggested a rule for ''optimal distribution'' of physicians based on the observed lack of correlation between distance and use of general practitioners in rural Pennsylvania. In the function

$$y = \frac{a}{x^b},$$

where y is frequency of use of service, a is a constant, and x is the distance, no correlation between distance and use of service was observed when the value of b was 2.3. This value of the exponent is suggested as a guide to ''optimal distribution'' (323, p. 31). Morrill and Earickson, on the basis of their own observations in an urban area, suggest a two-mile region of indifference in choosing among physicians (352, p. 131). Schneider has proposed that the ''ideal'' degree of spatial correspondence between the hospital and the patient residence distributions is when the standard distance of the first is about two-thirds that of the second (351, p. 32). The distances that persons say they are willing to travel for different types of services, as reported by Kane, might also be used as guides to the placement of these services (331). This assortment of simple-minded rules suggests that our current ability to plan with a view to locational efficiency is limited at best.

GEOGRAPHIC ACCESSIBILITY: ALTERNATIVE FRAMEWORKS. So far, we have used a particular framework in studying the locational effects and the locational efficiency of resources. This framework has assumed that as a general rule clients travel to the resource. Relatively little attention has been given to the possibilities that the resource may be mobilized so that it can be taken to the consumer. The traditional example of the latter has been the home call made by the physician. While this is a practice which is on the decline in the United States, other kinds of home service, including visiting-nurse service and organized home care, are becoming more prevalent. A variety of mobile clinics may also be organized. The considerations that apply to mobile resources are similar to those we have discussed for the more usual situation in which the resource is fixed while the client is mobile. However, there may be greater emphasis on the problem of losses in resource productivity due to time lost in travel and reduction in scale of operation. Certainly the direct and indirect costs and benefits of mobilizing the resource need to be compared with the same costs and benefits of mobilizing the client. One aspect of resource productivity under these circumstances is the factor of scheduling or programming travel so as to achieve greater shared use.

A more radical departure from conventional considerations of spatial analysis arises from the new technology for the conveyance of information rather than the moving of persons or equipment. The use of telephone, radio, or television to transmit information, and of computers to analyze it, opens new horizons in the spatial organization of resources. Distance still offers resistance, but the context is so radically different that the conventional dimensions of spatial correspondence will have to be radically altered.

Population and Area Served

In examining the relationship between supply, on the one hand, and need or demand, on the other, it may be useful or necessary to measure the population and identify the geographic area served by a given resource or cluster of resources. In this section we shall describe and evaluate the methods by which this information can be obtained and the uses to which it may be put.

POPULATION SERVED. Bailey has proposed a method for determining the size of the population served or the "effective population at risk" for a given hospital or group of hospitals (356). As described by Airth and Newell, the essential steps in the procedure are as follows (357, p. 20) :

1. Classify sample cases at the Survey hospitals by their home addresses.
2. For a sufficiently wide area, classify sample cases going to other hospitals by their home addresses.
3. From the above data, estimate for each local area the proportion of its cases treated in the Survey hospitals.
4. For each local area apply this proportion to its estimated population.
5. Add these numbers for all areas to obtain the total effective population served.

As described above, a case-load analysis of any given hospital defines the geographic area from which patients may go to a given hospital. The difficulty arises in finding out how many other hospital patients also arise in the population of this geographic area. This is why it is necessary to survey a large number of additional hospitals that are likely to serve this area, among others. The procedure described may be easier to understand if expressed in notational form as follows:

$$M = \frac{a}{a + b}(N),$$

where

> $M =$ effective population at risk or effective population served by hospital H;
> $a =$ number of patients from the area served by hospital H who go to hospital H;
> $b =$ number of patients from the area served by hospital H who go to other hospitals; and
> $N =$ population of area served by hospital H.

The fundamental assumption in the equation given above is that the proportion of persons (N) served by a hospital is equal to the proportion of patients $(a + b)$ served by that same hospital. For example, if a hospital attracts 10 percent of all *persons hospitalized* from a given area, it serves 10 percent of the *persons who live* in that area. This assumption is only an approximation since it does not recognize the considerably differentiated nature of hospital services and, consequently, the differences in drawing power of these different services. For example, for the group of hospitals studied by Airth and Newell, the population served by specialty ranged from 434,119 for ophthalmology to 600,906 for tuberculosis and diseases of the chest. The average for all specialties was 550,281 (357, Table 6, p. 20). Distortions are likely to arise to the extent that there are differences in service mix among hospitals and different levels of use by type of service among population subgroups.

In addition to comparability among hospitals, the population served by the several hospitals needs to be sufficiently homogeneous so that hospitalization rates are equal for the subpopulations served by each of the hospitals (389). This requirement that hospitalization rates be equal is easily demonstrable algebraically. If it cannot be met, or at least approximated, it will be necessary to conduct an actual population survey to determine which subpopulations are served by which hospitals. An additional feature, recognized by Bailey, is that the value for population served is a sample estimate subject to sampling error. Bailey describes the sources of sampling error and provides formulae for computing the variance of M (356, p. 148). The occurrence of sampling variability appears to account for the objections raised by Poland and Lembcke concerning a method, similar to that described by Bailey, for determining populations served, which does not depend on prior geographic subdivision into hospital districts. They conclude that such a method is "not recommended" because it does not include populations of geographic units from which no cases were reported during the study period (366, p. 42).

Generally, the effective population served by a hospital is derived from case-load data in the manner described above. It is possible, however, to begin with data about place of residence and place of hospitalization obtained from population surveys. The principles underlying the computation are the same as those described. The object is to obtain the number of hospital patients generated by a given population and the proportion of these patients that go to a given hospital. This proportion is applied to the total population in order to obtain the population served.

A determination of the population served is an essential prerequisite for epidemiologic studies based on case-load data. Without this information, case-load data cannot be used to construct rates, because it is not known what population they arise from. But given the "population base," one can conduct studies of hospital morbidity and mortality and of hospital use. Such studies, as well as the mere number of persons served, can serve to indicate demand, need, and possible unmet need.

GEOGRAPHIC AREA SERVED. The delineation of the geographic area served by a resource or group of resources contributes advantages over and above those that derive from mere quantification of the population served. Assumption of responsibility for a geographic area permits consideration of spatial dimensions such as location and travel, or other environmental factors, of aspects of social organization, and the like. It also permits more effective use of whatever data are available from other sources with respect to the areal units and their residents included in the geographic area served. According to Poland and Lembcke, "the outlining of mutually exclusive hospital service districts for existing hospitals is essential. Only after this has been done can comparisons between districts or comparison with a standard be made which reveal inequities between districts in the care available and which provide a basis for deciding whether and where new hospitals, more beds or services, or more skilled personnel are needed. Only after the district has been defined can the characteristics of the population served be studied. Only then can ratios between population and beds, population and patients, population and physicians and services be realistic'' (366, p. 105). More recently, de Visé has asserted that ''in the hospital planning field, it is now almost axiomatic that planning should be performed for specific geographically defined areas, and that it should be related to the needs, demands and patterns of use in those areas'' (368, p. 37). In the following pages we shall review the methods used for delineating service areas, discuss their underlying assumptions, and evaluate the extent to which the advantages mentioned above can be realized.

Several terms are used to indicate the linkage between a resource and the geographic area which it serves. These include the ''catchment area or basin,'' the ''draw,'' and the ''service area.'' The catchment area, or basin, and the draw are easy to define. They refer to the area within which resides the population from which the resource derives its case load. By contrast the term ''service area'' appears to have several meanings and is, by consequence, fraught with ambiguity. Some, including Drosness et al. (367) and Cherniak and Schneider (369), regard it as essentially similar to the catchment area or draw. United States Public Health Service regulations define a service area as

The geographic territory from which patients come or are expected to come to existing or proposed hospital or medical facilities, the delineation of which is based on such factors as population distribution, natural geographic boundaries, and transportation and trade patterns, and all parts of which are reasonably accessible to existing or proposd hospital or medical facilities (358, p. 30).

Ciocco and Altman offer the following definition:

A medical service area may be defined as one that is more or less self-contained with respect to the health demands of its population . . . The concept of medical service area is identical with that of the commercial trading area with which students of marketing have long been familiar, 361, p. 3).

It is clear that the notion of service area has the attribute of a mutual relationship between the resource and the area it serves, so that a large majority of the patients generated within the area use the resource and a large majority of the patients who use the resource come from within the area. The limiting case is where there is complete correspondence, so that one can delineate mutually exclusive service areas. Poland and Lembcke adopted this model as the basis for mapping ''hospital service districts'' in Kansas (366). They describe these districts as ''mutually exclusive'' and speak of the boundaries separating them as ''reminiscent of the line dividing watersheds and (that) may be thought of as the division between a 'population divide' although it is not as absolute as the divides between watersheds'' (366, p. 23). Dickinson, in his classic studies of physician service areas, adopted a model more realistically akin to the trade area. He saw the boundaries between two adjacent areas as a series of points, each being ''the breaking point, the 50 percent point—the point where the trade going to the two trade centers is approximately equal. This is one point on the boundary of the two trading areas served by two towns'' (365, p. 9).

There are two distinct, though interrelated, approaches to the delineation of service areas that have the property of mutually exclusive, or reasonably exclusive, relationship between resource and area served. One is predominantly empirical and the other normative. The empirical mapping of such areas is made possible because of the tendency, other things being equal, to utilize the nearest resource. Hence, mapping is easiest in rural areas where resources are few and dispersed and where the effect of distance is more sharply evident. In urban areas the multiplicity of adjacent resources and the ethnic, religious, or medical ties that modify the effect of spatial separation cause considerable overlap in catchment basins. Accordingly, the delineation of meaningful service areas may become very difficult. The mapping of normative service areas seldom occurs without prior established patterns of habitual use. Such mapping can, however, be somewhat more arbitrary since it depicts not what there is, but what should be, given certain political and administrative objectives. Theoretically, such areas can be *made* to be mutually exclusive, even though the power actually to make them so is seldom available or exercised.

The work of Mountin et al. is a classic example of the mapping of service areas based on a normative model—in this case, of the regional organization of hospitals (360). Underlying the spatial deployment is a concept of differentiation of health facilities by size and function into ''base,'' ''district,'' and ''rural'' hospitals, ''health centers,'' chronic disease ''institutions,'' and nursing homes. Corresponding to this functional scheme, a system is developed for aggregating counties within states into districts and regional areas. The districts, in turn, are differentiated into ''isolated,'' ''proposed secondary,'' ''secondary,'' and ''primary,'' depending largely on the number of hospital beds in each. The first step in districting was to assemble an inventory of hospitals, their size, functions, and location. Counties were then identified as possible nucleuses for primary, secondary, or proposed secondary districts according to the types of hospitals which they contained. The county with the largest number of beds was considered the nucleus, and adjacent counties were added to it to form a district. Geographic contiguity, rather than movements of those who seek care, determined the lines of cleavage. In this way the approach differed fundamentally from that based on the empirical delineation of medical trade areas. Another departure from the trading area concept was in the use of counties as the basic building stones for districts and in generally adhering to state boundaries in the construction of districts and regions. The justification for this is partly that data on population size and characteristics, and on the location of resources, are available by county. More important is the perceived need to link the system for providing care to the structure of political responsibility for financing and administration. We see here a deliberate effort to rationalize the system of institutional care by placing it within an essentially political mold. All this does not mean that the spatial configuration of districts and regions was unrelated to the flow of medical trade. It is reasonable to assume that geographic contiguity, and the scale of the hospital establishment in the nuclear counties, would correspond roughly to patterns of seeking care. Also, where there were alternative choices, trade areas were considered in drawing the district boundaries. In a few instances, districts were formed that straddled state lines.

Ciocco and Altman approached the task of determining service areas with a distinctly more empirical orientation (361). They conceived each service area as "more or less self-contained with respect to the health demands of its population" in a manner akin to the "commercial trading area" (361, p. 3). They included physician services in addition to hospital cases, and compared several methods for the delineation of service areas. In these respects their work set the pattern for much that was to follow and constituted the most important single contribution to the literature on medical service areas. However, like Mountin and his coworkers, Ciocco and Altman used the county as the primary unit for collecting data and constructing service areas, and remained within the boundary of the state (Pennsylvania) where they conducted their study.

Three distinct types of information were used for the delineation of service areas. The first was information on physician and hospital use obtained by household survey in 13 counties. The second was information on patients by place of residence obtained from physicians and hospitals. Physicians received mailed questionnaires that asked them to indicate the place of residence for all patients seen on one day (only 34 percent responded). Hospitals were asked to give place of residence for all admissions during one week. The third type of information consisted of data on place of residence of the mother and the place (hospital) of occurrence for all births to mothers in the study area, obtained from the National Office of Vital Statistics. The object was to test the extent to which data on births, which can be readily obtained from birth certificates, could substitute for more complete and costly studies of households or of case loads. These three methods—household surveys, case-load analyses, and analyses of birth certificates—represent all the approaches that have been used in the delineation of service areas. In each of the three, the basic datum is the linkage between place of residence and the location of care.

Ciocco and Altman accepted as given the patterns of movement within and among counties in the process of seeking care. Their task was to draw boundaries, always conforming to county lines, that would constitute areas that were ''self-contained with respect to the health demands'' of their population.

This definition implies that the movement into and out of a given area should be very small relative to the amount of movement among the counties within the area, and the amount of movement in the two opposite directions in the given area should tend to cancel out. The desired criteria must therefore be based on the quantitative expression of this definition. The mathematical formulation required for the purpose has not been developed as yet. Until it is worked out, we shall use an arbitrary level of magnitude, described below, to determine the dependent counties. It can be noted from the tables that the great majority of the counties which attract more patients than they lose, as measured by any of the indexes, do not have as much as 5 percent of their residents going to any one other county for medical care. Therefore we shall define as "dependent" the counties which have 6 percent or more of their residents going to some particular county. Thus, if county A has 6 percent or more of its residents going to county B and this is its highest percentage going to any one other county, then county A is dependent on county B and is considered as being in the same medical service area (361, pp. 12–13).

Tests were conducted to discover the degree of correspondence between the five items of information, from three sources, available for the delineation of service areas: location of physicians and hospitals as obtained by household survey; residence of patients as obtained from analyses of physician and hospital case loads; and residence of mother and location of birth as obtained from birth certificates. When percent of each of these events occurring within the county was used as the criterion, a high degree of correspondence was noted in the relative positions of counties, although there were a few aberrant cases. The delineation of service areas, as described above, using the physician, hospital, and birth indices respectively, also showed considerable correspondence. Ciocco and Altman also compared the areas obtained by their method with physician service areas obtained by Dickinson (to be described below) and the trading areas as shown in maps prepared by Rand, McNally. They considered the degree of correspondence to be "good." By contrast, agreement was less good with the regions envisaged by the Hospital Plan for Pennsylvania.

The use of birth data as a proxy for more detailed case-load or household survey studies has received further support since its early use by Ciocco and others (362, 363). Drosness and Lubin found that patient movements for maternity care in California counties corresponded closely to the use of hospitals for all other purposes combined (364). De Visé has documented essentially similar findings between birth data and patient origin studies from two hospital surveys in the Chicago area (368, pp. 26, 40).

One can see the progression from essentially administrative areas to the trade area concept as one compares the work of Mountin et al. with that of Ciocco and Altman. The trade area concept was applied in its purest form, without regard for political or administrative boundaries, in the classic work of Dickinson during his tenure as director of the Bureau of Medical Economic Research of the American Medical Association (365). Dickinson began his study because of dissatisfaction with the physician:population ratio by county as the measure of the adequacy of supply, as used by public health officials. He contended that medical care was spatially organized by trade areas rather than counties, and that the physician:population ratios within such areas were the more appropriate (or, as Dickinson put it, the "less worse") measure of the adequacy of supply (365, p. 1). According to Dickinson, the preferred method for delineating trade areas for physician services would have been to obtain case-load data by place of residence of patients. The dollar value of services, rather than the number of visits of patients, would serve to obtain a weighted aggregate of trade flow. The method actually adopted was to use the informed opinion of officials of local and state medical societies in delineating service areas.

The procedure began with identifying over 1051 "primary medical service centers" which draw medical trade from surrounding areas. Of these, 88 were designated "prime-primary centers" because they had "every type and kind of medical treatment and surgery." Every place with one or more active or inactive physicians was designated a "secondary center." The next step was to use opinion concerning the preponderant flow of trade, represented by estimated cash flow, to each of the primary centers, to draw service area boundaries. "The reader realizes, of course, that not all—perhaps very few—of these boundary lines constitute the ultimate in definitiveness either for the time they were drawn or for the present. There were then, and there are now, very few 'zero points'—points at which none of the residents of Area A shopped for physician's services in Area B and vice versa. Just as with any other economic goods (or services), some of the buyers of physician services are found to do their buying outside the circumscribed medical trading area'' (365, p. 17). The final step was the allocation of physicians and population to the service areas and the computation of physician : population ratios and other characteristics to be used in analysis. To the extent that total counties were included in the service areas, county data were used intact. To the extent that parts of counties were included, area was obtained from maps, using a planimeter (365, p. 19). The population in places as small as 100 persons could be precisely allocated. For intervening country the residual population was assumed to be evenly distributed, and was allocated in proportion to the area of the county included in the service area (365, p. 40). Physicians were allocated by postal address.

Some of the findings of the study remain of interest. There were 1,051 primary medical centers and 757 medical service areas, of which 212 straddled state boundaries. The primary centers were generally, but not always, larger towns, suggesting that medical trade may not always be congruent with other forms of trade. The large number of centers also suggests that ''medical trade is perhaps more localized than most forms of retail trade, and that the centers are more complementary, less mutually exclusive'' (365, p. 15). The service areas varied a great deal (see table on page 141 for a summary). In area they varied from 0.1 to 34.6 square miles, in population from 2,000 to 8,773,700, in number of physicians from 1 to 22,002, and in persons per active physician from 380 to 5,100. Seventeen percent of the land area of the United States was 25 miles or more from an active physician in April 1950. However, only 0.16 percent of the population was so located (365, p. 4). It would have taken only 361 physicians to bring all service areas to a level of, at most, 2,000 persons per physician. However, because there is no direct way to make physicians locate in under-doctored areas, Dickinson concluded that about 28,000 physicians (18 percent of all physicians) would have to be added to the national pool in order to bring about a general spatial redistribution that would achieve the goal of a maximum of 2,000 persons per physician in all service areas (365, pp. 104–105).

The distinctive characteristics of the method used by Dickinson were total disregard of political boundaries in the delineation of service area, the use of informed opinion to determine trade flow, and the use of estimated dollar value of trade flow in determining where boundaries were to be drawn. Contrary to the method used by Ciocco and Altman, there were no rules concerning the degree to which each area was self-contained with respect to the use of physician services. The boundary lines were drawn on maps at points where it was felt the preponderance of cash flow ceased to be directed to one primary center and began to be directed toward another.

Poland and Lembcke returned to the notion of self-contained areal units in their proposal for "mutually exclusive" "hospital service districts" in the state of Kansas (366). The geographic unit used for analysis and for constructing districts was the township, the smallest mutually exclusive administrative unit in Kansas. Data on patient residence were obtained from samples of the daily census of all general hospitals in the state. Each township which contained one or more hospitals was considered a district center. Data on percent of cases by hospital for the population of each adjacent township were used to add townships to the central township of each district. If less than 5 percent of patients from an adjacent township went to a hospital not in the central township, the adjacent township was included entirely in that district. If 5 percent or more went to another, but geographically contiguous, township, then the township where the patients originated was divided by area proportionate to hospital use, the parts being allocated among the townships to which it sent patients. The lines of division were arbitrary. The object was to get a visual equivalent of the proportionate division of the township rather than to define trade movement boundaries. In estimating the population of the district, the population of divided townships was allocated in strict proportion to the division of its hospital patients among adjacent districts. Admissions from a given township to hospitals in noncontiguous townships were ignored even when they constituted a considerable proportion of admissions originating in the township. In this manner it was possible to construct continuous district lines, without any "enclaves." The reader will note the affinities between this work and the work of Ciocco and Altman with respect to the concept of self-contained or mutually exclusive units and the application of the 5 percent rule. The method of allocating population in a manner proportionate to the distribution of patients is an application of the method used by Bailey for determining the effective population served.

The degree of success in attaining mutually exclusive service areas may be determined by examining two percentages: the percent of case load that arises within the service area and the percent of patients coming from within the service area who use resources located within the area. If separation between service areas is complete, both of these figures should be 100 percent. The districts drawn by Poland and Lembcke departed considerably from 100 percent in both respects, mainly because many patients traveled long distances to go to medical centers in noncontiguous townships. Poland and Lembcke report that no particular percentage—75 percent or 65 percent of whatever—was serviceable in determining district boundaries (366, p. 37). Drosness et al. have described a method, utilizing computer graphics, that facilitates the computation of the two percentages (367). The computer prints in the appropriate location on a map the number of hospital cases that originate in each census tract and the number of such cases that have gone to any specified hospital. Given the total case load of that hospital one can compute: (1) percent of case load of a specified hospital that comes from a given census tract, and (2) the percent of cases in any given census tract that have used a specified hospital. For each hospital-area linkage, two maps can be drawn, each showing census tracts by class intervals of each of the two percentages (see 367, Figs. 4 and 5). While such maps describe the relationships between hospitals and areal units they do not necessarily define "mutually exclusive areas." This is because, as we have seen, factors other than distance influence the use of service, especially in urban centers. For this reason, none of the studies that we have reviewed so far have attempted to dissect areas of population concentration into service areas. Indeed, their success in delineating service areas has rested to a large extent on the decision, where necessary, to cluster resources and to consider each cluster as related to a correspondingly large aggregate of people.

The problem of delineating service areas within urban concentrations remains a challenge to be faced. De Visé describes one approach as applied to the Chicago area, where there are 120 general hospitals and 200 communities from which they draw patients. Theoretically, it would be necessary to study all possible combinations between 120 hospitals and 200 communities to arrive at that set of groupings of hospitals and communities that maximizes the percent of a district's patients serviced inside the district and also minimizes "the inclusion within the same district of hospitals and communities between which there is little service linkage" (368, p. 26). In practice, a more "pragmatic" method was used. The first step was to obtain information on place of birth and place of residence for all maternity cases in one year. Using this information, two sets of maps were drawn. On hospital use maps, lines were drawn from communities of residence to each hospital, each line showing 100 maternity cases. On hospital case-load maps, similar lines were drawn, but each representing 5 percent of each hospital's case load. Thus one obtains a visual picture of the two parameters of the relationship between hospitals and communities. This pattern was used as a guide in delineating districts subject to certain guidelines. Three criteria were used:

1. The percentage of patients residing in a given area who go to hospitals in that area. This should be at least 50 percent.
2. Of all patients who use the hospitals in a given area, the percentage who live within that area. This should also be at least 50 percent.
3. The percent of communities within a district which have a "service linkage" with hospitals in that area. A "service linkage" is considered to exist between a hospital and a community when the community accounts for 1 percent or more of the hospital's maternity case load. For a given district which contains several communities and several hospitals, a "service linkage index" is computed. This is the percentage of instances in which the community–hospital linkages exceed the 1 percent of case load criterion. No particular cut-off point was used for the community service index, but it was stipulated that "the district be small enough to encompass hospitals serving most of the communities contained therein" (368, p. 29). It is this criterion that leads to the subdivision of the urban complex into subunits. The first two criteria would probably be best met by considering the urban conglomerate as one trading area.

In order to test the relative merits of alternative ways of grouping communities and hospitals a "composite score of best fit" was developed. Very simply this was:

> percent of local patients by hospital + percent of local
> patients by residence + service linkage index.

Using these criteria, 17 districts were delineated. The degree of success in meeting the three criteria may be judged from the summary in Table IV.81. It is clear that there has been only moderate success in achieving mutually exclusive separation. This, in spite of (1) clustering of hospitals and (2) assigning four "border hospitals" to district of service rather than district of location, and splitting the case loads of 10 border hospitals into 2 districts each.

Results such as these have led Cherniak and Schneider to question the utility of the notion of mutually exclusive service areas for hospitals, especially in a voluntary system such as that in the United States. They propose instead a concept very similar to that of the catchment area. They offer the "sectorgram" technique, which we have described in a previous section of this chapter, as a method for showing a service area for each hospital. The sectorgram gives a visual picture of the dispersion of the case load of each hospital around a "median center," which is the point of "minimum aggregate travel" to that hospital. The sectorgram

Table IV.81. Values for specified criteria for delineating service
areas in 17 such areas, Chicago 1963

Criteria Used for Delineating Hospital Districts	Values for Each Criterion Measured		
	Lowest Value	Highest Value	Average
Percent district hospital patients who reside in district	42	88	67
Percent of district patients who use district hospital	39	90	65
Hospital–community linkage index	52	100	79

SOURCE: Reference 368, Table 15, page 34.

does not, however, include the entire area from which patients come to
any given hospital (the catchment area), nor does it include any fixed
proportion of the case load or of the population that uses the hospital. It
is merely a standardized way of showing the extent of geographic dispersion, as well as the location and direction of that dispersion. The
proposed technique not only does not attempt separation into mutually
exclusive districts, but emphasizes, by showing sectorgrams of adjacent
hospitals superimposed over one another, the extent of overlap in catchment area.

READINGS AND REFERENCES

General

1. Klarman, H. E., "Supply of Personnel" and "Supply of Hospital Services," in
The Economics of Health (New York: Columbia University Press, 1965), pp. 74–125.
2. Feldstein, M. S., *Economic Analysis for Health Service Efficiency* (Amsterdam:
North-Holland Publishing Company, 1967). 322pp.

Specification and Classification

MANPOWER AND FACILITIES, GENERAL

3. National Center for Health Statistics, *Health Resources Statistics, 1968.* P.H.S.
Publication No. 1509 (Washington, D.C.: U.S. Government Printing Office, 1968),
260pp. Also see *Health Resources Statistics, 1969* and *Health Resources Statistics,
1970.*

4. Haug, J. N., and Roback, G. A., *Distribution of Physicians, Hospitals and Hospital Beds in the U.S., 1969.* Vol. I: *Regional, State, County;* Vol. II: *Metropolitan Areas* (Chicago: American Medical Association, Center for Health Services Research and Development, 1969. (This series began in 1963.)

MANPOWER, GENERAL

5. National Center for Health Statistics, *Health Resources Statistics*, 1965. P.H.S. Publication No. 1509 (Washington, D.C.: U.S. Government Printing Office, 1966). 182pp.
6. U.S. Public Health Service. *Health Manpower Source Book.* Public Health Service Publication No. 263 (Washington, D.C.: U.S. Government Printing Office).

a. Section 1   Physicians, 1952. 70pp.
b. Section 2   Nursing Personnel, 1953. 88pp. Revised 1966. 113pp.
c. Section 3   Medical Social Workers, 1953. 78pp.
d. Section 4   County Data from 1950 Census and Area Analysis 1954. 247pp.
e. Section 5   Industry and Occupation Data from 1950 Census, by State, 1954. 215pp.
f. Section 6   Medical Record Librarians, 1955. 43pp.
g. Section 7   Dentists. 158pp.
h. Section 8   Dental Hygienists, 1957. 87pp.
i. Section 9   Physicians, Dentists, and Professional Nurses, 1959. 80pp.
j. Section 10   Physicians' Age, Type of Practice, and Location, 1960. 199pp.
k. Section 11   Medical School Alumni, 1961. 319pp.
l. Section 12   Medical and Psychiatric Social Workers, 1961. 65pp.
m. Section 13   Hospital House Staffs, 1961. 43pp.
n. Section 14   Medical Specialists, 1962. 233pp.
o. Section 15   Pharmacists, 1963. 66pp.
p. Section 16   Sanitarians, 1963. 52pp.
q. Section 17   Industry and Occupation Data from 1960 Census, by State, 1963. 104pp.
r. Section 18   Manpower in the 1960's, 1964. 67pp.
s. Section 19   Location of Manpower in Eight Occupations, 1965. 167pp.
t. Section 20   Manpower Supply and Educational Statistics for Selected Health Occupations, 1968. 180pp.
u. Section 21   Allied Health Manpower, 1950–1980. 107pp.

7. U.S. Bureau of the Census, U.S. Census of Population, 1960. Subject Reports. *Occupation by Industry.* Final Report PC(2)-7C (Washington, D.C.: U.S. Government Printing Office, 1963). 146pp.
8. National Center for Education Statistics, *Summary Report on Bachelor's and Higher Degrees Conferred During the Year 1965–1966.* OE 54013A–66, Office of Education, U.S. Department of Health, Education, and Welfare (Washington, D.C.: U.S. Government Printing Office, 1968).
9. National Register of Scientific and Technical Personnel, *Reviews of Data on Science Resources, No. 11, Salaries and Selected Characteristics of U.S. Scientists, 1966* (Washington, D.C.: National Science Foundation, 1966).
10. Bureau of Labor Statistics, *Review of Occupational Employment Statistics: Employment of Scientific, Professional, and Technical Personnel in State Governments, January 1964.* Bulletin No. 1557, U.S. Department of Labor (Washington, D.C.: U.S. Government Printing Office, 1967). 29pp.
11. Bureau of Health Manpower, Public Health Service, Department of Health, Education and Welfare, and the American Hospital Association, *Manpower Resources in Hospitals, 1966* (Chicago: American Hospital Association, 1967).

12. Reed, L. S., *The Healing Cults*. Publications of the Committee on the Costs of Medical Care, No. 16 (Chicago: The University of Chicago Press, 1932). 134pp.

13. Scoville, J. G., "The Job Content of the U.S. Economy 1940–1970: An Attempt at Quantification" (unpubl. diss., Harvard University, Cambridge, Mass.: 1964).

14. Weiss, J. H., "A Job Classification Scheme for Health Manpower." *Health Services Research* 3:48–64 (Spring 1968).

15. Weiss, J. H., "The Changing Job Structure of Health Manpower" (unpub. diss. Harvard University, Cambridge, Mass., 1966). 267pp.

PHYSICIANS

16. American Medical Association. *American Medical Directory*. Chicago: The Association. 1906, 1909, 1912, 1916, 1918, 1921, 1923, 1925, 1927, 1929, 1931, 1934, 1936, 1938, 1940, 1942, 1950, 1956, 1958, 1961, 1963, 1967, 1969. The 1958 edition is the last to contain summary tabulations.

17. Advisory Board for Medical Specialties, *Directory of Medical Specialists, 1970–1971*. Vol. 14 (Chicago: Marquis—*Who's Who*, 1970). 2453pp.

18. Haug, J. N., Roback, G. A., and Martin, B. C., *Distribution of Physicians in the United States, 1970*. Regional, State, County, Metropolitan Areas. (Chicago: American Medical Association, Center for Health Services Research and Development, 1970). 329pp. (Prior publications in this series have appeared in two volumes, one for Regional, State, and County and another for Metropolitan Areas in 1963, 1964, and 1965.)

19. Theodore, C. N., Haug, J. N., Blafe, B. E., Roback, G. A., and Franz, E. J., *Reclassification of Physicians, 1968* (Chicago: American Medical Association, Center for Health Services Research and Development, 1968). 191pp.

20. Balfe, B. E., Lorant, J. H., and Todd, C., *Reference Data on the Profile of Medical Practice, 1971* (Chicago: Center for Health Services Research and Development, American Medical Association, June, 1971). 122pp.

21. American Medical Association, "Medical Licensure Statistics for 1969." *Journal of the American Medical Association* 212:1871–1948 (June 15, 1970). (A yearly summary published in the Medical Licensure number of the *Journal of the American Medical Association*.)

22. Stritter, F. T., Hutton, J. G., and Dube, W. F., "Study of U.S. Medical School Applicants, 1968–1969," *Journal of Medical Education* 45:195–209 (April 1970). (A yearly summary.)

23. Peterson, P. Q., and Pennell, M. Y. "Physician-Population Projections, 1961–1975: Their Causes and Implications," *American Journal of Public Health* 53:163–172 (February 1963).

24. Pennell, M. Y., "Statistics on Physicians, 1950–1963," *Public Health Reports* 79:905–910 (October 1964).

25. Stewart, W. H., and Pennell, M. Y. "Pediatric Manpower in the United States and Its Implications," *Pediatrics* 31:311–318 (February 1963).

OSTEOPATHIC PHYSICIANS

26. Pennell, M. Y., "Osteopathic College Alumni." *Journal of the American Osteopathic Association,* 61:755–762 (May 1962).

27. American Osteopathic Association, "Educational Supplement," *Journal of the American Osteopathic Association* 67:553–582 (January 1968).

28. American Osteopathic Association, *A Statistical Study of the Osteopathic Profession,* December 31, 1966 (Chicago: The Association, June 1967). 42pp.

DENTISTS

29. American Dental Association, Bureau of Data Processing Services, *1969 American Dental Directory* (Chicago: American Dental Association, 1969). 1256pp.

30. American Dental Association, *Distribution of Dentists in the United States by State, Region, District and County* (Chicago: The Association, 1969). 62pp.

31. Commission on the Survey of Dentistry in the United States, *The Survey of Dentistry: The Final Report* (Washington, D.C.: American Council of Education, 1962). 603pp.

PHARMACISTS

32. American Pharmaceutical Association, *A.Ph.A. Directory of Pharmacists* (Washington, D.C.: The American Pharmaceutical Association, 1964). 1741pp.

NURSES

33. American Nurses' Association, *Facts About Nursing: A Statistical Summary 1969 Edition* (New York: American Nurses' Association, 1969). 250 pp. (A yearly publication.)

SOCIAL WORKERS

34. Phillips, B., and Solon, J. A., ''Social Service for Private Patients: A Case Study,'' *Hospitals* 34:34–39 (October 1, 1960).

35. Pennell, M. Y., and Cooney, J. P., Jr., ''Social Service Departments in Hospitals: 1954–1964.'' *Hospitals* 41:88–92 and 97–100 (March 16, 1967).

FACILITIES, GENERAL

36. Bureau of the Census, *U.S. Census of Population: 1960. Subject Reports. Inmates of Institutions.* Final Report PC(2)–8A (Washington, D.C.: U.S. Government Printing Office, 1963). 303pp.

37. Division of Hospital and Medical Facilities: *Hill-Burton State Plan Data: A National Summary as of January 1, 1967.* P.H.S. Publication No. 930–F–2 (Washington, D.C.: U.S. Government Printing Office, 1968). 92pp.

38. Hatten, J., ''Health Insurance for the Aged: Participating Health Facilities, July 1968.'' *Social Security Bulletin* 32:12–19 (September 1969).

39. National Center for Health Statistics, *Development and Maintenance of a National Inventory of Hospitals and Institutions.* P.H.S. Publication No. 1000, ser. 1, no. 3 (Washington, D.C.: U.S. Government Printing Office, February 1965). 25pp.

40. National Center for Health Statistics, *Design and Methodology of the 1967 Master Facility Inventory Survey.* P.H.S. Publication No. 1000, ser. 1, no. 9 (Washington, D.C.: U.S. Government Printing Office, January 1971). 30pp.

41. Conference on Classification of Health Care Facilities, *Classification of Health Care Institutions* (Chicago: American Hospital Association, 1966). 26pp.

HOSPITALS

42. The American Hospital Association, *Hospitals,* Guide Issue, August 1, 1969, pt. 2.

43. Bureau of Health Insurance, Social Security Administration, Department of Health, Education and Welfare, *Directory of Medicare Providers of Services: Hospitals. Title XVIII, Health Insurance for the Aged* (Washington, D.C.: U.S. Government Printing Office, October 1968).

44. American Osteopathic Association, *Registry of Accredited Osteopathic Association Institutions*, 1967–1968 (Chicago, 1967).

45. Morrill, R. L., and Earickson, R., ''Variations of the Character and Use of Chicago Hospitals,'' *Health Services Research* 3:224–238 (Fall 1968).

NURSING AND PERSONAL CARE HOMES

46. Eagle, E., ''Nursing Homes and Related Facilities: A Review of the Literature.'' *Public Health Report* 83:673–684 (August 1968).

47. Solon, J., and Baney, A. M., ''General Hospital and Nursing Home Beds in Urban and Rural Areas,'' *Public Health Reports* 71:985–992 (October 1956).

48. Public Health Service, Division of Hospital and Medical Facilities, *Characteristics of Nursing Homes and Related Facilities: Report of a 1961 National Inventory*. P.H.S. Publication No. 930–F–5 (Washington, D.C., 1963). 46pp.

49. U.S. Department of Health, Education and Welfare, Public Health Service. *Nursing Homes and Related Facilities Fact Book*. P.H.S. Publication No. 930–F–4 (Washington, D.C., February 1963). 177pp.

50. National Center for Health Statistics, Reports of the Institutional Population Survey in Series 12 of the publications of the National Center for Health Statistics. So far the following numbers, relevant to nursing homes, have appeared:

No. 1. Institutions for the Aged and Chronically Ill, United States, April–June 1963. 46pp.

No. 2. Characteristics of Residents in Institutions for the Aged and Chronically Ill, United States, April–June 1963, 53pp.

No. 4. Utilization of Institutions for the Aged and Chronically Ill, United States, April–June 1963. 36pp.

No. 5. Employees in Nursing and Personal Care Homes, United States, May–June 1964. 34pp.

No. 6. Employees in Nursing and Personal Care Homes: Number, Work Experience, Special Training and Wages, United States, May–June 1964. 36pp.

No. 7. Chronic Illness Among Residents of Nursing and Personal Care Homes, United States, May–June 1964. 43pp.

No. 8. Prevalence of Chronic Conditions and Impairments Among Residents of Nursing and Personal Care Homes, United States, May–June 1964, 36pp.

No. 9. Charges for Care in Institutions for the Aged and Chronically Ill, United States, May–June 1964. 51pp.

No. 10. Nursing and Personal Care Services Received by Residents of Nursing and Personal Care Homes, United States, May–June 1964. 41pp.

No. 11. Uses of Special Aids in Homes for the Aged and Chronically Ill, United States, May–June 1964. 32pp.

No. 12. Marital Status and Living Arrangements Before Admission to Nursing and Personal Care Homes, United States, May–June 1964. 46pp.

51. *Report, National Conference on Nursing Homes and Homes for the Aged*. P.H.S. Publication No. 625 (Washington, D.C.: U.S. Government Printing Office, 1958). 85pp.

52. Bureau of Health Insurance, Social Security Administration, *Directory of Medicare Providers of Services: Extended Care Facilities, Title XVIII, Health Insurance for the Aged* (Washington, D.C.: U.S. Government Printing Office, October, 1968).

53. U.S. Department of Health, Education and Welfare, Social Security Administration, *Health Insurance for the Aged: Conditions of Participation for Extended Care Facilities* (Washington, D.C.: U.S. Government Printing Office, 1966). 60pp.

PSYCHIATRIC FACILITIES

54. The National Institute for Mental Health, *Patients in Mental Institutions, 1966,* pts. I, II, and III. P.H.S. Publication No. 1818 (Washington, D.C.: U.S. Government Printing Office, 1968).

55. The National Institute of Mental Health, *Outpatient Psychiatric Clinics: Data on Staff and Man-hours, 1965.* P.H.S. Publication No. 1448 (Washington, D.C.: U.S. Government Printing Office, 1968).

HOME CARE

56. Ryder, C. F., and Frank, B., ''Coordinated Home Care Programs in Community Heath Agencies: A Decade of Progress.'' *American Journal of Public Health* 57:261–265 (February 1967). (A summary of trends based on surveys in 1955, 1956, 1960, and 1964.)

57. U.S. Department of Health, Education and Welfare, Public Health Service, *Coordinated Home Care Programs: 1964 Survey.* P.H.S. Publication No. 1479 (Washington, D.C., December 1966). 72pp.

58. Bureau of Health Insurance, Social Security Administration, *Directory of Medicare Providers of Services: Home Health Agencies, Title XVIII, Health Insurance for the Aged* (Washington, D.C.: U.S. Government Printing Office, October 1967).

59. Public Health Service, Bureau of Health Manpower, Division of Nursing. *Services Available for Nursing Care of the Sick at Home.* P.H.S. Publication No. 1265 (revised 1967) (Washington, D.C.: U.S. Government Printing Office, 1968). 74pp.

EMERGENCY AND OUTPATIENT HOSPITAL SERVICES

60. Solon, J. A., ''An Overview of Outpatient Services.'' *Inquiry* 2:3–15 (November 1965).

61. Public Health Service, Division of Hospital and Medical Services, *Facts and Trends on Hospital Outpatient Services* (Washington, D.C.: U.S. Government Printing Office, 1964). 24pp.

62. American Hospital Association, *Outpatient Health Care: Report and Recommendations of a Conference and Follow-up Meeting of a Working Party* (Chicago, 1959). 58pp.

Also see the annual Guide Issue of *Hospitals,* Journal of the American Hospital Association.

GROUP PRACTICE

63. Hunt, G. H., and Goldstein, M. S., *Medical Group Practice in the United States.* P.H.S. Publication No. 77 (Washington, D.C.: U.S. Government Printing Office, 1951). 70pp.

64. American Medical Association, Committee on Medical and Related Facilities, ''Survey of Group Practice,'' *Journal of the American Medical Association* 164:1338–1348 (July 1957).

65. Altenderfer, M. E., and Raup, R. M., *Medical Groups in the United States, 1959.* P.H.S. Publication No. 1063 (Washington, D.C.: U.S. Government Printing Office, 1963). 172pp.

66. Balfe, B. E., and McNamara, M. E., *Survey of Medical Groups in the U.S.* (Chicago: American Medical Association, 1968). 135pp.

67. Balfe, B. E., ''A Survey of Group Practice in the United States, 1965,'' *Public Health Reports* 84:597–603 (July 1969).

68. Todd, C., and McNamara, M. E., assisted by Martin, B. C., *Medical Groups in the U.S., 1969* (Chicago: American Medical Association, 1971). 128pp.

69. Pomrinse, S. D., and Goldstein, M. D., *A Preliminary Directory of Medical Groups in the United States, 1959*. P.H.S. Publication No. 817 (Washington, D.C.: U.S. Government Printing Office, January 1961). 246pp.

NEIGHBORHOOD HEALTH CENTERS

70. Office of Economic Opportunity, *Directory of Comprehensive Neighborhood Health Service Programs*. Pamphlet No. 6128–1 (Washington, D.C.: The Government Printing Office, 1970). 54pp.

LABORATORIES

71. Bureau of Health Insurance, Social Security Administration. *Directory of Medicare Suppliers of Services: Independent Laboratories, Title XVIII, Health Insurance for the Aged* (Washington, D.C.: U.S. Government Printing Office, October 1968).

The Capacity to Produce Service

GENERAL

72. Klarman, H. E., "Selected Problems: Applications of the Medical Care Price Index," in *The Economics of Health*, (New York: Columbia University Press, 1965), pp. 147–162.

73. Strum, H. M., "Technological Developments and Their Effects Upon Health Manpower," *Monthly Labor Review* 90:1–8 (January 1967).

74. U.S. Department of Labor, Manpower Administration. *Technology and Manpower in the Health Service Industry, 1965–1975*. Manpower Research Bulletin No. 14 (Washington, D.C., May 1967). 109pp.

MEASURING PHYSICIAN OUTPUT

75. National Center for Health Statistics, *Health Survey Procedure: Concepts, Questionnaire Development, and Definitions in the Health Interview Survey*. P.H.S. Publication No. 1000, ser. 1, no. 2 (Washington, D.C.: U.S. Government Printing Office, May 1964). 66pp.

76. California Medical Association, *1964 Relative Value Studies* (San Francisco: Six Ninety Three Sutter Publications, Inc., 1964). 79pp.

77. Michigan State Medical Society, *1965 Michigan Relative Value Study* (revised 1968). (East Lansing, Michigan: The Society, 1968.)

78. Scitovsky, A. A., "Changes in the Costs of Treatment of Selected Illnesses, 1951–1965," *American Economic Review* 57:1182–1195 (December 1967).

79. Blendon, R. J., "An Attitude Scale for Evaluating Complexity of Surgical Procedures," *HSMHA Health Reports* 86:1025–1029 (November 1971).

80. Boyd, E. A. D., "DIFAM—A New Method of Medical Care Insurance Payment," *Medical Care* 5:334–342 (September–October 1967).

81. Kovner, J. W., "Measurement of Outpatient Office Visit Services," *Health Services Research* 4:112–127 (Summer 1969).

82. Kovner, J. W., *A Production Function for Outpatient Medical Facilities*. Doctoral dissertation, School of Public Health, University of California at Los Angeles, 1968. (Available from University Microfilms, Ann Arbor, Michigan.)

PRODUCTIVITY OF HEALTH MANPOWER : GENERAL

83. Fein, R., ''Productivity and Organization,'' in Fein, *The Doctor Shortage, an Economic Diagnosis* (Washington, D.C.: The Brookings Institution, 1967), pp. 90–129.

84. Berki, S. E., ''On the Measurement of the Output and Productivity of Physicians.'' Unpubl. manuscript (Ann Arbor: School of Public Health, The University of Michigan, October 9, 1970). 11pp.

85. Dickinson, F. G., *The Cost and Quality of Medical Care in the United States.* Bureau of Medical Economic Research, Bulletin 66 (Chicago American Medical Association, 1948). See section on ''Quality,'' pp. 16–19. Also see the section on ''Price and Quantity'' in the 1949 *Supplement to Bulletin 66.*

86. Dickinson, F. G., *Supply of Physicians' Services.* Bulletin 81 (Chicago: Bureau of Economic Research, American Medical Association, 1951). 16pp.

87. Dickinson, F. G., ''What We Get for What We Spend for Medical Care,'' in *Financing a Health Program for America,* vol. IV, of President's Commission on the Health Needs of the Nation, *Building America's Health* (Washington, D.C.: U.S. Government Printing Office, 1952), pp. 17–23.

88. Garbarino, J. W., ''Price Behavior and Productivity in the Medical Market,'' *Industrial and Labor Relations Review* 13:3–15 (October 1959).

89. Garbarino, J. W., ''Some Demand and Supply Considerations,'' in *Health Plans and Collective Bargaining* (Berkeley: University of California Press, 1960), pp. 45–48.

90. Commission on the Survey of Dentistry in the United States, ''Estimates of the Effects of Fluoridation, Improved Equipment, and Additional Auxiliary Personnel on Dental Manpower Requirements,'' in *The Survey of Dentistry: The Final Report* (Washington, D.C.: American Council on Education, 1962), App. A, pp. 475–482.

91. Weiss, J. H., ''The Changing Job Structure of the Patient Care—Dental Job Family,'' in *The Changing Job Structure of Health Manpower.* Doctoral dissertation, Harvard University, Cambridge, Mass., July 1966, pp. 120–156. (Processed.)

92. Penchansky, R., and Rosenthal G., ''Productivity, Price, and Income Behavior in the Physicians' Services Market—A Tentative Hypothesis,'' *Medical Care* 3:240–244 (December 1965).

93. Daniels, R. S., ''Physician Productivity and the Hospital: A Physician's View.'' *Inquiry* 6:70–78 (September 1969).

94. Johnson, E. A., ''Physician Productivity and the Hospital: A Hospital Administrator's View,'' *Inquiry* 6:59–69 (September 1969).

95. Roemer, M. I., ''Hospital Utilization and the Supply of Physicians.'' *Journal of the American Medical Association* 178:989–993 (December 9, 1961).

96. Pennell, E. H., ''Location and Movement of Physicians—Methods for Estimating Physician Resources,'' *Public Health Reports* 59:281–305 (March 3, 1944). See pp. 288–293 on ''A Physician's Capacity for Service.''

97. Jones, N. H., Struve, C. A., and Stefani, P., ''Health Manpower in 1975—Demand, Supply, and Price,'' in *Report of the National Advisory Commission on Health Manpower, Volume II,* App. V, pp. 229–263 (Washington, D.C.: U.S. Government Printing Office, November 1967).

98. Klarman, H., ''Economic Aspects of Projecting Requirements for Health Manpower,'' *Journal of Human Resources* 4:360–376 (Summer 1969).

PRODUTIVITY AND THE SCALE OF AMBULATORY CARE

99. Donabedian, A., *A Review of Some Experiences with Prepaid Group Practice.* Research Series No. 11 (Ann Arbor: Bureau of Public Health Economics, School of Public Health, The University of Michigan, 1965). 74pp.

100. Donabedian, A., ''An Evaluation of Prepaid Group Practice.'' *Inquiry* 6:3–27 (September 1969).

101. Boan, J. A., ''Productivity,'' in Boan, *Group Practice* (Ottawa, Roger Duhamel, 1966), pp. 23–31.

102. Yett, D. E., ''An Evaluation of Alternative Methods of Estimating Physicians' Expenses Relative to Output,'' *Inquiry* 4:3–27 (March 1967).

103. McCaffree, K. M., and Newman, H. F., ''Prepayment of Drug Costs under a Group Practice Prepayment Plan,'' *American Journal of Public Health* 58:1212–1218 (July 1968).

104. National Advisory Commission on Health Manpower, ''The Kaiser Foundation Medical Care Program,'' in *Report of the National Advisory Commission on Health Manpower*, vol. II, App. IV, pp. 197–228 (Washington, D.C.: U.S. Government Printing Office, 1967).

105. Bailey, R. M., ''Economies of Scale in Medical Practice.'' Paper presented at the Second Conference on the Economics of Health, Baltimore, Md., December 5–7, 1968). 28pp. Published in *Empirical Studies in Health Economics*, ed. H. E. Klarman (Baltimore: Johns Hopkins Press, 1970), pp. 255–273.

106. Bailey, R. M., ''A Comparison of Internists in Solo and Fee-for-Service Group Practice in the San Francisco Bay Area.'' *Bulletin of the New York Academy of Medicine* 44:1243–1303 (November 1968).

107. Bailey, R. M., ''Philosophy, Faith, Fact and Fiction in the Production of Medical Services,'' *Inquiry* 7:37–53 (March 1970).

108. Yankauer, A., Connelly, J. P., and Feldman, J. J., ''Physician Productivity in the Delivery of Ambulatory Care: Some Findings from a Survey of Pediatricians,'' *Medical Care* 8:35–46 (January–February 1970).

109. American Dental Association, Bureau of Economic Research and Statistics, ''1968 Survey of Dental Practice. II: Income of Dentists by Location, Age and Other Factors,'' *Journal of the American Dental Association* 78:342–346 (February 1969).

110. American Dental Association, Bureau of Economic Research and Statistics, 1968 Survey of Dental Practice. III: Income of Dentists by Type of Practice, Personnel Employed, and Other Factors,'' *Journal of the American Dental Association* 78:803–805 (April 1969).

111. American Dental Association, Bureau of Economic Research and Statistics, ''1968 Survey of Dental Practice. VII: Number of Patients and Patient Visits,'' *Journal of the American Dental Association* 79:378–380 (August 1969).

MEASURING HOSPITAL OUTPUT

112. Lave, J. R., ''A Review of the Methods Used to Study Hospital Costs,'' *Inquiry* 3:57–81 (May 1966).

113. Codman, E. A., ''The Product of a Hospital,'' *Surgery, Gynecology and Obstetrics* 18:491–496 (January–June, 1914).

114. Lytton, J. D., ''Recent Productivity Trends in the Federal Government: An Exploratory Study,'' *Review of Economics and Statistics* 41:341–359 (November 1959).

115. Saathoff, D. E., and Kurtz, R. A., ''Cost per Day Comparisons Don't Do the Job,'' *Modern Hospital* 94:14–16, 162 (October 1962).

116. American Hospital Association, ''A New Measure of Hospital Utilization,'' *Hospitals* 43:466–467 (August 1, 1969), pt. 2 (Guide Issue).

117. Feldstein, M., ''Hospital Cost Variation and Case-Mix Differences,'' *Medical Care* 2:95–103 (April–June 1965).

118. Rajgrodzki, P., ''Productivity in the Hospital Industry: A Preliminary Study,'' unpubl. manuscript, 1966. 21pp. and bibliography.

119. Collins, G. L., ''Cost Analysis and Efficiency Measures in Hospitals,'' *Inquiry* 5:50–61 (June 1968).

HOSPITAL SIZE AND PRODUCTIVITY

120. Hefty, T. R., ''Returns to Scale in Hospitals: A Critical Review of Recent Literature,'' *Health Services Research* 4:267–280, (Winter 1969).

121. Feldstein, P., *An Empirical Investigation of the Marginal Cost of Hospital Services* (Chicago: Graduate Program in Hospital Administration, University of Chicago, 1961). 77pp.

122. Carr, W. J. and Feldstein, P. J., ''The Relationship of Cost to Hospital Size,'' *Inquiry* 4:45–65 (June 1967).

123. Berry, R. E., Jr., *Competition and Efficiency in the Market for Hospital Services: The Structure of the American Hospital Industry* (Cambridge: Harvard University, Interfaculty Program on Health and Medical Care, August 1965).

124. Berry, R. E., Jr., *An Analysis of Costs in Short-Term General Hospitals.* Discussion Paper No. 30, Harvard Institute of Economic Research, Harvard University, Cambridge, May 1968. 20pp. (Mimeograph.)

125. Berry, R. E., Jr., ''Returns to Scale in the Production of Hospital Services,'' *Health Services Research* 2:123–139 (Summer 1967).

126. Berry, R. E., Jr., ''Product Heterogeneity and Hospital Cost Analysis,'' *Inquiry* 7:67–75 (March 1970).

127. Feldstein, M. S., ''Effects of Scale on Hospital Costs,'' in *Economic Analysis for Health Service Efficiency* (Amsterdam: North-Holland Publishing Company, 1967), pp. 56–86.

128. Cohen, H. A., ''Variations in Cost Among Hospitals of Different Sizes,'' *Southern Economic Journal* 33:355–366 (January 1967).

129. Cohen, H. A., ''Hospital Cost Curves with Emphasis on Measuring Patient Care Output.'' Paper presented at the Second Conference on the Economics of Health, Baltimore, Maryland, December 5–7, 1968. Processed. 20pp. Published in *Empirical Studies in Health Economics*, ed. H. E. Klarman (Baltimore: Johns Hopkins Press, 1970), pp. 279–293.

130. Ingbar, M. L., and Taylor, L. D., *Hospital Costs in Massachusetts: An Econometric Study* (Cambridge: Harvard University Press, 1968). 237pp.

OTHER FACTORS IN HOSPITAL PRODUCTIVITY

131. Commission on the Cost of Medical Care, *The Cost of Medical Care.* Vol. IV: *Changing Patterns of Hospital Care* (Chicago: American Medical Association, 1964). 173pp.

132. Revans, R. W., ''Research into Hospital Management and Organization,'' *The Milbank Memorial Fund Quarterly* 44:207–245 (July 1966), pt. 2.

133. Spencer, W. A., Vallbona, C., and Geddes, L. A., ''Requirements and Application of Automation in Hospital Functions,'' *Journal of Chronic Diseases* 17:469–481 (June 1964).

134. Weissman, O., and Sigmond, R. M., ''Is Separation of OB Cases Necessary?'' *Modern Hospital* 102:91–94 and 158 (January 1964).

135. Blumberg, M. S., ''The Effects of Size and Specialism on Utilization of Urban Hospitals,'' *Hospitals* 39:43–47, 130 (May 16, 1965).

Services Produced in Relation to Capacity to Produce

WORKLOAD OF PHYSICIANS AND OTHER HEALTH PERSONNEL: METHODS

136. Hill, A. Bradford, ''The Doctor's Day and Pay,'' *Royal Statistical Society Journal*, ser. ''A,'' 114:1–34 (1951).

137. Bevan, J. R., and Draper, G. J., "Sampling Problems in Studies of General Practice," *Medical Care* 3:168–178 (July–September 1965).

138. Backett, E. M., Shaw, L. A., and Evans, J. C. G., "Studies of General Practice (1): Patients' Needs and Doctors' Services: A Description of Method," *Proceedings of the Royal Society of Medicine* 46:707–712 (September 1953).

139. Peterson, O. L., Andrews, L. P., Spain, R. S., and Greenberg, B. G., "An Analytical Study of North Carolina General Practice: 1953–1954," *Journal of Medical Education* vol. 31, no. 12, pt. 2 (December 1956).

140. Van Deen, K. J., "Primary Medical Care: Analysis of the Work Load," *Milbank Memorial Fund Quarterly* 43:277–284 (April 1965), pt. 2.

141. Jeans, W. D., "Work Study in General Practice," *Journal of College of General Practitioners* 9:270–279 (May 1965).

142. Last, J. M., "Primary Medical Care. 1: Record Keeping," *Milbank Memorial Fund Quarterly* 43:266–276 (April 1965), pt. 2.

143. College of General Practitioners, Research Committee of Council, "The Records and Statistical Unit," *Journal of the College of General Practitioners* 6:195–224 (1963).

144. College of General Practitioners. *Present State and Future Needs.* Reports from General Practice, No. II (London, 1965).

145. Eimerl, T. S., "Organized Curiosity: A Practical Approach to the Problem of Keeping Records for Research Purposes in General Practice," *Journal of College of General Practitioners* 3:246–252 (1960).

146. Eimerl, T. S., "Organized Curiosity: An Outline of the Principles Underlying the Technique of Research in General Practice," *Journal of College of General Practitioners* 7:628–636 (1964).

147. Kuensberg, E. V., "Recording of Morbidity of Families: 'F' Book," *Journal of College of General Practitioners* 7:410–422 (1964).

148. Walford, P. A., "The Practice Index," *Journal of College of General Practitioners* 6:225–232 (1963).

149. Spenser, J. T., "A Diagnostic Work-Study Index: A Use of the E-Book to Measure Work Load in Relation to Morbidity," *Journal of College of General Practitioners* 13:39–54 (January 1967).

150. College of General Practitioners, Records and Research Advisory Service. "The 'L' Book," *Journal of College of General Practitioners* 14:289–293 (November 1967).

151. Jacob, A., "An 'Artificial Practice' as a Tool for Research into General Practice," *Journal of College of General Practitioners* 11:41–48 (January 1966).

152. Jacob, A., "Demand/Attendance Patterns in an 'Artificial Practice'," *Journal of College of General Practitioners* 11:174–183 (March 1966).

153. Jacob, A., "Delivery Patterns in a Real and Artificial Practice," *Journal of College of General Practitioners* 11:241–252 (May 1966).

154. LeRiche, J., and Stiver, W. B., "The Work of Specialists and General Practitioners in Ontario," *Canadian Medical Association Journal* 81:37–42 (July 1, 1959).

155. Rossiter, C. E., and Reynolds, J. A., "Automatic Monitoring of the Time Waited in Out-patient Departments," *Medical Care* 1:218–225 (October–December 1963).

156. Querido, A., "Direct Evaluation of the Work of Some General Practitioners," in *The Efficiency of Medical Care* (Leiden: H. E. Stenfert Kroese N. V., 1963), pp. 46–52.

157. White, M. J. B., and Pike, M. C., "Appointment Systems in Out-Patient Clinics," *Medical Care* 2:133–145 (July–September 1964).

158. Haussmann, R. K., "Waiting Time as an Index of Quality of Nursing Care," *Health Services Research* 5:92–105 (Summer 1970).

Services Produced in Relation to Capacity to Produce

WORK LOAD OF PHYSICIANS : U.S. AND CANADA

159. Ciocco, A., and Altman, I., ''Statistics on the Patient Loads of Physicians in Private Practice,'' *Journal of the American Medical Association* 121:506–513 (February 13, 1943).

160. Ciocco, A., and Altman, I., ''The Patient Load of Physicians in Private Practice: A Comparative Study of Three Areas,'' *Public Health Reports* 58:1329–1351 (September 3, 1943).

161. Ciocco, A., and Altman, I., and Truan, T. D., ''Patient Load and Volume of Medical Services,'' *Public Health Reports* 67:527–534 (June 1952).

162. Theodore, C. N., and Sutter, G. E., ''A Report on the First Periodic Survey of Physicians,'' *Journal of the American Medical Association* 202:516–524 (November 6, 1967).

163. Parrish, J. M., Bishop, F. M., and Baker, A. S., ''Time Study of General Practitioners' Office Hours.'' *Archives of Environmental Health* 14:892–898 (June 1967).

164. Last, J. M., and White, K. L., ''The Content of Medical Care in Primary Practice,'' *Medical Care* 7:41–48 (January–February) 1969.

165. Clute, K. F., ''Arrangements for Practice: Time,'' and ''Content of the General Practitioner's Work,'' in *The General Practitioner: A Study of Medical Education and Practice in Ontario and Nova Scotia* (University of Toronto Press, 1963), pp. 97–114, 227–261.

166. Wolfe, S., Badgley, R. F., Kasius, R. V., Garson, J. Z., and Gold, R. J. M., ''The Work of a Group of Doctors in Saskatchewan,'' *Milbank Memorial Fund Quarterly* 46:103–129 (January 1968).

167. Altman, I., Kroeger, H. H., Clark, D. A., Johnson, A. C., and Sheps, C. G., ''The Office Practice of Internists. II: Patient Load,'' *Journal of the American Medical Association* 193:667–672, (August 23, 1965).

168. Johnson, A. C., Kroeger, H. H., Altman, I., Clark, D. A., and Sheps, C. G., ''The Office Practice of Internists. III: Characteristics of Patients,'' *Journal of the American Medical Association* 193:916–922 (September 13, 1965).

169. Clark, D. A., ''The Office Practice of Internists, IV: Professional Activities Other than the Care of Private Patients,'' *Journal of the American Medical Association* 194:177–181, October 11, 1965.

170. Deisher, R. W., Derby, A. J., and Sturman, M. J., ''Changing Trends in Pediatric Practice,'' *Pediatrics* 25:712–716 (April 1960).

171. Bergman, A. B., Dassel, S. W., and Wedgwood, R. J., ''Time-Motion Study of Practicing Pediatricians,'' *Pediatrics* 38:254–263 (August 1966).

172. Bergman, A. B., Probstfield, J. L., and Wedgwood, R. J., ''Performance Analysis in Pediatric Practice: Preliminary Report,'' *Journal of Medical Education* 42:249–253 (March 1967).

173. Yankauer, A., Connelly, J. P., and Feldman, J. J., ''Pediatric Practice in the United States, with Special Attention to Utilization of Allied Health Worker Services,'' *Pediatrics* 45:521–554 (March 1970), pt. 2.

WORK LOAD OF PHYSICIANS : OTHER COUNTRIES

174. Logan, R. F. L., and Eimerl, T. S., ''Case Loads in Hospital and General Practice in Several Countries,'' *Milbank Memorial Fund Quarterly* 43:302–310 (April 1, 1965), pt. 2.

175. Stevenson, J. S. K., ''General Practice in Scotland—Why the Difference? A Comparative Study of Statistics from Practice in the United Kingdom,'' *British Medical Journal* 1:1370–1373 (May 23, 1964).

176. Lees, D. S., and Cooper, M. H., "A Preliminary Analysis of Research into General Practice," *Journal of College of General Practitioners* 6:233–241 (1963).

177. Lees, D. S., and Cooper, M. H., "The Work of the General Practitioner: An Analytical Survey of Studies of General Practice," *Journal of the College of General Practitioners* 6:408–435 (1963).

178. Cartwright, A., "General Practice in 1963: Its Conditions, Contents and Satisfactions," *Medical Care* 3:69–87 (April–June 1965).

179. Cartwright, A., *Patients and Their Doctors: A Study of General Practice* (New York: Atherton Press, 1967). 295pp.

180. Mechanic, D., "General Practice in England and Wales: Results from a Survey of a National Sample of General Practitioners," *Medical Care* 6:245–260 (May–June 1968).

181. Eimerl, T. S., Pearson, R. J. C., and the Merseyside and North Wales Faculty of the College of General Practitioners, "Working-Time in General Practice: How Practitioners Use Their Time," *British Medical Journal* 2:1549–1554 (December 24, 1966).

182. Crombie, D. L., and Cross, K. W., "The Use of a General Practitioner's Time," *British Journal of Preventive and Social Medicine* 10:141–144 (July 1956).

183. Fry, J., and Dillane, J. B., "Too Much Work? Proposals Based on a Review of Fifteen Years' Work in Practice," *Lancet* 2:632–637 (September 19, 1964).

184. Fry, J., "General Practice Tomorrow," *British Medical Journal* 2:1064–1067 (October 24, 1964).

185. Payne, E. M. M., "The Number of Items of General Medical Service Provided by a General Practitioner in One Year (1964)," *Journal of College of General Practitioners* 12:172–183 (September 1966).

186. Baker, C. D., "A Practice Pattern of Patient-Doctor Contact," *Journal of College of General Practitioners* 12:54–67 (July 1966).

187. Drury, M., "Work Load and the General Practitioner," *Lancet* 2:823–827 (October 14, 1967).

STUDIES RELEVANT TO MISUSE OF HEALTH PERSONNEL

188. Krass, I. M., "Is There Abuse in General Practice?" *Journal of College of General Practitioners* 10:124–132 (September 1965).

189. Hardman, R. A., "Late Calls in General Practice," *Journal of College of General Practitioners* 11:54–60 (January 1966).

190. Forbes, J. A., Mutch, L. M. M., Smith, G. T., and Tulloch, A. J., "Study of the Demand for Urgent Treatment in General Practice," *British Medical Journal* 3:856–858 (September 30, 1967).

191. Densen, P. M., Shapiro, S., and Einhorn, M., "Concerning High and Low Utilizers of Services in a Medical Care Plan, and the Persistence of Utilization Level, over a Three Year Period," *Milbank Memorial Fund Quarterly* 37:217–250 (July 1959).

192. Wamoscher, Z., "The Returning Patient: A Survey of Patients with High Attendance Rates," *Journal of College of General Practitioners* 11:166–173 (March 1966).

193. Kessel, N., and Shepherd, M., "The Health Attitudes of People Who Seldom Consult a Doctor," *Medical Care* 3:6–10 (January–March 1965).

194. Gaspard, N. J., and Hopkins, C. E., "Determinants of Use of Ambulatory Medical Services by an Aged Population," *Inquiry* 4:28–36 (March 1967).

195. Payson, J. E., Gaenslen, E. C., and Stargardter, F. L., "Time Study of an Internship on a University Medical Service," *New England Journal of Medicine* 264:439–443 (March 2, 1961).

196. Abdellah, F. G., Beland, I. L., Martin, A., and Metheney, R. V., *Patient-centered Approaches to Nursing* (New York: Macmillan, 1960). 205pp.

197. Christman, L. P., and Jelinek, R. C., "Old Patterns Waste Half the Nursing Hours," *Modern Hospital* 108:78–81 (January 1967).

198. Rosner, L. J., Pitkin, O. E., McFadden, G. H., Rosenbluth, L., and O'Brien, M. J., "Better Use of Health Professionals in New York City Schools," *Public Health Reports* 84:729–735 (August 1969).

WORKLOAD OF HOSPITAL EMERGENCY SERVICES

199. Skudder, P. A., McCarroll, J. R., and Wade, P. A., "Hospital Emergency Facilities and Services: A Survey." *Bulletin of the American College of Surgeons* 46:44–50 (March–April 1961).

200. Vaughan, H. I., and Gamester, C. E., "Hospital Emergency Room Utilization in Michigan," *Inquiry* 3:34–56 (May 1966).

201. Lee, S. S., Solon, J. A., and Sheps, C. G., "How New Patterns of Medical Care Affect the Emergency Unit," *Modern Hospital* 94:97–101 (May 1960).

202. Barry, R. M., Shortliffe, E. C., and Wetstone, H. J., "Case Study Predicts Load Variation Patterns," *Hospitals* 34:34, 38–42 (December 1, 1960).

203. Weinerman, E. Richard, and Edwards, Herbert R., "Triage System Shows Promise in Management of Emergency Department Load," *Hospitals* 38:55–62 (November 16, 1964).

204. Weinerman, E. R., Rutzen, S. R., and Pearson, D. A., "Effects of Medical 'Triage' in Hospital Emergency Service," *Public Health Reports* 80:389–399 (May 1965).

205. Weinerman, E. R., Ratner, R. S., Robbins, A., and Lavenhar, M. A., "Yale Studies in Ambulatory Medical Care. V: Determinants of Use of Hospital Emergency Services," *American Journal of Public Health* 56:1037–1056 (July 1966).

206. Kluge, D. M., "The Expanding Emergency Department," *Journal of the American Medical Association* 191:97–101 (March 8, 1965).

207. Reed, J. I., and Reader, G. G., "Quantitative Survey of New York Hospital Emergency Room, 1965," *New York State Journal of Medicine* 67:1335–1342 (May 15, 1967).

208. King, B. G., and Sox, E. D., "An Emergency Medical Service System—Analysis of Workload," *Public Health Reports* 82:995–1008 (November 1967).

HOSPITAL CAPACITY

209. Commission on Hospital Care, "Relation of Bed Occupancy Rate to Size of Hospital," in *Hospital Care in the United States* (New York: Commonwealth Fund, 1947), pp. 278–288.

210. Newell, D. J., "Provision of Emergency Beds in Hospitals," *British Journal of Preventive and Social Medicine* 8:77–80 (April 1954).

211. Bailey, N. T. J., "Statistics in Hospital Planning and Design," *Applied Statistics* 5:146–157 (November 1956).

212. London, M., and Sigmond, R. M., "Small Specialized Bed Units Lower Occupancy," *The Modern Hospital* 96:95–100 (May 1961).

213. Blumberg, M. S., " 'DPF Concept' Helps Predict Bed Needs," *The Modern Hospital* 97:75–81, 170 (December 1961).

214. Drosness, P. L., Dean, L. S., Lubin, J. W., and Ribak, N., "Uses of Daily Census Data in Determining Efficiency in Units," *Hospitals* 41:45–48, 106 (December 1, 1967), and 65–68, 112 (December 16, 1967).

215. Allemand, D. M., and Turney, W. G., "Simplified Statistical Approach to Hospital Planning," *Hospital Progress* 45:85–91 (December 1964).

216. Phillip, P. J., "Some Considerations Involved in Determining the Optimum Size of Specialized Hospital Facilities," *Inquiry* 6:44–48 (December 1969).

217. Isaacs, B., "Measuring the Demand for Geriatric Beds," *Medical Care* 4:194–196 (October–December 1966).

218. Querido, A., "Estimate of Need for Hospital Beds," in *The Efficiency of Medical Care* (Leiden: H. E. Stenfert Kroese, N. V., 1963), pp. 122–126.

219. Newell, D. J., "Provision of Emergency Beds in Hospitals," *British Journal of Preventive and Social Medicine*, 8:77–80 (April 1954).

220. Dowling, W. L., *A Linear Programming Approach to the Analysis of Hospital Production*. Unpubl. diss. The University of Michigan, Ann Arbor, 1970. 245pp.

STUDIES RELEVANT TO MISUSE OF HOSPITALS

221. State of New York, The Governor's Committee on Hospital Costs. *Report of the Governor's Committee on Hospital Costs* (New York, 1965). 128pp.

222. Feldstein, M. S., "Effects of Differences in Hospital Bed Scarcity on Type of Use," *British Medical Journal* 2:561–564 (August 29, 1964).

223. Feldstein, M. S., "Improving the Use of Hospital Maternity Beds," *Operations Research Quarterly* 16:65–76 (March 1965).

224. Feldstein, M. S., "Differences in the Intensity of Utilization of Capacity," in *Economic Analysis for Health Service Efficiency* (Amsterdam: North-Holland Publishing Co., 1967), pp. 128–163.

225. Feldstein, M. S., "An Aggregate Planning Model of the Health Care Sector." *Medical Care* 5:369–381 (November–December 1967).

226. Vaananen, I. S., Haro, A. S., Vauhkonen, O., and Mattila, A., "The Level of Hospital Utilization and the Selection of Patients in the Finnish Regional Hospital System," *Medical Care* 5:279–293 (September–October 1967).

227. London, M., and Sigmond, R. M., "How Weekends and Holidays Affect Occupancy," *The Modern Hospital* 97:79–83 (August 1961).

228. Lew, I., "Day of the Week and Other Variables Affecting Hospital Admissions and Discharges and Length of Stay for Patients in the Pittsburgh Area," *Inquiry* 3:3–39 (February 1966).

229. Crystal, R. A., and Brewster, A. W., "Selected Factors and Their Relationship to Day of Admission and Length of Stay." Paper presented at the Annual Meeting of the American Public Health Association, San Francisco, Cal., November 2, 1966. Processed. 11pp. plus 25 pages of charts and tables.

230. Weisbrod, B. A., "Some Problems of Pricing and Resource Allocation in a Non-Profit Industry—The Hospitals," *Journal of Business* 38:18–28 (January 1965).

231. Anderson, O. W., and Sheatsley, P. B., *Hospital Use—A Survey of Patient and Physician Decisions*. Research Series 24 (Center for Health Administration Studies, University of Chicago, 1967), 215pp.

232. Duff, R. S., and Hollingshead, A. B., "Route to the Hospital," in *Sickness and Society* (New York: Harper & Row, 1968). pp. 107–123.

233. Fitzpatrick, T. B., Riedel, D. C., and Payne, B. C., "Appropriateness of Admission and Length of Stay," in McNerney, W. J., and study staff, *Hospital and Medical Economics*, vol. I, pp. 471–494 (Chicago: Hospital Research and Educational Trust, 1962).

234. Morehead, M. A., Donaldson, R. et al., *A Study of the Quality of Hospital Care Secured by a Sample of Teamster Family Members in New York City*. Columbia University School of Public Health and Administrative Medicine, New York, 1964. 98pp.

235. Querido, A., "Indirect Evaluation of a Randomized Sample of the General Practitioners' Work (1954)," in *The Efficiency of Medical Care* (Leiden: H. H. Stenfert Kroese, N. V., 1963). pp. 52–58.

236. Mackintosh, J. M., McKeown, T., and Garratt, F. N., ''An Examination of the Need for Hospital Admission,'' *Lancet* 1:815–818 (April 15, 1961).

237. National Center for Health Statistics, *Persons Hospitalized by Number of Hospital Episodes and Days in a Year, United States, July 1960–June 1962*. P.H.S. Publication No. 1000, ser. 10, no. 20 (Washington, D.C.: U.S. Government Printing Office, June 1965). 42pp.

238. Roemer, M. I., and Myers, G. W., ''Multiple Admissions to Hospital,'' *Canadian Journal of Public Health* 47:469–481 (November 1956).

239. Lerner, M., and Fitzgerald, S. W., ''Three Complementary Multiple Admission Studies by Blue Cross Plans,'' *Inquiry* 1:3–20 (August 1963).

240. Solomon, M., and Ferber, B., ''Patterns of Repeated Hospital Admissions, Blue Cross and Blue Shield Federal Employees Program, July 1, 1960–December 1965,'' *Blue Cross Reports*, vol. 6, no. 3 (May 1968). 11pp.

241. Woosley, J. C., *A Study of Repeated Hospital Admissions Among Blue Cross Members*, unpubl. diss., University of Michigan, Ann Arbor, 1960.

242. Acheson, E. D., and Barr, A., ''Multiple Spells of In-Patient Treatment in a Calendar Year,'' *British Journal of Preventive and Social Medicine* 19:182–191 (October 1965).

243. Koplin, A. N., Hutchinson, R., and Johnson, B. K., ''Influence of a Managing Physician on Multiple Admissions,'' *American Journal of Public Health* 49:1174–1180 (September 1959).

244. Twaddle, A. C., and Sweet, R. H., ''Factors Leading to Preventable Hospital Admissions,'' *Medical Care* 8:200–208 (May–June 1970).

245. National Center for Health Statistics, *Hospital Discharge and Length of Stay: Short-Stay Hospitals, United States, July 1963–June 1964*. P.H.S. Publication, No. 1000, ser. 10, no. 30 (Washington, D.C.: U.S. Government Printing Office, June 1966). 66pp.

246. Altman, I., ''Some Factors Affecting Hospital Length of Stay,'' *Hospitals* 39:68–74 (July 15, 1965).

247. Nassau County Medical Society, Voluntary Insurance Committee, *Pilot Study of Hospital Use in Nassau County* (Garden City, New York: Nassau County Medical Society, November 1963). 76pp.

248. Querido, A., ''Analysis of Length of Stay,'' and ''Repeated Hospital Admissions of Children,'' in *The Efficiency of Medical Care* (Leiden: H. E. Stenfert Kroese, N. V., 1963), pp. 127–134 and 208–214.

249. Bailey, D. R., and Riedel, D. C., ''Recertification of Length of Stay: The Impact of New Jersey's AID Program of Patterns of Hospital Care,'' *Blue Cross Reports*, vol. 6, no. 4 (July 1968). 10pp.

250. Mikelbank, G., ''Approval of Individual Diagnosis (AID) Program New Jersey Blue Cross.'' Paper prepared for the Workshop on Medical Care Appraisal—Operational Aspects, American Public Health Association, Program Area Committee on Medical Care Administration, New York, November 11 and 12, 1966. 11pp. and appendices (mimeographed).

251. Zalk, M., ''Insurance Company's Gentle Persuasion Has Reduced Utilization,'' *Modern Hospital* 110:102–104 (February 1968).

252. Rosenfeld, L. S., Goldman, F., and Kaprio, L. A., ''Reasons for Prolonged Hospital Stay,'' *Journal of Chronic Diseases* 6:141–152 (August 1957).

253. Goldman, Franz, ''Prolonged Stay in General Hospitals. A Study of 200 Patients,'' *Geriatrics* 14:789–800 (December 1959).

254. Van Dyke, F., Brown, V., and Thom, A., *Long Stay Hospital Care* (New York: Columbia University School of Public Health and Administrative Medicine 1963). 112pp.

255. Wenkert, W., and Terris, M., ''Methods and Findings in a Local Chronic Illness Study,'' *American Journal of Public Health* 50:1288–1297 (September 1960).

256. Browning, F. E., and Crump, L., *Report to the Patient Care Planning Council on a Bed Utilization Study* (Rochester, New York: Council of Social Agencies, Undated). 20pp. and appendices. Mimeographed.

257. Berg, R. L., Browning, F. E., Crump, S. L., and Wenkert, W., "Bed Utilization Studies for Community Planning," *Journal of the American Medical Association* 207:2411–2413 (March 31, 1969).

258. Wenkert, W., Hill, J. G., and Berg, R. L., "Concepts and Methodology in Planning Patient Care Services," *Medical Care* 7:327–331 (July–August 1969).

259. Berg, R. L., Browning, F. E., Hill, J. G., and Wenkert, W., "Assessing Health Care Needs of the Aged," *Health Services Research* 5:36–59 (Spring 1970).

260. Berg, R. L., Hill, J. G., and Wenkert, W., "New Techniques in Evaluating High Quality of Care and Its Cost in an Aging Population," pp. 18–23 in Sirdić, M., Editor-in-Chief, *The 5th International Scientific Meeting of the International Epidemiological Association* (Belgrade: Savremena Administracija [The Publishing House], 1970). 592pp.

261. Preston, R. A., White, K. L., Strachan, J. E., and Wells, B., "Patient Care Classification as a Basis for Estimating Graded Inpatient Hospital Facilities," *Journal of Chronic Diseases* 17:761–772 (September 1964).

262. White, K. L., Wells, H. B., Preston, R. A., and Strachan, E. J., "Overnight Facilities for Ambulatory Patients: A Method for Estimating Potential Demand," *Hospital Management* 96:49–53 (October 1963).

263. White, R. P., Quade, D., and White, K. L., *Patient Care Classification: Methods and Application* (Baltimore: Department of Medical Care and Hospitals, School of Hygiene and Public Health, Johns Hopkins University, July 1967). 62pp. (Processed.)

264. Lowe, C. R., and McKeown, T., "The Care of the Chronic Sick. I: Medical and Nursing Requirements," *British Journal of Social Medicine* 3:110–126 (July 1949).

265. Lowe, C. R., and McKeown, T., "The Care of the Chronic Sick. II: Social and Demographic Data," *British Journal of Social Medicine* 4:61–74 (April 1950).

266. Garratt, F. N., Lowe, C. R., and McKeown, T., "Investigation of the Medical and Social Needs of Patients in Mental Hospitals. I: Classification of Patients According to the Type of Institution Required for Their Care," *British Journal of Preventive and Social Medicine* 11:165–173 (October 1957).

267. Garratt, F. N., Lowe, C. R., and McKeown, T., "Investigation of the Medical and Social Needs of Patients in Mental Hospitals. II: Type of Accommodation and Staff Required," *British Journal of Preventive and Social Medicine* 12:23–41 (January 1958).

268. McKeown, T., "The Concept of a Balanced Hospital Community," *Lancet* 1:701–704 (April 5, 1958).

269. Forsyth, G., and Logan, R. F. L., *The Demand for Medical Care*. (London: Oxford University Press for the Nuffield Provincial Hospitals Trust, 1960). 153pp.

270. Donabedian, A., *A Guide to Medical Care Administration*. Vol. II: *Medical Care Appraisal—Quality and Utilization* (New York: American Public Health Association, 1969). 221pp.

271. Payne, B. C., Editor, *Hospital Utilization Review Manual* (Ann Arbor: University of Michigan Medical School, Department of Postgraduate Medicine, February 1968). 117pp.

272. U.S. Office for Dependents' Medical Care, *Fifth Annual Report, Dependents' Medical Care Program* (Washington, D.C.: U.S. Government Printing Office, June 1962).

273. Acheson, E. D., and Feldstein, M. D., "Duration of Stay in Hospital for Normal Maternity Care," *British Medical Journal* 2:95–99 (July 11, 1964).

274. Innes, A., Grand, A. J., and Beinfield, M. S., ''Experience with Shortened Hospital Stay for Post-surgical Patients,'' *Journal of the American Medical Association* 204:647–652 (May 20, 1968).

275. Berg, R. B., Salisbury, A. J., and Kahan, R., '' 'Early' Discharge of Low-Birth-Weight Infants,'' *Journal of the American Medical Association* 210:1892–1896 (December 8, 1969).

276. Browning, F. E., '' 'The Record' in Hospital Bed Utilization,'' in *Utilization Review: A Handbook for the Medical Staff* (Chicago: American Medical Association, Department of Hospitals and Medical Facilities, 1965), pp. 77–82.

277. Zimmer, J. G., ''An Evaluation of Observer Variability in a Hospital Bed Utilization Study,'' *Medical Care* 5:221–233 (July–August 1967).

278. Zimmer, J. G., and Groomes, E. W., ''An Observer Reliability Study of Physicians' and Nurses' Decisions in Utilization Review of Chronic-Care Facilities,'' *Medical Care* 7:14–20 (January–February 1969).

HOSPITAL USE AND CONTROL THROUGH SCHEDULING

279. Young, J. P., ''Stabilization of Inpatient Bed Occupancy Through Control of Admission,'' *Hospitals* 39:41–48 (October 1, 1965).

280. Young, J. P., *A Queuing Theory Approach to the Control of Hospital Census*, unpubl. diss., Johns Hopkins University, Baltimore, 1962.

281. Goldman, J., Kanppenberger, A. H., and Eller, J. C., ''Evaluating Bed Allocation Policy with Computer Simulation,'' *Health Services Research* 3:119–129 (Summer 1968).

282. Parker, R. D., ''Variation of the Occupancy of Two Medical Units with the Amount of Sharing Between the Units,'' *Health Services Research* 3:214–223 (Fall 1968).

283. Robinson, G. H., Wing, P., and Davis, L. E., ''Computer Simulation of Hospital Patient Scheduling Systems,'' *Health Services Research* 3:130–141 (Summer 1968).

Capacity to Produce Service in Relation to Need and Demand

SUPPLY RELATED TO AGGREGATE NEED AND DEMAND

284. Boulding, K. E., ''The Concept of Need for Health Services,'' *Milbank Memorial Fund Quarterly* 44:202–221 (October 1966), pt. 2.

285. Butter, I., ''Health Manpower Research: A Survey,'' *Inquiry* 4: 5–41 (December 1967).

286. Friedman, M., and Kuznets, S., ''Demand and Supply Curves for Professional Services,'' in Friedman and Kuznets, *Income from Independent Professional Practice* (New York: National Bureau of Economic Research, 1945), pp. 155–173.

287. Friedman, M., ''The Supply of Labor in Different Occupations,'' in *Price Theory: A Provisional Text* (Chicago: Adline Publishing Company, 1962, 4th printing: rev. 1967), pp. 211–225.

288. Hansen, W. L., '' 'Shortages' and Investment in Health Manpower,'' in *The Economics of Health and Medical Care*, Proceedings of the Conference on the Economics of Health and Medical Care. (Ann Arbor: University of Michigan, 1964), pp. 75–91.

289. Fein, R., *The Doctor Shortage, an Economic Diagnosis* (Washington, D.C.: The Brookings Institution, 1967). 199pp.

290. Rayack, E., ''The Supply of Physicians' Services,'' *Industrial and Labor Relations Review* 17:221–237 (January 1964). (See also communications relevant

to this article in the same journal by Holtmann, vol. 18, April 1965, pp. 423–424, and Rayack, vol. 18, July 1965, pp. 584–587.)

291. Rayack, E., *Professional Power and American Medicine: The Economics of the American Medical Association* (Cleveland: World Publishing Company, 1967). 298pp.

292. Adams, R. E., *A Market Study of Hospital House Officers* (Chicago: Graduate Program in Hospital Administration, University of Chicago, 1961).

293. Ginzberg, E., "Physician Shortage Reconsidered," *New England Journal of Medicine* 275:85–87 (July 14, 1966).

294. Yett, D. E., "The Supply of Nurses: An Economist's View," *Hospital Progress* 46:88–102 (February 1965).

295. Yett, D. E., "The Nursing Shortage and the Nurse Training Act of 1964," *Industrial and Labor Relations Review* 9:190–200 (January 1966).

296. Yett, D. E., "Lifetime Earnings for Nurses in Comparison with College Trained Women," *Inquiry* 5:35–70 (December 1968).

297. Yett, D. E., "Causes and Consequences of Salary Differentials in Nursing," *Inquiry* 7:78–99 (March 1970).

298. Yett, D. E., *An Economic Analysis of the Nurse Shortage* (Washington, D.C.: U.S. Government Printing Office). Forthcoming.

299. Rice, D. P., and Horowitz, L. A., "Trends in Medical Care Prices," *Social Security Bulletin* 30:13–28 (July 1967).

300. Horowitz, L. A., "Medical Care Price Changes: Medicare's First Three Years," Social Security Administration, *Research and Statistics Note*, August 14, 1969. 8pp.

301. Monsma, G., *Notes on Methodology Used in Compiling Medical Expenditure Data—U.S. Departments of Commerce; Labor; and Health, Education and Welfare* (Washington, D.C.: Health Economics Branch, Division of Community Health Services, Public Health Service, 1963). 28pp. (Mimeographed)

302. Greenfield, H. J., and Anderson, O. W., *The Medical Care Price Index* (New York: Health Information Foundation, Research Series No. 7, 1959). 22pp.

303. German, J. G., "Some Uses and Limitations of the Consumer Price Index," *Inquiry* 1:137–154 (July 1964).

304. U.S. Department of Labor, Bureau of Labor Statistics, *The Consumer Price Index: History and Techniques*. Bulletin No. 1517 (Washington, D.C.: U.S. Government Printing Office, 1966). 118pp.

ACCESSIBILITY: GENERAL

305. Hawley, A. H., *Human Ecology: A Theory of Community Structure*, (New York: Ronald Press, 1950). 456pp.

306. Shannon, G. W., Bashshur, R. L., and Metzner, C. A., "The Concept of Distance as a Factor in Accessibility and Utilization of Health Care," *Medical Care Review* 26:143–161 (February 1969).

SOCIOECONOMIC ACCESSIBILITY

307. Gorwitz, K., and Warthen, F. J., "Effects of Desegregation of a State Mental Hospital System on Rates of Treated Mental Illness," *HSMHA Health Reports* 86:34–45 (January 1971).

308. Bashshur, R. L., Shannon, G. W., and Metzner, C. A., "Some Ecological Differentials in the Use of Medical Services," *Health Services Research* 6:61–75 (Spring 1971).

309. Morrill, R. L., Earickson, R. J., and Rees, P., "Factors Influencing Distances Traveled to Hospitals," *Economic Geography* 46:161–171 (April 1970).

GEOGRAPHIC ACCESSIBILITY : PRESENTATION AND MEASUREMENT

310. Marrinson, R., "Hospital Service Time Replaces Space," *Hospitals* 38:52–54 (January 16, 1964).

311. Moses, L. M., and Williamson, H. F., Jr., "Value of Time, Choice of Mode, and the Subsidy Issue in Urban Transportation," *Journal of Political Economy* 71:247–264 (June 1963).

312. Lubin, J. W., Drosness, D. L., and Wylie, L. G., "Highway Network Minimum Path Selection Applied to Health Facility Planning," *Public Health Reports* 80:771–778 (September 1965).

313. Bashshur, R. L., Shannon, G. W., and Metzner, C. A., "The Application of Three-Dimensional Analogue Models to the Distribution of Medical Care Facilities," *Medical Care* 8:395–407 (September–October 1970).

314. Kuhn, H. W., and Kuenne, R. E., "An Efficient Algorithm for the Numerical Solution of the Generalized Weber Problem in Spatial Economics," *Journal of Regional Science* 4:21–33 (Winter 1962).

315. Lefever, D. W., "Measuring Geographic Concentration by Means of the Standard Deviational Ellipse," *American Journal of Sociology* 32:88–94 (July 1926).

316. U.S. Bureau of the Census, *Census Use Study: Computer Mapping*, Report No. 2 (Washington, D.C.: U.S. Government Printing Office, 1969). 44pp.

317. Gabrielson, I. W., Siker, E., Sohler, K. B., and Stockwell, E. G., "Relating Health and Census Information for Health Planning," *American Journal of Public Health* 59:1169–1176 (July 1969).

ACCESSIBILITY AND CLIENT BEHAVIOR

318. Metzner, C. A., "Attractions and Blocks: The A and B of the Utilization of Dental Service," *Journal of the American Dental Association* 60:3–8 (January 1960).

319. Kauffman, H. R., and Morse, W. W., *Illness in Rural Missouri* (Columbia: Missouri AES Research Bulletin 391, August 1945).

320. Jehlik, P. J., and McNamara, R. L., "The Relation of Distance to the Differential Use of Certain Health Personnel and Facilities and to the Extent of Bed Illness," *Rural Sociology* 17:261–265 (September 1952).

321. Hoffer, C. R., Gibson, D. L., Loomis, C. P., Miller, P. A., Schuler, E. A., and Thaden, J. F., *Health Needs and Health Care in Michigan*, Special Bulletin 365 (East Lansing: Michigan State College, Agricultural Experimental Station, June, 1950). 94pp.

322. Koos, E. L., *The Health of Regionville: What People Thought and Did About It* (New York: Columbia University Press, 1954). 177pp. (Available in facsimile edition, Hafner Publishing Company, New York, 1967.)

323. Altman, I., *Distances Traveled for Physician Care in Western Pennsylvania.* Part II of Public Health Monograph No. 19. P.H.S. Publication No. 248 (Washington, D.C.: U.S. Government Printing Office, 1954), pp. 23–32.

324. Hodges, A., and Dörken, H., "Location and Outpatient Psychiatric Care," *Public Health Reports* 76:239–241 (March 1961).

325. Person, P. H., Jr., "Geographic Variation in First Admission Rates to a State Mental Hospital," *Public Health Reports* 77:719–731 (August 1962).

326. Sohler, K. B., and Thompson, J. D., "Jarvis' Law and the Planning of Mental Health Services: Influence of Accessibility, Poverty, and Urbanization on First Admissions to Connecticut State Hospitals," *Public Health Reports* 85:503–510 (June 1970).

327. Sohler, K. B., "Jarvis' Law and the Planning of Mental Health Services:

Role of Alternative Psychiatric Service in Connecticut," *Public Health Reports* 85:510–515 (June 1970).

328. Sohler, K. B., and Clapis, J. A., "Jarvis' Law and the Planning of Mental Health Services," *HSMHA Health Reports* 87:75–79 (January 1972).

329. Weiss, J. E., and Greenlick, M. R., "Determinants of Medical Care Utilization: The Effect of Social Class and Distance on Contacts with the Medical Care System," *Medical Care* 8:456–462 (November–December 1970).

330. Weiss, J. E., Greenlick, M. R., and Jones, J. F., "Determinants of Medical Care Utilization: The Impact of Spatial Factors," *Inquiry* 8:50–57 (December 1971).

331. Kane, R. L., "Determination of Health Care Priorities and Expectations Among Rural Consumers," *Health Services Research* 4:142–151 (Summer 1969).

332. King M. (Editor), *Medical Care in Developing Countries* (London : Oxford University Press, 1966). Unpaginated. See especially "Taking Services to the People," chap. 2, secs. 2:7 to 2:10.

333. Oxford Regional Hospital Board, Operational Research Unit, *Hospital Outpatient Services: A Statistical Analysis of Patients Attending the Outpatient Department During Three Months* (Oxford, 1963). 98pp.

334. Morrill, R. L., and Earickson, R. E., "Hospital Variation and Patient Travel Distance," *Inquiry* 5:26–34 (December 1968).

335. Simon, N. M., and Rabushka, S. E., *A Trade Union and Its Medical Service Plan* (St. Louis: Labor Health Institute, 1965). 47pp.

336. Freidson, E., *Patients' Views of Medical Practice* (New York: Russell Sage Foundation, 1961). 268pp.

337. Bashshur, R. L., and Metzner, C. A., "Patterns of Social Differentiation Between Community Health Association and Blue Cross–Blue Shield," *Inquiry* 4:23–44 (June 1967).

338. Shannon, G. W., *Spatial Diffusion of an Innovative Health Care Plan*, unpubl. diss., The University of Michigan, Ann Arbor, 1970. 178pp.

ACCESSIBILITY AND PROVIDER BEHAVIOR

339. Mountin, J. W., Pennell, E. H., and Nicolay, V., "Location and Movement of Physicians, 1923 and 1938. Effect of Local Factors upon Location," *Public Health Reports* 57:1945–1953 (December 18, 1942).

340. Terris, M., and Monk, M. A., "Recent Trends in the Distribution of Physicians in Upstate New York," *American Journal of Public Health* 46:585–592 (May 1956).

341. Dorsey, J. L., "Physician Distribution in Boston and Brookline, 1940 and 1961," *Medical Care* 7:429–440 (November–December 1969).

342. Marden, P. G., "A Demographic and Ecological Analysis of the Distribution of Physicians in Metropolitan America, 1960," *American Journal of Sociology* 72:290–300 (November 1966).

343. Lubin, J. W., Reed, I. M., Worstell, G. L., and Drosness, D. L., "How Distance Affects Physician Activity," *Modern Hospital* 107:80–82, 156 (July 1966).

344. Weiss J. E. ("The Effect of Medical Centers on the Distribution of Physicians in the United States") unpubl. diss., The University of Michigan, Ann Arbor, 1968. 239pp.

345. Williams, T. F., White, K. L., Andrews, L. P., Diamond, E., Greenberg, B. G., Hamrick, A. A., and Hunter, E. A., "Patient Referral to a University Clinic: Patterns in a Rural State," *American Journal of Public Health* 50:1493–1507 (October 1960).

346. Hopkins, E. J., Pye, A. M., Solomon, M., and Solomon, S., "The Relation of Patient's Age, Sex and Distance from Surgery to the Demand on the Family Doctor," *Journal of the Royal College of General Practitioners* 16:368–378 (November 1968).

347. Hobbs, M. S. T., and Acheson, E. D., "Perinatal Mortality and the Organization of Obstetric Services in the Oxford Area in 1962," *British Medical Journal* 1:499–505 (February 26, 1966).

STUDIES OF LOCATIONAL EFFICIENCY

348. Hodges, A., Fritz, K., and Fasso, T. E., "The Realities of Geographic Space in Rural Mental Health Programming," *Public Health Reports* 82:386–388 (May 1967).

349. U.S. Public Health Service, "Regulations. Community Mental Health Centers Act of 1963," *Federal Register*, May 6, 1964, p. 5952.

350. Schneider, J. B., "Measuring Locational Efficiency of the Urban Hospital," *Health Services Research* 2:154–169 (Summer 1967).

351. Schneider, J. B., "Measuring, Evaluating and Redesigning Hospital-Physician-Patient Spatial Relationships in Metropolitan Areas," *Inquiry* 5:24–42 (June 1968).

352. Morrill, R. L., and Earickson, R., "Locational Efficiency of Chicago Hospitals: An Experimental Model," *Health Services Research* 4:128–141 (Summer 1969).

353. Long, M. I., and Feldstein, P. J., "Economics of Hospital Systems: Peak Loads and Regional Coordination," *American Economic Review* 57:119–129 (May 1967).

354. Godlund, S., *Population, Regional Hospitals, Transport Facilities, and Regions: Planning the Location of Regional Hospitals in Sweden*. Lund Studies in Geography, Series B, Human Geography, No. 21. Lund (Sweden: The Royal University of Lund, Department of Geography, 1961). 32pp.

355. Abernathy, W. J., and Hershey, J. G., "A Spatial Allocation Model for Regional Health-Services Planning," *Operations Research* 20:629–642 (May–June 1971).

POPULATION AND AREA SERVED

356. Bailey, N. T. J., "Statistics in Hospital Planning and Design," *Applied Statistics* 5:146–157 (November 1965).

357. Airth, A. D., and Newell, D. J., *The Demand for Hospital Beds: Results of an Enquiry on Tees-side* (Newcastle upon Tyne: University of Durham, King's College, 1962). 91pp.

358. U.S. Department of Health, Education, and Welfare, Public Health Service, *Procedures for Areawide Health Facility Planning: A Guide for Planning Agencies*. P.H.S. Publication No. 930–B–3 (Washington, D.C.: U.S. Government Printing Office, September 1963). 118pp.

359. Mountin, J. W., and Greve, C. H., *Public Health Areas and Hospital Facilities: A Plan for Coordination*. P.H.S. Publication No. 42 (Washington, D.C.: U.S. Government Printing Office, 1950). 119pp.

360. Mountin, J. W., Pennell, E. H., and Hoge, V. M., *Health Service Areas*. Public Health Bulletin No. 292, Federal Security Agency, U.S. Public Health Service (Washington, D.C.: U.S. Government Printing Office, 1945). 68pp.

361. Ciocco, A., and Altman, I., *Medical Service Area as Indicated by Intercounty Movement of Patients*. Part I, Public Health Monograph No. 19, Public Health Service Publication No. 248 (Washington, D.C.: U.S. Government Printing Office, 1954). 20pp.

362. Ciocco, A., and Altenderfer, M., "Birth Statistics as an Index of Interdependence of Counties with Regard to Medical Services." *Public Health Reports* 60:973–985 (August 24, 1945).

363. New, P. K., "Use of Birth Data in Delineation of Medical Service Areas," *Rural Sociology* 20:272–281 (September–December 1955).

364. Drosness, D. L., and Lubin, J. W., "Planning Can Be Based on Patient Travel," *Modern Hospital* 106:92–94 (April 1966).

365. Dickinson, F. G., *Distribution of Physicians by Medical Service Areas.* Bulletin 94. Bureau of Medical Economic Research (Chicago: American Medical Association, 1954). 162pp.

366. Poland, E., and Lembcke, P. A., *Delineation of Hospital Service Districts, a Fundamental Requirement in Hospital Planning.* Publication No. 135 (Kansas City, Mo.: Community Studies, Inc., January 1962). 117pp. plus appendices.

367. Drosness, D. L., Read, I. M., and Lubin, J. W., "The Application of Computer Graphics and Patient Origin Study Techniques," *Public Health Reports* 80:33–40 (January 1965).

368. de Visé, P., *Hospital Study Districts for Metropolitan Chicago: A Geographic Analysis and Methodology.* Technical Report No. 21 (Chicago: Hospital Planning Council for Metropolitan Chicago, April 1966). 75pp.

369. Cherniak, H. D., and Schneider, J. B., *A New Approach to the Delineation of Hospital Service Areas.* Discussion Paper Series, No. 16 (Philadelphia: Regional Science Institute, August 1967). 41pp.

Additional References Cited

370. American Nurses' Association, *Facts About Nursing, 1966 Edition* (New York: American Nurses' Association, 1966). 252pp.

371. "M.D.-Population Ratio Increases," *A.M.A. News,* September 2, 1963, p. 1, and U.S. Public Health Service Press Release, September 6, 1968. Cited in *Public Health Economics,* vol. 20, October 1963, pp. 427–428.

372. American Nurses' Association, *Educational Preparation for Nurse Practitioners and Assistants to Nurses: A Position Paper* (New York: American Nurses' Association, 1965). 16pp.

373. Halberstam, J. L., and Dasco, M. M., "Foreign and U.S. Residents in University Affiliated Hospitals: An Investigation of U.S. Graduate Education," *Bulletin of the New York Academy of Medicine* 42:182–208 (March 1966).

374. Margulies, H., Bloch, L., and Cholko, F., "Random Survey of U.S. Hospitals with Approved Internships and Residencies: A Study of Professional Qualities of Foreign Medical Graduates," *Journal of Medical Education* 43:706–716 (June 1968).

375. Kosa, J., "The Foreign Trained Physician in the United States," *Journal of Medical Education* 44:46–51 (January 1969).

376. Ledley, R. S., and Lusted, L. B., "Reasoning Foundations of Medical Diagnosis," *Science* 130:9–21 (July 3, 1959).

377. Donabedian, A., "Evaluating the Quality of Medical Care," *Milbank Memorial Fund Quarterly* 44:166–206 (July 1966), pt. 2.

378. U.S. Department of Health, Education and Welfare, Division of Public Health Methods, *Chart Book on Health Status and Health Manpower* (Washington, D.C.: U.S. Government Printing Office, 1961). 52pp.

379. The Surgeon General's Consultant Group on Medical Education, *Physicians for a Growing America: Report of the Surgeon General's Consultant Group on Medical Education.* P.H.S. Publication No. 709 (Washington, D.C.: U.S. Government Printing Office, 1959). 95pp.

380. U.S. Department of Health, Education, and Welfare, Public Health Service, Bureau of Health Manpower. *Health Manpower. Perspective: 1967.* P.H.S. Publication No. 1667 (Washington, D.C.: U.S. Government Printing Office, 1967). 81pp.

381. Overpeck, M. D., "Physicians in Family Practice 1931–67," *Public Health Reports* 85:485–494 (June 1970).

382. Solon, J. A., Feeney, J. J., Jones, S. H., Rigg, R. D., and Sheps, C. G., "Delineating Episodes of Medical Care," *American Journal of Public Health* 57:401–408 (March 1967).

383. Solon, J. A., Rigg, R. D., Jones, S. H., Feeney, J. J., Linger, J. W., and Sheps, C. G., "Episodes of Medical Care: Nursing Students' Use of Medical Services," *American Journal of Public Health* 59:936–946 (June 1969).

384. Pocinki, L. S., Personal communication.

385. Donabedian, A., and Thorby, J. A., "The Systemic Impact of Medicare," *Medical Care Review* 26:567–585 (June 1969).

386. Hogarth, J., *The Payment of the Physician: Some European Comparisons* (New York: Macmillan, 1963). 684pp.

387. Hippocrates, "Waters, Airs and Places," in *The Medical Works of Hippocrates,* trans. John Chadwick and W. N. Mann (Oxford: Blackwell Scientific Publications, 1950), pp. 90–111.

388. Shiloh, A., "The Interaction Between the Middle Eastern and Western Systems of Medicine," *Social Science and Medicine* 2:235–248 (September 1968).

389. This condition of equality was brought to my attention by one of my students, Mr. Lawrence Clark.

390. Handschin, R., Group Health Cooperative of Puget Sound, Seattle, Washington; personal communication.

V

Estimating Requirements for Services and Resources

GENERAL FRAMEWORK

A dominant theme in this work has been the assessment of needs and resources and the correspondence between the two. To help the administrator go about this task in an insightful and orderly manner we have offered a model that helps classify the major considerations that are germane to the task and to point out interrelationships among them. Briefly, we have defined need primarily in terms of conditions and situations that require care. We have pointed out that, when so defined, need is not a unitary concept but is regarded somewhat differently by the several participants in the medical care transaction. We have, accordingly, postulated two major perspectives on need and the actions that flow from it: a professional perspective and a client perspective. One could usefully postulate a third—social perspective—that should embrace, arbitrate between, and reconcile the two.

In order for need to be met it is necessary that it be translated into services sufficient to it and to resources able to produce the services required. One can empirically measure the services produced and consumed and the resources that produce them. It is also possible to set up normatively a set of equivalences that attempt to specify the services that match the need and the resources that match the services. The norms that specify these equivalences are, as might be expected, most highly developed in the professional field. This, plus the professional identification of the administrator, accounts for the almost exclusive concern with this set of norms in the process of assessment. Nevertheless, the norms of clients, individually and collectively, continue to be expressed explicitly in their desires and aspirations, and implicitly in their demand for services and resources.

In addition to postulating a set of empirical transformations and normative equivalences that link needs, services, and resources, the model postulates a set of intervening factors that determine the capacity of resources to produce services and the ability of services to modify need. The former are discussed under the rubric of "productivity" and the latter under the rubrics of "potency" and "appropriateness."

The ability of services to modify need depends on the potency of medical science and technology and on the appropriateness of their application to the situations that require care. It is recognized that advances in medical science and technology increase the ability to modify need, but also reveal or create new needs for service. During any given period of development it is not clear which of the two effects dominates, nor is it possible to predict with any confidence for the future.

Assessment of the capacity of resources to produce service introduces a larger number of considerations and not a few ambiguities due to incomplete or imprecise knowledge. For example, it is necessary to ensure that there is correspondence between resources and services so that one does not include resources that make no contribution to the services under consideration. This matching of services to the resources that are relevant to them is increasingly complicated by functional differentiation among resources. It is also complicated by interdependencies among resources that make it difficult to specify the complex of resources that constitute the appropriate service-producing unit. The multiplicity of inputs in the production of any given service category and the qualitative and quantitative variations in such inputs make it difficult to specify and measure services in a manner that ensures comparability among situations and time periods. It also makes it difficult to specify the service-producing unit and to measure its capacity, since it is not usually known which among a set of inputs into the production of a given service places the limit on capacity. The specification of what is normative capacity depends on a number of additional factors. On the one hand there are certain characteristics of need and demand, such as temporal fluctuation and degree of urgency, that determine the extent to which use of service can be made predictable and amenable to control through scheduling. On the other hand, there are certain resource characteristics, such as size and compartmentalization, that influence the ability of the resource to accommodate fluctuations in demand. Other characteristics, such as the age of personnel or obsolescence in facilities, also influence normative capacity as well as actual production. Finally, assessment of capacity requires the determination of the degree to which a resource is used excessively, insufficiently, or inappropriately. In discussing excessive use we have distinguished "overload" from "overflow" and commented on the significance of the waiting list. Insufficient use is suggested by occupancy rates lower than made necessary by legitimate standby reserve and turnover-interval. Inappropriate use of a facility comes about through providing unnecessary care, through providing necessary care using a resource not suited for the level of care actually provided or required, and through less than complete use of time during the course of care. Such inappropriate use is responsible for hidden capacity ("latent service reserve") which, if released, would reduce or obviate the need for resource expansion.

Such are the bare bones of the model which we have used in the preceding two chapters as a tool to evaluate need and supply. This model, in all its detail, will also form the backdrop for the discussion, in this chapter, of estimating requirements for services and resources. This is because such estimates are, conceptually as well as operationally, only extensions of prior assessments of needs and resources. Their distinguishing characteristic is that they specify, in fairly precise quantitative terms, what are the requirements for services, for resources, or for both. The object is to conclude whether there is a deficit or an excess, and by how much. The administrator is always concerned with current requirements. Often he is also obligated to look further ahead and say whether, assuming certain trends, future resources will be adequate to meet future needs. Whether the task is to estimate current or future requirements, the administrator is concerned with the equivalences among need, services, and resources. This means that he should, ideally, take into account all of the intervening factors that we have discussed in our previous chapters, and briefly summarized in the introduction to this. Predictions call for these as well as additional considerations. First, it is necessary to predict the future magnitudes of need, demand, and resources and then to predict the future magnitudes and effects of the factors that influence the equivalences among them. All this is a counsel of perfection. In fact, transformations and predictions are usually made under simplifying assumptions. These are often so sweeping that one wonders about the meaning of the estimates that they yield. Accordingly, our discussion will emphasize the assumptions underlying the various methods of arriving at equivalences and predictions.

Before these methods are described it will be useful to present various "pathways" which transformations (whether contemporaneous or predictive) are likely to take. These pathways are easily visualized by a simplified diagram of the main components of our model, as shown in Fig. V.1. The major complete pathways are:

1. Need, to service equivalents, to service capacity, to resources.
2. Need, to demand, to service capacity, to resources.
3. Need, to resources, with or without service capacity estimates.
4. Demand, to resources, with or without service capacity estimates.

Fig. V.1.   Major transformation pathways among need, services, and resources.

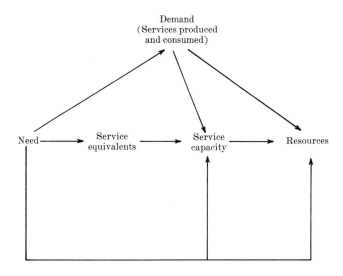

In many cases, transformations do not end in resource estimates, so that the pathway is incomplete. In fact, possibly the most frequent transformations of all are those that translate some measure of need into demand. Alternatively, need may be translated into service equivalents, with or without further comparison of these to effective demand. Some transformation pathways (not to be discussed in this chapter) may also proceed in a direction opposite to the arrows shown in Fig. V.1. The reader will recall that the chapter on the "assessment of supply" was concerned largely with the translation of resources into service capacity and actual services produced.

A major distinction is that the various pathways can be divided into those that originate in need and those that originate in demand. This distinction is sufficiently fundamental that we shall use it to organize the material in the chapter. It should become clear, however, that the two approaches are far from being totally unrelated, and that hybrid and combined forms exist.

To summarize our classification so far, our general concern in this chapter is with quantitative estimates of equivalences among need, demand, and resources. This involves transformations of any one of these into another. Such transformations may be contemporaneous or predictive. They may begin either with need or with demand, and they may take one of several possible pathways. The pathways themselves may be complete, ending in an estimate of resources, or incomplete, stopping short of such an estimate. We shall first discuss methods based primarily on demand and then proceed to those that are based primarily on need.

METHODS BASED PRIMARILY ON DEMAND

Classification and General Description

There are two options in selecting a measure of demand: to express demand in monetary terms (expenditures) or physical terms (visits, patient-days and the like). In this section, we shall discuss those studies, by far in the majority, that use the second type of measure. A study by Jones et al. (26), that used expenditures to predict demand will be described briefly in the concluding section of this chapter.

We have already discussed the many problems of measuring demand in physical terms so that there is product comparability. To the extent that differences in product are reflected in the productivity of service-providing resources, differences are taken into account if corrections are made for productivity. One seldom encounters anything more than very rough judgmental corrections for changes in the potency of the technology or the appropriateness of its application. In some instances, when trends in past demand are used to project future demand, the effects of changes in potency and appropriateness are implicitly included, even though they are not explicitly recognized. In such cases there is, of course, the assumption that changes in technology and professional performance will proceed in the future as in the past: in the same direction, at the same pace, and with the same effect. These assumptions become misleading to the extent that changes in medical science and medical care organization are rapid and unpredictable. Worse still, in many instances product comparability is either ignored or the product is assumed to remain unchanged. In almost all instances, therefore, the physical measures of demand are simple and traditional: visits for the services of physicians and admissions or patient-days for hospitals.

Having chosen the unit of measurement, the next step is to consider those factors that are likely to influence demand, currently and in the future. Here, there is a whole range of methods from the most simple to the fairly complex. The simplest method is to assume that demand varies linearly and directly with population size. Hence, one can express the current or projected relationship between demand and resources in terms

of fractions such as the physician : population—or the bed : population—
ratio. Such expressions could be taken to mean that "the average
person" represents a constant unit of demand or that he represents a
constant unit of need with a constant propensity to eventuate in demand.
These assumptions approach the reasonable to the extent that the transformation is contemporaneous and populations are comparable with
respect to characteristics that influence demand. The assumptions are
seldom warranted when the object is to predict for the future, although
the method has been widely used for this purpose. All that is needed for
the prediction of service and resource requirements, under these assumptions, is to predict the size of the population and apply to it the appropriate conversion ratio. Since this method has been used mainly within
the context of the need-oriented approach, we shall have more to say
about it in a subsequent section.

Next in the progression of methods are those that take into account not
only differences (or growth) in population size, but also differences (or
changes) in those characteristics of the population or its environment
that influence demand, through influencing need, the propensity of client
and care-providing system to act in response to need, or both. Hence, this
family of methods can be grouped under the rubric of "demand analysis." The category may be further subdivided according to (1) number
of characteristics taken into account, (2) the assumptions and methods
used to quantify the relationship between each of these characteristics
and demand, (3) the uses to which the analysis is put, and (4) the
assumptions made when the methods are used for estimation or prediction. Since the four categories of attributes of methods can appear in a
variety of combinations, they do not, unfortunately, result in a simple
classification of methods along any one axis.

The simplest methods that use demand analysis consider only one
variable and assume a linear relationship between that characteristic and
demand so that a percentage change in the characteristic is associated
with a constant percentage change in demand. Economists refer to a
relationship expressed in this form as "elasticity." The relationship need
not be rectilinear in form. A further refinement is to postulate a curvilinear relationship which is expressed in appropriate mathematical terms.
Of the single characteristics, health professionals have been most concerned with age, and economists with price or income. Both Klarman and
Paul Feldstein have reviewed the literature on demand analysis with
emphasis on economic variables (1, 3, 9). According to Klarman, the
findings concerning the percentage change in demand for physicians'
services with one percentage change in income, range from 0.21 to 0.62,

when demand is measured in visits, and from 0.17 to 0.82, when demand is measured in expenditures. He concludes: "It is fair to say that the values of this parameter have not yet been determined with exactitude" (3, pp. 363–364). It is further clear that there is no agreed-upon value that can be used as a conversion factor in estimating resource requirements. In contrast to the difficulties that are apparently connected with determining the relationship between income and use of service, the relationship between age and use of service is well understood, or perhaps accepted with less critical examination. Information about use of service by age group is not difficult to obtain. Given a statement or prediction of the size and the age structure of a population, and assuming use of service by age group remains stable, it is easy to estimate aggregate demand in that population. However, this method also involves the additional assumption that all the population characteristics that vary with age, and may also influence use of service (for example, sex, income, education, place of residence), are either of inconsequential effect as compared to the effect of age or will maintain an invariant relation to age. Using one or both of these assumptions, Navarro et al. have proposed a method that will predict the use of each of a range of medical services using what they have described as a "stochastic and deterministic model" based on the Markov process (16).

Next in a progression of complexity (and, ostensibly, of explanatory power) in demand analysis is to consider several characteristics that may influence demand. If each characteristic were truly independent of every other, it would be possible to estimate the effect of each on demand without regard to the others. Some methods do in fact make this assumption. Unfortunately, the several characteristics that influence demand are likely to be both correlated and interactive. Correlation refers to an association between two or more variables so that a difference in one is associated, in a regular way, with a change in the other. An example is the association in most populations between age and income, or income and color. Interactions occur when the effects of two characteristics are not simply additive, but may be synergistic or antagonistic. For example, both education and income tend to increase demand. Although education and income are associated in the population, there is reason to suspect that each has an independent effect and that their combined effect may be more or less than their added separate effects. In the presence of correlation and interaction, univariate methods of demand analysis are no longer appropriate. Reinke and Baker have classified the multivariate methods used for this purpose and briefly described their salient characteristics. The methods they mention are multiple regression, analysis of variance, "branching," a method developed by Sonquist and Morgan, and "multisort analysis" a method which Reinke and Baker have used (13, 14, 87). As we shall see, a point at issue in multivariate (as in univariate) analysis is whether the relationship between the several characteristics and demand is best expressed as a straight line or some mathematically definable curve. Another problem is that of choice of characteristics (independent or explanatory variables) for use in the analysis. The number of characteristics that may be postulated to have an effect on demand is very large. For example, Palmer was able to assemble 30 factors which were cited in the literature as possibly influencing hospital use (76). Beenhakker, in consultation with the staff of a hospital, was able to compile 117 factors (some of which were characteristics of the hospital and some of the community served) which were thought likely to influence the use of 17 services of the hospital. There was, however, much repetition, since similar factors were postulated to influence several of the services (10). One way to reduce the number of characteristics under consideration is to avoid assembling a grab bag of variables, but to begin instead with a theoretical model from which the relevant characteristics are derived. Unfortunately, our current understanding of demand is such that even this approach can yield a very large number of characteristics. For example, the social-psychological theoretical model used by Kalimo resulted in identifying 46 explanatory variables classified in 6 groups: illness, demographic, attitudinal, social stratification, availability, and background variables of municipality of domicile (15).

As Reinke and Baker emphasize, the choice of characteristics for demand analysis, and their reduction to a manageable set that significantly influences demand, is an important consideration that distinguishes the different methods of analysis (13). Kalimo used factor analysis to reduce his 46 variables into a smaller set. Beenhakker began by plotting each of 117 characteristics against the measure of demand (admissions to one of 17 hospital services) in order to gain a visual impression of whether there was a relationship and whether the relationship was best expressed by a function that was linear, quadratic, cubic, reciprocal, or exponential. Simple regression analysis was used for the same purpose if the relationship was not "immediately evident through the graph." In this way, the characteristics included in the analysis were reduced to 29, of which 22 proved to be significant (10). Wirick began with a theoretical formulation which yielded about 20 variables derived from the categories of need, realization of need, financial resources, motivation to obtain the needed care, and availability of service (12). He then used the Automatic Interaction Detector developed by Sonquist and Morgan (87). This is a method for identifying, among a number of independent variables, the one that contributes most to the variation in the dependent variable, which, in this case, is demand. Once the first variable is identified, the next in order is the one that contributes the next largest increment to variability in the dependent variable, and so on. The technique differs from the regular multiple regression analysis by using a "statistical process rather than human insight" in detecting interactions. However, it is fair to say that "human insight" was involved in the derivation and selection of independent variables, to begin with. Furthermore, as Reinke and Baker point out, "The sequential nature of the technique . . . causes later identification to be dependent upon the particular population classifications initially produced. Without independent evaluations of the several factors and interactions, one must question whether the unique importance of each has been revealed" (13, pp. 63–64). Reinke and Baker are partial to their own multi-sort method which helps identify, using reasonably simple computations, independent variables or interactive combinations of variables that are significantly related to the dependent variable (demand). The independent variables and interactions so identified can then be used in a multiple regression equation to specify the contribution of each to variation in the dependent variable (13, 14).

Two categories of variables are of particular interest in demand analysis, especially when the purpose is to estimate resource requirements. One is the use of services other than the one directly under study and the other is the presence and availability of resources. Other services are important because there are possibilities of substitution and complementarity among services, so that use of any one service may be associated with the use of more or less of the others. Wirick is among those who have included this factor in their analysis of demand (12). The prevalence and availability of resources are important because of a widespread belief, supported by some evidence (18–21), that the supply of resources promotes the use of such resources. This is particularly important in arriving at estimates of resource requirements because, to the extent that resources create their own use, such estimates have an aspect of self-fulfilling prophecies. Furthermore, an increase or decrease in level of resources could become the first step in a spiral that leads progressively to larger or smaller estimates of requirements, to the extent that demand behavior changes in response to resource availability. Obviously, there must be some limit to this progression, but it is not clear what that limit is. We shall return to this problem in estimating requirements in a subsequent section. The object of all the preceding analytic techniques is to determine what is the effect of each of several variables, or combination of variables, independently of all the others. Paul Feldstein has distinguished two purposes for such studies: "explanation" and "prediction" (9). The first has to do with an understanding of what are the factors that influence demand, in what way and to what extent. Such understanding may be put to use in formulating policy designed to influence use of service or in assessing the probable effects of policy. The second purpose, according to Feldstein, is to predict future demand. One might easily extend this category to include the prediction of demand in a specified population group, not in the future but in the present. The distinction being made, then, is not that between present and future estimates, but between understanding of demand and estimation of requirements. Obviously, these two are related. However, as Feldstein and German have shown, some methods may yield superior estimates without contributing much to understanding (17).

The distinction between "explanation" and "prediction" (including contemporaneous estimation) has some interesting ramifications. One has to do with the level of aggregation at which the analysis is to be conducted. Because data can be difficult to get for individuals or households that may reasonably be considered to constitute consumer units, states or other geographical divisions have been used as units of analysis (11, 17, 18, 20–22). As we have pointed out in a previous chapter, it is usually not possible to extrapolate to consumer behavior from such ecological correlations (88). It is not clear to what extent this may also compromise the predictive use of the relationships discovered on these grounds. Rosenthal, who used data at the state level to make estimates of requirements for general hospital beds, has pointed out some advantages and limitations of this level of aggregation. Among the limitations is the loss of much information that could be important. This includes, according to Rosenthal, the spatial disposition of hospitals, "the location of the segment of the population with high income and insurance coverage in relation to location of facilities," and "area differences within the state in insurance benefit coverage." "In general, the state level of aggregation prevents the refinement of data to reflect smaller qualitative differences which might be important to analysis." According to Rosenthal, there are also "strong advantages" to using states as the unit of analysis. States constitute reasonably self-contained service areas, and they are "the only level where there is now uniform planning and application of standards." Furthermore, there is the computational advantage of being able to express qualitative data (such as sex, race, degree of urbanization, and marital status) in quantitative terms (in this instance, proportions of the state population) "without resort to less acceptable methodology" (11, pp. 84–85).

The choice of independent variables is also related to whether explanation or prediction is sought. Some have selected the variables largely on the basis of whether they do or do not account for significant amounts of the variance in the dependent variable (use of service) among units (individuals, households, states). This is a practice more suited to prediction than explanation. Rosenthal has argued that, on the contrary, the independent variables should be selected because they have some "logical" relationship to use of service and should be retained even though they do not help in accounting for variation in the statistical sense (11).

When demand analysis is used to estimate current requirements the procedure is first to obtain a measure of the relationship between one or more characteristics and demand in a standard or reference population. These relationships are then used to estimate demand in another population, provided two things are known about it: its size and its characteristics. The assumption is made that the relationships between characteristics and demand in the reference population hold also for the population for which estimates are to be made. In contemporaneous estimates this assumption is reasonable but not completely without risk of error. The estimates can be wide of the mark if important characteristics have been omitted from the analysis and if the two populations are not comparable with respect to the characteristics that were omitted. Needless to say, all the coefficients used in estimating demand are also subject to sampling error which, however, can be specified. The error due to noncomparability of populations cannot be specified and is usually not even suspected.

When demand analysis is used to estimate future requirements it is, once again, necessary to know population size and characteristics. This requires a double prediction—first of population growth and second of all the characteristics of the population and of its environment that are postulated to influence demand. The problems of arriving at valid predictions of this kind need no emphasis. Given such predictions about the population, it is possible to proceed under one of two assumptions. Most frequently, relationships revealed through current demand analysis in a given population are assumed to hold for the future date. In other words, it is assumed that the characteristics of the population and of its environment change, but that relationships between these characteristics and demand do not. Intuitively one has reason to be suspicious of such an assumption. On the basis of retrospective empirical study, Paul

Feldstein and Jeremiah German have shown that relationships between hospital demand and characteristics of states are not always stable even over the relatively short period of 10 years. They found, for example, that "in 1951 the effect of income on utilization was much more important than it was in 1961. Conversely, the effect of insurance on utilization increased from 1951 to 1961 . . . The effect of the hospital room rate also declined from 1951 to 1961" (17, p. 30). Rosenthal has also examined the relationship between demand for general hospital services and population attributes at the state level. Comparing 1950 and 1960, he found that a "change in structural demand relationships has taken place" and surmised that such change will continue to occur. However, he also found that during this period the relative position of each state was not significantly affected. He concluded that the relationships are sufficiently stable to be used if the object is to determine the optimal relative distribution of national resource estimates (using criteria that we shall describe below) (11).

If there is reason to believe that the relationships between population (including environmental) characteristics and demand are not stable, the consequence is that one must take account of such instability in arriving at predictions of future requirements. Under these most realistic of all the assumptions so far described, one would need to predict (1) population size (2) population and environmental characteristics, and (3) the relationship between such characteristics and demand. All this, merely to arrive at predictions of demand. Still to be predicted are changes in the capacity of resources to provide service and the level of resources likely to be available. For all these predictions, the best guide appears to be the projection of past trends, with or without modifications based on informed judgment. One important safeguard is to make several projections based on a variety of assumptions about the trends in the variables involved. For example, it is customary to offer several projections of population size depending on several expected levels of the birth rate. Similarly, as an example, it is possible to postulate several levels of increase in resource productivity and to examine the hypothetical effect of each level on the expected adequacy of resources.

So far, we have dealt with methods which center on consumer demand without distinction as to the sector of the economy within which demand originates. Several studies have used information on institutional demand—that is, demand by producers of service—to supplement their estimates and predictions. Baker and Perlman have introduced still another distinction by explicitly separating private from public sector demand for the services of health personnel (25). When institutional demand is used, the measure of current demand is usually the budgeted position. Budgeted vacancies are taken to mean a deficit between institutional demand and the availability of resources. However, budgeted vacancies may simply mean a need perceived by the institution in the absence of willingness to bid for resources at competitive prices. In line with this reasoning, Baker and Perlman defined public sector demand as "simply the number of health professionals, àt all levels, employed by government services. It does not include budgeted vacancies, for these indicate that the public sector is unable to meet the estimated need by providing adequate salaries" (25, p. 4). Furthermore, to the extent that institutional demand is derived from consumer demand, care should be taken not to double-count in the process of arriving at estimates by proceeding as if the two segments of demand were independent and additive. Both institutional demand and public sector demand are often more conveniently expressed in terms of units of resources (personnel, beds) or expenditures. In line with our comment on the meaning of budgeted vacancies, the appropriate staffing of institutions and public services is often based on professional estimates of need and is consequently more often a feature of the methods that fall under the category: "Need-oriented."

In the preceding pages we have discussed briefly the attributes of the different methods that have been used to estimate demand. Several of these attributes could be used as means of classifying methods. For example, the units that are used to measure demand classify methods into those that use (1) services, (2) resources, (3) expenditures. Using the determinants of demand as the classifier, the methods of estimation could be classified as those using (1) population size, (2) population size plus one or more characteristics, assuming a constant relationship between characteristic(s) and demand, and (3) population size plus one or more characteristics, assuming a changing relationship between characteristic(s) and demand. According to the number of characteristics considered and the technique used for analysis, the methods of estimating demand could be classified as (1) univariate or (2) multivariate. The relationship between one or more characteristics and demand could be postulated to be (1) rectilinear or (2) curvilinear. According to the units of analysis one distinguishes methods that use (1) consumer units or (2) geographic units. According to source of demand, one distinguishes (1) consumer demand and (2) institutional demand. Finally, according to purpose, the methods of demand analysis could be classified as (1) explanatory or (2) predictive. Because many of these attributes appear in a variety of combinations, it has not been possible to arrive at a fully satisfactory simple classification. The following is offered as a reasonably useful one:

Methods based primarily on demand
  1. Consumer demand
    a. Differences in population size, with:
      (1) A constant demand-population ratio
      (2) A demand-population ratio extrapolated from past trends (94)
    b. Differences in population size and one or more characteristics: "demand analysis"
      (1) Constant relationships between characteristics and demand
      (2) Changing relationships between characteristics and demand

  2. Institutional demand
    a. Resources employed or owned
    b. Budgeted positions

Illustrative Studies Based on Demand Analysis

Our discussion of the methods for estimating resource requirements based on demand for service have so far been rather general and abstract. A review of some illustrative studies should give the methods greater specificity and concreteness. We shall begin by reviewing briefly two studies of manpower requirements, one by Fein (24) and the other by Baker and Perlman (25).

Fein tackled the job of projecting demand for physicians' services and the supply of physicians for the United States during the period 1965–1975. The prediction of demand began with data on use of physicians' services by population subgroup as reported by the National Health Survey for the period 1963–1964. The population characteristics used were age, sex, region, and urban-rural residence, color, education, and income. In making predictions of demand, two basic assumptions were made : (1) "We assume that persons with given characteristics in 1975 will visit physicians as often as persons with these same characteristics visit physicians today"; and (2) "various prices, which if changed would induce a greater or smaller consumption of medical services, are assumed unchanged (or alternatively, as bearing the same relative relationships to each other and to income as now prevails). So too are tastes that would attract individuals to consume more or to consume less services than they now do'' (24, pp. 23 and 27). Fein was, of course, aware of the existence of correlations among several of the characteristics listed above. He isolated the effect of each variable essentially through a process of cross-tabulation. For example, the effects of color and income were separated by obtaining data on the number of visits by color for each of several income groups. In addition to arriving at quantitative estimates for the effects of predicted changes in population characteristics listed above, Fein arrived at a quantitative estimate of the possible effects of Medicare (but not of a more general national health scheme). He also offered some qualitative estimates of the effects of factors such as new discoveries, new social standards and higher expectations, changes in the proportion of the physicians' time occupied by hospital care, reduction in unsatisfied demand, and the institution of new programs. Table V.1 describes the methods in greater (though not complete) detail.

The preceding summary shows that the methods used by Fein are characterized by simplicity of computational technique and a heavy application of informed judgment to formulate a range of estimates and choose a most likely value within the range. It is also clear that population growth is the single most important factor among those responsible for the change in aggregate demand between 1965 and 1975. It accounts for more than half the quantitatively predicted increment. The second most important factor is income, which accounts for more than a quarter of the increment.

Population estimates, as we shall illustrate in a subsequent section, are subject to large margins of error, mainly due to variability in the birth rate. Income changes, whose effects pervade the entire population, can also be rapid and unpredictable, as Fein himself points out. Thus, inaccuracies in predicting population and income place a serious limit on the precision of demand predictions.

Baker and Perlman took on the task of predicting requirements for physicians and other health personnel in Taiwan for the years 1973 and 1983, departing from a baseline in 1963 (25). One step in accomplishing this task was the prediction of demand for physicians' services in each of the private and public sectors. As we have already said, demand in the public sector was defined simply as physicians employed by government services. However, 50 percent of the time of physicians in public service is given to private practice. To avoid double counting, this proportion was allocated to the private sector in the form of ''full-time equivalents.'' The prediction of future demand by the public sector consisted, in essence, of judgments about future governmental policy. The major

Table V.1   Predicted changes in use of physicians' services attributed to changes in specified population characteristics that influence demand, U.S.A., 1965–1975

Characteristics that Influence Demand	Percent Increase in Total Visits, 1965–75	Comments Relating to Method
Population growth	12.2–14.6	Based on two intermediate projections out of four made by the Bureau of the Census. The extreme values are 10.0 and 16.9.
Age and sex	1.0	Obtained by adjustment of visits for age and sex; shows effect of a projected greater proportion of older persons and of females in 1975.
Region and urban-rural residence	0.2	"Even if all persons on farms moved to SMSA's and then had utilization rates equal to present per person utilization rates in SMSA's, total utilization would be raised by about 0.2 percent per year over the decade . . . Total utilization would increase by only 0.8 percent if 10 percent of the population left the South, the region of lowest utilization, and used medical services to the same extent as Westerners do" (pp. 34 and 35). Migration is not likely to be so great, nor changes in use patterns of migrants so marked, partly because past habits persist. Furthermore, the effect of region plus residence must be separated from the effect of associated characteristics (color, income and education) which are partly responsible for the increments cited above.
Color	0.5	Growth in the "nonwhite" segment is more rapid and use of service levels are lower. Hence, if changes in composition by color are included in the estimates of population growth, the increments in visits would be somewhat lower: 13.2–15.6 versus the 12.2–14.6 cited above. Color and income are associated, so the effect of income needs to be separated out. If nonwhites in 1975 will have the same income distribution as whites in 1965 and will use services at the same

Table V.1.   (*continued*)

Characteristics that Influence Demand	Percent Increase in Total Visits, 1965–75	Comments Relating to Method
Color	0.5	rate as whites, in the corresponding income groups do in 1965, there would be a 3.8 percent increase in total demand (Whites plus nonwhites). If nonwhites in 1975 will have the same income distribution they do in 1965, but if use of service changes so that nonwhites in 1975 use service at the same rate as whites in the corresponding income groups use service in 1965, the increment in total use would be 3.7 percent. If income distribution changes so that income of nonwhites in 1975 is the same as income of Whites in 1965, but use of service is unchanged so that nonwhites in 1975 use service at the same rate as nonwhites in corresponding income groups do in 1965, the increment in total use would be 0.7 percent. The factor selected (0.5 percent) is the author's "best guess" of "the additional contribution to the total demand not taken account of in the income calculated as a result of changes in the characteristics of the total population (including nonwhites)" (pp. 156 and 38).
Education and income	7.0–7.5	Education, age, and income are associated, and each has an effect on use of service. If it is assumed that within each educational group, the distribution by age and income in 1975 will be the same as in 1965, the effect of improvements in educational state would be 1.5 percent. If the population is divided into 5 income classes (under $2,000, $2,000–3,999, $4,000–6,999, $7,000–9,999 and $10,000 and over) and it is assumed that: (1) by 1975 all persons will have moved up one income class, and (2) in 1975 persons will visit physicians as often as persons in the equivalent income groups do in 1965, and (3) within each income group the distribution by age and

Table V.1.   (*continued*)

Characteristics that Influence Demand	Percent Increase in Total Visits, 1965–75	Comments Relating to Method
Education and income	7.0–7.5	education in 1975 will be the same as in 1965, the total number of physician visits will increase by about 7.6 percent. On this basis, the author's estimate of the effect of change in education is an increment of 6.5–7.5 percent. However, because education and income are associated, the effect of education and income combined is somewhat less than the sum of the effects attributed to each separately.
Medicare (Title XVIII)	1.0–2.0	Insufficient data on the impact of Titles XVIII and XIX were available at the time the estimates were made. However, even if all individuals 65–74 years old were to use services at the maximum rate found for any income group of the same age, the result would be increase in total demand of only 1.0 percent.
Total of characteristics for which quantitative estimates were made	21.9–25.8	Sum of increments attributed to each characteristic.
New discoveries	Increased demand	Certain discoveries reduce demand through disease prevention, while others increase demand through creating new professional standards. (Effect on life span included under changes in age structure of population.)
New social standards and higher expectations	Increased demand	
New patterns of hospital care	No effect	The definition of "visits" in the national Health Survey does not include hospital visits. However, it is assumed that changes in patterns of hospital care will not occur or, if they occur, will be balanced by increases in the productivity of physicians.

Table V.1.   (*continued*)

Characteristics that Influence Demand	Percent Increase in Total Visits, 1965–75	Comments Relating to Method
Reduction of unsatisfied demand	Increased demand	The quantitative estimates cited above rest on the assumption that whatever difference exists in 1965 between the number of visits that persons make and the number of visits that they would like to make, the same difference would also exist in 1975.
New programs	Increased demand	New programs that increase the ability of persons to obtain service are likely to be instituted.

share, however, was contributed by the requirements for staffing future hospital services, inpatient and outpatient. Prediction of these involved, first, a projection of hospital supplies "on two broad assumptions: first, that the construction outlined in the Ten Year Plan will actually take place and second that the total number of hospital beds will keep pace with population growth" (25, p. 168). The second step was to predict demand to staff these beds on the basis of certain assumptions about staff-bed and staff-outpatient visit relationships (25, pp. 169–172). The translation of hospital beds to staff requirements represents a category of method: the conversion of one resource to its equivalent (or complement) in terms of another resource with implicit or explicit normative assumptions. Further examples will be cited in a subsequent section. The attempt to predict demand in the private sector came up against some interesting (and instructive) difficulties. It was discovered, for example, that persons differing widely in preparation and practice provided medical care, so that a decision had to be made as to their inclusion in the estimates. A more difficult problem was the lack of acceptable information necessary for the estimation of requirements. Accordingly, the investigators had to launch several surveys of their own, including household interviews to obtain information about population characteristics and use of service. Six population attributes were considered: morbidity, age, sex, income, education, and urban-rural residence. "Multisort analysis" (13, 14) was used to identify correlations among the above variables and their influence on demand. Morbidity was shown to be the primary factor that influenced demand; other variables had much smaller influence, independently of morbidity. Baker and Perlman recognize morbidity as the "biological basis of demand for medical care" and assert that "for clear understanding of health manpower analysis familiarity with the major disease patterns of a nation is essential'' (25, p. 113). Nevertheless, they conclude that demand and not need is the relevant criterion for estimates of manpower requirements.

Of the five remaining variables, sex and education had no significant relation to use of service. The three other variables—age, income, and urban-rural residence—were associated with one another. There was, in addition, an interaction between age and income so that ''the age differential in doctor usage was especially pronounced among those of higher income.'' Having identified the relevant variables (age, income, residence, and the age-income interaction) multiple regression was used to quantify the contribution of each element to variation in use of service. The equation showing this is:

$$\text{Predicted } V = 1.039 - 0.987A + 0.223A^2 + 0.156W + 0.060R - 0.035AW,$$

where V = visits per person per month,

A = age,

W = income or economic level, and

R = residence.

Age is obviously the most important variable and shows a quadratic (U-shaped) relation to use of physicians' services.

To predict demand it was assumed that population characteristics might change but that the relationships between characteristics and visits, embodied in the equation described above, would persist. Although residence influences use, it was judged that the urban-rural distribution of the population would not alter appreciably during the relevant period. Consequently, the task of prediction was reduced to (1) a projection of the total population by age and economic status and (2) application of the demand coefficients to the predicted population.

These procedures involved a large number of assumptions, many of which are cited below to give the reader a feel for the firmness of the ensuing predictions.

—Current age-specific mortality rates will continue.
—The range between two estimates of age-specific fertility rates (one high and one low) will include the true value.
—Real per capita income will increase 20 percent during each of two successive decades.

—The per-capita income increase will be the same with either high or low population projection.

—The per-capita income increase will be distributed uniformly over all economic levels.

—Each economic group will reflect the same general pattern of age distribution as now prevails in relation to economic groups.

—The death rate of one economic group will not change in relation to that of another.

—The age-specific fertility rate of one economic group will not change in relation to that of another.

—Persons who move from one economic level to another will purchase medical care at the same rate as persons now in the latter group.

—Prices for medical service will not rise faster than the general price increase.

—Doctors will provide the same amount of service irrespective of price.

Under these assumptions, Baker and Perlman estimated the effect of demographic shifts on the estimate of resource requirements. The changes in age and economic level accounted for 15 percent of the total estimate of requirements. ''This difference in doctor demand is larger than the difference caused by the two extremes of population projection'' (25, p. 143). This finding should be compared with the situation in the United States as revealed by Fein. According to Fein's estimates, the single largest increment in demand (and hence, in requirements for physicians) is attributable to population growth with income change holding second place and change in age structure making a much smaller contribution. This illustrates what one would expect a priori: that predictions in one locale cannot be transferred to another where social and economic conditions are so different.

A review of the two methods reveals the kinship between the methods used by Fein and by Baker and Perlman in spite of the more sophisticated techniques of multivariate analysis used by the latter. Both take into account the effect of projected population characteristics on use of service. Both assume that present relationships between such characteristics and use of service will also hold in the future. This is not to say that they do not realize the weaknesses in this and their other assumptions. Baker and Perlman comment as follows:

We are only too well aware of the hazards of using cross-sectional analysis for long-term purposes. In the case of our general study of the supply of and demand for professional medical personnel in Taiwan, we have had no earlier data to permit examination of changes over time. We have thus been obliged to use cross-sectional analysis and have taken care to consider the various components of demand in order to speculate on the likelihood of their stability over a decade or so in the future. In sum, we think that, despite its limitations, the disaggregated approach we have adopted is better than the simple enumeration of ratios and the projections stemming from them" (25, p. 125).

Among the methods that use only one variable to predict demand, that proposed by Navarro et al. deserves special mention (16). This is a method that will predict the use of each of a range of medical services using what the authors describe as a "stochastic and deterministic model" based on the Markov process. Needed are (1) a specification of the various use states, such as no care, physician care, hospital care, nursing home care, etc.; (2) the assumption that a person must be in one and only one state at any given time; (3) a specification of the probability that a person will move from one use state to another during a period of time that is shorter than the minimum length of stay in any state; (4) the Markovian assumption that the "transitional probability" of moving from a current state to another depends solely on the patient's current state and not on any previous states; (5) the assumption that the transitional probabilities remain stable; (6) an estimate of the birth rate; and (7) an estimate of the death rate by age group. If desired, the effect of migration on population change can also be introduced into the computation. Of the several events under consideration, aging is totally predictable (deterministic) whereas births, deaths, migration, and use of service occur in various probabilities (stochastic). Given the assumptions, a succession of matrices are used to arrive at the use of the entire range of services during a given period of time. Obviously, the population constructed is a somewhat theoretical one in a steady state, brought about by specified birth and death rates and stable probabilities of transition from one use state to another. Furthermore, the basic assumption that the present use state fully determines the probability of occurrence of the next state may be open to question. For example, Fetter and Thompson examined experience in a hospital organized according to the "progressive patient care" principle. They found that the probability of movement among units in the patient care progression "does vary a great deal not only with where the patient is in a system at a given-time, but according to what zone of care he occupied before then and the zone of care to which he was originally admitted. The Markov model was therefore discarded" (45, p. 455). Finally, the method described by Navarro et al. also involves the assumption that all population characteristics that vary with age, and may also influence use of service (for example, sex, income, education, place of residence), are either of inconsequential effect as compared to the effect of age or will maintain an invariant relation to age. A similar comment could be made about all methods that use a single characteristic in demand analysis. Of course, even when several characteristics are used, one is not certain that some important variable has not been overlooked. However, if the proper statistical techniques have been used, one can have an estimate of how much of the variability in use of service remains unaccounted for by the characteristics included in the analysis.

Among the studies that have attempted to estimate requirements for hospital beds, perhaps the most interesting, in concept and method, is that by Rosenthal (11). Unlike the three studies we have already reviewed, Rosenthal is concerned with contemporaneous rather than predictive estimates, even though his method could be used for prediction. Furthermore, the nature of his concern and the availability of data lead him to use characteristics of states, rather than attributes of families or households, to specify the demand function—thereby raising the question of "ecological correlation" (88). Rosenthal is also more concerned with critically testing certain features of the method he uses: for example, the assumptions of linearity and of the stability of coefficients that measure the relationships between state characteristics and demand. The major distinction, however, is the presence of a normative core to Rosenthal's work. He is not content, as other demand analysts are, with the question, "What will be?" He is fundamentally concerned with "What should be?" As we shall point out in a subsequent section, the methods that use demand as the basis for estimating resource requirements are almost never as value-free as they seem to be. In Rosenthal's work the value questions are central.

Rosenthal is concerned with the proper distribution of nonfederal general and special short-term hospital beds among jurisdictions. He selects states partly because they are reasonably self-contained service areas, but mainly because current planning for hospital resource distribution is largely at the state level. Rosenthal begins with a profound dissatisfaction with ratios that assume need-demand to be totally proportional to population size. He insists that these ratios must take into account characteristics of the population that are likely to influence demand through influencing either need or the propensity to seek care in response to need. The first order of business, then, is to construct such ratios. This Rosenthal does by selecting a small set of variables that he believes, on the basis of plausibility and of findings reported in the literature, to be the most important ones in determining use of hospital resources. Having made the selection on these grounds, he believes that each variable must be retained in the mathematical expression of the demand function, even though it may contribute little to the statistical variation in demand. This is a curious position for an empirical analyst to take. It may represent intuitive recognition of the possibility that the contribution of a factor known to be operative in consumer demand may happen to be masked at the state level of analysis (88). The dependent variables that Rosenthal uses are admissions, average length of stay, and patient-days per 1000 persons. The independent variables are divided into sociodemographic and economic variables as follows:

Sociodemographic variables:
1. The proportion of population over 64 years of age.
2. The proportion of the population under 15 years of age. (Two age groups were used to account for higher use at two ends of the age span.)
3. The proportion of females aged 14 and over who are married.
4. The proportion of the population 14 years old and older who are male.
5. The proportion of the population who reside in areas classed as "urban" by the Bureau of the Census.
6. The proportion of the population that is "nonwhite."
7. The proportion of the population over 25 with 13 or more years of schooling.
8. Persons per dwelling unit.

Economic variables:
1. The mean of the most frequent charges for a two-bed hospital room.
2. The proportion of families and unrelated individuals with annual incomes over $5,999.
3. The proportion of families and unrelated individuals with annual incomes under $2,000. (Two income groups are selected to account for the possibility that both high income and low income groups may have higher levels of use than those in the middle.)
4. The proportion of the population covered by some type of hospital insurance.

Having selected and specified the variables, a least-squares linear multiple regression model was used to quantify the contribution of each characteristic to variation in demand. "Although theoretical considerations imply that the demand relationship is curvilinear, over any narrow range of observation the curve is slight and may be reasonably approximated by a linear model'' (11, p. 22). An alternative curvilinear model that assumed a linear relationship between the logarithm of utilization and the logarithms of the independent variables yielded results which did not differ significantly. In the curvilinear model the ''constraining effect of a greater proportion of low incomes'' was less, and the influence of insurance coverage in 1950 was more. ''However, there do not seem to be any clear-cut grounds for preferring one model over the other for purposes of this study'' (11, p. 94).

Using demand as the criterion, the simplest rule for resource allocation is that resources should be proportionate to demand as *empirically observed* in the several states. For reasons that, in the opinion of the author, are never made clear, Rosenthal does not consider this alternative. Instead, he proposes, as his first rule, that resource allocation be proportionate to demand as *computed* from the demand function, which itself is derived from observation of variations in demand among the several states as ''explained'' by state characteristics. The implicit assumption is that the demand equation yields a measure of what demand should be, since it yields a measure of what demand would be if the effects (coefficients) of the independent variables were equal (for each variable) in all the states. Given this partly normative estimate of average demand within each state, Rosenthal allocates to each state that complement of hospital beds that equalizes ''occupancy pressure'' in all states. The considerations that underlie this adjustment for occupancy pressure have been described in a previous chapter and will be raised again in a subsequent section. Briefly, Rosenthal assumes (1) that demand is Poisson-distributed; (2) that all hospitals in a state are equal in size to the mean hospital size for that state; (3) that the mean hospital size for each state is not to be changed or will not change; and (4) that there should be enough beds so the bed complement of the average hospital is not fully occupied more than once in each 100 days.

The first of Rosenthal's rules for hospital bed allocation assumes no particular upper limit to the hospital beds that may be provided for the United States as a whole. The aggregate number of beds is arrived at by summing the number of beds in each state. An alternative situation is one in which there is an upper national limit so that allocation among the states is to be made in a manner that uses up, but does not exceed, the total. Here the rule, once again, is that resource allocation be proportionate to demand so that occupancy pressure is equal in all states. The difference between this second formulation and the first is that, by the first rule, occupancy pressure was normatively defined as full occupancy one day out of 100. In the second instance, the occupancy pressure is to be equal, but the level at which it is equalized is set by the total number of beds to be provided nationally. Depending on how generous is the total provision of beds, this could be more or less stringent than the "1 in 100" level. The method for both situations may be made clearer by a stepwise summary of the procedure as follows:

1. Estimate patient-days of care in each state using the regression equation.

2. Determine the empirically observed average bed size in each state. This is the capacity that should not be exceeded more than once in 100 days. (If data are available, the computation from here on could be made for each of narrower classes of hospital size.)

3. Using Poisson probability tables determine the normative average daily census that will permit the hospital of average size to meet the condition that its capacity be not exceeded more than once in 100 days.

4. $$\frac{\text{Normative average daily census}}{\text{Empirically observed average hospital size}} = \text{Normative average occupancy}$$

   The numerator of the fraction is given in item 3 and the denomator in item 2. Rosenthal refers to the quotient as "maximum average occupancy".

5. $$\frac{\text{Patient days of care per year}}{365} \times \frac{1}{\text{average occupancy}} = \text{beds needed}$$

   Patient days of care per year are given in item 1 and average occupancy in item 4. The beds needed satisfy what we have called Rosenthal's first rule.

6. Add all beds required in all states, as given in item 5.

7. Express bed needs in each state as percent of the total (which is given in item 6).

8. Take an aggregate number of beds which is to be distributed among the states. Rosenthal applied Hill-Burton guidelines to arrive at the total number of beds for the United States.

9. Multiply the total number given in item 8, by the ratios given in item 7. This yields the number of beds in each state according to what we have called the second of Rosenthal's rules.

The first two rules of allocation that we have described are based on demand. Rosenthal also offers several "need-oriented" procedures for allocation. He begins by assuming that, in his equation, sociodemographic variables roughly represent "need," whereas the economic variables represent "demand." If so, it is possible to compute "need-oriented" estimates by introducing certain assumptions into the prediction equation, such as: (1) hospital prices in all states are the same as in the lowest; (2) insurance coverage is the same as in the highest;

(3) both the above; (4) specified shifts in income distribution. Changes such as those envisaged in assumptions 1, 2, and 3 can be brought about reasonably quickly, so that they represent short-term effects. Assumptions concerning income distribution take much longer to realize. In general, the "need-oriented" assumptions result in higher requirements for beds. However, assuming hospital prices in all states to be equal to those in the state with lowest prices results in further lowering (as compared to demand-oriented estimates) of requirements in the states with lowest demand and raising the requirements in those with the highest demand. This is because the low demand areas begin with having the low prices. A paradoxical result such as this indicates the limitations in this method of analysis and this definition of "need." It is also interesting to note that when all economic variables (price, insurance coverage and income) are set at levels that reveal "need," the requirements that result are higher than those generated by the Hill-Burton guidelines.

Table V.2 shows three of Rosenthal's bed requirement estimates by state for 1960. The second estimate, which assumes that the total number of beds available for distribution among the states is set by Hill-Burton standards, results in about a 36 percent increase in the bed population ratio in each state. The "need-oriented" estimate was computed on the assumption that all states have (1) hospital charges equal to the lowest charge observed among the states, (2) insurance coverage equal to the highest coverage observed among the states, and (3) income equal to the states having the highest proportion of population with income over $5,999 and the lowest proportion with income under $2,000. This estimate results in an increase in requirements over the second (demand-oriented) estimate in every state except two. The range is from no increase for West Virginia and Wyoming to 67 percent increase for Mississippi. This corresponds to a 37–130 percent increase over the first, more conservative, demand-oriented estimate. Inspection of the appropriate scatter diagrams (in which each point represents a state) shows that there is a rather weak positive relationship between beds per 1000 population as given by the demand-oriented and the need-oriented estimates. This is because the need-oriented estimate is never below and almost always above the demand-oriented one, but the difference between the two estimates differs greatly among states with comparable demand-oriented estimates. However, there is a negative relationship between the demand-oriented estimate of a state and the percent increase in that estimate which is brought about by the particular need-oriented demand function described above. Of course, this means that the states with lower

Table V.2.   Nonfederal, general and special hospital beds per 1000 population under three allocation procedures, by state, U.S.A., 1960

States	Allocation Procedures[a]		
	A	B	C
Alabama	2.5	3.4	5.3
Arizona	2.5	3.4	5.3
Arkansas	2.7	3.7	5.8
California	3.0	4.1	5.8
Colorado	3.8	5.2	5.5
Connecticut	3.4	4.6	5.0
Delaware	2.9	4.0	4.6
D.C., Md., Va.[b]	3.3	4.5	5.2
Florida	2.7	3.7	5.1
Georgia	3.0	4.1	5.2
Idaho	2.8	3.9	5.7
Illinois	3.8	5.2	5.4
Indiana	3.3	4.5	4.9
Iowa	3.7	5.0	5.7
Kansas	3.7	5.0	5.6
Kentucky	3.1	4.2	5.9
Louisiana	2.8	3.8	5.3
Maine	3.8	5.2	6.5
Massachusetts	3.7	5.0	6.1
Michigan	3.1	4.2	4.8
Minnesota	4.0	5.5	6.1
Mississippi	2.6	3.6	6.0
Missouri	3.6	4.9	5.5
Montana	4.3	5.9	6.6
Nebraska	3.9	5.3	6.1
Nevada	3.3	4.5	6.1
New Hampshire	3.7	5.1	6.1
New Jersey	2.9	4.0	4.7
New Mexico	2.6	3.6	5.1
New York	3.6	4.9	5.3
North Carolina	2.8	3.8	5.1
North Dakota	4.6	6.3	6.9
Ohio	3.3	4.5	4.8
Oklahoma	3.6	4.9	5.8
Oregon	3.1	4.2	5.5
Pennsylvania	3.7	5.0	5.1
Rhode Island	3.6	4.9	5.9
South Carolina	3.2	4.4	5.7

Table V.2. (*Continued*)

States	Allocation Procedures[a]		
	A	B	C
South Dakota	3.8	5.2	6.5
Tennessee	2.8	3.8	5.2
Texas	3.1	4.2	5.4
Utah	2.8	3.8	4.8
Vermont	4.1	5.6	6.7
Washington	3.2	4.4	6.0
West Virginia	4.0	5.5	5.5
Wisconsin	4.1	5.6	5.7
Wyoming	4.1	5.6	5.6

SOURCE: Reference 11, Tables 7, 12, and 17, pp. 51, 73, and 80.
[a] The three allocation procedures were
   A: Demand-oriented estimate with no limit on total beds
   B: Demand-oriented estimate with total determined by Hill-Burton guidelines
   C: Need-oriented estimate with all economic variables adjusted to optimal values.
[b] The District of Columbia, Maryland, and Virginia were combined because they were considered as one hospital service area.

levels of demand are favored more by a change to a need-oriented estimate. But here, also, variability around the trend line appears, by inspection, to be large, as shown by the following tabulation which summarizes features of both types of comparisons described above.

The entries in Table V.3 are the ranges of values of beds per 1000 for a group of several separate jurisdictions. The total number of jurisdictions is 45 because 2 jurisdictions are omitted from the tabulation. Both of these had a demand-oriented estimate of 3.4 beds per 1000 and a need-oriented estimate of 5.3 beds per 1000.

Table V.3. Ranges in the estimates for hospital[a] beds per 1000 persons, according to criteria for estimation, U.S.A., 1960

Number of Jurisdictions	Beds/1000: Demand-oriented Estimate B	Beds/1000: Need-oriented Estimate	Percent Increase from First to Second Estimates
18	3.5–4.4	4.6–6.0	67–12
20	4.5–5.4	4.8–6.5	49– 2
7	5.5–6.4	5.6–6.9	20– 0

SOURCE: Reference 11, Tables 7, 12 and 17, pages 51, 73, and 80.
[a] Nonfederal, General, and Special Hospitals.

Rosenthal is well aware of the many limitations of his method and discusses several in his monograph. These include the assumptions concerning the use of states as the unit of analysis, the assumption of linearity in the demand function, the question of stability in the demand coefficients, and the use of average hospital size, rather than the distribution of hospital sizes, to compute occupancy pressure. The first three features have already been discussed. The use of average hospital size in the determination of occupancy pressure was dictated by absence of information. It may have lowered the estimates for requirements in certain states where a few large hospitals may have outweighed many very small hospitals in computing the mean. Another major limitation, which Rosenthal concedes, but which also applies to all the other demand-oriented studies that we have described, is the assumption that current use of resources is appropriate. Rosenthal does deal with what we have called "manifest service reserve" when he corrects for occupancy pressure. None of the studies we have described so far deals with the more difficult question of "latent service reserve" due to patient misclassification and inefficient use. Related to this is the substitutability among resources of various kinds which Rosenthal recognizes, but which is not taken into account in his estimates.

A final criticism particularly germane to demand-oriented estimates is that they do not account for the effect of supply on demand. Rosenthal points out, quite correctly, that if supply were the sole determinant of demand, any allocation of resources among the states would be economically, though not socially, as good as any other. Since this assumption would strike at the very foundations of traditional demand analysis, Rosenthal takes pains to examine it in detail. He points out that to demonstrate a simple relationship between demand and supply does not mean that supply creates demand, since it is equally likely that demand creates supply. He argues that if supply fully determines demand, the pressure on beds should be uniform among geographic areas. In fact, the states differ widely in this respect. Rosenthal also computed correlation coefficients between occupancy pressure and demand and between occupancy pressure and supply (beds per 1000) without regard to the 12 state characteristics, and then computed the corresponding partial correlation coefficients, which hold the effect of the 12 characteristics constant. The raw correlation coefficients showed that occupancy pressure was positively related to demand but weakly or ambiguously related to supply. The partial correlation coefficient showed a positive relationship between occupancy pressure and demand, but a negative relationship between occupancy pressure and supply. However, none of the raw or partial coefficients was very large, and the relationship between demand and occupancy pressure was largely explained by longer stays rather than by more admissions. According to Rosenthal, "This exercise has cast considerable doubt on the theory that exogenous changes in supply will automatically generate a demand for that supply. It has also suggested that a distribution of facilities based on demand would make possible their most effective utilization and therefore would represent the economically optimal allocation" (11, pp. 61–62).

The assumption that supply fully determines demand is likely to be a straw man. The more realistic assumption is that supply influences demand together with other factors. Martin Feldstein, who has examined the data assembled by Rosenthal, concludes that supply ought to be included as a factor (22).

So far, we have concentrated on that category of demand-oriented predictions of resource requirements that include consideration of change in population and population characteristics but assume that current relationships between population characteristics and demand remain constant. The author has encountered no instance of a study that bases its predictions on quantitative (as contrasted to qualitative) estimates of changes in all three factors: population size, population characteristics, and the demand coefficients of these characteristics.

Empirical Verification of Predictions Based on Demand

We have already had occasion to comment on the numerous sources of error that are likely to afflict predictions of demand, including the many simplifying assumptions that add unreality to the estimates. At least two studies have investigated the accuracy of predictions based on specified methods and their associated assumptions. The device used in both studies is to find out what would have happened if a specified method were used at some past date to predict demand for services and resources in the present. This constitutes a kind of hypothetical retrospective verification. In a subsequent section we shall describe briefly actual historical experience with the predictive accuracy of need-oriented methods.

As part of his larger study, Fein constructed a retrospective prediction of the current (1964) rate of physician visits by applying 1959 utilization rates to the actual population changes between 1959 and 1964 (24, pp. 113–181). Since this assumes perfect prediction of population size and characteristics, all that is being tested is the stability of the relationships between characteristics and demand and the effect of characteristics not used in the prediction. The method predicted a 12.0 percent increase in visits during the 5-year period (1959–1964), whereas the actual increase was only 3.8 percent, which was less than the rate of population growth! This large discrepancy over so short a period, under partial testing stress, is disturbing, to put it mildly. Fein offers several explanations. In large measure these read like a recapitulation of the reservations concerning concept and method that we have already raised. First, visits may not be the proper measure of the physician's product. Second, there may have been less readiness on the part of physicians to offer service accompanied by a sufficient increase in prices to lessen demand. Third, while the aggregate number of physicians (or their readiness to provide service) may not have changed, there may have occurred a larger degree of geographic maldistribution. Fourth, there may have been substitution of physician's services in favor of others, such as drugs and hospital care, and, finally, the population may have become healthier. Fein is careful to point out that the lower-then-predicted increase in physicians' visits does not necessarily mean less than adequate care. If this interpretation is correct, then the prediction is not only empirically inadequate, but also without normative utility.

Paul Feldstein and Jeremiah German have subjected demand-based predictions to a more exhaustive, but still partial and inconclusive, test (17). They obtained "predictions" of hospital demand in 1961, which was known to them, by using present and past characteristics of hospitals or populations in 47 states. The rule adopted was that, for each year between the present and the future time for which a prediction is to be made, one needs to use data for an equal number of years in the past. Accordingly, data for 1952–1956 were used to "predict" or "explain" hospital demand in 1961. The three major hypotheses tested were that current demand is best predicted or explained by (A) past hospital demand, (B) past hospital supply, (C) current population characteristics, or (D) a combination of current population characteristics and past demand. Subsidiary hypotheses resulted in testing 12 variants, as shown in Table V.4.

There are several components in testing the predictive accuracy of the several methods. One is to measure the standard error of the estimate of the dependent variable (patient-days). Another is to measure the standard error of the net regression coefficients of each of the independent variables in the demand equation, in order to determine how reliable these coefficients are. A third is to determine the coefficient of correlation. The square of this coefficient (R^2) measures the proportion of variation in the dependent variable that is accounted for by all the independent variables combined. By all these tests, the accuracy of prediction varied

Table V.4.   Specified independent variables used by Feldstein and German to predict specified measures of hospital utilization (dependent variable)

Dependent Variable	Independent Variable
(A) 1. Patient-days/1000 in 1961	Patient-days/1000 for each of 5 years, 1952–1956
2. Patient-days/1000 in 1961	*Average* patient-days/1000 1952–1956
3. *Change* in patient-days per 1000, 1961–1956	*Change* in patient-days/1000 in each of 5 adjacent pairs of years, 1956–55 to 1952–51
4. *Change* in patient-days per 1000, 1961–1956	*Average change* in patient-days/1000 in 5 adjacent pairs of years 1956–55 to 1952–51
(B) 5. Patient-days/1000 in 1961	Beds/1000 for each of 5 years, 1952–56
6. Patient-days/1000 in 1961	*Average* beds/1000, 1952–56
7. *Change* in patient-days per 1000, 1961–1956	*Change* in beds/1000 in each of 5 adjacent pairs of years, 1956–55 to 1952–51
8. *Change* in patient-days per 1000, 1961–1956	*Average change* in beds per 1000 in 5 adjacent pairs of years 1956–55 to 1952–51
(C) 9a. Patient-days/1000 in 1961	Measures of income, insurance coverage, urbanization, color and price in 1961
9b. Patient-days/1000 in 1951	Measures of the above in 1951
10. *Change* in patient-days per 1000, 1961–1956	Change in above measures 1961–51
(D) 11. Patient-days/1000 in 1961	Measures of the above (9a) in 1961, plus patient-days/1000 in 1956

SOURCE: Reference 17.

widely among the different methods. For example, R^2 varied from 0.198 for Method 4 to 0.94 for Method 11. The methods that use average values or changes in values tend to give less accurate predictions than those that use absolute values for each of the 5 years. The value of R^2 for the major methods was as shown in Table V.5.

In spite of the exhaustiveness of the tests described above, they do not offer direct evidence on the ability to predict for future years, as yet unknown. This is because the tests do not involve predictions for years

Table V.5. Measures of correlation between predicted and observed values of hospital utilization using spefied methods[a]

	R^2
1. Patient-days/1000 for each of 5 years, 1952–1956	0.89
5. Beds/1000 for each of 5 years, 1952–56	0.73
9a. Measures of income, insurance coverage, age, urbanization, color, and price in 1961	0.73
11. The above measures plus patient-days/1000 in 1961	0.94

SOURCE: Reference 17.

[a] The numbers before the methods are keyed to those in Table V.4.

that were not used in the development of the equations themselves. Also, because all the terms in the equations are in the form of rates, it would not be possible to arrive at absolute estimates without first having a prediction of future population size. In fact, the authors "assume that the problem of population prediction has been solved" (17, p. 14). This includes predicting not only size, but also population characteristics that influence demand. Furthermore, there is the question whether present or past relationships will remain unchanged in the future. In fact, by determining the relationships between demand and population characteristics by state for two years a decade apart (1951 and 1961), Feldstein and German reveal significant instability. Recognizing these limitations, a subset of methods, those that use past demand to predict future demand, was used by Feldstein and German to predict demand in 1962 and 1963. The findings were not "very different" from those obtained for 1961. In other words, the equations derived from the relationship between demand in 1952–56 and demand in 1961 were still serviceable to predict demand in 1962 and 1963. The authors do concede, however, that "undoubtedly, the predictive ability will begin to decline as equations over a given period are used further in the future" (17, p. 351). One wishes that the authors would take advantage of the lapse of a decade to test once again the predictive or explanatory power of their initial formulations.

Feldstein and German discuss the utility of the different methods they have used by distinguishing prediction from explanation. They feel that although past demand or supply may have been the best predictor according to these tests, they do not help us understand what the factors are that bring about changes in demand. Consequently, exclusive reliance on demand and supply trends may leave us unprepared to meet the consequences of changes in population characteristics. Rosenthal has also expressed a similar viewpoint in offering his approach to demand analysis (11). One could argue, however, that past demand may be the best predictor of future demand because it is the most accurate representation of the joint effect of the factors that bring it about, factors that are only partially represented in the demand equation. The trends also reflect changes in the levels of these factors, as well as changes in the independent, correlated, and interactive effects of these factors on demand. Thus they represent the closest approach to a method that accounts not only for population change but also for change in the demand coefficients. It is true, however, that all these factors are included implicitly rather than explicitly. Hence, though the method offers prediction, it does not provide understanding.

Adjustment of Demand to Service Capacity

Estimates of demand take us only halfway to estimates of resource requirements. Demand has still to be translated into its equivalents in resources. This requires some estimate, empirically or normatively derived, of the service capacity of the corresponding resources. It may also involve an assessment of the extent to which current demand and current service capacity are in or out of balance. Different methods of estimation differ in the degree to which they take into account the several facets of service capacity. In some studies the question of service capacity is not raised at all, the assumption being that it will remain constant. This is true when a resource : population ratio is used to estimate requirements. Other studies make a variety of adjustments with varying degrees of sophistication and precision. In this section we shall review some of these studies classified according to the major aspect of service capacity taken into account. Since some methods take account of several aspects of service capacity, a decision will be made as to what feature is most distinctive of the method. Where possible, the methods will be arranged in a progression of increasing sophistication and/or comprehensiveness with respect to adjustments to service capacity. The progression will be as follows: (1) productivity in general, (2) expected or desirable capacity, (3) expected or desirable occupancy, (4) occupancy pressure, (5) occupancy pressure taking account of compartmentalization, (6) waiting time, (7) waiting lists, (8) unsatisfied demand, (9) latent service reserve, (10) patient classification. A feature of some of these adjustments is their strong normative content. In fact, when one considers unsatisfied demand, one gets quite close to concepts of "need." Studies of patient classification are so obviously based on estimates of need for service that one could easily challenge their inclusion in this progression of demand-oriented methods. They have been placed here mainly for convenience in presentation.

PRODUCTIVITY IN GENERAL. Aspects of defining and measuring productivity have been discussed in detail in a previous chapter. Even some of the relatively early need-oriented estimates of resource requirements were cognizant of the relevance of productivity to the estimates that were constructed. For example, the Report of the Surgeon General's Consultant Group on Medical Education considered explicitly "factors affecting efficiency of medical practitioners" and concluded that further increases in services per unit time would probably not occur without loss to a meaningful patient-physician relationship (71, pp. 11–12). But in this, as well as in other studies of its type, productivity was considered in a qualitative, judgmental manner, with no attempt to quantify it. One exception is the study of requirements for dentists, which we shall describe in a subsequent section (66). An obstacle to the use of quantitative estimates of productivity in drawing the balance between demand and service-producing resources, is the difficulty of defining and measuring this term. Klarman has recently compiled a listing of estimates of physician productivity reported in the literature for the years 1936–65 which range from 1.9 to 4.5 per annum, or from 20.7 to 55.3 over a decade (3). Among the demand-oriented studies that we have already described, Fein compares the minimum estimates of 21.9 to 25.8 percent increase in demand with the estimated 19 percent increase in the number of physicians over the same time period. He then speculates on whether or not the difference can be made up through increases in productivity. Baker and Perlman make no estimates of productivity change in predicting manpower requirements in Taiwan, but they do offer a standard of service capacity. Increasingly, productivity is becoming recognized as the key element in the balance between need-demand and resource supply. However, one must avoid falling into the trap of defining productivity in such a manner that demand and supply are seen to be always in balance, with productivity changes serving as the balancing factor.

EXPECTED OR DESIRABLE SERVICE CAPACITY. A specified capacity to provide service, which is derived from experience or offered as a desirable standard, is necessary to change estimates of demand into equivalents in service-producing resources, or the reverse. For example, Baker and Perlman converted data on number of visits per month into number of physicians by dividing by 1000, which was the average monthly number of visits observed to be provided by physicians. The application of this factor to the projected number of visits assumes that there will be no changes in productivity when the product is measured in visits. On the contrary, "In Taiwan, as in other developing regions, where doctors see from 50 to 100 patients in an office session, technological changes which improve patient care would tend to lower, not raise, the number of patients seen per doctor" (25, p. 125). However, if this is the case, the visit one decade hence is likely to be different in potency from the visit today, so that one must question the use of current demand experience to project future demand. Further examples of empirical or normative standards of service capacity will be encountered in subsequent descriptions of methods.

EXPECTED OR DESIRABLE OCCUPANCY. Expected or desired occupancy rates are simply one variant of service capacity measures which is applicable to hospitals. Perhaps the simplest of all examples is one encountered in a study of hospital requirements in Metropolitan St. Louis (28, p. 36). The projections are based on only 4 items of information:

P_1 = Current population size,
D = Current hospital demand in total patient days,
P_2 = Future population size,
O = Desirable occupancy ratio: for example 0.85.

It is assumed that the current hospital utilization rate will hold for the future. The computations are exceedingly simple, as shown in Table V.6.

The Division of Hospital and Medical Facilities, Public Health Service, has offered a method for estimating hospital requirements based on the application of desirable occupancy rates, but which also introduces a number of important refinements (29). The major steps in the method are described in Table V.7. One interesting feature is the use of separate estimates of demand by type of service. The basis for estimation also differs by type of service. For total short-time hospital use the basis is the projected age-sex composition of the population and a projected rate of use by age and sex. Utilization of pediatric beds is separated out from the

Table V.6. Procedure for computing requirements for hospital beds using changes in population size and a desirable occupancy ratio

1. Current patient-days	÷	Current population	=	Patient-days per person
2. Projected population	×	Patient-days per person	=	Projected patient-days
3. Projected patient-days	÷	365	=	Projected average daily census for all hospitals combined
4. Projected average daily census for all hospitals combined	÷	Desirable occupancy ratio	=	Projected bed requirement, all hospitals

SOURCE: Reference 28, page 36.

In symbols: Projected bed requirements $= \dfrac{D}{P_1} \times P_2 \div 365 \div O$

total by applying the appropriate rate to the pediatric age group. A component of long-term facility care is added by projecting the age group most at risk, those 65 and over, and predicting what percent would be in a long-term facility on a given day. The projection for obstetrical care uses a method of which there are several examples in the literature (40, 79). It requires, explicitly or implicitly, successive prediction of (1) the population subject to pregnancy, (2) the risk of pregnancy, (3) the likelihood of being admitted to the hospital for complications of pregnancy and for childbirth, and (4) the average length of stay. All of these factors are subject to change, except that in the United States admission to the hospital for childbirth is almost universal. McEwen has shown how the maternity-bed population ratio for England will change as the proportion of births that occur in hospitals increases and the average stay per case goes down (79).

Another interesting feature of the method proposed by the Division of Hospital and Medical Facilities is the use of several desirable occupancy ratios, one for each type of service. These differences reflect the average size of hospital unit devoted to each type of care, as well as the different characteristics of demand for these services: for example, the unpostponable or emergent nature of obstetric and pediatric care and the low turnover in long-term facilities. The method is also capable of further refinements. To estimate use of service, current levels of demand are applied to future populations. It is recognized, however, that this is a simplification and that changes in the demand coefficients may need to be

Table V.7. A Procedure for estimating requirements for short-term general hospitals and long-term facilities

Type of Requirement	Symbols	Items and Steps in Computation	Method of Computation[a]	Numerical Example
Total short-term hospital use	$A_1, A_2 \cdots$	Projected population by sex and age groups (in thousands)		250,000
	$B_1, B_2 \cdots$	Patient-days of short-term hospital use per 1000 per year for each sex and age group. (Current use, with or without modification to account for changes in other factors that may influence use.)		See p. 24 of ref. 29 for age-sex distribution and hospital use by age and sex
	C	Total projected patient-days per year	$A_1B_1 + A_2B_2 \cdots$	208,708
Obstetrical bed use, short-term hospitals	D	Projected number of females aged 15–44, in thousands (from A, above)		55.2
	E	Deliveries per 1000 females aged 15–44, per year (current or projected rates)		95.6
	F	Length of stay, in days, per delivery (current or projected values)		4.5
	G	Projected patient-days of obstetrical care per year	$D \cdot E \cdot F$	23,747
Pediatric bed use, short-term hospitals	H_1, H_2	Males and females under 15, respectively, in thousands (from A)		41.9 40.9

Table V.7. *Continued*

Type of Requirement	Symbols	Items and Steps in Computation	Method of Computation[a]	Numerical Example
	I_1, I_2	Patient-days per 1000 per year for H_1 and H_2, respectively (current or projected).		315.1 274.2
	J	Projected patient-days of pediatric care per year	$H_1 I_1 + H_2 I_2$	24,418
Medical-surgical bed use, short-term hospitals	K	Projected patient-days of medical-surgical care per year	$C - (G + J)$	160,543
Average daily census, by type of service, short-term hospitals	L	Projected average daily census for obstetrical care	$G \div 365$	65.1
	M	Projected average daily census for pediatric care	$I \div 365$	66.9
	N	Projected average daily census for medical-surgical care	$K \div 365$	439.8
Beds by type of service, at specified occupancy ratios, short-term hospitals	O	Projected beds for obstetrical care at 75% occupancy	$L \div 0.75$	87
	P	Projected beds for pediatric care at 75% occupancy	$M \div 0.75$	89
	Q	Projected beds for medical-surgical care at 85% occupancy	$N \div 0.85$	517

Type of Requirement	Symbols	Items and Steps in Computation	Method of Computation[a]	Numerical Example
	R	Total projected beds	$L + M + N$	693
Long-term facility beds for the aged	S	Projected persons 65 and over, in hundreds (from A)		176
	T	Percent of persons 65 and over who are in a long-term facility on any given day (current or projected)		5
	U	Projected average daily census in long-term facilities	$S.T$	880
	V	Projected long-term facility beds at 95% occupancy	$U \div 0.95$	926

SOURCE: Reference 29, pp. 24–26.

[a] The letters in the arithmetic operations identify the quantities shown by the symbols in Column 2 of the table.

considered. Unfortunately, no specific method of predicting such change is offered. By contrast, a method is offered (as we shall describe toward the end of this section) for making adjustments for patient misclassification. Finally, it is recognized that the desirable occupancy rates can be further refined to reflect factors such as hospital size and empirically observed patterns of demand. A quantitative adjustment of this kind would move the method into the next category to be described below.

OCCUPANCY PRESSURE. The considerations that go into adjustments for occupancy pressure have been discussed in some detail in the preceding chapter. Briefly, what is involved is (1) obtaining a temporal distribution of demand, (2) knowing the capacity of the facility that must meet the demand, and (3) deciding how frequently it is acceptable for the capacity to be fully occupied. The distribution of demand may be obtained by observation over a sufficiently long period of time. When only the average demand is known, it has been reasonably realistic, provided certain precautions are observed, to assume that the temporal distribution of demand is well represented by a Poisson distribution. This means that the mean of the distribution is equal to its variance. Since this is so, if the average demand (or the average daily census) is known one can compute, or obtain from appropriate tables, the probability of any given daily demand (average daily census) being exceeded. Knowledge of the capacity of the facility is important because the smaller the facility the larger is the proportion of total capacity that has to be set aside to meet fluctuations in demand, and yet stay within the limit of the acceptable probability that the capacity will be exceeded. One aspect of the determination of relevant capacity is the extent to which the facility is internally subdivided into compartments with little or no exchange of patients among compartments (32). Another is the extent to which the facility is required to be totally self-sufficient or has possibilities of patient exchange with other similar facilities in an area. The larger the capacity of the pool within which exchanges may occur the smaller the proportion of that capacity that has to be set aside as "stand-by reserve." When corrections have to be made for occupancy pressure in planning for hospitals of varying size in a geographic area, the question arises as to what is the representative hospital size to be used in computing stand-by reserve, and therefore average occupancy. In a previous section we have described the study by Rosenthal which assumed all hospitals within an area (in his case, a state) to be equal (11). A preferable method would be to obtain the frequency distribution of hospitals by size and compute stand-by reserve or occupancy rate for each class.

Further refinements would include (1) adjustments to different charac-teristics of demand (for example, of urgency), (2) different patterns of compartmentalization, and (3) different degrees of isolation or mutual exchange, provided it is shown that these characteristics are related to size, as they are likely to be. For example, the normatively acceptable levels of stand-by reserve (and hence, of occupancy) are not likely to be the same in a metropolitan area as in a rural area with many small hospitals that are very far apart.

The method that we have described above rests on precise theoretical assumptions supported by a fair amount of empirical observation. Less formally developed, and simpler, expressions of the relationship between hospital size and occupancy have been available for some time. The Commission on Hospital Care, assuming that the distribution of daily censuses exhibited a "normal curve pattern," proposed two standards of occupancy, brought about by providing sufficient beds to accommodate the average daily census (C) plus a multiple of the average daily census, as follows:

$$\text{``Low level occupancy''} = C + 4\sqrt{C}$$
$$\text{``High level occupancy''} = C + 3\sqrt{C}$$

The Commission offered no guidelines about which of the two standards might be applicable, beyond remarking that the lower standard "is not a rigid mathematical law" and that "some hospitals will find that they can have higher occupancy rates without great inconvenience" (30, pp. 279–281). Blumberg has pointed out that application of the "square root approximations" given above yield results "materially different" from those obtained using the Poisson probability tables. This is because "the probability of a full facility varies not only with the square root formula used, but also with the size of the facility" (32, footnote to Table 2, p. 79).

Additional examples of studies that have used quantitative adjustment to occupancy pressure, almost always under the assumption that demand is Poisson-distributed, will be described when we consider patient classi-fication toward the end of this section.

OCCUPANCY PRESSURE, TAKING ACCOUNT OF COMPARTMENTALIZATION. We have already pointed out that estimates of stand-by reserve, and hence of desirable occupancy, become more realistic if one takes account of the fact that a facility (such as a hospital) is not one reservoir of capacity but is usually subdivided into compartments with limits on transfer of patients among compartments. Blumberg has emphasized this feature of hospitals and has given examples of how estimates of hospital bed requirements are computed with this feature in view (32). In essence, one needs a separate estimate of average demand for each hospital service (compartment). Assuming this demand to be Poisson-distributed, and adopting an acceptable probability of full occupancy, one can estimate the size of each service (compartment). The size of the hospital is merely the sum of all its independent parts.

An example, based on one given by Blumberg, may help clarify some of the points made above. Assume an area which is to be served by one hospital and in which there is predicted to be an average daily census of 300 hospital patients. The simplified Poisson probability table cited by Blumberg (32, p. 78) gives the values shown in Table V.8 for total bed

Table V.8. Occupancy ratios expected and hospital beds needed under specified assumptions[a]

Predicted Average Daily Census	P = 0.01		P = 0.001	
	Beds	Percent Occupancy	Beds	Percent Occupancy
300	340	88	354	85

[a] See text.

size necessary if the hospital is to be filled on an average of 1 day in 100 (P = 0.01) and 1 day in 1000 (P = 0.001), respectively. This assumes that all beds in the hospital are freely interchangeable. If, however, one considers the hospital to be divided into 3 major services, the bed requirements (as shown in the Poisson probability table) and the occupancy rates, will be as shown in Table V.9. The hospital may be further

Table V.9. Occupancy ratios expected and hospital beds needed to accommodate an average daily census of 300 patients under specified assumptions[a]

Hospital Service	Predicted Average Daily Census	P = 0.01		P = 0.001	
		No. of Beds	Percent Occupancy	No. of Beds	Percent Occupancy
Medical-surgical	200	235	85	245	82
Pediatric	55	74	74	80	69
Obstetric	45	62	73	68	66
All services	300	371	81	393	76

[a] See text.

subdivided into private and ward accommodation and the predicted average daily censuses taken to be as in Table V.10. In this case the bed complements required and the occupancies would be as shown in Table

Table V.10.   Average daily census distributed by type of service and accommodation in a hypothetical hospital with a total average daily census of 300 patients

| Hospital Service | Total Census | Accommodation | |
		Private	Ward
Medical-surgical	200	160	40
Pediatric	55	40	15
Obstetric	45	35	10
All services	300	235	65

V.11, if a full occupancy on an average of 1 in 100 days were acceptable. A similar table can be constructed under the assumption that the acceptable probability of complete occupancy is 1 day in 1000. Table V.12 summarizes the total number of beds required under the several preceding assumptions. All the estimates in Table V.12 assume that there is no

Table V.11.   Occupancy ratios expected and hospital beds needed to accommodate an average daily cenusus of 300 patients under specified assumptions.[a]

| Hospital Service | Total Census | | Private | | Ward | |
	Beds	Percent Occupancy	Beds	Percent Occupancy	Beds	Percent Occupancy
Medical-surgical	247	81	191	84	56	71
Pediatric	82	67	56	71	26	58
Obstetric	69	65	50	70	19	53
All services	398	75	297	79	101	65

[a] See Table V.10 and text.

transfer of patients among hospital subparts. To the extent that such transfer occurs, the estimates of bed requirements would be reduced and occupancy increased. Furthermore, it is assumed that all patients who need admission will be accepted. As we shall see below, to the extent that some admissions are elective and patients can be made to wait, bed requirements are further reduced.

Table V.12.   Occupancy ratios expected and hospital beds needed to accommodate an average daily census of 300 patients under specified assumptions.[a]

| | Acceptable Probability of Full Occupancy | | | |
| | 0.01 | | 0.001 | |
Assumptions About Hospital Beds	No. of Beds	Percent Occupancy	No. of Beds	Percent Occupancy
All beds interchangeable	340	88	354	85
Three services	371	81	393	76
Three services, two types of accommodation	398	75	432	69

WAITING TIME. A further refinement in adjusting requirements for
hospital beds to demand is to allow for waiting times of varying length,
depending on type of case. Querido has reported a computational procedure, developed by de Wolff, that allows for this under certain assumptions (33). In Holland, requests for admission to municipal hospitals are
scrutinized by screening physicians. The cases approved for admission in
this manner were taken to represent demand. The daily demand by
specialty, excepting epidemics, was found to constitute a normal distribution, so that a value 1, 2, and 3 standard deviations above the mean is
equal to, or is larger than, 84, 97, and 99.8 percent respectively of the
values in the distribution. Thus, a value of 3 standard deviations above
the mean will include all but 0.2 percent of all cases that are approved for
admission each day.

In the following discussion let

B = number of beds;
I = daily average number of approved requests for admission
during period V; and
V = average length of stay in days.

If there were no fluctuations in daily approved requests (I) and the
length of stay per case were equal to V days, the number of hospital
patient days of demand generated each day would be IV. This means
that this number of beds would have to be provided if all approved
requests were to be admitted on the same day and the hospitals were
capable of operation at full occupancy. Under these circumstances the
number of beds (B) required would be:

$$B = IV$$

However, daily approved requests fluctuate in the manner described above. This being the case, if it is desired to provide hospital beds sufficient to meet demand 99.8 percent of days (998 days out of 1000), the hospital beds required would be as follows, assuming no impediment to full occupancy other than fluctuations in demand:

$$B = IV \left(1 + 3\frac{\sigma_I}{I} \times \frac{1}{\sqrt{V}} \right)$$

It is not necessary, however, to admit all approved requests immediately. Consultation with experts resulted in the formulation of "rather arbitrary" permissible waiting times before admission. "It was decided that ideally a non-acute patient should not wait more than 3 weeks after admission was deemed necessary. A waiting time of less than 6 days has no appreciable effect on the case flow. The permissible waiting time was therefore fixed between these values" (33, p. 123). If all approved requests for admission are required to wait the full length of the permissible waiting time, at the end of a period of time equal to the permissible waiting time, there will be generated a waiting list which is the maximum permissible. This waiting list equals IT, the product of approved daily requests for admission (I) and the permissible waiting time (T). Any excess over this means that one or more cases have waited more than the permissible waiting time. Given a fixed bed complement and a fluctuating daily demand (I), actual daily admissions can be above or below demand, as a consequence of which the daily waiting list will fluctuate. However, it is required that the waiting list should not exceed a certain limit, IT. A reasonable rule is to provide enough beds so that the specified limit is not exceeded more than 2 days in a thousand. Given the properties of the distribution of daily demand, this value is given by the following equation (see source for derivation) :*

$$B = IV \left[1 + \frac{9}{4} \left(\frac{(\sigma_I)^2}{I} \right) \cdot \frac{1}{\frac{T-W_0}{I}} \right],$$

where B = number of beds required
I = daily number of approved requests for admission;
V = average length of stay in days;
σ_I = standard deviation of I;
T = permissible waiting time in days;
O = daily number of admissions;
W_0 = the waiting list at any given time.

* The author has not been able to verify the derivation of this equation.

Although W_0 may fluctuate depending on fluctuations in I and O, in the long run, if the system is to remain in equilibrium, the average of W_0 cannot exceed IT which itself must not exceed OT. In other words, on the average, admissions must be at least equal to requests for admission, if an infinite waiting list is to be avoided. Another assumption implicit in the above formulation is that there is no obstacle to full occupancy other than fluctuations in demand. In other words, B = OV. This means that turnover interval is essentially equal to zero, since beds are reoccupied within 12 or 24 hours, at the latest (34).

Querido has given normative standards and bed requirements, by specialty, for Amsterdam in 1949. The figures, shown in Table V.13, are

Table V.13.   Requirements for hospital beds, by specialty, under specified assumptions, Amsterdam, Holland, 1949

Specialty	Beds Sufficient for Average Need	Beds Necessary	Average Percent Occupancy	Permissible Waiting List	Permissible Waiting Time in Days
Internal medicine	640	831	77	70	7
Surgery	868	960	90	215	10
Infectious diseases	93	129	77	0	0
Obstetrics	151	212	71	104	10
Gynecology	144	160	90	77	8
E.N.T.	195	215	91	226	20
Psychology and Neurology	290	340	85	27	7
Eye disease	66	76	86	43	20
Dermatology	71	100	71	14	7
Pediatrics	137	166	80	0	0

SOURCE: Reference 33, Table 52, page 126.

interesting. "Beds Sufficient for Average Need," cited in column 1 of the table, represent average daily approved demand plus an increment for incomplete occupancy even at constant demand (34). The waiting lists are much shorter than expected, given the permissible waiting time. No doubt this is because not all cases approved for admission fall in the category of patients who can wait. The variability in percent occupancy results in part from the need to accommodate to nonpostponable demand and is brought about by differences in mean unpostponable demand and variability around the mean. In part, variability in occupancy results from accommodation to postponable demand and is brought about by differences in the mean and variability of that demand, and the permissible waiting time. According to Querido, the major portion of the variability is due to fluctuation in demand which may result in the bed requirements being as much as 30 percent above average daily demand. "The augmentation due to the permissible waiting list figure is small, and amounts to a few percent" (33, p. 125). It is not known to what extent other factors that influence occupancy have been included in the figures cited in the table. These additional factors would include hospital and hospital sub-unit size in Amsterdam as well as length of stay and turnover interval by specialty.

Querido concludes by asserting that requirements in the present are the best guide for future hospital requirements.

An extrapolation on the base of estimates of future population figures would be as doubtful as an estimate of present necessity based on beds per thousand inhabitants. Furthermore, it was felt that an increase or shift in population would be less consequential for future needs than changes in medical procedure which are quite unforeseeable. There is no reason to suppose that changes in the need for bed capacity due to new medical inventions or new insights in medical procedure would be met by planned over-capacity. These changes might just as well have the effect of decreasing the need of beds. Therefore, responsibility in planning for the future would be absolved by exact determination of present needs, and furthermore by devising a highly flexible system of hospital organization, since unexpected changes will be more qualitative than quantitative (33, p. 127).

WAITING LIST. The presence of a waiting list is generally taken to mean that the capacity of a resource to provide service has been exceeded. If, on more careful scrutiny, this assumption is sustained, and the waiting list is accepted as a true representation of demand, estimates of resource requirements will have to include the increment necessary either to eliminate the waiting list or reduce it to an acceptable length. In the preceding section we discussed the utility of developing, by design, waiting lists of controlled length. In this section we are concerned with the elimination of waiting lists that are unintended and uncontrolled. The variants of methods that deal with this situation have been developed most formally by N. T. J. Bailey (35–38). The basic premise is almost self-evident: that over any given period of time the average capacity to provide service must be at least equal to the demand for service. The critical point is where capacity and demand are in precise balance. Any sustained excess of average demand will result, according to the theory of queues, in a waiting list of infinite length and an infinite average waiting time. At any point below the critical point of precise balance, waiting time and length of queue depend on the capacity of the resource, the interval between cases demanding service, the length of stay in service, and the fluctuations in rate of demand and length of stay. Under the assumption that both demand for service and the length of stay are Poisson-distributed, it is possible to compute average waiting time and length of queue (35). Such computations, would obviously be an alternative way of determining required capacity, given certain characteristics of demand and length of stay, and a normatively acceptable average waiting time. However, neither Bailey nor those who have applied his thinking, have used specifications of waiting time in the determination of resource requirements (35–41). Instead, they have proceeded on the assumption that a small excess of capacity over demand results in waiting times (and lists) of acceptable length. Furthermore, although the basic method applies to both ambulatory and hospital services, it has been applied mainly to hospitals.

The critical number of hospital beds may be determined using information either on yearly or daily demand. The general description which follows will be phrased in terms of daily demand. A specific example using yearly data, and introducing further refinements, will be given later in the section.

1. Average daily ad- + Average daily additions = Average demand per day
   missions   to the waiting list minus
                       removals from the wait-
                       ing list

2. Average demand × Average length of stay = Patient-days generated
   per day   of hospitalized cases   each day

3. Patient-days   = Average daily census   = Critical number of
   generated each   effective beds
   day

The value of the critical number of effective beds is almost always based on observed values of daily admissions and length of stay and is therefore subject to sampling error. The variance of the critical number is given by the equation (36) :

$$\mathrm{Var}\ (c) = c^2 \left(\frac{1}{n} + \frac{1}{n'} \right),$$

where c = the critical number;
         n = the number of observations from which the estimate of
               average demand per day is derived;
         n' = the number of observations from which the estimate of
               average length of stay is derived.

To account for sampling error, two times the standard error of the critical number must be added to it. If an additional one or two beds are provided, estimated capacity will in most instances be sufficient to meet demand within reasonable limits of waiting time. The estimated requirements for effective hospital beds, therefore, are:

critical number + twice standard + 1 or 2 beds
of beds   error of criti-
                     cal number

These are the bare bones of the "critical number" method. More careful examination is necessary to understand its uses and limitations. These arise from certain implicit or explicit assumptions concerning (1) the manner in which hospital capacity is used, and (2) the characteristics of hospital demand. With respect to the use of hospital capacity, the major feature of the method, as originally formulated by Bailey, and as shown above, is that the critical number is the number of beds at 100 percent occupancy (35). It is clear, therefore, that allowance must be made for minimum turnover interval and for what Bailey sees as "deficiencies due to administrative difficulties in filling beds" (35, p. 139). For these reasons, and others to be described below, the critical number must be adjusted for occupancy ratios of less than 100 percent. In some studies, more than one estimate of requirements is cited assuming alternative desirable occupancy rates (37, 39, 40). It is not clear, however, what is the basis for selection. Forsyth and Logan are particularly emphatic in condemning the application of a uniform occupancy rate, which would seem to assume that higher occupancies represent overcrowding rather than increased efficiency (41, p. 100). They also criticize the "implicit assumption that beds constitute the proper measure of capacity, or are the initial limiting factor as demand rises." They point out that the waiting list for surgery may be due to insufficient operating room facilities rather than surgical beds and, if so, is not remediable by additional beds. In support of this contention, Airth and Newell found, in their survey of Tees-side, that there was a surplus in beds allocated to ophthalmology in the presence of a long, and even growing, waiting list. They suggest that in this instance a shortage of staff placed a limit on bed use (40, pp. 36–37). A final implicit assumption—that all persons who are in the hospital need to be there—has been examined and found to be unwarranted by Forsyth and Logan, among many others, as we have described in a previous chapter. It is only fair to say, however, that the assumptions concerning bed capacity and appropriateness of use are not peculiar to the criterial number method, but are implicit in all the methods we have described so far. However, there is one adjustment made in some of these methods that the critical number method generally does not make: namely, the division of aggregate demand and capacity into individual hospitals and of hospitals into compartments. We have already discussed the relationship between the size of these subdivisions and the observed as well as the desirable capacity. However, when the critical number is determined for individual hospitals, or services within hospitals, an adjustment to size of facility is made implicitly because the standard error of demand is larger in relation to the mean when demand is small. As the reader will recall, twice this standard error is added to the critical number as one element in arriving at bed requirements.

A large number of considerations arise from the assumptions concerning demand and the actual properties of that demand. First, the procedure for deriving the critical number, as described above, makes it clear that concern is with current demand. Thus, additions to the waiting list are added to average daily admissions, but removals from the waiting list are subtracted. Second, there are certain assumptions about the distributional properties of current demand: that it is random, that seasonal fluctuations are absent or small, and that there is no secular trend. Thus, the method does not provide for epidemics. Seasonal fluctuations, if slow and not very large, "would lead to a build-up of a long waiting list when the demand was above the critical value, which would gradually be worked off when the demand fell again" (35, pp. 140–141). If seasonal fluctuations are "marked," the only efficient solution is to arrive at estimates for the different seasons and provide for corresponding differences in the bed complement. Perhaps more realistic is to accept some inefficiency by providing a larger bed complement. Bailey, who was statistician to the Northampton and Norwich Surveys, concludes as follows: "Until further investigations are made into the effect of a fluctuating level of demand, the best plan seems to be to estimate the critical numbers on the basis of a year's results and, unless there are marked seasonal variations, to provide a few extra beds" (38, p. 153). Trends in demand, which are almost always on the increase, would obviously lead to a periodic reassessment of the critical number. As we shall see below, growth between reassessments could possibly be adjusted to by changes in average length of stay.

The assumptions concerning length of stay are important and appear to have attained greater prominence in the later thinking of Bailey (37). One such assumption is that persons on the waiting list, when admitted to the hospital, would have an average length of stay equal to that of the current mix of patients. This may not be the case. During the period when the waiting list is being rather rapidly depleted through admissions, the observed length of stay may change in a direction that is not predictable on a priori grounds. More important than this, however, is whether normative or empirical standards are to be used in the computation of the critical number. As we have seen above, the critical number at 100 percent occupancy is the product of daily demand and length of stay. Both of these terms are generally measured empirically, thereby ignoring the likelihood of inappropriate use. However, there is no reason why both demand and length of stay could not be normatively defined in arriving at the critical number. Bailey offers one such example, which also includes adjustments for a normatively defined turnover interval (and, therefore, of a less than 100 percent occupancy). The example is based on demand for general surgery in the United Oxford Hospitals, England, 1959 (37). It is given in Table V.14, in modified form, because it may help the reader to see the method in more concrete form. In the example of Table V.14 the observed length of stay was considered by the surgeons to be too low, hence the bed requirements were to be increased. The reverse situation would probably be more common in the United States.

In addition to introducing adjustments for normative length of stay and turnover interval, Bailey has come to regard purposive variations in length of stay as a major, perhaps necessary, feature in the application of the critical number method, particularly in bringing about adjustments to rising trends in demand and, possibly, seasonal variation as well. In his own words:

We have based our calculations on attempting to supply exactly the number of beds needed to meet demand. Now in the mathematical theory of queueing (and it is essentially a queueing situation that we are dealing with) it usually happens that when supply and demand are *exactly* equal, the average length of the queue, or waiting list in our context, is infinite. But a reasonably short queue can be achieved merely by adding one or two units to the so-called "critical" number calculated as described above. This distinction has often been regarded as important in small specialties where the number of beds involved is also rather small. However, I now incline to the view that this small adjustment, though theoretically important, may easily fail to be effective in practice if the demand increases appreciably. It is probably better to have about the right number of beds but to ensure that a long queue does not build up by making the average length of stay at any time depend inversely on queue length . . . The question arises, of course, of how best to implement such a recommendation. While exact mathematical investigation would reveal the basic properties of the queueing process, it would probably be unnecessary in practice to employ any very elaborate methods of control. Indeed, it is my belief that, if the consultant [responsible physician] knew the exact state of affairs each day with regard to current waiting list,

Table V.14. Procedure for computing hospital bed requirements using the "critical number" method

---

1. Data
   - A. Number of "available" beds 183
   - B. Number of discharges, 1959 5,583
   - C. Number of waiting list, Dec. 31, 1958 1,413
   - D. Number on waiting list, Dec. 31, 1959 1,650
   - E. Average stay in days 9.8
   - F. Turnover interval in days 2.2
   - G. Percent occupancy 82

2. Standards
   - H. Desirable length of stay, in days 15
   - I. Desirable turnover interval, in days 2

3. Calculations
   - J. Change in waiting list, 1958–1959 $D - C = +237$
   - K. Total demand, 1959 $B + J = 5,820$
   - L. Critical number at 100 percent occupancy

   $$\frac{K \times E}{365} = \frac{5,820 \times 9.8}{365} = 156$$

   - M. Critical number using observed length of stay and turnover interval (yields an observed occupancy ratio of 82 percent)

   $$\frac{K\,(E + F)}{365} = \frac{5,820 \times 12}{365} = 191$$

   - N. Critical number using normative length of stay and turnover interval (yields an occupancy ratio of 88 percent)

   $$\frac{K\,(H + I)}{365} = \frac{5,820 \times 17}{365} = 272$$

SOURCE: Reference 37.

average length of stay, turnover interval etc., an adequate control could be effected on the basis of personal judgment alone. The information required could easily be produced by a fairly streamlined hospital records system, and a small number of control charts showing the present state of the service in each specialty should enable the consultant in charge to make the appropriate administrative adjustment needed (37, pp. 59, 64–65).

In order to deal with a large existing list, the critical number would be computed using the optimal length of stay, but the length of stay put into operation would initially be shorter than optimal and would gradually be increased to the optimal length. Thereafter, as demand increases, the length of stay could be progressively shortened, of course up to a limit. Although Bailey does not say so, a logical extension would be also to deal with seasonal variations in this manner. Bailey's proposals are hypothetical. As we have discussed in a previous chapter, empirical studies have, in fact, shown that length of stay may change as demand rises in relation to capacity. However, as Martin Feldstein has observed, both in England and in the United States, the response to increased demand seems to be more in the curtailment of admissions than in the reduction of length of stay (20, 22).

Another consideration of fundamental importance to the application of the critical number method is the handling of demand for emergency admissions. The method as described by Bailey, and applied by him and by others, makes no separate provision for those cases that require immediate admission, except indirectly, through allowing for lower levels of occupancy. However, at the suggestion of Bailey, Newell came up with a method that represents, to our knowledge, the first formal application of the properties of the Poisson distribution to the solution of this problem (31), antedating, by many years, the work of Blumberg (32). It would seem reasonable, therefore, to treat the demand for emergency care separately from other demand in applying the ''critical number method.'' Incidentally, this would further reduce the normative occupancy rate, since enough beds have to be provided so the risk of turning away an emergency patient is reduced to a specified limit. In the context of the critical number method, there can be no waiting list for emergency cases. Commentators on the critical number method, including Bailey himself, have recognized that this property applies also to other segments of demand, such as that for infectious disease and obstetrical services (37, 40). According to Airth and Newell, ''In certain specialties, no inpatient waiting list in the normal sense exists. Where none is possible, as in Infectious Diseases, the method degenerates into identification of 'demand' with 'supply.' Where, as in Obstetrics, no waiting list is possible, but a list of unsatisfied applicants is conceivable, the method might work. It would, however, need modification to use such a test, and in any case the routine characteristic of the method disappears since no such list is maintained in our hospitals'' (40, pp. 85–86). This characteristic of obstetrical demand was recognized by Bailey who, in the Norwich Survey, took demand for obstetrical care to be the same as the number admitted (38, p. 166).

In using the critical number method, the significance of the waiting list needs to be carefully considered. In a previous chapter we have commented on the validity of the waiting list and pointed out that many persons normally on the waiting list may no longer need (or demand) care because they have died, have moved, have recovered, have received care elsewhere, or are no longer desirous of receiving care. On the contrary, persons who have applied for care may have not been placed on a list or may have had their names prematurely removed. In certain, admittedly unusual, situations the waiting list may be generated by factors unrelated to bed capacity per se. For example, Airth and Newell have reported that the suspension of tonsillectomies during epidemics, particularly of poliomyelitis, can result in long waiting lists in the presence of an adequate supply of beds (40, p. 35). Perhaps more important is the situation to which we have alluded already, in which bed capacity is adequate but insufficient staff or ancillary services results in less than complete use of beds.

Several additional aspects of demand require careful evaluation. One point made by Airth and Newell is that the demands for the several specialties are not totally independent of each other, presumably because care in one can generate care in another or be substituted for another. This introduces inaccuracies when the critical number is estimated separately for each specialty, but not if all specialties are combined (40, p. 86). More important are inaccuracies in estimating the relationships between a population and the demand that it is likely to generate. Bailey has described two variants of his method: one adapted to estimation of current demand in an existing catchment area and another to estimating future demand in an area that has been newly defined. When current demand in an existing area serves as the basis for estimates of the critical number to be applied to estimating future requirements for that area, there arises the question of what Bailey has called "edge effects" (37, pp. 62–63). This is because the flow of patients into and out of the catchment basin, at its periphery, can change sufficiently to alter the demand for any given group of hospitals. This difficulty is more troublesome when planning is done piecemeal, by small areas, and is relatively less troublesome when the areas included are large. When demand is to be predicted for a catchment area that has been newly defined, it is necessary first to estimate the population served (as we have described in the preceding chapter) and then to apply to it some rate of expected demand. When the population served is itself derived from a sample estimate, the variance of this estimate has to be included in computing the variance of the critical number (see 36, p. 149, for method of computation).

Perhaps the most fundamental feature of the critical number method is that it is based on current demand which, by and large, is accepted to be legitimate and to reasonably represent need. One result of this, as Newell has shown, is that the estimated bed requirements in the several British Surveys that have used this method differ widely, but are closely correlated to the existing supply of beds in each of the areas surveyed (27, Table 1, p. 754). As Forsyth and Logan succinctly conclude, "It appears that the number of beds used is the number available!" (41, p. 101). One consequence of this observation is to question whether additions to the waiting list and, for that matter, admissions to the hospital, actually require the care that they seek. Alternatively, one may question, especially in areas of low bed supply, whether there is a portion of unexpressed demand that remains hidden or unsatisfied. However, when one questions whether a portion of expressed demand is legitimate and whether some demand remains unexpressed, it must be recognized that one has moved away from basing estimates on demand and has introduced some overriding concept of need, a position in which we have found ourselves repeatedly in our development of the critical number method.

UNEXPRESSED OR INAPPARENT DEMAND. Several of the studies that have used the critical number method have broadened their concern to include a survey of unexpressed or inapparent demand. Demand may remain unexpressed because, as Airth and Newell have pointed out, "the 'threshold' for admission may well depend upon the general practitioner's and consultant's knowledge of the availability of beds" (40, p. 75). Demand may be expressed, but inapparent, if, for example, patients are referred for care outside the hospital group and service area under study. One feature of the Norwich Survey was a poll of general practitioners "to discover whether the need for hospital care was being adequately met." Also,

the medical advisors sought the opinion of each consultant on the correct medical interpretation of the recorded demand on his department . . . As a result of these inquiries among the general practitioners and consultants it was believed that a true picture had been gained of the demand during 1951. The inquiry among general practitioners established the fact that from their point of view there was little unsatisfied demand for hospital care . . . the majority of cases requiring hospital care in fact received it; the discussions with the consultants confirmed that all the patients who received hospital care were properly hospital cases (38, p. 160–161).

Barr has reported a similar survey of family doctors in connection with the study of hospitals in the county borough of Reading, England. The physicians who responded did report some difficulty in having patients admitted and also having to refer patients to hospitals outside the group, both occurrences varying by whether the physicians practiced within the city or in the surrounding area (39). Airth and Newell have also reported expressions of dissatisfaction by general practitioners concerning access to beds, but were unable to interpret these in "numerical terms" (40, p. 78). Forsyth and Logan report that in Barrow there was no evidence that "waiting-lists (which are short anyway) were in any way suppressing demand" (41, p. 99). It appears that, in general, surveys of general practitioners have not revealed unexpressed or inapparent demand sufficiently large to influence estimates of bed requirements. However, Forsyth and Logan have questioned the validity of the results obtained.

It is difficult to know what value to give to enquiries of this kind. These enquiries are really opinion polls and attitude surveys, and as such are valuable if deficiencies are so marked that general practitioners are immediately conscious of them; but in none of the areas where these enquiries have been carried out has this proved to be the case. General practitioners are no more able than anyone else to think outside the confines of their everyday task and environment (41, pp. 99–100).

The same criticism can be made of the too facile conclusion that all admissions to hospital are justified.

LATENT SERVICE RESERVE. In the preceding chapter we have discussed in detail the general issue of defining and measuring unnecessary resource use and the "misclassification" associated with it. All we need to do here is to point out that to the extent that there is concealed or inapparent capacity of this kind, estimates for additional resources can be reduced, provided misused capacity can be released for more appropriate use. This condition is very important. In many instances it may be more realistic to assume that current levels of misclassification will continue. On the other hand, overuse of a given resource may increase owing to the reduction of financial and other barriers, or decrease owing to provision of and providing access to substitute services.

Forsyth and Logan have reported that in the Barrow group of hospitals there was sufficient unnecessary hospital use in general medicine, general surgery, and pediatrics to permit reduction of the critical number of beds for these services by 15 percent and the total bed requirements for all services by 8 percent (41, pp. 95, 99). While Forsyth and Logan describe the manner in which unnecessary use was identified, they do not give the details of the computation that convert their measure of patient misclassification into a corrected estimate of bed requirements. Two computational approaches are possible: one is to obtain data on the number of patient-days of necessary or unnecessary use, and the other to obtain a revised estimate of the daily census. Data on patient-days require longitudinal study. Cross-sectional studies of misclassification, such as those that determine the proportion of patients who need to be in the hospital on a given day, do not provide data on patient-days of unnecessary care. They can, however, provide estimates of a corrected daily census.

The Division of Hospital and Medical Facilities of the U.S. Public Health Service suggests a method that assumes knowledge about patient-days of unnecessary use but does not describe how this information is obtained. The method for arriving at a revised estimate of bed requirements is an extension of the one already described in a previous section and summarized in Table V.7 (29, p. 27). The following steps are involved.

1. It has been determined that 90 percent of patient days in the medical-surgical and pediatric services are appropriate and that practically all the patient-days in obstetrics are appropriate.

2. Reduce by 10 percent the estimated yearly patient days for the pediatric and medical-surgical services (items J and K, Table V.7).

3. Use these new estimates of patient-days to obtain a revised estimate of average daily census (by dividing by 365).

4. Convert average daily census figures to beds, by dividing by the desirable occupancy ratio (0.75 for pediatrics and 0.85 for the medical-surgical services).

   If it is assumed that all the patient days of care that do not require general hospital resources do, nevertheless, require the services of a long-term facility, the following further adjustments are made.

5. Convert patient-days of care that do not require general hospital care (10 percent of items J and K, Tables V.7) into the corresponding daily census (by dividing by 365).

6. Convert this average daily census figure to beds by dividing by the desirable occupancy ratio for long-term facilities (0.95).

7. Add this number of beds to the original estimate of requirements for long-term facility beds (item V, Table V.7).

An alternative method, using average daily census data and the properties of the Poisson distribution will be illustrated below.

PATIENT CLASSIFICATION. An extension of the studies that attempt to separate ''necessary'' from ''unnecessary'' care are those that adopt some system for classifying patients by level of care and corresponding resource, thus matching the needs of patients to the resources equipped to meet these needs. We have discussed this category of studies, in fair detail, in a previous chapter. In this section we shall focus on procedural aspects of arriving at estimates of resource requirements by describing studies that illustrate variants of method.

White et al. (42) and Preston et al. (43) have described facets of a survey that attempted to estimate bed requirements for a university hospital to be organized, by level of care, into the following units: intensive care, intermediate care, self-care, long-term care, observation ward care, and overnight care. The problem was to examine current demand for the services of the hospital, both inpatient and outpatient, and to translate these, first into normatively defined categories of demand, and then to corresponding bed equivalents for inpatient care. To achieve the first objective, a 9-week survey was conducted. On each of 63 successive days there were taken (1) a 10 percent random sample of hospital beds stratified by ward; (2) a 10 percent sample of patients in the larger outpatient clinics and a 50 percent sample of those in the smaller clinics; and (3) a 10 percent sample of the emergency-room case load. For each patient in the sample, those persons ordinarily responsible for making decisions about the disposition of the patients (generally the resident or intern) indicated the appropriate level of care. Conversion of the resulting data, on the daily sample or roster of number of patients by level of care, into bed-estimates involved some of the following considerations. In the hospital sample, "The items sampled each day were 'patient care days'; the same bed and the same patient occasionally recurred in several samples. This was assumed to reflect the true distribution of patient care needs and bed utilization in the hospital" (42, p. 49). In other words, the daily sample of hospital beds was considered to yield an equivalent sample of partial daily censuses for each level of care (partial because it was yet to be supplemented by admissions from the ambulatory care sample). As to the daily ambulatory care (outpatient and emergency services) samples, the patients who each day were thought to need overnight care were considered to be equal to the daily census of the overnight facility. Presumably, this is because the overnight facility may be considered to have an average length of stay of one day. There is some ambiguity about how the daily demand for the other inpatient facilities that was generated from the ambulatory care samples was converted to its equivalent in daily census. This is because each patient identified in the daily ambulatory care sample is sampled only once (unlike the hospital beds), but each patient who is considered to require care in any level of facility other than overnight care, generates days of care, and an average daily census, equal to the average length of stay in days, for that category of care. Hence, one either needs information about average length of stay or must admit patients from the ambulatory case load to the hospital and include them in the hospital sample. In any event, the procedures described above yield 63 partially hypothetical daily censuses for each category of inpatient service. These censuses can then be transformed into bed requirements if one specifies some normative level of occupancy. One could conceivably apply a ''desirable occupancy rate'' for each facility. One might use the actual distribution of daily censuses observed to set a level of probability of each inpatient unit being filled not more often than a specified number of days out of 100 or 1000. One might compute the mean of 63 observations for each category of beds and, assuming each distribution to be Poisson in type, use the appropriate probabilities to set the kind of limit described above. White et al. found that, in fact, the daily demand for the overnight facility was not significantly different from a Poisson distribution (42). There is no information on the shape of the distribution for the other subcategories of demand that collectively constitute the ''progressive care'' spectrum in this study.

The Division of Hospital and Medical Facilities of the U.S. Public Health Service has offered a method for determining estimated bed requirements in each unit of a hospital organized along the lines of ''progressive patient care'' (44). In addition to assuming that demand for almost all the subunits is Poisson-distributed, an important feature of the method is the provision of ''flexible care zones'' which reduce compartmentalization and, correspondingly, increase the capacity of any one unit to handle fluctuations in demand for the level of care it provides. The publication describes a method for conducting a survey of hospital patients that results in data on daily census by three levels of care: intensive care, intermediate care and self-care. Given these estimates of average daily census, the conversion to bed requirements proceeds as follows:

A. The size of the intensive care unit is equal to the estimated average census for this unit. This yields approximately 90 percent occupancy.

B. The size of the intermediate care unit equals the estimated average daily census for this unit. This also yields approximately 90 percent occupancy.

C. Provide for a "flexible care zone" between intensive and intermediate care units (using a Poisson probability table) that adds beds sufficient to contain the daily census of the intensive care unit on all but one day a month.

D. Provide for "flexible beds" for the entire hospital based on the average daily census of the intensive and intermediate care units combined, using the same rule and procedure as in C.

E. The number of "flexible beds" between the intermediate and self-care units equals D minus C.

F. The number of beds in the self-care unit equals total hospital capacity minus (average daily census of intensive care unit plus average daily census of intermediate care unit plus total flexible beds). This equals Totals beds— $(A + B + C + E)$. It is clear that the number of self-care beds is a residual. In the words of the report, "The number of basic self-care beds is somewhat arbitrary. Since this segment of the census is largely elective, the laws of probability which affect the other census are not operative and administrative policy can dominate" (44, p. 10).

In summary, what this method yields is a redistribution of the current case load of a hospital. It is assumed that there is no waiting list and no unexpressed or inapparent demand. However, modifications could easily be introduced to meet these features should they exist.

Fetter and Thompson have used a simulation technique to reconstruct the daily censuses in the several units of a "progressive care" hospital (45). An additional important feature of their approach is that it goes beyond the estimation of bed requirements by dealing with the problem of allocation, given scarce resources—which is a matter of considerably greater complexity that we shall not discuss. To set up the simulation, data were obtained from Manchester Hospital, a pioneer of the "progressive care" mode of organization. The object was to determine empirically the frequency with which patients were admitted to each of the several units in the progressive care spectrum and the paths they followed as they moved from unit to unit, until discharge. There were 129 such paths, but a network of 22 paths was found to be sufficient to model patient flow. In fact, in most instances, patients experienced care in only one or very few units. It was also found that holding time in each unit was a function of both the patient path and the unit. That is, "the probability of change does vary a great deal, not only with where the patient is in the system at a given time, but according to what zone of care he occupied before then and the zone of care to which he was originally admitted" (45, p. 455). Since the probabilities of moving from one unit to another were not independent of prior states, a Markovian model could not be used to predict the census in each unit. However, "such a hospital can be described by a network of patient paths where the holding time at each node is a probability distribution which is a function of both the patient path and the node" (45, pp. 455–456). A simulation using the 22 most frequent paths produced probabilities of occupancy of the beds in each unit. By setting up the simulation without limits on the possible number of beds in each unit, the results represented "the maximum number of beds which would ever be used.'' However, since data from an actual hospital were used, it would seem that the characteristics of that hospital, and the manner in which it is used, have introduced constraints that have shaped the observed pathways and the probabilities of their occurrence. The applicability of the findings to other communities and hospitals can therefore be questioned. But the study, in addition to illustrating a method for estimating bed requirements through simulation, constitutes a valuable contribution to our understanding of how ''progressive patient care'' actually works.

Normative Content of Estimates Based on Demand

In setting the stage for the discussion in this chapter we recognized two major orientations that guide the preparation of estimates for service and resource requirements: one based on demand and the other on need. In theory, the demand approach is empirical, geared to what is or is likely to be, while the need approach is normative, concerned with what ought to be, now and in the future. In practice, one finds in the estimates based on demand varying degrees of normative concern that should be recognized if one is to arrive at a proper appreciation of these methods.

At the most fundamental level, the argument that demand should determine the aggregate level as well as the distribution of services and resources is itself a value position linked to the tenets of laissez-faire economics and the libertarian tradition, as we have discussed in our opening chapter. But what is more interesting, is that over this foundation one may find layers that modify or contradict the foundation. For example, when it is assumed that future services and resources will bear the same relationship to population characteristics as they do now, or have done in the recent past, except that there shall be no change in relative prices, a value assumption may have been made. The assumption is that the present relationship between demand and the supply of services shall be, or should be, maintained. This may be because the present situation is regarded as at least acceptable, or perhaps, adequate. Unless one wishes to preserve the present situation as at least tolerable, there is no reason why one may not postulate that prices will rise steeply so as to suppress a portion of potential demand and significantly alter its distribution (86). Another example of the confounding of normative and empirical considerations, in arriving at estimates of resource requirements is the proposal by Rosenthal that the aggregate number of hospital beds might be set through the application of some standard of adequacy, but that the distribution of beds among states should be in accordance with demand. As Rosenthal himself has recognized, the need and demand orientations become even more openly confounded when one retains demand as the criterion for estimating requirements, but sets out to alter the level and distribution of demand through manipulations of income, price, or both (11).

Further normative considerations are very likely to come into the estimates at the point where demand and resource capacity are adjusted to one another. The values that are introduced do tend to be technical, but are not without important social implications. For example, when it is required that capacity be fully used and that unnecessary care be curtailed or eliminated, the standards introduced are those of efficiency and appropriateness. But these are also social values that pertain to the prudent use of social capability and the pursuit of individual and collective welfare.

It is clear that the separation between demand-oriented and need-oriented methods is far from absolute. Notions of need creep into methods ostensibly based on demand. As we shall see in our next section, considerations more or less rooted in empirical observations of demand are often part of methods apparently based on need.

METHODS BASED PRIMARILY ON NEED

Classification and General Description

The distinguishing characteristic of the methods we are about to describe is that they explicitly or implicitly take as their point of departure some notion of need and pursue the social objective of bringing about satisfaction of that need. They must begin, therefore, with some measure of need. What is taken to be the measure of need varies considerably and may serve to classify the various studies. We have defined need, fundamentally, in terms of conditions and situations requiring care. Estimates of service and resource requirements may, in fact, begin with data on the occurrence of such conditions and situations, including morbidity, mortality, pregnancy, childbirth, and the like. Very frequently, in the cruder methods of estimation, need is measured in a summary or proxy fashion. As in measurements of demand, the aggregate number of people may be taken to represent need. Somewhat more refined are the methods that account for different levels of need among different population subgroups. Thus, the population may be subcategorized by age, sex, occupation, and so on. For example, Rozenfeld suggests that different estimation standards might be developed for preschool children, school children, adolescents, and athletes, and proceeds to estimate the service and resource requirements of children in crèches and children's homes (5). The institutional linkage is of particular interest because it represents a category of studies in which need is defined in institutional rather than personal terms—a form of what might be called "derived need," analogous to the well-established notion of derived demand. In fact, the analogies between the indirect measures of need and of demand are clearly apparent. Some of the same things may be taken to represent potential to generate either need or demand, depending on which orientation one wishes to impose upon the procedures that follow.

Since need is fundamentally a normative concept, a major differentiating aspect of need-oriented methods is the nature of the standards used to convert measures of need into their equivalents in services and resources. Perhaps the most important distinguishing characteristic of standards is their derivation. In this context, the first question might be: Whose standards? The answer is that, almost invariably, the standards are those defined by professionals with little attention to the perceptions, wishes, and desires of clients. Thus, though the methods based on need are more egalitarian than those based on demand, in the process of paying more attention to client welfare they may give less attention to the hierarchism in client preferences. In their derivation, the professional standards used in need-oriented studies may be normative or empirical. Normatively derived standards rest on what professionals who are regarded to be qualified, or authoritative, believe or assert to be the service or resource equivalents of need. Empirically derived standards rest on observed experience in which need is judged to be appropriately satisfied, again using mainly professional judgment to make the determination.

Normatively derived estimates of service equivalents of need are a feature of many studies that we shall describe later. Here we shall discuss some general features of such standards. One important feature is the extent to which the judgments are representative, on the one hand of professional norms, and on the other hand of the nature of need in the real world. The first kind of representativeness has to do with the choice of professional judges and the validity and reliability of their estimates, subjects to be discussed below. The second kind of representativeness has to do with the manner in which conditions or situations that represent need are selected prior to the application of professional judgments to them. In one category of studies actual samples of persons or patients, more or less representative, are examined by experts who arrive at estimates of need and of service equivalents. Several of the studies that we shall describe subsequently are of this kind. These include the study of general service needs of population samples by the Commission on Chronic Illness (46), the study of home nursing needs by Mickey (56), and the study of post-hospital care by Greenlick et al. (47). In a second category of studies, estimates are based on the professional person's recollection of some average patient or a representative mix of patients, a kind of recollected composite, or memory sample. The distinction we are making is well illustrated by two separate studies of the requirements for renal dialysis, one by Lipworth (50) and the other by Hallan and Harris (51). In the first, information was collected about an actual sample of deaths, and expert judgments made on the suitability of each case for dialysis. In the second, panels of physicians were asked to estimate, for each of a list of diagnostic designations, (1) upper- and lower-bound estimates of the percent who might have had irreversible uremia among those who die from the disease, and (2) the percent of those with uremia who had a primary condition or complications that precluded dialysis. Other studies that have used such essentially hypothetical, though not necessarily unrealistic, samples include the classic work of Lee and Jones (59), its more recent replication and considerable further development by Falk, Schonfeld, and their associates (60–65), and the study by Kalimo and Sievers (58), in which they develop a scale of need. Lee and Jones, as well as Kalimo and Sievers, give estimates of need or of service equivalents for some average patient based on memory. The Falk and Schonfeld reports give, on the same basis, frequency distributions of service equivalents as well as measures of central tendency. This represents a distinct advance over the prototype Lee-Jones study. Only Schonfeld has dealt explicitly with the characteristics of what we have called the "recollected or memory sample" and pursued its implications for arriving at estimates of requirements (65). In the studies that he reports, physicians were given a choice of four categories of patients, any one of which they could use as a basis for constructing normative standards. As it turned out, almost all the primary physicians who dealt with disease in adults, and the majority of those who dealt with disease in children, constructed standards of service that related to a recollected population of new cases who had not hitherto received care and who had actually sought medical attention. Obviously, this is only part of the spectrum of disease as we have discussed it in a previous chapter. Furthermore, there may be a bias based on the individual physician's experience, since each physician may see a different "average" patient or range of patients. Needless to say, when standards differ by category of patients, one must know the mix of patients before one can apply the standards to any actual population group. Schonfeld describes a method for converting normative standards for specified categories of patients to standards for a population in a steady state with respect to the categories in question (65). Another problem in dealing with recollected samples of need is the difficult one of arriving at standards for the care of more than one illness that might occur simultaneously. The effect of such co-presence could be partially additive, additive, or more than additive. (Neither Lee and Jones nor Falk, Schonfeld and their associates have dealt with this matter.) Quite arbitrarily, Kalimo and Sievers assigned to such situations the normative service equivalents of the condition with the highest equivalents. This was on the assumption that care for the lesser condition would be included in the care of the major one (58).

In all normative standards, whether based on empirically observed or on recollected samples, there are serious questions of reliability and validity. These are quite analogous to considerations of reliability and validity of patient classification judgments that we have discussed in the preceding chapter, and the judgments of appropriateness of care that the author has reviewed in another publication (89, pp. 81–93). These issues are relevant at the very outset when the professionals who are to formulate standards are selected. Should these be representative professionals or professionals who are unusually qualified? The choice is generally in favor of the second alternative, although attempts may also be made to include attributes that are thought to improve the validity or generalizability of the standards. Lee and Jones appear to have sought some safety in numbers by polling more than 125 physicians (59, p. vii). Kalimo and Sievers used both numbers (10 physicians) and representation of several specialists on their team of judges. The physicians found the task of converting diagnostic categories into estimates of need for care "relatively difficult," but incomplete estimates were very few. Average intercorrelation between the estimates of 10 judges was about 0.50, with a range, by type of need, from 0.19 to 0.59. The reliability of the final scores (which will be described below) rose to a level exceeding 0.90 (58). Falk, Schonfeld, et al. took pains to combine expertise with realism by selecting physicians who were affiliated with a university medical center but were also in private practice. They do recognize, nevertheless, that their standards might not be universally applicable. In their first paper they describe the care they took to obtain what they considered valid estimates. For each condition, several physicians were interviewed at length, the number varying according to the nature of the disease. "The results are reviewed and composited, presenting areas of consensus and retaining diversities of opinion where these are regarded as well founded, justified and significant by the senior review physician" (60, p. 1122). The retention of data on variability of opinion represents another advance over the prototype Lee-Jones study. Several representative examples are cited. Among five physicians interviewed, the estimate of the percent of patients with myocardial infarction who required only one visit for diagnosis ranged from 90 to 70 percent, with a mean of 82 percent and a standard error of 4 percent (60, p. 1122). The importance of using several judges is illustrated by the observation that one out of five internist primary physicians said that 50 percent of cases with cancer of the large intestine and rectum should be referred to a chemotherapist, whereas the average for all five was 10 percent (62). In addition to such idiosyncratic variability, there were systematic differences in perspective. For example, internist primary physicians felt they could handle 97 percent of myocardial infarction and 98 percent of essential hypertension. By contrast, internist cardiologists believed that only 80 percent of cases in each category could be handled fully by the internist primary physician without referral to a cardiologist for diagnosis or treatment (62). Such differences are not confined to physicians. Mickey, in her study of home nursing needs, arranged for "double interviews" for a portion of her sample, during which one nurse would conduct the interview while another would listen and record independent judgments. This procedure, which may not constitute completely independent replication, demonstrated that there was "remarkable agreement on judgments for intensity of need and capacity to cope," but that "there was significant difference between interviewers on whether to refer the families for nursing service" (56, p. 1049). Differences were much more marked between the judgments of the research team and the nurses in the service agency, the degree of agreement varying by category of need. "For the most part, in nearly all categories, the interviewers judged needs to be more serious than the staff nurses." In cases where needs were judged by the former to be moderate, serious or critical, there was only 55 percent agreement. The rest were judged by the service nurses to be "slight" (56, pp. 1055–1056). These discrepancies may represent the differences between the research and service perspectives. In any event, these and similar findings demonstrate the problems of between-observer variability, and of validity, in the formulation of normative standards, whether on the basis of recollected or actually observed samples. In none of the studies reviewed has the author encountered data on within-judge reliability.

A consideration, related to that of validity, is the stability of normatively derived standards, or any other kind of standard. Those who have developed such standards have recognized their essentially temporary and contingent nature. Lee and Jones, for example, express this thought as follows. ''The need for medical care is compounded of two constantly changing factors: the science and art of medicine on the one hand; on the other, the changing expectancy of disease . . . It is therefore impossible to determine once and for all time the services which will represent an adequate application of medical knowledge and skill to the needs of the people'' (59, p. 10). Falk, Schonfeld, et al. include an even wider range of factors that may alter current standards and estimates when they say: ''Nor do we at this time attempt to anticipate the future impacts of changes in composition of population, morbidity, technology, insurance practices, health education, economic resources, or social policies on either need or provision of medical care'' (60, p. 1133). Although instability is a feature of all standards, whether normatively or empirically derived, the latter are generally easier to revise or to keep current.

Unlike normatively derived standards which rest on what experts believe ought to be done, empirically derived standards flow from what is observed to occur under situations that are defined as, or judged to be, acceptable or optimal. In other words, they rest on demand, but within a normative or evaluative context. The simplest such standard is to postulate that current levels of demand, or of supply, are acceptable, and that they should be maintained in the future. Under this premise the need-oriented and demand-oriented studies almost coincide. They do not fully coincide because of differences in basic assumptions. For example, when the Surgeon General's Consultant Group on Medical Education (Frank Bane, chairman) recommended that the physician population ratio in 1975 be maintained so it equalled that in 1959, it considered many of the factors that might influence need, demand, and the capacity to provide service, but hoped that the changes in these would cancel each other, so that the same physician : population ratio would still be reasonably satisfactory (72).

Another way of deriving an empirical standard is to postulate that the higher segment in an observed range of demand is both preferred and demonstrably possible of attainment, and therefore should be the standard for all. For example, demand in the highest quartile of states or in the highest socioeconomic group in a population may be set as a standard, even though it is known that, normatively speaking, there is likely to be increase in inappropriate as well as appropriate utilization as the aggregate level of demand rises. One encounters many examples of this procedure for setting standards, especially in the older studies of manpower and hospital bed requirements. One standard proposed by the

National Health Assembly was that the physician : population ratio in 1960 be equal to the average physician : population ratio in the highest 12 states in 1940 (69). Among the goals for 1960 proposed by the President's Commission on the Health Needs of the Nation was "to bring the lower regions of the country to the 1949 national average of 131 per 100,000 civilian population." Another, more ambitious goal, was to provide for the United States in 1960, the same physician : population ratio (166 per 100,000) that prevailed in the New England and Central Atlantic States in 1949. This assumed "that the over-all physician-population ratio achieved by a wide area with a long history of generally high economic and education levels and with a relatively good supply of health facilities is a reasonable goal for the rest of the country" (71, pp. 184–185). As Dickinson pointed out many years ago, a deficit in resources is certain to be found when this method is used to formulate the standard, since some states have their provision of resources raised, but none have it reduced (4). According to Klarman : "This is not erroneous per se, if there are acceptable reasons for designating the selected point as the standard. But what do we know of the adequacy of medical care at the selected points, A, B, or C? There have been no detailed studies of their medical resources, how they are employed and the extent to which they are kept busy, on the one hand, and need, on the other hand" (2, pp. 637–638). The answer is that more physicians may be assumed to be better than few physicians until one considers how well additional physicians are being used and what has been given up in order to make possible the increment in physician supply.

Klarman has reviewed the arguments that bear on whether need or demand should be the basis for estimates of service and resource requirements and has concluded that the basis should be neither a normatively and abstractly defined need, nor simply demand, but something in between, namely an operationally or empirically defined level of need. According to Klarman, demand measured under specified conditions yields such a measure of need.

The standard of need is best measured under these conditions : (1) services are comprehensive in scope; (2) they are available to a population of known age and sex composition; (3) they are fully used by patients, because there are no obstacles to the recipient of an additional individual service; (4) total services are subject to over-all supervision by physicians; (5) the limit on total services rendered is set by the available medical resources that can be purchased at reasonable prices by a known outlay; (6) the size of the outlay must be related to the economic capacity of the population served. These conditions are met when a medical group renders comprehensive services to subscribers of average means who prepay for their care (2, pp. 636–637).

Accordingly, Klarman suggests that the physician : subscriber ratio in the Health Insurance Plan of Greater New York (HIP), which at that time was 125 physicians per 100,000, might serve as a standard of requirements, after corrections were made for the time such physicians gave to patients who were not plan subscribers. Some important projections of manpower requirements have, in fact, used experience in prepaid group practice, or comparable situations, as the basis for estimation. One example is included in the projections made in 1953 by the President's Commission on the Health Needs of the Nation. According to the Commission's report, "Data from prepayment plans and other studies indicate that to provide adequate medical care to individuals requires on the average about one physician for each 1,000 people . . . Los Alamos . . . provided full dental care to 10,000 people, including children, with nine dentists, two hygienists, one dental technician, one dental roentgenologist, and nine dental assisants" (71, pp. 183–184, 185–186). More recently, the Public Health Service proposed staffing patterns in prepaid group practice as one standard of manpower requirements, as shown in Table V.15 (73). The application of such standards to the general population raises some questions because the number of physicians is influenced by the particular mode of financing and organization in the group practice setting.

It is interesting to note the degree of correspondence between our classification of the derivation of standards and that offered by others. Burkens believes that methods for estimating service and resource requirements are most highly developed in Russia (6). If so, the classification by Popov is of special interest (7). First, Popov distinguishes "public health norms" from "public health estimating standards," in line with a recommendation of the Eighteenth World Health Assembly of 1965. Norms are "arrived at by scientific research," whereas "standards are empirically established" (7, p. 42). In this context "empirical" appears to mean "arbitrary" rather than "based on experience," as we have used the term. Popov goes on to say that norms may be derived in one of three ways: "the statistical method," "the expert method," and the "experimental method." The "statistical method" uses practice or experience in "so-called 'pilot towns' or districts . . . in which the community's out-patient and hospital requirements are most fully met." Obviously, this corresponds to our category of empirical standards derived under near-optimal conditions. Under the "expert method" two variants are recognized, which may also represent a sequence (7). The first variant, or stage, consists in collecting data on known morbidity and use in a specified population and making adjustments for "unsatisfied

Table IV.15. Average number of physicians per 100,000 persons in six medical groups, by specialty

Specialty	Average Number of Physicians per 100,000[a]	
	Mean	Median
All specialties	109.4	
Internal medicine	45.2	44.9
Allergy	1.6	1.4
Dermatology	2.8	2.5
Pediatrics	18.0	15.8
Obstetrics	9.1	8.0
Orthopedics	3.2	3.0
Ophthalmology	3.7	3.3
Otolaryngology	4.6	3.5
Surgery	6.5	6.7
Urology	1.9	1.5
Radiology	4.4	4.0
Physical medicine	1.3	1.0
Anesthesiology	1.5	1.5
Pathology	1.8	1.6
Neurology	1.0	1.0
Psychiatry	2.8	1.5

SOURCE: Reference 73, Appendix Table 6, page 75.

[a] Numbers of physicians exclude interns and residents in hospitals. The table is based on unpublished information for different years from the Kaiser Foundation (2 groups), HIP, Montefiore, Group Health Association (D.C.), and Rip Van Winkle. Data for physical medicine based on 3 groups, anesthesiology on 2 groups, and pathology and neurology on 4 groups. These services are provided in the remaining groups in other ways.

demand." The second variant, or stage, involves actual examination of population samples and estimation of need by "practising doctors" and "qualified specialists brought from the outside." It is quite clear that Popov's "expert method" corresponds to our category of normatively derived standards using actual samples. Popov's third category, the "experimental method," apparently has to do with extrapolating from restricted experimental or demonstration programs to larger populations. It would appear to fit in our category of empirically derived norms and could well correspond to the extrapolation from the experience of a group practice to the population at large (7, pp. 44–45).

To return to our own classification, the reader will have noted that the distinction we have drawn between normatively derived and empirically derived standards, while useful, is not absolute. Empirically derived standards appear to rest on demand under normatively defined situations.

Analogously, there are often implicit empirical elements in normatively derived standards. Such standards are seldom formulated, as Klarman seems to have feared, in terms that accord health needs unrealistically complete primacy over all other needs (2). For example, Lee and Jones aimed

to present a conservative and reasonable standard which members of the medical profession regard as sufficient and appropriate. No attempt has been made to catalogue all desirable medical services which might be rendered in a society exclusively devoted to the pursuit of health; nor have the requirements of good practice been kept to an absolute minimum. "Luxury" services now widely consumed are omitted; on the other hand, some services which are not at present demanded even by very wealthy people are included as essential to good medical care. Our standards call for no more than a general application of good current practice (59, p. 11).

Perhaps to assure realism, Lee and Jones obtained not only the opinions of experts, but also records of their practice. The fact that the Lee-Jones estimates revealed a relatively small deficit in aggregate physician supplies and an excess in nursing manpower supports the realism of their standards. Similar emphasis on realism, or empirical experience, is to be found in the work of Falk, Schonfeld, et al. In their words:

Each physician is asked not to describe ideal or extravagant care. He is asked to consider, but not to be bound to, the care presently given—which may be influenced and modified by many interfering factors such as costs and ability to pay, convenience to the patient or to the physician, acceptability by the patient, the organizational patterns of the services, or the actual availability of personnel and facilities . . . This may be described as the type of care that can be offered in urban communities with, or within convenient reach of, comprehensive facilities and resources for medical care; maybe this is the same as saying 'practical ideal' rather than 'idealistic' medical care (60, pp. 1122 and 1135).

Somewhat similarly, in the study by Kalimo and Sievers, "The physicians were requested expressly to base estimates upon what they considered to be an average Finnish patient's need for medically motivated and recommendable care in each diagnostic category. Their decisions were to be based on experience. It was emphasized particularly that the estimates should *not* be based on *patients'* usual behavior in seeking care" (58, pp. 2–3). In spite of such instructions, it is likely that physicians set their standards at varying levels in the continuum between "practical" and "ideal."

The experiential content of normatively derived standards relates, of course, to a more general characteristic that applies to all standards, namely, the level at which they are set. Russian planners, perhaps faced with the problem of allocating limited resources in a systematic manner, appear to have given the greatest explicit attention to this matter. Popov distinguishes two levels of norms: "optimal" and "intermediate," or "limited" (7). Rozenfeld, another Russian, recognized three categories: "optimal," "limited," and "average" (5). The last category appears to be a statistical rather than an ordinal or hierarchical concept. It simply recognizes that the level of resources in a region may include optimal provision in some areas and much less than optimal levels in others. In the United States the notion of standards at several levels of stringency finds expression in studies that have made alternative estimates of requirements under different sets of assumptions. In 1949 the National Health Assembly offered estimates of physician requirements for 1960 using three different goals. The highest estimate was 11 percent higher than the lowest (68). A few years later, the President's Commission on the Health Needs of the Nation offered as many as six levels of objectives, resulting in estimates of physician requirements for 1960 that ranged from 227,000 to 292,000, a difference of 13 percent (71). Mountin et al. were able to divide the United States into 126 "provisional health service regions" which, when arrayed from high to low, revealed that about one-fourth of persons lived in regions with a physician : population ratio of 146 per 100,000 or more, one-third lived in regions with a physician : population ratio of 136 per 100,000 or more, and one-half lived in regions with a physician : population ratio of 118 per 100,000 or more. Using these figures (146, 136, and 118) as alternative standards, requirements for 1960 for active nonfederal physicians were estimated to be 241,172, 229,785, and 213,532 respectively, the highest estimate exceeding the lowest by about 11 percent (70).

Germane to the notion of graded standards is the possibility of attaching priorities to normative estimates of need equivalents, so that they can be implemented in a stepwise fashion. Cordero has shown how "minimum adequate" standards can be formulated and translated into arrangements for the staffing and operation of ambulatory care services when resources are very limited (8). However, no multilevel set of weighted standards has been encountered in the literature. This may be because physicians are more comfortable in assuming that patients should always receive all that medical science can offer, even though many would agree that in the real world this is not always the case.

There are two characteristics of standards that are often related, though they are conceptually separate. One is the degree of detail in the standard and the other the extent of prior validation. An example of detailed standards, which have also been subjected to a fair degree of validation, are those that convert disease categories into service requirements and the latter into requirements for resources. This detailed procedure can, of course, eventuate in a summary index—for example, that 142 physicians and 462 general hospital beds are needed per 100,000 of a population with specified characteristics (59). There are other standards of a summary nature that do not rest on any validated base but simply represent custom or convention. Often, their origin and rationale are obscure, undefined, or insufficiently validated. Generally, they are used to convert persons into their equivalents in resources, omitting in the process the intermediate stage of service equivalents. The original Hill-Burton standards for general hospital beds might serve as an example. The number of beds per 1,000 persons differed by type of area and density of population, as shown in Table V.16. It would be

Table V.16.   Proposed Hill-Burton guidelines for the provision of general hospital beds, type of areas, and density of population, U.S.A., 1946

Type of Area	Persons per Square Mile		
	12.0 or more	6.1–11.9	6.0 and less
Base	4.5	5.0	5.5
Intermediate	4.0	4.5	5.0
Rural	2.5	3.0	3.5

SOURCE: Reference 80, page 19.

useful to have an accepted terminology that differentiated the several kinds of standards that result from combinations of degree of detail and validation. As we have seen, Popov uses "norms" for those standards that are "arrived at by scientific research," and "estimating standards" for those that are "empirically established" (7). One might also refer to these categories as "validated" versus "arbitrary," or "rule-of-thumb." The other dimension—of detail—has also been recognized. Burkens, for example, speaks of "global methods" such as those that use a bed:population ratio to arrive at requirements for hospitals (6). In this context one might speak of "detailed" versus "summary" standards. All this is somewhat tentative, and is made more uncertain by the observation that the distinctions being made are sometimes not in the standard but in the manner in which the standard is used. For example, the Lee-Jones or the Hill-Burton summary standards might be shown to rest on valid foundations, but be used in an "arbitrary," or "rule-of-thumb," manner in situations where they do not properly apply.

A final characteristic of standards is their prescriptive aspect—that is, the extent to which they are taken to be compelling rules or merely guidelines for planning. Reed and Hollingsworth point out that the Hill-Burton standards were only intended to be "limits beyond which the Federal Government would not participate in hospital construction in any State." However, "the ceilings have, through force of Federal regulations and instructions to State agencies, tended to become established as definite and fixed standards of bed needs" (80, pp. 1–2). As Burkens puts it, "Russian authorities are convinced that with elaborate research, definite standard requirements can be formulated, and that these requirements are definitely determined by social and economic laws, as they are by morbidity patterns." This is in contrast to the "orientation indices" which are used in Czechoslovaka, apparently only to guide the planning of health services (6, p. 113).

So far, we have suggested that need-oriented methods for estimating service and resource requirements can be differentiated according to (1) the phenomena that they use to measure need, and (2) the characteristics of the standards that they use to convert need into its service or resource equivalents. Standards can be differentiated according to representativeness, derivation, degree of detail and validation, level and prescriptiveness. Need-oriented methods can also be differentiated according to the paths they traverse in arriving at their estimates. The reader will recall our discussion of the major "transformation pathways" in the introductory section of this chapter. A review of that discussion will show that when need, rather than demand, is the point of departure, there are many more pathways potentially open than when one begins with demand. Hence, the greater utility of this attribute to classify need-oriented methods. Accordingly, we shall use the following classification to order our description and discussion of illustrative need-oriented methods: (1) need to services, (2) need to services to resources, (3) need to resources, (4) services to resources, and (5) resources to resources. If we conceive of these five categories as rows in a table, one could attempt further categorization by constructing columns each of which corresponds to characteristics of standards. However, such a classification might prove too complex and will not be used here. Instead, as the several studies are discussed we shall have occasion to refer to the measures of need and the characteristics of standards that they use. In addition, as need or services are translated to resources we shall consider adjustments to service capacity, using as a framework our previous discussion of this subject under the heading of methods primarily based on demand. Since the general principles of adjusting to resource capacity are the same, regardless of whether one departs from need or demand, this topic will not receive separate consideration.

Illustrative Studies of Estimates Based on Need

In this section we shall describe and discuss a selection of studies that estimate requirements for services and resources primarily based on data or assumptions concerning need. This will provide an opportunity to illustrate more concretely certain points made in our more general discussion, to describe additional aspects of method and to evaluate the estimating procedures now available. As we have already said, transformation pathways will provide the major categories for classification.

CONVERSION OF NEED TO SERVICE. Taking need as the point of departure, the smallest step is to estimate the service equivalents of need. However, even this one step can be smaller or larger and can be taken in a variety of ways. We shall accordingly distinguish two major subcategories: (1) a set of studies that convert some measure of need to proportions of persons that require specified services, and (2) another set that proceeds further by specifying the actual volume of services provided. The distinction is of some importance since it may be easier to convert the volume of services to resource equivalents than to do the same for percentage of persons requiring particular services. A third category will consist of one unusual study that constructs a weighted index of service needs.

The first subcategory of studies—those in which need is converted to the percentage of persons requiring specified services—can be further subdivided by the measure of need used as the starting point. Many such studies begin with measures of morbidity. One such study, conducted by the Commission on Chronic Illness, obtained samples of urban and rural populations and measured need in these samples by a variety of means, including household interviews and clinical examinations (46). As we have described in our third chapter, these multiple determinations offered an unusual opportunity to compare different definitions and measures of need. However, the Commission felt that it was not sufficient to measure need in terms of disability and morbidity; that it was necessary to "translate these figures into terms with which a community deals." The Commission recognized explicitly that there was a choice of how to proceed. "The estimates could be expressed in terms of the 'people' needed, the 'services' required, or the 'facilities' needed to provide the care." The decision was to use "categories of services needed," including not only those that are traditionally regarded as medical care services, but also supportive services such as "financial aid," "adjustment of living conditions" and "social, cultural or recreational opportunities or outlets." (Reference 46, pages 123, 127 and 128.) The procedure used for estimation was as follows. At the time of the clinical evaluation, the examining physicians made estimates of services needed for the care of all chronic conditions identified in each of those examined. Later, a subsample of persons who had "maximum disability" or one of a set of diseases (diabetes, diseases of the central nervous system, neoplasms, heart disease, arthritis and rheumatism), were re-evaluated by a team composed of physicians, a public health nurse, a social worker, a vocational counselor and other members of the study staff. Needs for additional categories of service were established by this team. The Commission emphasizes that the resulting estimates are only for chronic conditions as a whole, or for only a subset of these. The major service needs for the "high disability group" were as shown in Table V.17 arranged in order of frequency. These figures are cited not because they necessarily possess generalizable validity, but because they illustrate the

Table V.17. Percent of disabled persons[a] estimated to need care of specified types, Baltimore, Md., 1953

Type of Care	Percent of Persons
General medical supervision and care	90
Diet therapy	65
Aid in financing medical care	38
Specialist consultation	32
Nursing care	27
Social needs (unmet)	27
Aid in financing subsistence	24
Personal services	20
Appliances	15
Modification of living arrangement	14
Psychiatric care	13
Care of the home	13
Surgical treatment	7
Self-help devices	7
Occupational therapy	2
Institutional care	1

SOURCE: Reference 46, Figure 6, page 178.

[a] Persons who have "maximum disability" or one of the following diseases: diabetes, diseases of the central nervous system, neoplasms, heart disease, arthritis, and rheumatism.

kinds of services taken into account and the relative prevalence of need for the several services.

In further discussing their procedure, the authors of the Commission's report comment on some important aspects of method. First, they distinguish the estimates of need that professionals are constantly engaged in making during the clinical management of individual patients from the representative, standardized, and reproducible estimates required for research or planning. Second, they recognize that estimates need to be standardized with respect to the health goals to be attained and the period over which service needs are to be projected. The period selected was six months after the time at which the examination was made. The health goals were as follows. For "disabling conditions the progress of which can be expected to be controlled, arrested, reversed, or eliminated" the goals were for the individual to be "self-sufficient," "productive," and "economically independent." When "the disabling condition is such that no predictable progress toward restoration of lost ability can be expected," the goal was for the individual to be "free from pain; nourished; clean; and free from worry" (46, p. 126). A final factor in improving the estimates was that variability in the "background and philosophy" of individual judges was "tempered by the team process," so that the resulting estimates represent majority opinion. In spite of all this, the Commission recognizes that the judgments are subjective, that the judges have sometimes changed their views in line with prior experience, and that "the estimates are far from precise and cannot be used for anything more specific than guides or 'pointers' " (46, p. 124).

The Commission on Chronic Illness was indeed ambitious in attempting to estimate need for a whole range of services, even though the volume of service needed was generally not specified. A much larger number of studies have attempted to assess needs for specific services. Greenlick et al. have reported what they consider to be an "objective" method for identifying those patients who are highly likely to require skilled nursing care after discharge from the hospital (47). The most distinctive feature of the method used is the specification of the criteria as well as of the decision rules to be used in arriving at the judgment of high risk—hence the rather ambitious claim of "objective measurement." A panel of 15 physicians representing "all the medical and surgical specialties" set the criteria to be used. An interesting feature of the criteria is that they identify five dimensions of patient disability: (1) mobility, (2) continence, (3) need for rehabititative services such as physical or occupational therapy, (4) mental state, particularly with regard to agitation, confusion, and coma, and (5) need for special procedures and equipment such as parenteral fluids, irrigation, suction, catheterization, respirator or oxygen equipment, and the like (see 47, p. 1194, for a detailed list of criteria). Thus, the criteria are only partly stated in terms of morbidity. To a considerable extent, need is stated in the form of requirements for service. The decision rules specify that there is a "high probability" of need for post-hospital skilled nursing care if (1) the patient has "two or more sets of disability on discharge," or (2) the patient has "only one area of disability," but has "no one in the home to constantly care" for him. Given the criteria and decision rules, the attending physicians were easily able to make the necessary determinations using the patients' hospital records, even though 2–6 months had elapsed from the time of discharge. It was found that 7 percent of all discharges, and 18 percent of discharges of persons 65 or older, belonged in the group with a high probability of requiring post-hospital skilled nursing care. The authors make no claim that the findings can be generalized, since the figures cited would vary by type of case load and hospital policy governing status at discharge. The authors are also aware that the validity of the judgment concerning risk and the quantification of the risk remain to be established by prospective observation. No data on reliability of estimates are given, so that the claim for "objectivity," although reasonably well-founded, cannot be established.

Similar to the study by Greenlick et al., except that the criteria used are not so clearly spelled out, is the survey of welfare clients to determine need for home health aides, reported by Lemon and Welches (49). A "public health physician" and two public health nurses who reviewed the social service records of part of the case load of a public welfare agency, were able to determine need for home health aides and to distinguish need for "personal" services from that for "domestic" services. Visits by a public health nurse to a subsample of patients confirmed the estimate of need in 35 out of 40 cases. Other studies that belong in this category (translation of morbidity or health status into requirements for specified types of service) include the many studies of patient classification that we have reviewed in the preceding chapter.

Next, we shall briefly review two studies both of which emphasize mortality as the measure of need and set out to estimate need for the same service: renal dialysis. These similarities make the differences between the two methods even more instructive. Lipworth began his quest with a one-third sample of deaths, during a period of two years, of San Francisco residents who were 15–64 years old (50). Information concerning each death was obtained fom an examination of hospital records, including autopsy reports, and from a visit to the relatives or friends of the deceased. The object was to determine whether the death was associated with chronic renal failure that would have benefited from dialysis and whether there were physical or psychological reasons that would have rendered dialysis unsuitable. As it turned out, information obtained from relatives and friends was not useful in identifying disqualifying behavioral attributes, so that the decision of suitability was made on physical factors alone. The samples yielded 13 patients suitable for dialysis. This corresponded to 41 persons per million, with 95 percent confidence limits of 18 to 63 per million. Assuming a true value of 18 per million, and survival for an average of 5 years per case, there would be a build-up to a steady level of 90 cases per year per million, or about 10,000 for the United States. This assumes, of course, that all cases of chronic renal failure end in death; that dialysis is suitable only for chronic failure in persons between 15 and 64; that the incidence of conditions leading to chronic renal failure will remain unchanged; and that the technology of dialysis will remain such that suitability and survival characteristics will not alter.

The study by Hallan and Harris, as we have pointed out, did not begin with a concrete sample (51). Instead, a list was made, from the ICDA classification, of diagnostic categories likely to be associated with kidney failure. Each of a panel of physicians, consisting of three urologists and one epidemiologist, was then asked to estimate for each disease condition upper- and lower-bound values of (1) the percent of those persons who die from the disease who have irreversible kidney failure, and (2) the percent of those with kidney failure who are not suited to dialysis. The "Delphi method" was used to obtain convergence and stability of opinions among panel members (90). In this procedure, initial opinions of panel members are relayed back to all members and revised opinions requested, together with justification for extreme responses. Several repetitions may be used to narrow down differences. Eventually, a representative value (mean or mode) is used to indicate the collective position of the group. The values obtained as above were then applied to data on actual mortalities by age group (within the broad range of those 15–54) in order to obtain the numbers of persons within each age group who, based on expert predictions, would require dialysis. The answer turns out to be 6665 persons between the ages of 15 and 54 in the United States, during 1968. The authors identify the following limitations in their method: (1) "These estimates are based upon training, experience, and intuitive judgment and represent a first approximation"; (2) "estimates . . . are based only upon mortality data"; (3) "estimates are made only for the age group 15–54"; and (4) "no consideration is given . . . to those potential candidates who are rejected for therapy because of psychiatric complications'' (51, p. 216). Hallan and Harris also review the literature on estimates of requirements for dialysis. It is a reflection on the state of the art that estimates for the United States have varied from 2,000 to 60,000 (51, Table 4, p. 212). It is true, however, that most estimates are near the lower end of this range.

We shall conclude our discussion of this group of studies by describing briefly a method for estimating need for family planning services. The procedure was developed by Dryfoos, Polgar, and Varky, and has been described by Jaffe (52, 53). We shall use the version given in a report by the Center for Family Planning Program Development (54). The object of the so-called ''DPV formula'' is to estimate the number of women who are at high risk of having an unwanted pregnancy according to a standard set by others, even though the women in question might neither perceive the need nor demand the service. We encounter here the concept of professionally defined need in almost its purest form. The number of women at risk of having a not wanted (actually, ''not needed'') pregnancy is the product of:

(Number of women 18–44) (0.87) (0.86), which is
(Number of women 18–44) (0.75).

If the additional notion of eligibility for publicly financed services is introduced, further reductions are necessary, depending on the criteria for eligibility. The translation of ''need'' to demand would further deplete the number. Table V.18 gives the factors that go into the estimation of professionally defined need and eligibility, and the derivation of the values for the terms. As an illustration, the number of women who are estimated to need family planning services in a county in which 50 percent of families have incomes below $3,000 and 15 percent live on farms would be

$$\left(\begin{array}{c}\text{Number of}\\\text{women 18–44}\end{array}\right) \quad (0.87) \quad (0.86) \quad (0.50) \quad (1.12).$$

In this formula, the number of women 18–44 and the proportion living on farms are data pertaining to the locality for which estimates are being made. The other terms (0.87, 0.50, and 1.12) are extrapolations from national data. Siegel et al., on the basis of a survey of a sample of addresses in 23 low-income census tracts in Charlotte, N.C., raise some questions about the general applicability of the quantitative factors of the DPV formula to local situations. Data obtained through the survey

Table V.18.   Procedure for estimating percent of women who require publicly provided family planning services

Factor	Explanation and Derivation
1. Women 18–44	Women of childbearing age; although about 5% of childbearing occurs outside this age range.
2. 0.87	13% of deduction from number of women of childbearing age for estimated prevalence of natural or postoperative sterility. Mere subfecundity is not considered a reason for removal from the population at risk.
3. 0.86	14% deduction from the remaining population to allow for the time needed by a women to have an average of three "wanted children." Each live birth makes contraception unnecessary for an average of 6 months of seeking pregnancy and a further 9 months until term. A fetal death accounts for 6 months of seeking pregnancy and another 3 months until fetal death. Assuming fetal deaths to be 15% of live births, each live birth corresponds to 16.35 months during which contraception is not needed, or a total of 49.05 months for 3 live births. Since about 5% of all births occur outside the age range 18–44, only 95% of 49.05 months is to be deducted from the period of 27 years (324 months) between the ages of 18 and 44, which is about 14%.
4. Proportion of families with income below $3,000	A family income below $3,000 is considered to represent eigibility for publicly financed services.
5a. $(1.2)/F^{0.11}$, if the proportion of families living on farms is equal to or greater than 0.020; or	F is the proportion living on farms as given in the census reports for the area for which an estimate is to be made. The adjustment is necessary to allow for the observation that the same cash income represents a higher real income for a farm family than a nonfarm family.
5b. 1.12, if the proportion of families living on farms is less than 0.020	

SOURCE: Reference 54.

made possible a more precise measurement of need for the locality in question (55).

So far, we have described studies that begin with actual or hypothetical samples of persons who are ill or disabled, who have died, or who are exposed to some risk, and recast them into estimates of persons who are deemed to require a range of services, or some particular service. Next in line for discussion are studies that attempt to estimate the actual volume of needed service. In this category, a study that includes some interesting features of method is the survey of extra-hospital nursing needs by Mickey (56). Sample households were visited by one of four qualified nurses, who administered a "tight interview schedule" concerning "18 categories of potential health problems present on the day of the interview." In addition to specifying categories of need, the method distinguished two further aspects of need: "intensity of need" and the "family's capacity to cope with this need." As we have seen, the ability of the family to care for its members was also a factor in the estimates for post-hospital home care as formulated by Greenlick et al. (47). In the study by Mickey, "intensity" and "ability to cope" were each rated with the use of a five-point scale, and had a bearing on the estimates made of the number of nursing visits and the length of time, up to six months, required to deal with the specific needs that were identified. It is obvious that multiple needs might be present and that, if this is so, the requirements for service may not be simply additive. The findings showed a large reservoir of professionally defined need, most of it not known to the local health department. With respect to intensity of need, 3 percent of familes had no need; in 61 percent need was rated "slight"; in 30 percent, "moderate"; in 6 percent, "serious"; and in none "critical". Ability to cope was excellent or good in 68 percent, "moderate" in 29 percent, "slight" in 2 percent, and "none" in 1 percent. Based on the presence of need, its intensity and the ability of the family to cope with it, 33 percent of households were referred for nursing service. The visits needed averaged 1.6 per household, to be provided during the period of six months following the interview. No visits were needed in 67.1 percent of families, 1–3 visits were needed in 19.2 percent, 4–8 visits in 8.5 percent, and 9 or more visits in 5.2 percent. Two further considerations intervened between these initial estimates of need and actual receipt of service. One was concurrence of the service-providing agency with the estimate of need, and the second, the acceptability of the service to the family. The first was of a relatively low order, so that only two-thirds of recommended visits were made. The second was of a relatively high order, so that 83 percent of families fully accepted the services and an additional 9 percent admitted the nurses, but the visits were felt to be unsatisfactory. To summarize, in this study, the factors intervening between the presence of a professionally defined health problem and demand were the intensity of need, the ability of the family to cope, an undefined set of service agency priorities and perceptions, and the potential client's own priorities and perceptions. Thus, the presence of several partially overlapping definitions of need is elegantly demonstrated. The findings concerning reliability between judges have been discussed in a previous section.

Ast et al. have developed estimates for needed dental services among children, with the added interest of a comparison between two communities, with and without a fluoridated water supply (57). By examining and treating each child, first during the kindergarten or first grade, and then every 9–14 months during an additional period of three years, it was possible to estimate "initial, accumulated" need and "incremental" need, expressed in terms of services, in mean chair time in minutes, and in cost. Table V.19 may be of interest since it shows the several measures

Table V.19. Specified measures of need for dental care in school children as observed initially and during three-year period in two communities with and without fluoridated water supplies, New York State, 1962–1965

	Initial Accumulated Need		Incremental Need	
Measure of Need	Fluoridated	Not	Fluoridated	Not
Services	810	1549	292	582
Mean chair time in minutes	52.4	82.8	21.0	37.5
Cost	$11.92	$27.61	$6.17	$11.51

SOURCE: Reference 57.

of need per person, their relative magnitudes and their relationship to fluoridation. The three measures of requirements are not fully comparable. Services and costs exclude clinical examinations, x-rays and prophylaxis, but the time estimates include these. The cost data are based on arbitrary, but reasonable, prices. More detailed estimates by type of service are cited in the paper. It is clear that in this study, as well as in the study of nursing needs by Mickey, we have moved much closer to concrete estimates of resource requirements. Visits, services and especially time estimates, should not be too difficult to convert to requirements for manpower (nurses and dentists, for example). Mickey hoped that, with some further work, her method would permit the development of "formulas" that could be used to convert demographic characteristics into service needs. If so, we would witness the progression from detailed estimation procedures to a reasonably well-validated summary standard or conversion factor.

The final subgroup under our category of studies that convert need to service requirements is a study by Kalimo and Sievers which eventuates in the construction of a weighted index of need (58). A household interview survey was made of a sample of 16,715 persons aged 15 and over, representing the adult population of Finland, but excluding those in institutions. Information on health status was obtained using four questions concerning (1) current defect or injury that diminished ability to work, (2) most recent sickness that caused confinement to bed for three successive days, (3) sickness that caused last contact with a physician, and (4) any current ailment additional to the above for which the respondent wished to undergo medical examination or to obtain medical treatment. The answers to the foregoing questions were used to construct an inventory of health status expressed in diagnostic categories. All diseases were grouped into 97 categories based on the International Classification of Diseases. Some categories were designated "acute" and others "chronic," "depending on the estimated proportion of long-term patients in the category in question." A group of ten physicians representing general practice and several specialties were asked individually to estimate the likelihood of need for medical care for the "average Finnish patient" who fell in any of 97 categories of disease. For each of the categories, each physician estimated the likelihood of the need for 5 types of care: (1) hospitalization, (2) care by a physician, (3) x-ray or laboratory examination, (4) medicines, and (5) other care. Thus, there were 5 need estimates for 97 categories of disease by each of 10 physicians: a total of 5x97x10, equalling 4850 estimates. The likelihood of need for care was not always expressed in the same way. For all types of care in all disease categories designated as "acute," the physician–judge was asked to estimate the precent of cases with that disease who would require each kind of care. The likelihood for "medicines" and for "other types of care" in diseases designated as "chronic" was also expressed as above. But need for "hospitalization," "care by a physician" and "x-ray and laboratory examination" was expressed in terms of the frequency during a year that such care would be necessary. For all services and all categories of disease the likelihood of needing service was converted into a four-point scale: 0–3. The estimates of 10 physicians were then averaged. A scaling procedure was used that would express the likelihood of each of 5 types of need for each of 97 categories of disease in terms of another four-point scale: 0–3. The total need for medical care for each category of disease was obtained by adding the five component scores, giving equal weight to each. Thus, the total score of need could vary from a minimum of 0 to a maximum of 15. For example, the scores, by type of care needed, assigned by each of ten physicians, averaged and standardized for the category of "rheumatoid arthritis, arthritis" were as shown in Table V.20. The need for medical care in the population was

Table V.20.   Proposed weights for requirements for specified types of care for the diagnostic category of "rheumatoid arthritis, arthritis"

Type of Need	Score
Hospitalization	1
Care by a physician	2
X-ray or laboratory examination	2
Treatment with medicines	3
Other care (surgical, physical, etc.)	2
Total	10

SOURCE: Reference 58, page 17.

estimated by applying the scores listed in Table V.20 to the volume of illness reported in the survey, by age and sex group. Where more than one illness was reported for any person, the highest score of any need was taken to represent that particular need, and the sum of these highest scores to represent total need. This was justified on the assumption that "at times of utilization of medical services, more than one sickness can be treated."

The findings of the study can be divided into substantive and methodological categories. The major substantive finding was that "the differences in morbidity between age groups and sexes are accentuated when attention is paid to the need for care of the diseases" (58, p. 9). The findings relevant to method concerned mainly the ability of physicians to make reliable estimates of the likelihood of need for care. The average intercorrelation between the initial estimates was about 0.50, with a range by type of need from 0.19 to 0.59. The reliability of the final scores of each type of need rose to a level exceeding 0.90. We have commented, in previous sections, on this and other aspects of the method. We have pointed out the hypothetical nature of the "average" patient for whom estimates of need were made, and the problems of fixing the level at which the standard of care is to be put. The validity of the method depends on (1) the validity of the information about disease as obtained from respondents, (2) the validity of the opinions of physicians about the need for care, and (3) the validity of the assumptions used in the construction of the scoring system. The scoring system does not seem to quantify need fully. For example, there is a judgment on the likelihood of hospitalization but none on the length of time in hospital. The assigning of the highest score for any category of need, when more than one disease is present, is also open to question. The relation may not be one of total inclusivity, but may be additive or even synergistic to a greater or lesser degree. The summation of scores for each need into a total score giving equal weight to all components constitutes an important feature, also open to serious question. Finally, interactions between demographic factors and illness are ignored. The same illness, identified by name may require more care when it occurs in one age group (for example, the aged) than in another. All these criticisms notwithstanding, the method holds a great deal of theoretical and practical interest. It yields an index which is probably a more precise measure of need for service than the much less differentiated proxy measures of age or sex. This, however, is all that it can do. In its present form it cannot be used to derive estimates of requirements for resources. To see how that can be done, we shall have to move on to our second category of methods.

CONVERSION OF NEED TO SERVICES, TO RESOURCES. In this section we shall describe the most ambitious, the most detailed, and the most conceptually satisfying of all methods for the estimation of requirements. These represent the U.S. counterparts of the "scientific" application of the "expert" method as perceived by Russian authors such as Rozenfeld and Popov (5, 6, 7), with the exception that the U.S. studies in this category have used what we have called "hypothetical samples" rather than actual samples of persons with need, as the Russians seem to envisage and prefer. The two major U.S. studies in this category are the classic work by Lee and Jones carried out about 40 years ago under the auspices of the Committee on the Costs of Medical Care (59), and its recent, and current, replication and further development by Falk, Schonfeld, and their associates at Yale (60–65).

The work of Lee and Jones represents a monument in medical care literature not only because of the stunning scale of their undertaking and the care which they took in its execution, but also because of their thorough conceptual grasp of the major issues relevant to what they had set out to do. One finds here no evidence of the naïveté that later critics have attributed to them, possibly because these critics have not read their source with sufficient care. On the contrary, one finds hardly a qualification emphasized by subsequent scholars that Lee and Jones have not themselves explicitly recognized. If so, why attempt something so thickly hedged about with caveats? The answer seems to be that Lee and Jones, as many before and since, were passionately convinced that professional standards of adequate medical care were definable, and that they could be set as a goal to which at least certain societies might aspire. This, then, is the essential characteristic of the "Lee-Jones method": that it rests on professional norms, but with certain important qualifications. First, the perspective is not narrowed down, as is the case with that of many clinicians, to the technical management of illness in individual patients primarily by physicians. On the contrary, Lee and Jones deal with the broadest range of medical care functions and concerns, emphasizing prevention as well as treatment, community health as well as individual health, the contribution of other health professionals as well as those of physicians. Second, the standards formulated, though normative, are not pie-in-the-sky estimates untempered by experience. Finally, in presenting and evaluating their method and in interpreting their findings, Lee and Jones take pains to set out clearly the context within which their work is relevant and the situations under which it is not. Thus, a large portion of their book consists of specifying what they postulate and assume to be the "functions of modern medicine" (pp. 3–6), the "concept of good medical care" (pp. 6–10), the characteristics of the major resources that they perceive to constitute the care providing apparatus (pp. 16–28), what constitutes appropriate patient behavior in the pursuit of health (pp. 26–28), and what are the "fundamental procedures" in preventive medicine, in the diagnosis and treatment of physical and mental illness, and in dental care (pp. 31–90). Notable among all these, are the eight "articles of faith" which collectively define "good medical care" as follows: (1) "good medical care is limited to the practice of rational medicine based on the medical sciences"; (2) good medical care emphasizes prevention"; (3) "good medical care requires intelligent cooperation between the lay public and the practitioners of scientific medicine"; (4) "good medical care treats the individual as a whole"; (5) "good medical care maintains a close and continuing personal relation between physician and patient"; (6) "good medical care is coordinated with social welfare work"; (7) "good medical care coordinates all types of medical services"; and (8) "good medical care implies the application of all the necessary services of modern, scientific medicine to the needs of all the people" (59, pp. 7–10).

A major feature of the Lee-Jones approach is that it sets out to construct the whole from smaller elements, proceeding, with some exceptions, from some measure of service requiring potential to service equivalents and, finally, to resource equivalents. We shall briefly describe this stepwise progression, as well as the aggregation of elements, giving special attention to the measures of need, services, and resources, and to the factors that enter into the conversion from one to the other. Four categories of need and of corresponding services were considered to constitute the whole. These were (1) services for community health preservation, (2) preventive services for the individual, (3) services in dentistry, and (4) medical diagnosis and treatment of physical and mental illness. "Community health preservation" was a function allocated to the health department. The measure of need was a "standard population" of 100,000, representative of the United States as a whole. No attempt was made to translate people into services. Instead, indices were used to translate persons to health personnel, using as conversion factors personnel : population ratios. The derivation and validity of these conversion indices is not examined in detail. Hence they would fall in the category of arbitrary, summary indices that we described in our general discussion of standards. For example, around 1933, for each 100,000 of the standard population, expert opinion would recommend that the health department employ : 1 health officer, 2 physicians, 1 epidemiologist, 1 bacteriologist, 1 chemist, 1 sanitary engineer, 8 inspectors, 1 statistician, 1 educational director, 7 clerks, 1 technician, 1 director of nursing, 3 supervisors of nursing, 25 public health nurses, and 2 medical social workers. The reader will note that agency staffing is the immediate consideration and that institutional need, or what we have called "derived need," is at issue. Lee and Jones also give personnel requirements for the standard population by type of "function" (p. 131) and for the United States as a whole (Table A-1, p. 132).

Need for "preventive services for the individual" is expressed in terms of 100 persons, in each of six age groups. For each 100 persons, estimates were developed of the number of (1) x-rays, (2) immunizations, (3) laboratory procedures, and (4) visits to the physician. For physician visits there were, in addition, estimates of minutes per visit and total hours per 100 persons. Given these standards, and the age composition of the United States, it was an easy matter to arrive at service estimates for a standard population of 100,000 persons (Table A-4, p. 134). Hours of physician time were converted to number of physicians using a procedure to be described below. As far as we can determine, the other service needs remain unconverted to their resource equivalents.

Need for dental care was also expressed, as a first step, in terms of 100 persons in each of four age groups, rather than in terms of specific diseases, which Lee and Jones would have preferred. This was done because there were at that time no "comprehensive data on the incidence of the various forms of dental defects in the general population" (p. 134). There was, however, considerable detail in the estimates of service equivalents for each 100 persons in each of the age groups. Three types of dental practitioners were distinguished: general dental practitioner, exodontist, and orthodontist. The services for which separate estimates were made included examinations, treatment of gums, orthodontia, fillings, crowning, bridges, dentures, extractions, and postoperative care. For each of these, the estimates included number of services, minutes per visit, and total hours for that category. For some services (orthodontia and dentures) a distinction was made between chair hours and laboratory hours. Estimates were also made for number of x-rays, time per procedure, and total hours. The conversion of personnel time requirements to personnel requirements will be described later in this section.

The estimation of requirements for medical diagnosis and treatment of physical and mental illness constitutes, as one might expect, the major portion of the work, and represents what is usually meant by the "Lee-Jones approach." Here, persons who have specified illnesses, or illness categories, represent the measure of need. For each of 10 age groups, empirical data were assembled, from various sources, concerning "annual expectancy rates for pathological conditions which require diagnosis and treatment." Data for 95 detailed disease conditions were grouped into 19 categories (see Table 3, p. 97–100). The diseases exclude "minor disorders shown by the prevalence studies to be almost 'normal,' such as constipation and postural defects," which are presumed to receive attention during the periodic health examination, as well as "irremediable afflictions such as total blindness," for which medicine can do nothing (p. 101). The diseases considered include self-limiting acute diseases as well as incurable chronic diseases which are believed to "require medical attention" (p. 100).

The process of standard formulation is most precisely described for this category of need. Because it is such a critical feature of the method it may be best to describe it in the words of the authors themselves.

The quantitative estimates of the services required for the diagnosis and treatment of diseases and physical and mental defects presented in this report are based upon sample opinions and case records of leading practitioners of medicine. The physicians were asked to give their opinions or, if possible, the records of their practice to indicate the amount of service necessary in each broad disease category (e.g. digestive diseases or respiratory diseases). For each of the representative diseases within the category (e.g. appendicitis or influenza) similar data were requested concerning the amount of service of various kinds required in the treatment of 100 typical cases, with such considerations as the average duration of the disease and the normal proportion of severe to mild cases. The physicians' replies were made the basis of arbitrary estimates of the services required (p. 102).

In making the quantitative estimates of the services required in view of the present expectancy of diseases and conditions, the aim of the study has been to present a conservative and reasonable standard which members of the medical profession regard as sufficient and appropriate. No attempt has been made to catalogue all the desirable medical services which might be rendered in a society exclusively devoted to the pursuit of health; nor have the requirements of good practice been kept to an absolute minimum. "Luxury" services now widely consumed are omitted; on the other hand, some services which are not at present demanded even by very wealthy people are included as essential to good medical care. Our standards call for no more than a general application of good current practice (p. 11).

The application of these standards results in estimates for fairly detailed categories of service. For physicians, estimates were made of the services of general practitioners, consultants, and specialists—specifying the type of specialty. Some visits were categorized, by type, into pre-operative, operative, postoperative and follow-up. The estimates for visits included number of cases (out of the hypothesized, "typical" 100) who required care, the number of visits, minutes per visit, and total hours for all visits. For services by nurses, estimates were made of the number of cases requiring care, the days of nursing attention per case, and the total nursing days. Attendants were classified into full-time and part-time, and estimates made of the number of cases, days per case, and total days. For hospital care, estimates were for cases, days per case, and patient-days, by type of hospital or service: maternity, medical, surgical, psychiatric, nervous and mental, and tuberculosis. Diagnostic procedures and x-ray examinations were estimated by type and number required. The definitions adopted for the several measures of service illustrate some of the problems in defining and measuring the relevant products. The "physician-hour" comprises only time spent with patients. It excludes time waiting for patients and for traveling. These latter segments of time become factors to be considered in determining service capacity. "A nursing day" consists of 12 hours of duty, excluding regular hospital nursing, which is included in the "hospital day." A "full-time attendant day" consists of 8 hours of duty. A "hospital day" includes staff nursing, excludes physician services in general hospitals, but includes physician services in special hospitals, such as tuberculosis and mental hospitals (see 59, footnote to Table 4, p. 104).

Conceivably, Lee and Jones could have decided at this point to develop a measure or index of need analogous to that constructed by Kalimo and Sievers (58). Instead, they move on to the final step in their procedure: the estimation of the resource equivalents of need. The process involves primarily the conversion of services quantified in units of time to corresponding resources, postulating norms of service capacity. These norms are, of course, very important. In addition to helping to determine the level of resource requirements, they must be taken into account in interpreting seeming deficits or excesses in current resources. A deficit is created to the extent that the norms of capacity are below current average practice, and an excess to the extent that they are above. The capacity norm for physicians was a working time of 8 hours a day for 6 days a week and 48 weeks a year, from which are deducted 300 hours for necessary travel, resulting in an average annual "production" of 2,000 physician hours. Although this norm was "something less than the present heroic working schedule," it did not make an allowance for time consumed in continuing professional education and "in the inevitable waiting time between calls, due to the fact that patients do not become ill in turns and do not demand services in even, uninterrupted sequence" (p. 114). Under the capacity norm that was adopted, requirements for physicians were estimated to be 141.57 physicians per 100,000, actively engaged in "preventive services for the individual," "the care of the "puerperal state," "diagnosis and treatment," and "refraction" (Table 7, p. 115). For dentists the capacity norm was 8 hours of work, for 5½ days a week, for 48 weeks, resulting in a total of 2112 hours. The rationale for assigning shorter working hours to the dentist is not clear, especially since the greatest discrepancy between requirements and supplies was for dentists. Lee and Jones recognized that the productivity of physicians and dentists would depend to a significant extent on the contributions of paraprofessional personnel and other features of the organization of service. However, only in the case of dentists were these factors taken into account in arriving at quantitative estimates. For dentists, estimates were made under four different assumptions, ranging from the dentists doing all their own laboratory work, x-ray work, and scaling and cleaning, to the dentists doing nothing but chair work and hygienists doing the scaling and cleaning. Requirements ranged from 178.7 per 100,000, under the first assumption to 98.6 per 100,000 under the last (59, Table 11, p.126). For hospitals, the norms selected were 300 days of care per bed per year for general hospitals, equivalent to a normative occupancy rate of 80 percent. For chronic disease, tuberculosis and mental hospitals, the production norm was 340 days per bed per year, or an occupancy of 90 percent. This yields an estimated requirement of 4.62 general hospital beds per 1000 persons (Table 9, p. 119). The manner in which such norms influence the final estimates of deficit or excess is illustrated by the observation that the current average occupancy for general hospitals was only 66 percent. However, since observed hospital occupancy includes a significant segment of "unnecessary" use, the scale of both manifest and latent service reserve in the hospital establishment becomes abundantly clear. It must be pointed out, however, that Lee and Jones specifically excluded social reasons for the use of the hospital from their estimates of service requirements, (p. 120), and that they did not adjust for size, isolation, and other factors that influence occupancy. The estimates for nurses are interesting because they derive from several sources, including hospital beds. Using recommendations of the American College of Surgeons, it is envisaged that there should be one nurse for each eight general hospital beds, or 58 per 462 beds per 100,000 population. To meet needs for home and special nursing, it is assumed that nurses work 300 days a year—more than either physicians or dentists—and that their days are 12 hours long, as against 8 for physicians and dentists. Under these almost punitive norms, an additional 180 nurses would be required to provide an estimated 54,000 days of home and special care per 100,000 population, making a total of 238 per 100,000. Lee and Jones also consider the possible effects of an organized visiting nursing service in reducing the needs for days of nursing home care and the needs of the community for 25 public health nurses per 100,000. In summary, it is concluded that 220 nurses per 100,000 are required, a figure lower than the approximately 240 per 100,000 then available!

Lee and Jones have a sharp appreciation of the conceptual underpinning of their study, and of its uses and limitations. They base their estimates on professionally defined need. They see "need for medical care as compounded of two constantly changing factors: the science and art of medicine on the one hand; on the other, the changing expectancy of disease . . . The real need for medical care is a medical, not an economic concept" (pp. 10, 12). Thus, it is distinguishable from demand and has relevance only where a society espouses the values, and has the means necessary to convert it into demand. "Against an entirely different background, as for example in modern India, need would represent merely the expression of a narrow professional opinion and would bear no relation to the needs of society. Since, however, modern America values health and has accepted the science and art of medicine as the proper instrument for its advancement, a definition of the need for medical care in the terms of the capacities of modern medicine would seem both relevant and useful'' (p. 12). Thus, Lee and Jones regard the specification of need to have an important social component and recognize that ''health can be achieved only as part of a high standard of living, in which good medical care is only one of a number of essential elements'' (p. 15). Finally, the distinctions between need and demand lead Lee and Jones to draw a fine distinction between deficit and shortage which few estimates oriented to need have made. They conclude that the small ''relative numbers'' of a resource do not mean a shortage unless there is demand for more services than can be provided (p. 118).

As to the standards that they formulated and used, Lee and Jones emphasize that these are set at a ''conservative and reasonable'' level; that they are related to the actual practice of actual, though not representative (in the sense of average) physicians; that they are ''frankly founded on arbitrary judgment; and that they are ''impossible to determine once and for all time.'' Lee and Jones also recognize that their assumptions concerning the ''typical'' 100 patients, in the ''typical year'' in the ''standard community,'' yield estimates of need that are too general to be applied to a particular population. The characteristics of the specific community should be taken into account. Further, ''this study provides an *a priori* definition of adequate medical care. The needs of any particular community can only be determined inductively—by continued experimentation in ways and means of supplying medical services'' (p. 14). As we have seen, Lee and Jones are also aware of several characteristics of service capacity and of productivity that are germane to conversion from services to resource equivalents. They are aware of the complementarity and substitutibility of resources, and point out that disproportionate reduction in one service may result in waste in another (p. 14). Lee and Jones emphasize that features of organization, such as ''group clinic service,'' may influence materially the productivity of resources (p. 103). They are aware, in particular, of the contribution of ''subsidiary personnel'' in increasing manpower productivity. As we have seen, the estimates for dentists are explicitly based on four different assumptions concerning the division of labor in providing dental services. Similarly, the estimates for nursing manpower consider the substitution of visiting nurse services for a certain proportion of days of home and special nursing, each nursing visit being considered equal to one-half nursing day (p. 122). Lee and Jones also know that such aggregate estimates as theirs are not sufficient to evaluate resources, and that the problem may be in geographic distribution (pp. 117–118). Finally, Lee and Jones are among the few who have recognized that the provision of resources and services to meet need is likely to alter the nature and magnitude of that need, and that estimates of future requirements must be modified accordingly. Unfortunately, because medical science also changes, Lee and Jones find themselves unable to clearly predict what the resultant of these two forces will be. They do, however, introduce a guessed-at downward adjustment in the requirements for dental services to allow for reduction in dental morbidity under more adequate care (p. 137).

Lee and Jones did their work for the Committee on the Costs of Medical Care under the general direction of I. S. Falk. More than thirty years later, in the face of considerable skepticism and some opposition, Falk was able to get started at Yale Medical School a similar study that would set, for another time, a new benchmark of "good" medical care and perhaps become a fitting capstone for his own long and remarkably fruitful career. The philosophy and general approach of the new study are admittedly the same as those of the original. There are, however, some important differences, most of them for the better. One difference that may be both a strength and a weakness, is that all the expert judges were selected from the faculty of Yale-New Haven Medical Center, rather than being "selected physicians in various and diverse communities," as was true of the Lee-Jones study (60, p. 1120). While this may have reduced the representativeness and general applicability of the norms, it has also permitted greater formalization of, and control over, the process of developing standards. The method for obtaining opinions from physicians has been more standardized. The reliability of estimates has been looked at. As a result, the standards show not only areas of consensus, but also "diversities of opinion where these are regarded as well founded, justified and significant by the senior review physician" (60, p. 1122). The nature of what we have called the "hypothetical sample" has also received detailed attention, to our knowledge for the first time in studies of this kind (65). As one might expect, the kinds of services concerning which information has been sought are considerably expanded over the original. This has made it necessary to use as judges not only physicians and dentists but "later, others such as nurses, dental hygienists, and so on" (64, p. 2098). This should improve the validity of the standards in the relevant specialized fields, whether the standards are used for the auditing of care or the estimation of resource requirements: their two separate but related uses. Finally, much of the information concerning service requirements was obtained not in terms of some average value, but as frequency distributions of cases in specified categories by classes of volume of service. Thus, the new standards reflect much better than before two kinds of variability: that in states of nature and that in judgments concerning these states. In previous sections we have discussed and evaluated other general and special features of the work of Falk, Schonfeld, and their associates. Rather than repeat these, we shall give one example of how the standards can be used to yield requirements for services and resources. The illustration selected is one offered by Schonfeld et al. and deals with requirements for diagnostic visits at home or in the office for "influenza" in children below the age of six. The procedure is summarized in Table V.21.

This procedure is repeated for (1) this age group, influenza, other services, (2) this age group, other conditions, all services, and (3) other age groups, all conditions, all services. The manner in which final estimates emerge through the piecemeal aggregation of parts should become clearly evident. In just the category described above (influenza in children) there would be four additional subgroups of service: diagnostic phone calls, treatment and follow-up phone calls, treatment and follow-up office visits, and treatment and follow-up hospital visits. The major steps in the process should also be clear:

Population base:	item A
Morbidity expectation:	item B
Equivalents in services:	items D, E, and F
Equivalents in time:	items G and H
Service capacity:	item I
Equivalent in resources:	item J

An interesting feature of the procedure cited is the introduction of a factor specifying the proportion of children with influenza who are expected to seek care (item C). This is based on an empirical observation, and so introduces an element of demand into the estimates. It is made necessary because the large majority of physicians who made estimates of service requirement took as their point of reference ("hypothetical sample") children who had sought care (65). To maintain a consistent need-oriented approach, factor C would have given the proportion of children who *should* seek care, rather than those who *do*. Several subsequent factors (for example, D, E, and G) might, in that case, also have been different. Another possibly empirical element has been introduced in the form of the standard for service capacity, Factor I. The value given is merely illustrative and represents 48 weeks of 40 hours per week devoted to patient care. Thus, it excludes travel, study time, waiting for patients, and the like. We have already discussed the consequences of setting this value above or below average observed practice. The hypo-

Table V.21.   Procedure for estimating requirements for pediatricians to provide diagnostic visits at home or in the office, for "influenza," in children below the age of six

Nature of Information	Factors or Standards	Computations
A. Number of children under 6	1,000	
B. Proportion who have influenza during year (empirical epidemiological data)	0.472	$1,000 \times 0.472 = 472$ persons
C. Proportion of those with influenza who seek care (empirical observation)	0.490	$472 \times 0.490 = 231$ persons
D. Proportion of those who seek care who require pediatric diagnostic visits at home or in the doctor's office (normative standard)	0.720	$231 \times 0.720 = 166$ persons
E. Average number of visits for each person requiring service (normative standard)	1.4	
F. Number of visits per 1,000 children under age 6		$166 \times 1.4 = 232$ visits
G. Average time in minutes per unit of service (normative standard)	19 minutes	
H. Time needed per 1,000 children under age 6		$232 \times 19 = 4408$ minutes
I. Amount of time worked by a pediatrician per year in minutes (normative or empirical standard)	115,200 minutes	
J. Number of pediatricians needed for diagnostic visits at home or in the office for care of influenza in 1,000 children under 6		$4408 \div 115,200 = 0.0383$ pediatrician

SOURCE: Reference 64, note 2, page 2106.

thetical physician used in the example represents a primary physician for children. He could very well be a person with some other form of training suited to this particular function. As professional roles are redefined it might turn out that 30 percent of the time the pediatrician devotes to this category of care could be replaced by the services of a nurse, without loss, or even with gain, in quality. If so, 0.0268 pediatrician would suffice for the performance of this function for 1,000 children under 6. An increment of hours would then have to be added to the work of the nurse. It may be that as many hours are added to the nurse's service as are removed from the pediatrician's. But the value could be more or less, depending on relative skills, self-imposed or other-imposed standards of performance, work planning or organization, and possibly other factors. These rates of exchange, so to speak, and the factors that influence them, would be an important area of research in medical care organization.

In our discussion of methods of prediction, as distinct from contemporaneous transformation, we have so far, and shall in subsequent sections, repeatedly come up against the question of estimating the probable magnitude of the effect of changes in technology and medical care organization. We shall next describe an exercise that illustrates an attempt to deal with some aspects of this problem as they affect predictions of requirements for dentists (66). Although difficult to classify, this exercise is discussed in this section because we see it as primarily oriented to need, and because it includes transformation of need to services to resources. However, as we shall see, these are not the only transformations involved. Furthermore, the approach is a little roundabout. The object is not to predict what is going to be required, but to predict how many dentists are *not* going to be required, because (1) fluoridation can be expected to reduce cavities; (2) improved dental equipment, especially that for high-speed cutting, can be expected to reduce time needed for certain dental procedures; and (3) utilization of additional auxiliary personnel is expected to increase productivity of the dentist. To estimate the effect of fluoridation at some estimated target date (in this instance, 1970) the procedure is as follows.

A. The number of relevant persons effectively exposed to fluoridation by 1970.

These were defined as persons who, in 1970, are 34 years or less in age and were first exposed to fluoridation prior to their fourteenth birthday. Their number depends on (1) the size and age composition of the yearly increment of population exposed to fluoridation due to its introduction into community water supplies; (2) births and deaths, by age, in communities with fluoridation; and (3) migration, by age, in and out of these communities. Based on historical data concerning the spread of fluoridation, it was estimated that 2 million persons of all ages would be newly exposed each year between 1960 and 1970 due to water supply treatment. This is less than the yearly average of about 3.5 million during the decade 1949–59, but more than would be indicated by the declining trend in yearly increases. The age composition of this yearly increment of exposed persons was, of course, unknown, but was assumed to correspond to that of the nation as a whole, in each of the years 1960–1970. Bureau of the Census population projections were used to estimate natural population increase. There was no information on inmigration or outmigration or on the effect on dental caries of temporary exposure to fluoridation as a result of population mobility. To deal with these factors it was "assumed that the cumulative effect on the national caries rate of sporadic exposure of a large number of children in a mobile population will be equal to the effect of a smaller stable population receiving an equivalent number of years of exposure to fluoridation" (66, p. 477). Thus, the effect of population mobility need not enter the computations, which yield an estimate of a little over 28 million persons in 1970 exposed to fluoridation prior to their fourteenth birthday.

B. Reduction in yearly volume of dental caries due to exposure to fluoride in the relevant population.

This depends on the yearly incidence of caries by age in nonfluoridated communities and the yearly incidence of caries by age and length of exposure, in communities with fluoridated water supplies. Without giving full documentation, it is estimated that the relevant population would have 38,236,000 cavities each year as against an expected 76,472,000—a reduction of 50 percent due to fluoridation.

C. Reduction in yearly volume of fillings due to exposure to fluoride in the relevant population.

The reduction in the incidence of dental caries cannot be translated directly into a corresponding reduction in requirements for service because not all persons who have caries seek care. Again without providing documentation, it is assumed that "not more than one-third of all new cavities will be filled each year." Thus the reduction in need and service equivalents of need brought about by fluoridation is estimated to be 50 percent, but the reduction in the demand equivalents only one-third of 50 percent, or 12.7 million fillings (76 million × ½ × ⅓).

D. Reduction in time input of dentists during a year due to reduction in demand for fillings in the relevant population.

Assuming each filling to take 25 minutes, this amounts to 5.3 million dentist-hours (12.7 million $\times$ 25 $\div$ 60).

E. Reduction in requirements for dentists due to reduction in demand for fillings in the relevant population.

Assuming each dentist puts in 1,600 hours a year of effective working time, 5.3 million hours of dental time equals 3,300 dentists.

It is concluded that 3,300 fewer dentists would be required in 1970 than would otherwise have been the case. This is the consequence of the projected spread of fluoridation and the effect of that on the incidence of dental caries. Needless to say, the estimate reflects the assumptions on which it rests. It does not include the effect of other forms of fluoride application. Nor does it include consideration of effects other than those on the demand for fillings. It has been suggested, for example, that the saving of teeth due to fluoridation may increase the need for care for diseases of the gums later in life. Should the demand for fillings correspond to two-thirds rather than one-third of cavities, the entire expected savings would be wiped out.

The estimates for the effect of improved equipment are for 1975, as compared to 1950, and concern the effect of high-speed cutting apparatus on three services: fillings, bridges, and crowns. The key assumptions are that (1) in 1975 there will be 235 million persons, each of whom will require, in that year, 1.0 filling, 0.0124 bridge, and 0.0155 crown; (2) high-speed cutting equipment will cause a reduction of 4 minutes per filling, 15 minutes per bridge and 10 minutes per crown; and (3) dentists will put in 1670 hours of effective work each year. The bases for these assumptions, which are critical, are so imperfectly documented in the source that they cannot be discussed. The computations, which are simple, are as follows:

A. Persons $\times$ Services per person per year $\times$ Time saved per service $=$ Total time saved per year

B. Total time saved in hours per year $\div$ Service capacity in hours per year per dentist $=$ Number of dentists not required

It is concluded that 1741 fewer dentists would be required in 1975 than would have been the case in the absence of improved cutting equipment.

The estimates of the effect of using additional auxiliary personnel are for 1975 as compared to 1950. The basic data come from periodic surveys of dental practice by the American Dental Association. The estimation procedure fundamentally involves (1) the prediction of the distribution of dentists by number of auxiliary personnel in 1975; and (2) measuring

the effect of this distribution on productivity using current (1955) relationships between gross income and number of auxiliary personnel as the
measure of productivity. The estimation of future distribution of dentists by number of auxiliary personnel appears to be based on past
trends, modified by informed judgment concerning prospects of acceptability and suitability. The relationship between productivity and the
number of auxiliary personnel is expressed as a "production index"
which sets 1955 gross income for the category of dentists with no auxiliary personnel equal to 1, and gross income in each of the other
categories as multiples of 1. Application of these values to the corresponding categories of the percentile distribution of dentists by number
of auxiliary personnel, in 1950 and 1975 respectively, yields a "weighted
index of production" which is 162.2 for 1950 and 225.2 for 1975, indicating a productivity increase of 39 percent attributable to predicted
changes in the frequency of use of auxiliary personnel. The presentation
of the data in Table V.22 will make it easier to understand the verbal

Table V.22.   Data used for adjusting requirements for dental manpower to predicted increases in productivity[a]

Number of Auxiliaries	Percent of Dentists		Production Index 1955	Weighted Index of Production	
	1950	1975 (Predicted)		1950	1975 (Predicted)
0	34.4	8.0	1.00	34.4	8.0
1	54.3	45.0	1.75	95.0	78.8
2	8.5	32.0	2.57	21.8	82.2
3	1.9	12.0	3.43	6.5	41.2
4+	0.9	3.0	5.01	4.5	15.0
All	100	100	—	162.2	225.2

SOURCE: Reference 66, Index Table A-5, page 481.
[a] See text for description of data and computations.

description and will also indicate the magnitude of changes envisaged at
the time the predictions were made. The values in the last two columns
are obtained by multiplying the values in column 4 (production
index) by those in the corresponding cells of columns 2 and 3, respectively. This assumes, of course, that gross income is a reasonably good
measure of productivity and that the relationships between productivity
and number of auxiliary personnel observed in 1955 will be unchanged in
1975. In particular, this means that whereas more dentists will use more

auxiliary personnel, the functions of the auxiliaries—that is, the manner in which the division of labor occurs—will not change. The absolute impact of the 39 percent increase in productivity that is predicted to occur under these assumptions, depends on the aggregate number of dentists expected to be available in 1975. If this is assumed to be 61,500, and each dentist can produce 39 percent more work, the equivalent of 24,000 dentists has been added to the working capacity of 61,500. This means that the work of 84,500 can be done by 61,500, or a saving of 24,000 dentists. Compare this to a saving of 1,741 brought about by the effect of improvements in high-speed equipment between 1950 and 1975, and the saving of 3,300 brought about by the effect of the spread of fluoridation between 1950 and 1970 on the demand for fillings. Admitting less than complete comparability, one must still conclude that organization of service emerges as the dominant factor.

CONVERSION OF NEED TO RESOURCES. Perhaps the most common practice in arriving at current or future requirements for resources is to begin with some simple proxy measure of need and use some summary conversion factor to change it to a corresponding measure of resources. The proxy measure most frequently used is the person, who is seen to represent a standard capacity to generate need or to consume services, or both. Thus, as we have already pointed out, need and demand can be ambiguously intertwined in conversions of this kind. Sometimes a death, rather than a person, has been used as the proxy measure of need-demand. Thus, we have conversion factors or standards phrased as physician : population, bed : population, and death : bed ratios. But the ratio may take any other form that serves the purpose—for example a case : bed ratio, if it is asserted that a given number of cases of illness require a specified number of hospital beds to care for them. Needless to say, many assumptions are implicit in such transformations, so that the derivation of the conversion index and its validity become questions of prime concern. As we have already shown, a summary conversion factor such as these could derive from prior detailed evaluations of need, service equivalents of need and of service capacity of resources. Thus, the Lee-Jones studies could be considered to have yielded requirements per 100,000 persons of 142 physicians, 462 general hospital beds, 1158 hospital beds of all types, 240 nurses, and 99–179 dentists, depending on degree of work delegation to dental auxiliaries (59). Needless to say, these ratios have validity only under specified assumptions, that is, for a given population at a given time. Their wide and indiscriminate use calls their validity into question and characterizes their use as arbitrary. The conversion standard may sometimes represent nothing more than average observed relationships or, as we have described before, the situation in a particularly favored segment of the population or of the country. Sometimes the origins of the standards remain undefined and must be accepted as representing the best judgment of those who propose them.

The National Advisory Commission on Health Manpower has published a brief review of 14 major studies of manpower requirements that were done between 1930 and 1965 (67). Hansen has commented on some of the more recent projections of manpower requirements (86). Palmer has reviewed the literature on measuring need for general hospital beds (76). Out of 225 references reviewed, 74 were included in an annotated bibliography. Reed and Hollingsworth reviewed a smaller selection of these studies and offered some new estimates of their own (80). While all these studies taken together represent a very mixed bag indeed, the majority of them do use need : resource ratios as the method for determining requirements. Palmer identified only three studies, one of them the work of Lee and Jones, in which requirement for resources derived from studies of morbidity. A few studies used the death : bed ratio which we shall describe below. Most used population : bed ratios, regarding persons as generators of need, demand or some unspecified mixture of both. In some studies there was no awareness of the distinction between need and demand. A few, considered the bed-ratios as "gospel," but most were aware of the provisional nature of the estimates, offering them as guides that should be used when taking into account local conditions influencing need and demand. One also finds awareness of many factors that modify requirements for resources through influencing need, demand, and the capacity to produce service. Palmer has assembled 30 such factors, which she has grouped under the headings of (1) availability and quality of medical care, (2) attitudes toward medical care, (3) ability to procure needed service, (4) level of utilization of facilities, (5) population characteristics, (6) industrial, occupational, and recreational hazards, and (7) climate and topography (76, pp. 4–5). Several studies take account of urban-rural differences, including the effects of regionalization and the influence of population sparsity on travel distance, propensity to seek care, and lower bed occupancy (80). Thus, though the physician : population or bed : population ratio is a crude device, it has often been used with a reasonable understanding of its limitations and of the factors that must modify its arbitrary and uniform application. In some studies the resource : population ratio is supplemented by expectations of meeting needs expressed in terms of institutional staffing, such as meeting the needs of health departments, federal health agencies, the armed forces, hospitals, mental institutions, medical schools, industrial health services, and the like (68, 71). Another interesting feature is that more than one standard may be offered representing a gradation of successively more ambitious goals. As we have already described, Mountin et al. (70) and The National Health Assembly (68) each offered three such standards, and the President's Commission on the Health Needs of the Nation offered six (71).

The study of hospital requirements by Reed and Hollingsworth is of particular interest because it compares several bases for the derivation of the bed:population ratio and highlights the many problems of interpreting the ratio (80). Six derivations were considered, of which five were used. The first was the hospital utilization rate observed in the nine states in which over 98.5 percent of births occurred in hospitals. It was argued that "if the people in these states receive as much hospital care as is needed for childbirth, it is likely that they also receive close to an adequate volume of hospital service for other conditions" (80, p. 43). The second standard was the hospital utilization rate observed in the quarter of the states (12 in number) with the highest average per capita income during 1949–51. The third was utilization experience under Blue Cross insurance plans with adjustments for (a) limitations on duration of hospitalization provided, (b) under-utilization due to partial benefits, (c) under-representation of low-income groups, (d) under-representation of the aged, (e) care for Blue Cross eligibles in Veterans' Hospitals, and (f) care for Blue Cross eligibles under Workmen's Compensation. The fourth and fifth standards were experience under the Saskatchewan and British Columbia hospital plans, respectively. These plans had the advantage, from the viewpoint of standard formulation, of offering very extensive benefits. Finally, the authors considered, but did not use, experience under prepaid group practice as a possible sixth standard.

The five standards that were considered, gave a wide range of requirements for hospital service, as in Table V.23. Reed and Hollingsworth are aware of the problems in using the six sources of data as standards. The adjustments that had to be made in the Blue Cross data show the importance of taking into account noncomparability of populations (proportion of poor and aged), barriers to the translation of need to demand (limitations in benefits), and artifacts in the data (use of Veterans' Hospitals and Workmen's Compensation). All together, these adjustments increased by 39 percent the reported data for use under Blue Cross. There is also an insightful discussion of why the Saskatchewan data cannot be transposed, without modification, to the United States. Important peculiarities of Saskatchewan include rurality, severe climatic con-

Table V.23.   Estimated requirements for general hospital service using specified standards of need, U.S.A., c. 1950

Standard Population	Days of Hospital Care per 1,000		
	Short Term	Long Term	All
9 States where over 98.5 percent of births take place in hospitals	1,128	262	1,390
12 states with highest per capita income	1,064	246	1,310
Blue Cross, adjusted	1,256	—	—
Saskatchewan	—	—	2,021
British Columbia	1,550	—	—

SOURCE: Reference 80, page 58.

ditions, use of hospitals in part as nursing homes, a large supply of beds, the method of paying hospitals, and the (then) absence of coverage for physicians' services. Reed and Hollingsworth are also aware of the need to vary hospital occupancy by type of hospital care, hospital size, and population density. Hence they adopt for formulating their own recommendation an occupancy of 75 percent for general hospitals (77 percent in urban and 65 percent in rural states) and 85 percent for long-time beds. Their estimate of requirements for general hospital beds is, accordingly, 4.3–4.6 per 1,000 population in urban states and 5.1–5.5 in rural states, with an overall ratio of 4.4–4.7 beds per 1,000. For long-term care, Reed and Hollingsworth suggest that the number of aged be used as the measure of need and that a provision be made of 28–32 beds per 1,000 persons 65 or over, which amounts to 2.3–2.6 per 1,000 persons in the general population. To see these estimates in historical context, one notes that, according to Palmer, most estimates of the need for general hospital beds in combined urban and rural populations have been between 4.5 and 5.0 beds per 1,000 persons. However, the range has extended from 2.5 to 9.0 beds per 1,000, with no secular trend evident. The highest ratios, between 7.0 and 9.0 beds per 1,000, were reported from England and Canada. The estimates for urban populations have ranged from 3.8–8.0 and for rural areas from 1.0–7.0 (76, pp. 4–7). Reed and Hollingsworth emphasize that their own estimates are provisional and that they need to be modified to account for local conditions, including the ability to pay for care and the availability of substitutes to the hospital. They also stress the importance of making the estimates conservative so as to avoid over-building.

The bed : death and the bed : birth ratios are interesting variants in the category of methods that convert need to resources. The bed : death ratio was introduced by the Commission on Hospital Care in its landmark report on *Hospital Care in the United States* (77). It was considered to be a new method which was "a significant departure from conventional methods" in (1) having its "emphasis entirely on need," rather than some combination of need and demand, and (2) being based on "vital statistics rather than the general population." The bed-death ratio derives from the empirical observation of an essentially constant relationship between occupied beds and deaths in hospital as well as between patient days and deaths in hospital, by state. For each 250 days of general hospital care there was one death in hospital which meant an average daily census of 0.685 (about 0.7) occupied beds per year for each hospital death (including infants). At the time of the study (1944), 38 percent of deaths occurred in hospitals. If one assumed that a desirable proportion would be 50 percent of deaths to occur in the hospitals (or any other desired proportion), one could arrive at an estimate of needed beds as follows:

$$\left(\begin{array}{c}\text{death rate}\\\text{per 1,000}\end{array}\right) \times \left(\begin{array}{c}\text{proportion of deaths expected}\\\text{or desired to occur in hospital}\end{array}\right) \times 0.7$$

= average daily census of occupied beds per 1,000 persons.

The average daily census of occupied beds can then be corrected for average observed or desirable occupancy rates. The projection can be refined by separating out deaths in the newborn. This is not necessary, however, because in most states "newborn mortality is not greatly different from the adult hospital death rates" (p. 8). If it is assumed that the average length of stay per maternity case is 11 days, each such case would require a bed for 0.03 of a year. This is the bed : birth ratio. The bed : death ratio, excluding obstetrical care, is 0.6. Therefore, the total bed requirements using both ratios would be:

[(yearly nonobstetrical deaths) × (proportion of such deaths that occur or should appropriately occur in hospital) × (0.6)] + [(yearly births) × (proportion of births that occur or should appropriately occur in hospital) × (0.03)] = occupied hospital beds on any given day.

The occupied hospital beds are adjusted for observed or desired occupancy ratios by dividing by the occupancy ratio. For any given geographical area, adjustments have to be made for hospitalization in the area of persons from outside and hospitalization outside the area for persons who live in it.

There are some interesting features to this approach. The quantity of the bed : birth ratio depends on prior decisions about the appropriate proportion of births that occur in the hospital and the appropriate average length of stay. The ratio itself is analogous to a "critical number" in the absence of a waiting list, as described in our section on methods oriented to demand. The death : bed ratio is somewhat different because it rests on an empirically observed constant relationship between fatal and nonfatal cases, so that knowing one, the other is also known. The death : bed ratio is therefore one way of knowing total demand, given only a portion of it—namely, demand by fatal cases. The normative (or need-oriented) element arises from the statement concerning the proportion of all deaths that should take place in the hospital. The fixity of the relationship between fatal and nonfatal patient-days, so to speak, is a curious observation that invites further study. During 1940–43, the use of hospital beds per unit population in the several states was such that as overall use increased, it was so partitioned between fatal and nonfatal cases, that the ratio of deaths to beds remained constant. This was so, even though deaths in hospital, by state, varied during 1943 from 1.7 per 1,000 population to 6.3 per 1,000; occupied beds in 1940 varied from 1 to 5.2 per 1,000; and patient-days varied in 1943 from 466 to 2,253 per 1,000. Theoretically, the death :bed ratio must be determined by (1) the propensity to admit potentially nonfatal cases and the length of stay of such cases, (2) the propensity to admit potentially fatal cases and the length of stay of such cases, and (3) the propensity to allow patients to die in the hospital as against allowing them to go home, or to send them to another facility, before death occurs. It is hard to believe, therefore, that as the scale of the hospital establishment and its functions change, the death : bed ratio will remain unchanged. Nevertheless, it would be interesting to reassess the situation in the light of experience since 1940.

The bed : death ratio has been a traditional device in estimating requirements for tuberculosis hospitals. The original Hill-Burton standards specified tuberculosis beds equal to 2.5 times the average number of deaths from tuberculosis in the state during the period 1940–44 (80, p. 2). Lee and Jones used expert estimates of service needs and a service capacity standard of 90 percent to arrive at a requirement of 138 tuberculosis beds per 100,000. Lee and Jones comment that "this corresponds roughly with the standards of the Committee on Administrative Practice of the American Public Health Association, an average of 2 beds per annual death from tuberculosis, or between 100 and 200 beds per 100,000, population'' (59, p. 120). Since then, the revolutionary changes in the treatment of tuberculosis must have radically altered the death-bed relationship for this disease.

CONVERSION OF SERVICES TO RESOURCES. We have chosen to illustrate this category of studies, the method for estimating manpower requirements as described by Rozenfeld, partly because it provides us with a look at practice within the Soviet Union, where the organization of health services both demands and permits a greater degree of standardization and central planning (5). As we have already noted, Rozenfeld emphasizes that because means are limited it may not be possible to achieve everywhere within a country the same provision of services and resources. For example, the number of students now in medical school places an upper limit on the supply of physicians for the next several years. Consequently, Rozenfeld distinguishes ''optimum'' from ''limited'' standards and points out that the coexistence of both in different parts of a larger territory leads to the formulation of an ''average standard'' that characterizes the overall situation. Rozenfeld also distinguishes ''short-term'' from ''long-term'' estimates. For short-term estimates one may use standards or norms established by the Ministry of Public Health. It appears that official standards have been formulated to cover every conceivable aspect of the supply and operation of health resources. These standards are considered to be ''optimal.'' For long-term estimates, Rozenfeld advocates, where possible, a method that allows more flexibility by taking into account changes in factors that influence demand for medical care and the manner in which resources are used. The approach is fundamentally normative: the object being to meet the population's requirements for service. Conceptually, the estimate of requirements depends on three factors: (1) states of morbidity, (2) the state of medical technology and of the organization of health services, and (3) the propensity of the population to seek care. Thus, it is similar to the Lee-Jones approach in including the first two factors. It differs in placing more emphasis on demand, which Lee and Jones also considered, but somewhat peripherally. It also differs in not operationally beginning with morbidities but with normative estimates of use of service, which are presumably related to morbidity states and needs for preventive service. Once service equivalents are established, the next step is to translate them to resource equivalents. Here, norms are used which define service capacity in terms of days worked per year, hours worked per day, and the normal quota of cases seen per hour. As might be expected in a system that uses salaried physicians, these norms are highly developed and detailed, quite unlike the situation in the United States. The unit of supply is not the physician, but the "medical allocation." This is a normatively defined full-time medical post. Since, within limits, physicians are allowed to work overtime, and to hold more than one post, the number of physicians required is less than the number of "medical allocations." Conversion from medical allocations to physicians is made by using "coefficients of multiplicity." These coefficients appear to be empirically derived; in other words, they represent current practice. Normatively, the eventual aim is to have one physician hold only one post: a coefficient of 1. Rozenfeld describes methods for estimating requirements for urban and rural populations, for clinical and nonclinical functions, by specialty, by institutional locus, and so on. The example to be cited deals only with requirements for "basic specialized types" of hospital and outpatient clinical services in an urban population. The joint consideration of these services recognizes their interrelatedness and also makes possible the use of hospital staffing norms as part of the estimation procedure. In the interests of simplicity, the estimates are for all physicians combined, but the source tables also give requirements by specialty.

Table V.24 shows procedure for estimating requirements for physicians in the basic specialties, including stomatology, in outpatient clinical and hospital services, for 10,000 persons in an urban locality.

Since none of the examples we have cited so far, including the Lee-Jones study, have concerned manpower requirements for laboratory and x-ray services, it might be of interest to see how Rozenfeld handles this matter. The estimates per 10,000 urban inhabitants are arrived at as shown in Table V.25.

The estimates in Table V.25 give only a part of total requirements. Rozenfeld provides estimates for physicians who are needed to perform additional functions, which are "augmenting groups," "auxiliary types of service," "sanitary-preventive institutions," "crèches and children's homes," "nursing homes," "forensic medicine," and "institutes of scientific research, for training personnel and for administration." These add up to the remarkable figures of 438 "allocations" which equal 365 physicians per 100,000 urban inhabitants. When these figures are compared to the Lee-Jones estimates of 142 physicians per 100,000, it becomes dramatically clear how different assumptions lead to very different conclusions.

CONVERSION OF RESOURCES TO OTHER RESOURCES. In many situations, data are not available to permit conversion of consumer need to requirements

Table V.24   Procedure for estimating requirements for physicians,[a] based on specified assumptions, urban locality, U.S.S.R.

A. Normatively defined number of outpatient visits: 100,000

This comprises 5–6 visits per person per year for the care of disease and 4–5 visits for preventive purposes: a total of 10 visits per person per year.

B. Number of visits per "medical allocation":   6,300

This figure is based on norms that establish the number of days per year worked, the number of hours per day and the number of visits per hour. For physicians in general medicine and pediatrics, an allowance is made for home visits. For all physicians, an allowance is made for time spent on activities other than direct outpatient care ("work in hospital, night duties, committees, consultations, sanitary-educational work, etc.").

C. Number of "medical allocations" for outpatient clinic services: 15.7

A ÷ B

D. Number of hospital beds required: 112

Involves estimates of the percent of persons that require hospitalization (by specialty) during a year, and norms governing the intensity of use of the hospital plant. The figure cited represents 20 percent of the population hospitalized during a given year and 17 patients ("turnovers") per bed per year.

E. Number of hospital beds per "medical allocation":   19

Based on norms for the adequate staffing of hospitals

F. Number of "medical allocations" for hospital services: 5.8

D ÷ E

G. Number of "medical allocations" held by department heads: 2.75

Based on a standard of "10–15% of the total number of posts for house-physicians in hospital and outpatient clinic services."

H. Total number of "medical allocations":   24.25

C + F + G

Table V.24 (*continued*)

I. "Coefficient of Multiplicity":	1.25
Based on actual number of posts ("medical allocations") held by each urban physician. The normative optimum (and hence the goal for long-range planning) is a coefficient of 1.	
J. Total number of physicians:	19.45
H ÷ I	

SOURCE: Reference 5, Tables 52, 53, 54, 55 and on pages 87, 88, 91, 93 and 126.

a Physicians in the basic specialties, including stomatology, in outpatient and in hospital services, per 10,000 persons.

for services and resources. Needs expressed by agencies and institutions are then used in place of, or as a supplement to, requirements estimated by other means. Such needs are almost always expressed in terms of manpower or other resources. Frequently, it is easier, or seems easier, to predict needs for hospitals or other facilities. In those instances the staffing requirements of such facilities can be used to estimate one seg-

Table V.25.   Procedure for estimating personnel for specified laboratory services per 10,000 urban inhabitants, U.S.S.R.

Steps in Procedure	Laboratory Services	X-ray Services
A. Units per hospital patient	8	6
B. Units per bed at 20 turnovers per year	160	120
C. Units per 100 beds per 10,000 persons	16,000	12,000
D. Units per outpatient visit	0.1	0.05
E. Units per 100,000 visits per 10,000 persons	10,000	5,000
F. Total units (C + E)	26,000	17,000
G. Units per medical allocation:	8,600	11,000
1. For laboratory services, the work norm is 32 units per day for 289 working days per person in a team of 1 physician and 2 workers; includes "small losses in working time."		
2. For x-ray services, "the physician-roentgenologist averages 11,000 ($40 \times 277 = 11,080$) units per year."		
H. "Medical allocations" (F ÷ G)	3	1.5

SOURCE: Reference 5, pp. 92–95.

ment of manpower requirements. Here again, one kind of resource, the hospital bed, is being converted to another resource, professional manpower. As we have already pointed out, this approach amounts to the estimation of a "derived need" analogous to the category of derived demand, which we discussed in the appropriate section of this chapter.

There are many examples. Bases I and II of the estimates of the National Health Assembly assume "that (a) Federal agencies will be staffed to meet their estimated requirements, (b) that an adequate number of physicians will be serving in state and local health departments and hospitals for tuberculosis and mental disorders, (c) that the hospital construction program will call for additional physicians" (68, p. 8). Premise 4 of the President's Commission on the Health needs of the Nation reads, in part as follows: "That in 1960 we would need enough physicians to: (1) give direct care to the civilian population at a rate of 1 physician per 1,000 population—which would require about 188,000 physicians . . . ; and (2) maintain present levels of intern and resident training and service in hospitals, meet standards for public health, industrial service, mental and tuberculosis hospitals, and medical schools, and meet the requirements of the Armed Forces at present staffing levels, which would require another 75,000 physicians" (71, p. 184). As we have described, the Lee-Jones estimates for services for "community health preservation" are based on the desirable staffing of local health departments (59, pp. 131–133). Perhaps the most extensive use of staffing as a basis for estimating manpower requirements has been by the Surgeon General's Consultant Group on Nursing (75). The Consultant Group points out two major phenomena: (1) the prevalence of substantial proportions of vacancies for nurses on the staffs of many service and educational institutions, and (2) the low and dwindling participation of professional nurses in the care of patients in hospitals. The first could be interpreted to represent both demand and need. The second is asserted to represent poor quality, since it is estimated to have exceeded legitimate levels of substitution of nonprofessional for professional nursing service. In essence, then, the approach adopted rests on the enunciation of normative standards of staffing and of work allocation among professional nurses and others. For general hospitals, "it is the judgment of the Consultant Group that a general ratio of 50 percent of direct patient care provided by professional nurses, 30 percent by licensed practical nurses, and 20 percent by nursing aides would provide an adequate level of patient care" (75, pp. 15–16). For nursing homes, the requirement is that "each nursing home should have at least one professional nurse plus three practical nurses for 24-hours' coverage, with nursing aides providing supervised services" (p. 16). For public health agencies, "an accepted minimum standard for public health work in local areas is one public health nurse to 5,000 population, a figure which does not provide for care of the sick at home . . . And as many more professional nurses would be needed by public health agencies for care of the sick at home'' (p. 17). Given data on projected numbers of general hospital beds, nursing homes, and persons in the population, it is an easy matter to convert these into requirements for professional nurses using the standards given above. Unfortunately, one must still question the validity of (1) the estimates of hospitals, nursing homes, or population size, and (2) the staffing standards themselves. The Consultant Group appears to accept the first as given. It does, however, give a small amount of attention to the second. The general hospital standard appears to derive mainly from a study by Abdellah and Levine in a sample of hospitals which showed that patients were most satisfied when 50 percent of direct care was given by professional nurses (91). However, the Consultant Group offers its own parallel recommendation as provisional, pending further study of more efficient ways of dividing work among nursing personnel, without prejudice to quality.

The use of staffing norms to compute manpower requirements is an important part of the methods advocated by Rozenfeld for use in the Soviet Union. We have already seen an example in the estimation of the hospital component of physician requirements for urban populations. For rural populations, the norms that specify the services to be demanded and the capacity of physicians to generate services, are apparently poorly developed in the Soviet Union. Hence, major reliance has to be placed on staffing the hospital establishment as the method for estimating physician requirements. It is estimated that for each 10,000 rural inhabitants, 2 hospital beds are needed at the first or subdistrict level, 2 at the second or district level, and 1.5 at the third level, in the city to which rural people go for care. There are norms for the staffing of hospital beds at each of these levels, the total number varying by size of hospital. The smaller the rural hospital, the larger the relative number of physicians to unit number of beds. Taking this phenomenon into account, Rozenfeld estimates a total requirement per 100,000 rural inhabitants of 50 physicians at the first level, 60 at the second and 40 at the third, a total of 150 physicians per 100,000 (5, pp. 98–113).

PREDICTING SUPPLIES AND COMPARING THEM TO REQUIREMENTS

The prediction of requirements for resources is almost always a preliminary to some judgment as to whether there will be ''enough'' of any particular resource at the time for which predictions are made. To make such a judgment it is necessary to predict not only requirements, but also to predict the stock of resources at the specified time. This is true, of course, whether need or demand underlies the approach to estimating requirements. We shall, later in this section, discuss the significance of comparisons between predicted requirements and predicted supplies. First, it might be useful to examine briefly some aspects of predicting the latter.

In our chapter on the "assessment of supply" we developed a detailed framework for the analysis of supply that is relevant also to the problem of prediction, since it calls for the specification of what is being predicted. The reader will recall that the first step is to specify the units that have the potential to produce service and to determine their relevance to the task at hand. For example, neurosurgeons are hardly worth counting when the object is to determine the potential to provide family services. As we shall see, most predictions are made in terms of rather crudely defined units of resources, such as physicians or beds, with only minimal adjustment for the factors that we have included under the rubric of "relevance." At a higher level of refinement, the predictions would be in terms of service equivalents rather than units capable of producing service. Here one might want to distinguish services potentially forthcoming from services expected to be forthcoming. The first involves the application of normative standards of service capacity. The latter is based on empirically derived expectations of how the units of supply will in fact perform. Expectation may be lower or higher than normatively defined potential. Finally, the "potency" of services in neutralizing need is a vital issue in the balance between predicted requirements and predicted stocks of resources. Under some definitions of "productivity," this term includes all, or most, of the factors that intervene between the service-producing unit and the neutralization of need. If so, one can say that the comparison of predicted requirements, stated in terms of units of resources and of predicted supplies, stated in the same units, cannot be made without adjustments for productivity. As we have already indicated, the adjustments can be made to the estimate of requirements. Contrariwise, the adjustment could be made to the predicted supplies. It is immaterial which of the two is done as long as the correction is made before the balance is struck between predicted requirements and predicted supplies.

Almost all the predictions of supplies that we have encountered in the literature have to do with manpower. This may be because such resources as hospital beds are assumed to be easy to produce once the requirement for them is established. This is certainly not true for manpower, especially where an immense investment in educational institutions and lengthy training are involved. Jones et al. have estimated the supply of hospital beds on the assumption that growth rates in number of beds during the decade 1965–75 would be the same as those during 1955–65 (about 2.6 percent per year) and that hospital beds are "retired" at the rate of 3 percent per year. Comparing their predictions of supplies and demand they concluded that 490,000 to 540,000 nonfederal short-term hospital beds would need to be constructed between 1965 and 1975, assuming past trends in occupancy rates continue into the future (26, p. 254).

Predictions of physician manpower tend to be more complex, but also center around the same three basic components: (1) the present stock, (2) additions, and (3) depletions. Information about current stock is obtained from sources such as those we described in our chapter on supply, generally one of the professional directories. Additions derive from graduates of U.S. medical schools, immigration of graduates of foreign medical schools, and reactivation of persons who have been temporarily inactive in the profession. For purposes of prediction, data on past graduations from medical school need to be modified by what is known about plans for expansion in enrollment of existing schools and in building of new schools. Plans for shortening or lengthening the medical curriculum are also important. The annual Medical Education issue of the *Journal of the American Medical Association* is a good source of information concerning these matters. Some studies have also looked at the segments of the population from which applicants to medical school are derived, the number of applicants to medical school, the proportion of those who are selected for admission, and the proportion of those admitted who fail to complete their education. The degree of government and other support of medical students, and medical education in general, is a relevant factor in estimating applications, admissions, and completions. For example, Fein concludes that the supply of young men and women from among whom the medical schools may select will be adequate in both quantity and quality (24, pp. 81–84). Peterson and Pennell, in order to arrive at estimates of graduates of medical schools, used past enrollment figures with allowances for depletion as follows: first year, 7.8 percent; second year, 3.0 percent; third year, 1.4 percent; and fourth year 0.4 percent (83). Rozenfeld estimates that 8–10 percent of entrants to medical schools in the Soviet Union do not complete their education (5, p. 132). Graduates of U.S. medical schools are only one part of the additions to the stock of physicians in the United States. A further substantial addition is made by graduates of foreign medical schools, some of whom are U.S. citizens. Some of these "foreign medical graduates," as they are called, are a temporary addition who provide care while they train in our hospitals. Others continue here, or return after a short stay abroad, to constitute a permanent increment to the pool of physicians in the United States. The numbers involved are not precisely known. Butter has estimated that for the two-year period, December 1966 through December 1968, as many as 12,072 foreign medical graduates were admitted to the United States, and that 3,172 such graduates left, leaving a net inflow of 8,900, of whom about 50 percent are estimated to be a permanent addition to U.S. supplies (92). The Surgeon General's Consultant Group on Medical Education estimated that 750 foreign medical graduates would be added to the supply of U.S. physicians each year between 1969 and 1975. This was less than trends should have indicated to the Consultant Group, but the lower figure may have been an expression of what ought to be rather than what was likely to be true (72, pp. 1–3). Peterson and Pennell estimated a somewhat more realistic 1,200 per year between 1964 and 1974, inclusive (84, Table 1, p. 165). Fein assumed that between 1965 and 1975 there would be a yearly addition of 200 graduates of Canadian medical schools and 1,600 graduates of other non-U.S. medical schools, a yearly total of 1,800 (24). Jones et al. also used an increment of 1,600 graduates of foreign medical schools each year between 1965 and 1975 (26). Rozenfeld points out that migration is not an issue in manpower supplies for the Soviet Union as a whole. It is, however, a very important consideration for regional planning within the U.S.S.R. "There are at present some regions . . . and republics . . . where the number of physicians leaving per year is greater than the number of physicians entering" (5, p. 134).

This brings us to the third factor in predicting number of physicians: that of depletions. Depletions are due to outmigration, change of occupation, inactivity, retirement, and death. Outmigration has not, to the author's knowledge, been a factor in estimates of supply for the United States. However, the study by Butter suggests that it may deserve some attention (92). It is certainly a factor in local and regional manpower supply in the United States as it is in the U.S.S.R. Inactivity and retirement, on the other hand, are major factors that have received considerable attention. Inactivity is a particularly important factor in health occupations, such as nursing and dental hygiene, in which there is a preponderance of women. By the same token, the potential for returning to active status remains an important, though imperfectly quantified, element in predictions of supplies for these professions. Initial choice of, or subsequent entry into, a field such as teaching, research, or administration, which does not directly contribute to patient care raises the question of relevance in the count of units for purposes of prediction. Some have advocated that such persons be considered inactive insofar as patient care is concerned. Hansen, on the other hand, has suggested that research physicians, by contributing to medical advances that increase productivity, also contribute to service capacity (86). It would seem, however, that if productivity is included in the estimate, the further inclusion of research or administrative personnel would represent double counting. As to deaths, the usual practice has been to apply to present stock and subsequent additions, current death rates, by age, for white males (83, 84). A notable exception is the work of Baker and Perlman in Taiwan. They believed that general death rates were not applicable to physicians, ''for physician age-specific death rates are uniformly lower than general population age-specific death rates. In studies as widely separated in time as 1925 and 1951, and as widely separated in space as the United States and Japan, the lower mortality for physicians holds true'' (25, p. 65). Accordingly, Baker and Perlman collected their own information on deaths among health professionals, by age.

Several studies have examined the relationship between age or time since graduation and inactivity or retirement. Among the earliest is the work of Burgess, who used information obtained from directors of 423 out of 1630 hospital schools of nursing to construct a ''professional life table'' of nurses expected to be alive and active (during 1927) at specified periods of years after graduation from nursing school (81). This showed an unexpectedly rapid rate of depletion soon after graduation so that more than one-quarter of nurses had dropped out by the end of the third year and more than one-half by the end of the eighth year following graduation. Activity status then became stabilized until about 35 years following graduation, when a rapid rate of repletion set in, probably due to permanent retirements and deaths (see Fig. V.2). Burgess used the trend line of past graduations to predict yearly additions to the stock of nurses and, by applying current inactivity rates by years since graduation to current stock plus yearly additions to that stock, was able to predict nursing supplies in 1960. The prediction was for 54,595 graduates and 626,202 active nurses, whereas contemporary data for 1960 cite 30,267 graduates and 504,000 active nurses (93). It appears that the predictions of yearly graduations were an overestimate, whereas the activity ratios were underestimated. In 1949 West used an essentially similar technique to predict nurse supplies for 1960, except that information on activity status was obtained from published directories. As shown in Fig. V.2, the general configuration of what Burgess called the ''pro-

Fig. V.2.   Percent of physicians and professional nurses who are active in their respective professions at specified years following age 25–26 for physicians, and following graduation for nurses, specified years. U.S.A.

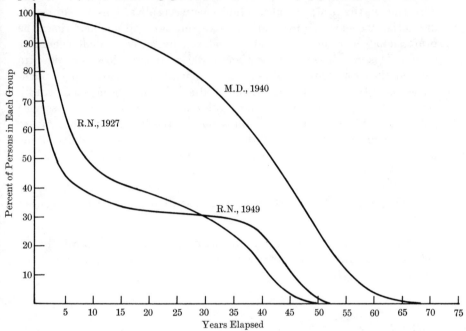

SOURCE: References 81, 82 and 83, Table 6, Column 4.

fessional life table'' was also similar to that found by Burgess, except that early depletion was even more rapid than that observed in 1927 (82). Pennell constructed a professional life table for physicians which indicated the separate effects of death and retirement and added the expectancy of service by age for those physicians who were alive and active (83). Mortality data were those of white males as of 1930–39. Estimates of being ''gainfully employed'' were derived from entries of ''retired'' or ''not in practice'' in the American Medical Association's *Directory* for 1940. The relationship between age and the expectancy of providing service was derived from survey findings on the number of weekly visits per physician. The data were tabulated not by years follow-ing graduation, but by age, beginning at 25–26, which represents reason-ably well the age at graduation from medical school. Assuming these data and assumptions to be valid, the manner in which the potential of a cohort of physicians to provide service is depleted by death, inactivity, and reduced service production associated with age, is shown in Fig. V.3. The validity of the findings concerning service expectancy as related to age has been discussed in a previous chapter. As shown in Fig. V.2, the difference in the professional life tables between physicians and nurses is dramatic. A cohort of physicians offers about two and one-half times the professional years of work that are offered by an equivalent cohort of nurses. This may be an exaggeration, however, since it does not take into account the propensity of physicians in private practice to report themselves as active even though their productivity has been considerably reduced by age. Pennell used his tables to predict the future service potential of the current stock of physicians rather than to predict future stock. Regardless of which of the two is done, the implications of his findings are very clear, whether supplies are to be predicted in terms of active physicians or full-service equivalents.

Finally, in this account of studies relevant to occupational attrition, Folk and Yett have recently reviewed several methods that have been

Fig. V.3.   Stationary population of physicians, physicians gainfully employed and full-service physician equivalents, by years following age 25–26, U.S.A., c. 1940

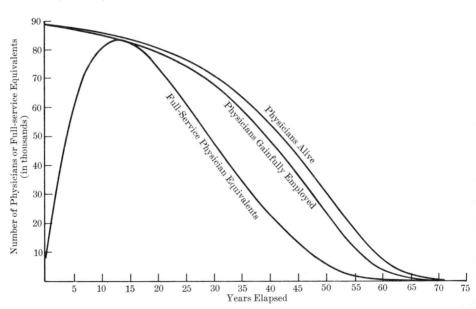

SOURCE: Reference 83, Table 6, pp. 299–230.

used to quantify the phenomenon (85). According to Folk and Yett, "the simplest framework of the employment of a particular type of skilled labor is to assume that the initial stock of persons employed in the occupation . . . grows at a gross compound growth rate . . . and is subject to attrition at a compound rate . . . over a period of N years" (84, pp. 297–298). Given (1) existing stock, (2) additions each year, mainly graduates, who are all assumed to be employed, and (3) stock at the end of a given period, it is possible to compute attrition rate, using one "exact" and several approximate methods. Folk and Yett describe these methods and compare results obtained using data on nursing as well as a variety of engineering specialties. The authors believe that such overall attrition rates may not be as good predictions for the future as might be age-specific employment rates, such as those used by Burgess (81), West (82), and Pennell (83). The age specific rates are thought to be more stable. This is because "many factors that cause an individual to leave an occupation at a given age are practically constant in the short run and subject only to relatively smooth trends in the long run. Death and retirement rates at a given age are outstanding examples. To a lesser extent, marriage rates for college-educated women, and rates of promotion from professional to managerial positions, are also both age-dependent and relatively stable for a given age" (85, p. 300). To compute age-specific employment rates it is necessary to have information on (1) the number of persons, by age, employed in the occupation, and (2) the number of persons, by age, qualified for the occupation. The employment rates are a ratio of the two series. As we have seen, one factor that can be separately identified are losses due to death. "If the stock of qualified persons is weighted by survivor rates, the resulting age-specific employment rates should yield improved projections . . . To make projections of supply, the stock of qualified persons used to estimate unemployment rates is 'aged' to the target date, and augmented by the number of expected graduates to yield a new stock of qualified persons by age. The age-specific occupational-employment rates are then applied to this stock in order to obtain employment projections for the occupation" (85, p. 300). Folk and Yett apply this method to predictions of nursing supply in 1960, comparing these to predictions obtained by other methods as well as to the actual reported figures for 1960. The average attrition methods, based on attrition experienced during 1950–56, yield estimates of 455,490 to 461,110 nurses for 1960. The age-specific method yields 501,162 nurses. There are two reports of actual numbers for 1960. The Bureau of the Census reports 550,162, and the Interagency Conference on Nursing Studies reports 501,000. The authors conclude that "the predictive superiority of the age-specific method is not clearly demonstrated'' (p. 302). However, the differences between what purport to be actual numbers of active nurses are so great that it is difficult to quibble about differences among methods of prediction!

Hansen discusses the problem of the utility of manpower projections in general (86). Three separate considerations are involved: (1) the accuracy of the prediction of supplies, (2) the validity of the prediction of requirements, and (3) the interpretation of the deficit or excess found to exist between the prediction of supplies and the prediction of requirements. The first of these, the accuracy of the prediction of supplies, is always subject to empirical verification, provided one waits long enough. One might contend, however, that lack of agreement between eventually observed and historically predicted values does not necessarily reflect on the validity of the prediction. This is because a major objective of the original prediction is usually to create concern about predicted deficits and bring about change in supplies. Such predictions are necessarily in the nature of self-negating prophecies. With this reservation in mind, it would be useful to look at some past predictions of requirements and supplies and compare them with actual conditions as they turned out. Table V.26 cites four such predictions for 1960 and points out differences between predicted and actual values. All the predictions cited underestimated the growth in population, perhaps the most important generator of increased requirements, as well as the growth in supplies. These two errors tended to cancel each other out, so that the deficits predicted are not as erroneous as they might otherwise have been. Nevertheless, actual supplies in 1960 vary in relation to predicted requirements, under various assumptions, from an excess of 20,257 to a deficit of 44,743. In the face of such findings one is forced to wonder, as does Hansen, about the utility of manpower projections. Hansen has reviewed the findings of six projections for 1975. Although these do not have the advantage of historical verification, they do reveal a very large range in the difference between supplies and requirements, from an excess of 21,700 to a deficit of 65,000.

We have already discussed in fair detail the many assumptions inherent in the several methods for predicting requirements for resources and the implicaton of such assumptions for the validity of the ensuing predictions. All that remains to be done is to discuss briefly the possible meaning of the deficits or excesses revealed by comparing predicted supplies to predicted requirements. When need has served as the basis for estimating requirements, the interpretation is quite simple, since the framework has been normative throughout. Subject to limitations in the

Table V.26. Comparisons among specified predictions of physician supplies and requirements for the U.S.A. in 1960 and actual supplies for 1960

	Predictions for 1960				Actual 1960
	National Health Assembly, 1948	Ewing, 1948	Mountin et al., 1949	President's Commission, 1953	
PREDICTIONS					
Population	153,375,000 to 162,011,000 (4)	169,418,000[b]	158,286,000	171,176,000	does
Supplies	212,356[a]	212,000	227,119[a]	233,000[c]	not
Requirements	227,500 to 260,700 (3)	254,000	244,532 to 272,172 (3)	227,000 to 292,000 (6)	apply
Difference: predicted supplies minus predicted requirements	−15,144 to −48,344	−42,000	−17,413 to −45,053	+6,000 to −59,000	
ACTUAL FOR 1960					
Population	does not apply	does not apply	does not apply	does not apply	185,369,000
Supplies					247,257[a]
DIFFERENCES:					
Actual population minus predicted population	+31,994,000 to +23,358,000	+15,951,000	+27,083,000	+14,193,000	does
Actual supplies minus predicted supplies	+34,901	+35,257	+20,138	+14,257	not
Actual supplies minus predicted requirements	+19,757 to −13,443	−6,743	+2,725 to −24,915	+20,257 to −44,743	apply

SOURCE: References 68, 69, 70, 71, 93.
[a] Active Federal and non-Federal Physicians. [b] Computed from (Requirements) × (Physician : Population Ratio). Numbers in parentheses indicate numbers of estimates. [c] Activity not specified.

validity of estimates, one can say that, according to professional judgment, there ought to be more or less of any given resource: physicians,
hospital beds, and so on. If the estimate of requirements has been based on
demand, the interpretation is not so clear because, as Hansen has pointed
out, the deficit or excess results from separate estimates of demand and
supplies, ignoring the interaction between them through the intermediacy of changes in price. Hansen contends that there is considerable
flexibility in the ability of a given stock of resources to supply services,
as well as in the expression of need in the form of demand. Therefore,
with suitable changes in price, it is possible to so adjust supply and
demand that a new point of equilibrium is attained. Hence a ''deficit'' in
the normative sense does not necessarily mean a ''shortage'' in the
market sense.

Few predictions have dealt with the supply of services as distinct from
the presence of a stock of resources, with or without adjustments for
productivity. One exception has been the work of Jones et al. for the
National Advisory Commission on Health Manpower (26). According to
Jones et al., between 1965 and 1975 there is an expectation of 9–18
percent increase in the number of physicians in private practice, predicted on the basis of (1) ''programmed increases in medical school
facilities,'' (2) some shortening of the medical curriculum, (3) con-
tinuation of the current inflow of foreign graduates, and (4) attrition
due to death. In terms of service capacity, the increase in manpower will
be greater because of increases in productivity. Productivity is measured
by expenditures for physician services per physician, deflated by price.
Jones et al. note that from 1959 to 1964 physician visits, as measured by
the National Health Survey, increased by only 4 percent, whereas expenditures per physician, after deflation by price, increased by 17 percent. They conclude that more is being done for patients per service. In
other words, the discrepancy between services and expenditures is attributed to productivity rather than to errors in the data on use, price, or
expenditures. Changes in productivity (including visits per physician)
are therefore by definition changes in expenditures that are not explained by changes in price. On the demand side, the authors estimate
visits in 1975 by assuming that 1963–64 age-specific visit rates will
remain the same throughout 1965–1975. If so, there will be a 13.5 percent
increase in visits, presumably on the basis of population projections by
age group, although this is not made explicit. However, during this same
time period, expenditures are predicted to increase by 130–135 percent.
The authors suggest that this will come about, as in the past, by a 3
percent annual increase in prices and a 4 percent annual increase in
everything else, this latter being subsumed under the rubric of ''produc-

tivity.'' If so, the situation will remain unchanged. And since it is accepted that in 1965 consumers were willing to buy more services than physicians were willing to supply at prevailing prices, it is concluded that a shortage, in the economic sense, will continue to exist. The crux of the argument is that neither changes in price nor changes in productivity will be sufficient to bring demand and supply into equilibrium. It would seem, however, that so many things were assumed to remain unchanged in constructing the predictions that no other conclusion was possible.

The argument, so far, is that in an interactive system it is unrealistic to consider demand and supply as separate things that can be predicted separately and then compared to see if there is a deficit or an excess. This argument raises again the issue of whether the presence of unused resources creates demand for the use of these resources, thus nullifying, at least partially, what would otherwise have appeared to be an ''excess.'' Feldstein has proposed a method to take account of this circularity (22, 23). This is done by constructing an ''econometric model,'' which is a set of equations that describe the effect of certain ''explanatory variables'' on selected features of the medical care system, including use and supply of specified resources. Among the variables that determine present use and supply levels of physicians and hospital beds are past levels of physician and hospital bed supply. Thus it is possible to estimate the direct as well as indirect effects of policies that propose to change supply or other variables in the set of equations that represent the properties of the medical care system as a whole.

Correcting demand to reflect changes in supply that are themselves responses to demand, represents awareness of complex feedback mechanisms within an interactive system. It is likely that the level of supply also influences normative judgments made by professionals about desirable levels of use of service, thus influencing estimates of need. Most important, however, is the effect of providing service on health and on future need or demand for medical care. We have speculated on this matter in earlier sections of this chapter and, in greater detail, in a previous chapter on the ''Assessment of Need.'' We have suggested that the provision of service may in fact increase future need for service by revealing illness that has been hitherto undetected, by allowing the survival of unhealthy people who might otherwise have died, and by prolonging average life span so that more people live to be aged and, consequently, to experience higher levels of illness. Against this must be put the effect of early care in preventing and ameliorating disease. What the net effect of these opposing forces is likely to be, no one seems to know.

Another limitation in projections of need, demand, and resources stems from the level of aggregation at which such studies are usually made. Estimates at the national level do little to reveal what is often the major problem: the maldistribution of resources both spatially and socially. Even if deficits at the aggregate level were to be made good, the likely consequence in a free market is for the increment of resources to be attracted to those areas where resources are already closest to adequate. It would seem that the determination of aggregate deficits is of little value unless a society is prepared to deal with the problem of maldistribution by creating purchasing power where it does not now exist, by creating in currently deprived areas, the social and professional environment that attracts and retains professional manpower, and, if necessary, by imposing some degree of control on the location of facilities and personnel.

All these limitations in the validity of contemporaneous and predictive estimates of need and demand, in the accuracy of projections of resource supplies, and in the interpretation of comparisons between requirements and supplies, raise serious questions about the social utility of the effort that goes into studies of this kind. As Hansen concludes: "All too often . . . it appears that projections are produced largely to help solidify support for public programs and policies which are seen as beneficial by their promoters. Many of these programs and policies can stand on their own—we should not have to rely upon projections to frighten us into pursuing objectives we should be pursuing anyway" (86, p. 106). It may well be that doomsday predictions are a social and political necessity as a spur to action. In any event, the insistent call for such predictions should stimulate more critical thinking about the relationship between need, demand, and supplies, leading to more precise measurement of the several phenomena involved. In this way they would contribute to knowledge. Furthermore, to the extent that such studies reveal aggregate deficits and spatial or social maldistributions, they serve to create the climate of opinion necessary to bring about orderly change.

Thus we end—hoping that our exposition of social values, objectives, need, demand, and supply has not been only an intellectually engaging and challenging exercise, but also a preparation for more clearly reasoned, and hence more appropriate, social action.

READINGS AND REFERENCES

Need and Demand for Resources: General

1. Klarman, H. E., *The Economics of Health* (New York: Columbia University Press, 1965), 200pp.
2. Klarman, H. E., "Requirements for Physicians," *American Economic Review* 4:663–645 (May 1951).
3. Klarman, H. E., "Economic Aspects of Projecting Requirements for Health Manpower," *Journal of Human Resources* 4:360–376 (Summer 1969).
4. Dickinson, F. G., *The Alleged Shortage of Physicians* (Chicago: American Medical Association, Bureau of Medical Economic Research, Bulletin M–31, 1950. Also appeared in the *Journal of the American Medical Association* 145:1260–1264 (April 21, 1951).
5. Rozenfel'd, I. I., *Planning and Allocation of Medical Personnel in Public Health Services.* Gosudarstvennoe Izdatel'stvo Meditsinskoi Literatury (Medgiz): Moscow, 1961. Translated from Russian by M. Roublev. Published for the National Science Foundation, Washington, D.C., by the Israel Program for Scientific Translations, Jerusalem, 1963. 139pp.
6. Burkens, J. C. J., "The Estimation of Hospital Requirements," *World Hospitals* 2:110–118 (April 1966).
7. Popov, G. A., "Some Aspects of the Use of Norms and Standards in Studying the Efficiency of Medical Care," in *The Efficiency of Medical Care* (Copenhagen: World Health Organization, Regional Office for Europe, 1967), pp. 39–48.
8. Cordero, A. L., "The Determination of Medical Care Needs in Relation to a Concept of Minimal Adequate Care: An Evaluation of the Curative Outpatient Services of a Rural Health Center," *Medical Care* 2:95–103 (April–June 1964).

Identifying and Measuring Factors that Influence Demand

9. Feldstein, P. J., "Research on the Demand for Health Services," *Milbank Memorial Fund Quarterly* 54:128–165 (July 1966), pt. 2.
10. Beenhakker, H. L., "Multiple Correlation—A Technique for Prediction of Future Hospital Bed Needs," *Operations Research* 1:824–839 (October 1963).
11. Rosenthal, G. D., *The Demand for General Hospital Facilities.* Hospital Monograph Series, No. 14 (Chicago: American Hospital Association, 1964). 101pp.
12. Wirick, G. C., "A Multiple Equation Model of Demand for Health Care," *Health Services Research* 1:301–346 (Winter 1966).
13. Reinke, W. A., and Baker, T. D., "Measuring Effects of Demographic Variables on Health Services Utilization," *Health Services Research* 2:61–75 (Spring 1967).
14. Reinke, W., "The Multisort Analysis," in T. D. Baker and M. Perlman, *Health Manpower in a Developing Economy: Taiwan, A Case Study in Planning* (Baltimore: Johns Hopkins Press, 1967). App. I, 187–194.
15. Kalimo, E., *Determinants of Medical Care Utilization* (Helsinki, Finland: Publications of the National Pensions Institute, Ser. E: 11, 1969). 47pp. (Reprint: The English Summary and the main tables of *Lääkintäpalvelusten Kayttöön Vaikuttavat Tekijät* by E. Kalimo. Publications of the National Pensions Institute, Finland—Ser. A:5, Helsinki, 1969, 235–253).
16. Navarro, V., Parker, R., and White, K. L., "A Stochastic and Deterministic Model of Medical Care Utilization," *Health Services Research* 5:342–357 (Winter 1970).

17. Feldstein, P. J., and German, J. J., "Predicting Hospital Utilization: An Evaluation of Three Approaches," *Inquiry* 2:13–36 (June 1965).

The Effect of Supply on Demand

18. Shain, M., and Roemer, M. I., "Hospital Costs Relate to the Supply of Beds," *Modern Hospital* 92:71–73 (April 1959).
19. Roemer, M. I., "Bed Supply and Hospital Utilization: A Natural Experiment," *Hospitals* 35:36–42 (November 1, 1961).
20. Feldstein, M. S., "Effects of Differences in Hospital Bed Scarcity on Type of Use," *British Medical Journal* 2:561–564 (August 29, 1964).
21. Feldstein, M. S., "The Supply and Use of In-Patient Care," in *Economic Analysis for Health Service Efficiency* (Amsterdam: North-Holland Publishing Co., 1967), chap. 7, pp. 187–228.
22. Feldstein, M. S., "An Aggregate Planning Model of the Health Care Sector," *Medical Care* 5:369–381 (November–December 1967).
23. Feldstein, M. S., "An Aggregate Planning Model for the Health Care Sector," in *Economic Analysis for Health Service Efficiency* (Amsterdam: North-Holland Publishing Co., 1967) chap. 9, pp. 261–294.

Demand for Manpower

24. Fein, R., *The Doctor Shortage: An Economic Diagnosis* (Washington, D.C.: The Brookings Institution, May 1967). 199pp.
25. Baker, T. D., and Perlman, M., *Health Manpower in a Developing Economy: Taiwan, A Case Study in Planning* (Baltimore: Johns Hopkins Press, 1967). 203pp.
26. Jones, N. H., Jr., Struve, C. A., and Stefani, P., "Health Manpower in 1975—Demand, Supply and Price," in *Report of the National Advisory Commission of Health Manpower*, Vol. II. (Washington, D.C.: U.S. Government Printing Office, November 1967), App. V, pp. 229–263.

Demand for Hospitals

GENERAL

27. Newell, D. J., "Problems in Estimating the Demand for Hospital Beds," *Journal of Chronic Diseases* 17:749–759 (September 1964).

EXPECTED OR DESIRABLE OCCUPANCY

28. Metropolitan St. Louis Hospital Planning Commission, *Facilities and Services for Long-Term Chronic Illness and Convalescent Care in the Metropolitan St. Louis Area* (St. Louis, Missouri: Metropolitan St. Louis Hospital Planning Commission, Inc. November, 1963). 63pp. + appendices.
29. Public Health Service, Division of Hospital and Medical Facilities, "Estimating Need," in *Procedures for Areawide Health Facility Planning: A Guide for Planning Agencies*, P.H.S. Publication No. 930–B–3 (Washington, D.C.: U.S. Government Printing Office, September 1963), chap. IV, pp. 22–29.

OCCUPANCY PRESSURE

30. Commission on Hospital Care, "Relation of the Bed Occupancy Rate to Size of Hospital," in *Hospital Care in the United States*, (New York: The Commonwealth Fund, 1947), chap. 20, pp. 278–288.

31. Newell, D. J., ''Provision of Emergency Beds in Hospitals,'' *British Journal of Preventive and Social Medicine* 8:77–80 (April 1954).

32. Blumberg, M. S., '' 'DPF' Concept' Helps Predict Bed Needs,'' *Modern Hospital* 97:75–81, 170 (December 1961).

WAITING TIME

33. Querido, A., ''Estimate of Need of Hospital Beds,'' in *The Efficiency of Medical Care*, (Leiden, Holland: H. E. Stenfert Kroese N. V., 1963), pp. 122–127.

34. Personal communication from the author.

WAITING LISTS AND THE ''CRITICAL NUMBER''

35. Bailey, N. T. J., ''Queuing for Medical Care,'' *Applied Statistics* 3:137–145 (November 1954).

36. Bailey, N. T. J., ''Statistics in Hospital Planning and Design,'' *Applied Statistics* 5:146–157 (November 1956).

37. Bailey, N. T. J., ''Calculating the Scale of Inpatient Accomodation,'' in Davies, J. O. F., Brotherston, J., Bailey, N., Forsyth, G., and Logan, R., *Towards a Measure of Medical Care: Operational Research in the Health Services, A Symposium* (London: Oxford University Press, for the Nuffield Provincial Hospitals Trust, 1962), chap. III, pp. 55–65.

38. Nuffield Provincial Hospitals Trust, ''Planning to Meet Demand,'' in *Functions and Design of Hospitals*, (London: Oxford University Press, 1955), chap. 7, pp. 149–185.

39. Barr, A., ''The Population Served by a Hospital Group,'' *Lancet* 2:1105–1108 (November 30, 1957).

40. Airth, A. D., and Newell, D. J., *The Demand for Hospital Beds: Results of an Enquiry on Tees-side* (Newcastle-upon-Tyne: University of Durham, King's College, 1962). 91pp.

LATENT SERVICE RESERVE

41. Forsyth, G., and Logan, R. F. L., *The Demand for Medical Care: A Study of the Case-Load in the Barrow Furness Group of Hospitals* (London: Oxford University Press, for the Nuffield Provincial Hospitals Trust, 1960). 153pp.

PATIENT CLASSIFICATION

42. White, K. L., Wells, H. B., Preston, R. A., and Strachan, E. J., ''Overnight Facilities for Ambulatory Patients: A Method for Estimating Potential Demand,'' *Hospital Management* 96:49–53 (October 1963).

43. Preston, R. A., White, K. L., Strachan, E. J., and Wells, H. B., ''Patient Care Classification as a Basis for Estimating Graded Inpatient Hospital Facilities,'' *Journal of Chronic Diseases* 17:761–772 (September 1964).

44. Public Health Service, Division of Hospital and Medical Facilities, *The Progressive Patient Care Hospital: Estimating Bed Needs*. P.H.S. Publication, No. 930–C–2. (Washington, D.C.: U.S. Government Printing Office, 1963). 17pp. This is a summary of an unpublished report by Charles D. Flagle, Howard Lockward, John Moss, and Josephine Strachan. A shortened version was published as ''How to Allocate Progressive Care Beds'' in *Modern Hospital* 100:78–83 (February 1963).

45. Fetter, R. B., and Thompson, J. D., ''A Decision Model for the Design and Operation of a Progressive Patient Care Hospital,'' *Medical Care* 7:450–462 (November–December 1969).

Conversion of Need to Service

46. Commission on Chronic Illness, ''Estimating Needs for Care,'' ''Estimated Needs for Care of a High Disability Group,'' and ''Estimated Needs of a Representative Sample of Three Items of Care,'' chaps. 6, 9, and 10, in *Chronic Illness in the United States*. Vol. IV: *Chronic Illness in a Large City: The Baltimore Study* (Cambridge: Harvard University Press, 1957).

47. Greenlick, M. R., Hurtado, A. V., and Saward, E. W., ''The Objective Measurement of the Post-Hospital Needs of a Known Population,'' *American Journal of Public Health* 56:1193–1198 (August 1966).

48. Scutchfield, F. D., and Freeborn, D. K., ''Estimation of Need, Utilization, and Costs of Personal Homes and Home Health Services.'' *HSMHA Health Reports* 86:372–376 (April 1971).

49. Lemon, G. M., and Welches, L., ''Survey of Welfare Clients to Determine Need for Home Health Aides,'' *Public Health Reports* 82:729–734 (August 1967).

50. Lipworth, L., ''Estimating the Need for Facilities for Renal Dialysis,'' *Public Health Reports* 83:669–672 (August 1968).

51. Hallan, J. B., and Harris, B. S. H., ''Estimation of a Potential Hemodialysis Population,'' *Medical Care* 8:209–220 (May–June 1970).

52. Jaffe, F. S., ''Financing Family Planning Services,'' *American Journal of Public Health* 56:912–917 (June 1966).

53. Jaffe, F. S., Dryfoos, J. G., and Lerner, R. C., ''Planning for Community-Wide Family Planning Services,'' *American Journal of Public Health* 59:1339–1354 (August 1969).

54. Center for Family Planning Development, ''Need for Subsidized Family Planning Services,'' in *Need for Subsidized Family Planning Services: United States, Each County, 1968* (Washington, D.C.: U.S. Government Printing Office, 1969), pp. 238–240.

55. Siegel, E., Tuthill, R., Coulter, E., Chipman, S., and Thomas, D., ''Measurement of Need and Utilization Rates for a Public Family Planning Program,'' *American Journal of Public Health* 59:1322–1330 (August 1969).

56. Mickey, J. E., ''Findings of Study of Extra-Hospital Nursing Needs,'' *American Journal of Public Health* 53:1047–1057 (July 1963).

57. Ast, D. B., Cons, N. C., Carlos, J. P., and Polan, A., ''Time and Cost Factors to Provide Regular, Periodic Dental Care for Children in a Fluoridated and Non-Fluoridated Area: Progress Report II,'' *American Journal of Public Health* 57:1635–1642 (September 1967).

58. Kalimo, E., and Sievers K., ''The Need for Medical Care: Estimation on the Basis of Interview Data,'' *Medical Care* 6:1–17 (January–February 1968).

Conversion of Need to Services to Resources

59. Lee, R. I., and Jones, L. W., *The Fundamentals of Good Medical Care*. Publication of the Committee on the Costs of Medical Care, No. 22 (Chicago: The University of Chicago Press, 1933). 302pp.

60. Falk, I. S., Schonfeld, H. K., Harris, B. R., Landau, S. J., and Milles, S. S., ''The Development of Standards for the Audit and Planning of Medical Care, I. Concepts, Research Design and the Content of Primary Care,'' *American Journal of Public Health* 57:1118–1136 (July 1967).

61. Schonfeld, H. K., Falk, I. S., Sleeper, H. R., and Johnston, W. D., ''The Content of Good Dental Care: Methodology in a Formulation for Clinical Standards and Audits, and Preliminary Findings,'' *American Journal of Public Health* 57:1137–1146, (July 1967).

62. Schonfeld, H. K., Falk, I. S., Lavietes, P. H., Milles, S. S., and Landau, S. J., "The Development of Standards for the Audit and Planning of Medical Care: Pathways Among Primary Physicians and Specialists for Diagnosis and Treatment," *Medical Care* 6:101–114 (March–April 1968).

63. Schonfeld, H. K., Falk, I. S., Sleeper, H. R., and Johnston, W. D., "Professional Dental Standards for the Content of Dental Examinations," *Journal of the American Dental Association* 77:870–877 (October 1968).

64. Schonfeld, H. K., Falk, I. S., Lavietes, P. H., Landwirth, J., and Krassner, L. S., "The Development of Standards for the Audit and Planning of Medical Care. Good Pediatric Care—Program Content and Method of Estimating Needed Personnel." *American Journal of Public Health* 58:2097–2110 (November 1968).

65. Schonfeld, H. K., "Standards for the Audit and Planning for Medical Care: A Method for Preparing Audit Standards for Mixtures of Patients," *Medical Care* 8:287–297 (July–August 1970).

66. Dollar, M. L., "Estimates of the Effects of Fluoridation, Improved Equipment, and Additional Auxiliary Personnel on Dental Manpower Requirements," App. A, pp. 475–482, in American Council on Education, Commission on the Survey of Dentistry in the United States, *The Survey of Dentistry: The Final Report.* S. Hollingshead, Director (Washington, D.C.: American Council on Education, 1961).

Need for Manpower

67. National Advisory Commission of Health Manpower, "Major Studies of Manpower Requirements for Health Services, 1930–1965," in *Report of the National Advisory Commission of Health Manpower, Vol. II* (Washington, D.C.: U.S. Government Printing Office, November 1967), App. VI, pp. 265–277.

68. The National Health Assembly, "What is the Nation's Need for Health and Medical Personnel," in *America's Health: A Report of the Nation* (New York: Harper and Brothers, 1949), chap. I, pp. 1–38.

69. Ewing, O. R., *The Nation's Health: A Ten Year Program* (Washington, D.C.: U.S. Government Printing Office, September 1948). 186pp.

70. Mountin, J. W., Pennell, E. H., Berger, A. G., *Health Service Areas: Estimates of Future Physician Requirements.* Public Health Bulletin No. 305 (Washington, D.C.: U.S. Government Printing Office, 1949). 89pp.

71. President's Commission on the Health Needs of the Nation, (Paul B. Magnuson, Chairman), "Improved and Increased Health Personnel," in *Building America's Health, Volume 2: America's Health Status, Needs and Resources,* (Washington, D.C.: U.S. Government Printing Office, 1953), pp. 183–191.

72. The Surgeon General's Consultant Group on Medical Education (Frank Bane, Chairman), "How Many Physicians are Needed?" in *Physicians for a Growing America.* P.H.S. Publication, No. 709 (Washington, D.C.: U.S. Government Printing Office, 1959), chap. I, pp. 1–13.

73. Public Health Service, Bureau of Health Manpower, *Health Manpower Perspective: 1967.* P.H.S. Publication No. 1667 (Washington, D.C.: U.S. Government Printing Office, 1967). 81pp.

74. United States Department of Labor, *Health Manpower 1966–1975: A Study of Requirements and Supply.* Report No. 323 (Washington, D.C.: U.S. Government Printing Office, June 1967). 50pp.

75. The Surgeon General's Consultant Group on Nursing (A. C. Eurich, Chairman), *Toward Quality in Nursing: Needs and Goals.* P.H.S. Publication No. 992 (Washington, D.C.: U.S. Government Printing Office, 1963). 73pp. See especially chap. IV, pp. 15–19, on "Needs for 1970."

Need for Hospitals

76. Palmer, J., *Measuring Bed Needs for General Hospitals: Historical Review of Opinions with Annotated Bibliography* (Washington, D.C.: Department of Health, Education, and Welfare, Public Health Service. Division of Hospital and Medical facilities, October, 1956). 32pp. (Mimeographed)

77. Commission on Hospital Care, "Measuring Need for Hospital Facilities," in *Hospital Care in the United States* (New York: Commonwealth Fund, 1947), chap. 21, pp. 289–301.

78. The National Health Assembly. "What Is the Nation's Need for Hospital Facilities, Health Centers, and Diagnostic Clinics?" in *America's Health: A Report to the Nation* (New York: Harper, 1949), chap. II, pp. 39–59.

79. McEwan, E. D., "The Case for a New Maternity Bed Ratio," *Lancet* 1:489–490 (March 1967).

80. Reed, L. S., and Hollingsworth, H., *How Many General Hospital Beds Are Needed? A Reappraisal of Bed Needs in Relation to Population.* P.H.S. Publication No. 309 (Washington, D.C.: U.S. Government Printing Office, 1953). 73pp.

Predicting Supplies

81. Burgess, M. A., "How Far Is It Going?" in *Nurses, Patients, and Pocketbooks,* (New York City: Committee on Grading of Nursing Schools, 1928), chap. 3, pp. 48–65.

82. West, M. D., "Estimating the Future Supply of Professional Nurses," *American Journal of Nursing* 50:656–658 (October 1950).

83. Pennell, E. H., "Location and Movement of Physicians—Method for Estimating Physician Resources," *Public Health Reports* 59:281–305 (March 3, 1944).

84. Peterson, P. Q., and Pennell, M. Y., "Physician—Population Projections, 1961–1975: Their Causes and Implications," *American Journal of Public Health* 53:163–172 (February 1963).

85. Folk, H., and Yett, D. E., "Methods for Estimating Occupational Attrition," *Western Economic Journal* 6:297–302 (September 1968).

86. Hansen, W. L., "An Appraisal of Physician Manpower Projections," *Inquiry* 7:102–113 (March 1970).

Additional References Cited

87. Sonquist, J., and Morgan, J., *The Detection of Interaction Effects* (Ann Arbor: University of Michigan, Survey Research Center, Monograph No. 35, 1964). 292pp.

88. Robinson, W., "Ecological Correlations and the Behavior of Individuals," *American Sociological Review* 15:351–357 (June 1950).

89. Donabedian, A., *A Guide to Medical Care Administration, Volume II: Medical Care Appraisal* (New York: American Public Health Association, 1969). 176pp.

90. Helmer, O., "Analysis of the Future: The Delphi Method." In J. R. Bright (Editor), *Technological Forecasting for Industry and Government: Methods and Applications* (Englewood Cliffs, N. J.: Prentice-Hall, 1968). 484pp.

91. Abdellah, F. G., and Levine, E., *Effect of Nurse Staffing on Satisfaction with Nursing Care.* Hospital Monograph Ser. No. 4. (The American Hospital Association, Chicago, 1958). 82pp.

92. Butter, I., "The Migratory Flow of Doctors to and from the United States," *Medical Care* 9:17–31 (January–February 1971).

93. National Center for Health Statistics, *Health Resources Statistics, 1965.* P.H.S. Publication No. 1509 (Washington, D.C.: U.S. Government Printing Office, 1966). 182pp.

94. The need to include this category was brought to my attention by one of my students, Mr. David Rogoff.

Index

Specialists
American Boards of, 234
distribution among population, 580
income, 413
productivity of, 281
travel time to, 440, 452
workload of, 279, 281
Speed and productivity, 277
Staff nurses, levels of activity, 400
''Standard deviation ellipse,'' 432, 433
''Standard distance circle,'' 432, 433
State hospitals; *see* Hospitals, mental
Statistics, vital, 126
Supply
assessment of, 208–508
model for, 209
model for, and productivity, 253
excess of, 405
physician, 631
conventions used in reporting, 219
prediction, and comparison to requirements, 622–634
shortage of, 405
units of, specification of, 211–246
Surveys
continuous local, 115–117
household interview, 92–115
use in medical care administration,
114
partial, 115–117
self-administered, 124–126
''symptom,'' 117–124
''Symptom'' survey, 117–124

Teeth; *see* Dental
Time-intensity gradient in disease, 71, 73
Time-intensity relations in disease, 72
Transformation pathways among need,
services and resources, 512
Travel distance; *see also* Accessibility
to general practitioners, 440
to hospitals, 432
admissions related to, 442, 446

general practitioners' use of
hospitals and, 451
mental, and first admission rates, 446
for maternity care, specialist, 452
outpatient treatment and, 443
patients' willingness to travel, 445
to physicians, 438, 439
to specialists, 440
maternity care, 452

Urgency in office visits of general
practitioners, 396

''Validity,'' 97
Values; *see* Social values
Visits, physician
home, 259
office
categories of, 259
general practitioner, degree of
urgency, 396
pediatricians, per hour, 317
non-hospital, 273
pediatricians, 317
for cases of influenza in children, 606
Vital statistics, 126
''Vulnerability,'' to control, disease, 186
classification of, 186

Waiting list for hospital beds, 557–565
Waiting time for hospital beds, 554–557
Women; *see* Females
Workload
of dentists, 303
of general practitioners, 308
by age, 272
comparisons of actual and desired
workloads, 359
seasonal changes in, 355
of internists, 273
of physicians, 278, 311
age and, 276
of specialists, 279, 281